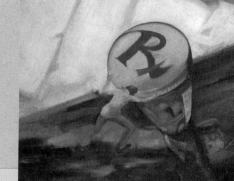

The Pharmacy Technician Series

PHARMACOLOGY

Series Author
Mike Johnston, CPhT

Contributing Authors
Jeanetta Mastron, BS, CPhT
Robin Luke, CPhT

PEARSON
Prentice
Hall

Upper Saddle River, New Jersey 07458

Library of Congress Cataloging-in-Publication Data

The pharmacy technician series. Pharmacology / [edited by] Mike Johnston.
   p. ; cm.
Includes bibliographical references and index.
ISBN 0-13-114764-1
1. Pharmacology. 2. Pharmacy technicians. I. Title: Pharmacology. II. Johnston, Mike, CPhT.
[DNLM: 1. Pharmacology—methods. 2. Pharmaceutical Preparations—metabolism. 3. Pharmacists' Aides.
QV 4 P5368 2006]
RM300.P5265 2006
615'.1—dc22
                                                2005045921

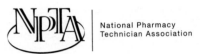

National Pharmacy
Technician Association

The NPTA logo is a trademark of the
National Pharmacy Technician Association

straden-schaden, inc.

RxPRESS
PUBLICATIONS

The Straden-Schaden and RxPress logos are
both trademarks of Straden-Schaden, Inc.

Publisher: Julie Levin Alexander
Assistant to Publisher: Regina Bruno
Acquisitions Editor: Joan Gill
Developmental Editor: Triple SSS Press Media Development, Inc.
Editorial Assistant: Bronwen Glowacki
Director of Marketing: Karen Allman
Marketing Coordinator: Michael Sirinides
Channel Marketing Manager: Rachele Strober
Director of Production and Manufacturing: Bruce Johnson
Managing Production Editor: Patrick Walsh
Production Liaison: Christina Zingone
Production Editor: Rosaria Cassinese/Prepare, Inc.
Manufacturing Manager: Ilene Sanford
Manufacturing Buyer: Pat Brown
Design Director: Cheryl Asherman
Interior Designer: Amy Rosen
Cover Designer: Mary Siener
Cover Illustrator: Edward Sherman
Compositor: Prepare, Inc.
Printer/Binder: Courier/Westford
Cover Printer: Phoenix Color Corp.
Cover Illustration: © 2006 by Edward Sherman

Notice: The author and the publisher of this volume have taken care to make certain that the doses of drugs and schedules of treatment are correct and compatible with the standards generally accepted at the time of publication. Nevertheless, as new information becomes available, changes in treatment and in the use of drugs become necessary. The reader is advised to carefully consult the instruction and information material included in the package insert of each drug or therapeutic agent before administration. This advise is especially important when using, administering, or recommending new and infrequently used drugs. The author and publisher disclaim all responsibility for any liability, loss, injury, or damage incurred as a consequence, directly or indirectly, of the use and application of any of the contents of this volume. It is the responsibility of the reader to familiarize himself or herself with the policies and procedures set by the federal, state, and local agencies as well as the institution or agency where the reader may be employed. It is the reader's responsibility to stay informed of any new changes or recommendations made by any federal, state, and local agency as well as by his or her employing institution or agency.

Pearson Education Ltd.
Pearson Education Singapore Pte. Ltd.
Pearson Education Canada, Ltd.
Pearson Education—Japan

Pearson Education Australia Pty. Limited
Pearson Education North Asia Ltd.
Pearson Educación de Mexico, S.A. de C.V.
Pearson Education Malaysia Pte. Ltd.

PEARSON
Prentice
Hall

10 9 8 7
ISBN 0-13-114764-1

Dedication

To Jody & Wendy . . . *I consider it a privilege to have you as my mentors. I consider it an honor to have your trust and respect. Above all, however, I consider it a joy to have you as my friends.*

"I have learned that success is to be measured not so much by the position that one has reached in life as by the obstacles which he has overcome while trying to succeed."—Booker T. Washington

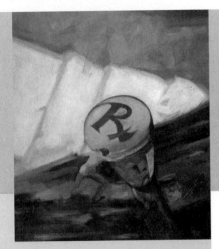

Contents

Preface   xxi

About the Authors   xxiii

About NPTA   xxiv

Acknowledgments   xxv

Contributor   xxvi

Reviewers   xxvii

1   Introduction to Pharmacology   1

Introduction   1
Studying Pharmacology   2
Basic Terminology   3
Major Areas of Pharmacology   5
Summary   5
Chapter Review Questions   6

2   The Realm of Pharmacology   7

Introduction   7
Classification of Drugs   8
Drug Names   12
Routes of Administration   13
   Oral Administration   13
   Buccal and Sublingual Absorption   15
   Topical Administration   16
   Rectal and Vaginal Administration   17
   Inhalation Administration   17
   Nasogastral Administration   18
   Parenteral Administration   18
Summary   19
Chapter Review Questions   20

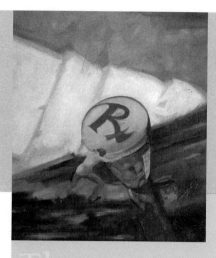

3   The Body and Drugs   21

Introduction   21
Structure of the Human Body   22
    Cardiovascular System   22
    Respiratory System   25
    Renal System   27
    Gastrointestinal (GI) System   28
    Endocrine System   30
    Hematologic System   32
Summary   34
Chapter Review Questions   35

4   Pharmacodynamics   37

Introduction   37
Receptor Complex   38
Site of Action   39
Mechanism of Action   39
Receptor Site   39
Agonists and Antagonists   40
The Dose–Response Curve   41
    Potency   42
    ED50   42
The Time–Response Curve   43
Pharmacodynamic Mechanisms   43
Summary   45
Chapter Review Questions   46

5   Pharmacokinetics   48

Introduction   48
Plasma Concentration (Cp)   49

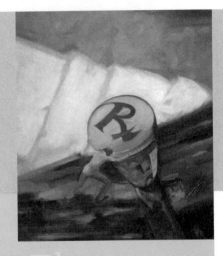

Drug Absorption   49
Drug Distribution   50
Membrane Transport Mechanisms   50
   Passive Diffusion   51
   Facilitated Diffusion   51
   Active Transport   51
   Pinocytosis   51
The Quality of Drugs—Solubility   52
Drugs and Their Ionization   53
Summary   53
Chapter Review Questions   54

6   **Drug Distribution and Metabolism**   **56**

Introduction   56
The Path   57
Plasma Binding Protein   58
   What Do You Really Need to Know
     about Pharmacokinetics? 59
Equilibrium   59
Absorption   60
   Salt Forms   60
Rate of Administration   60
Volume of Distribution   60
   Important Note about "Two Compartments" 61
Clearance   61
Half Life   61
Information Resources   62
Summary   62
Chapter Review Questions   63

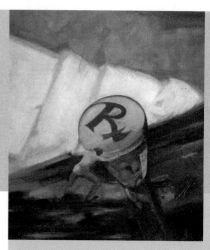

7   **Addiction**   **64**

Introduction   64
The Disease   65
Characteristics   66
Causes   66
The Criteria for Addiction   67
The Roots of Drug Abuse   68
Alcohol   68
    Alcohol, Other Drugs, and the Brain   69
    Treatment for Alcoholism   71
Summary   71
Chapter Review Questions   72

8   **Drug Dependency**   **74**

Introduction   74
The Problem   75
Controlled Medications   75
Addiction Versus Dependence   77
Summary   77
Chapter Review Questions   78

9   **The Skin**   **79**

Introduction   79
Anatomy   80
Diseases and Conditions of the Skin   81
Drugs versus Cosmetics for the Skin   85
Pharmaceutical Treatment of Various Skin Diseases   85
No Pharmaceutical Treatment   89
Summary   89
Chapter Review Questions   90

The
Pharmacy
Technician
Series

The
Pharmacy
Technician
Series

The
Pharmacy
Technician
Series

The
Pharmacy
Technician
Series

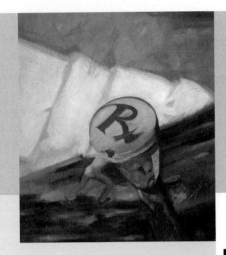

10	**Eyes and Ears**	**94**
	Introduction	94
	Anatomy and Physiology of the Eye	95
	How the Eye Works	96
	Diseases of the Eyes	97
	Infections of the Eye and the Pharmaceutical Treatment	97
	Stye	97
	Blepharitis	98
	Conjunctivitis	98
	Eye Disorders that Affect Vision	104
	Glaucoma	104
	Cataract	106
	Vascular Retinopathies Retinopathy	106
	Cycloplegic, Mydriatic Drugs, Lubricants	113
	Basics of Using an Ophthalmic Product	113
	How to Apply an Ophthalmic Ointment	114
	How to Instill an Ophthalmic Solution	114
	The Ear	115
	Anatomy and Physiology of the Ear	115
	Eustachian Tube	116
	Cochlea	116
	Vestibular Labyrinth	116
	Complications of Earwax Buildup	117
	Types of Hearing Loss	118
	Conductive Hearing loss	118
	Sensory Hearing Loss	118
	Drug Induced	118
	Neural Hearing Loss	118
	Presbycusis	118
	Otitis Media	119
	Summary	120
	Chapter Review Questions	121

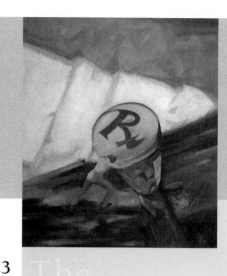

11 The Gastrointestinal System 123

Introduction 123
Anatomy and Physiology of the Digestive System 124
Function of Digestion 125
The Digestive Process 125
    The Mouth 125
    The Stomach 126
    The Small Intestine 127
    The Large Intestine or Colon 128
Disorders of the Digestive System 129
    GERD or Gastric Esophageal Reflux Disease 129
    Nausea and/or Vomiting 130
Ulcers 132
    NSAIDs 133
    Causes and Treatments 135
Nutrition 137
Basic Nutrition 138
    Macronutrients 138
    Carbohydrates 138
    Fats 139
    Protein 140
    Vitamins 141
    Minerals 146
    Water 147
Food Guide Pyramid 147
    Food Allergies 147
Total Parenteral Nutrition 147
    Indications 148
    Two Types of TPN Lines 150
    TPN Solutions for Special Disease
        State Dietary Needs 152

The
Pharmacy
Technician
Series

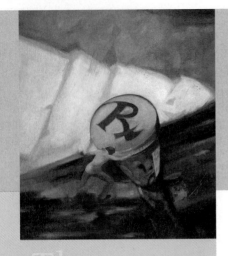

	Compatibility	153
	Stability	153
	Summary	155
	Chapter Review Questions	156
12	**The Musculoskeletal System**	**158**
	Introduction	158
	Anatomy of the Muscles	159
	Muscle Action	159
	The Bones	160
	Long Bones	160
	Bone Marrow	161
	Anatomical Vocabulary	163
	The Functions of Bones	163
	Musculoskeletal Disorders	164
	Osteomyelitis	165
	Osteoporosis	166
	Paget's Disease	168
	Bursitis	168
	Tendonitis	168
	Myalgia	168
	Bone Marrow Disorders	168
	Anemia	168
	Leukemia	168
	Arthritis	168
	Rheumatoid Arthritis	169
	Osteoarthritis	169
	Gout	169
	Treatment of Arthritis	170
	Disease Modifying Anti-Rheumatic Drugs (DMARDs)	170
	Gold (Ridaura®)	171

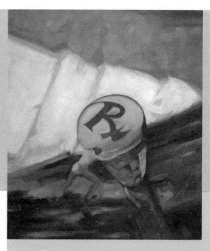

Penicillamine	171
Sulfasalazineis	171
Hydroxychloroquine (Plaquenil®)	171
Leflunomide (Arava®)	171
Second Line of Therapy	172
Inflammation	172
Treatment for Inflammatory Diseases	173
Salicylates	173
Nonsteroidal Anti-inflammatory Drugs (NSAIDs)	174
Cox-2 Inhibitors	174
Skeletal Muscle Relaxants	176
Adverse Actions	178
Treatment of Weak, Fragile, or Soft Bones	178
Bisphosphonates	180
Calcitonin	181
Selective Estrogen Receptor Modulators	181
Nonpharmacologic Treatments of Osteoporosis	181
Treatment of Gout	184
Drugs of Choice	184
Preventative Treatment	184
Spastic Diseases	186
Multiple Sclerosis	186
Cerebral Palsy	186
Summary	187
Chapter Review Questions	188

13   The Respiratory System   191

Introduction	191
Anatomy of the Respiratory System	192
Function of the Respiratory System	192
A Difference between Air and Oxygen	194
Actual Respiration and the External Exchange	194

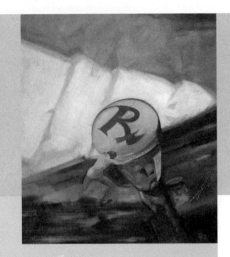

The Diaphragm	195
The Lung and the Conducting Airways	195
How We Breathe	195
Disease States of the Respiratory Tract	197
Cough and Colds	197
How a Cold Virus Becomes a Disease	198
Cough as a Symptom and a Complication of the Common Cold	198
Treating the Common Cold with Drugs	200
Antihistamines for the Common Cold	201
Decongestants	203
Cough Medications	205
Nondrug Treatment of the Common Cold	205
Asthma	207
Bronchoconstriction	208
Allergic Asthma	208
Treatment	208
Emphysema	209
Cystic Fibrosis	211
Treatment of APAP OD	212
Allergies	212
Antihistamines	212
Mast Cell Stabilizers Used to Prevent Allergies	213
Treatment of COPD	215
Bronchodilators	215
Xanthines	215
Anticholinergics	216
Anti-inflammatory Agents	216
Mast Cell Inhibitors	217
Anti-leukotriene Drugs	219
Summary	221
Chapter Review Questions	222

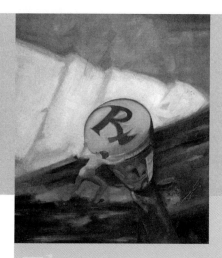

14 **The Cardio, Circulatory, and Lymph Systems** **226**

Introduction	226
Anatomy of the Heart	227
The Function of the Heart	228
Pumping of Blood	228
Blood	229
Blood Flow	229
The Conduction System	232
Nerve Supply to the Heart	233
Diseases of the Heart	233
Congestive Heart Failure (CHF)	233
Complications of CHF—Ischemia, Myocardial Infarction, and Arrhythmias	234
Types of Arrhythmias	234
Coronary Artery Disease (CAD)	237
Treatment for Diseases of the Heart	237
Cardiac Glycosides	238
Diuretics	238
Vasodilators	240
ACE Inhibitors	241
Beta-Adrenergic Blockers	243
Hypertension	244
Treatment of Coronary Artery Disease	245
Antiplatelet Agents	245
Anticoagulants	245
Tissue Plasminogen Activators	248
Stages of Clot Formation	249
Stage I	249
Stage II	249

The Pharmacy Technician Series

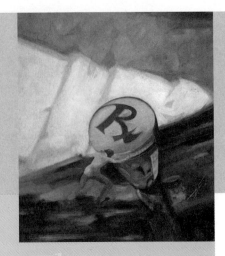

Stage III		250
Stage IV		250
Antidotes for Overdose of Antiplatelets or Anticoagulants		250
New Direct Thrombin Inhibitors		251
Antihyperlipidemics or Hypolipidemics		251
Adrenocorticosteroids		252
Cholesterol		252
Triglycerides		253
Treatment of Arrhythmias		255
Class I Anti-arrhythmic Agents		256
Class II Anti-arrhythmic Agents		256
Class III Anti-arrhythmic Agents		256
Class IV Anti-arrhythmic Agents		256
The Lymphatic System		256
Structural Components		256
The Lymphatic Route		259
Diseases of the Spleen		260
Summary		261
Chapter Review Questions		262

15 The Immune System   **264**

Introduction		264
Anatomy and Physiology of the Immune System		265
The Body's Defense Mechanisms		265
Nonspecific Defense Mechanisms		265
Specific Defense Mechanisms		266
Lymphocytes		267
Specific Mechanism of Defense		270
Cell Structure and Function		271
Types of Infectious Organisms		271

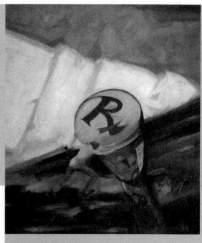

Animal Microorganisms	271
HIV/AIDS	274
Progression of HIV to AIDS to Death in Five Stages	275
Retroviral Replication	275
The HIV Replication Process in 11 Stages	275
HIV/AIDS Drugs	276
Autoimmune Diseases	279
Rheumatoid Arthritis	279
Plant Microorganisms	283
Antifungals	284
Amebicides/Antiprotozoal	284
Prions	287
Gram Staining	287
Methods of Transmission	288
Anti-infectives	288
Resistance	288
Antibacterials	295
MOA of Cephalosporins	298
Antivirals	304
MOA of Antivirals	304
Vaccines	305
Various Infectious Disease States	306
Cancer	310
Drugs Used to Treat Cancer	311
Summary	315
Chapter Review Questions	316

16   The Renal System   318

Introduction	318
Anatomy and Physiology of the Renal System	319
The Bladder and Urine	321

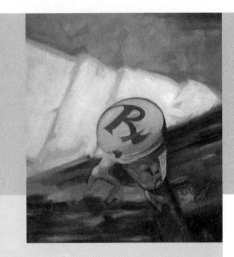

Diseases of the Urinary System and Treatment   322
   Urinary Incontinence   322
   Urinary Retention   323
   Urinary Tract Infections   324
   Kidney Stones   327
   Edema and Hypertension   328
   Diabetes Mellitus and the Kidneys   328
Diuretics   329
Summary   331
Chapter Review Questions   332

17   The Endocrine System   336

Introduction   336
Anatomy of the Endocrine System   337
Glands, Organs, and Secretions   338
Hormones   340
The Glands   342
   Hypothalamus   342
   The Pituitary Gland   343
   Thyroid and Parathyroid   343
   Adrenal   345
Glucocorticoids   347
   Administration of Glucocorticoids   347
Mineralcorticoids   348
The Gonads   349
Female Sex Hormones   349
Male Sex Hormones   350
Estrogen Replacement Therapy and Menopause   351
   Contraindications   354
Testosterone Hormonal Replacement   354
   Contraindications   355
   Side Effects of Anabolic Steroids   356

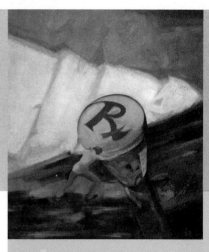

Precautions   357
Glandular Disease States   357
  Examples of Cancers that Benefit
    from Endocrine Therapy   357
Endocrine System Disorders
  and Pituitary Abnormalities   358
  Pituitary Gigantism   358
  Pituitary Dwarfism   358
  Acromegaly   359
Diabetes   359
  Insulin   361
  Diabetes Insipidus   362
Abnormalities of the Adrenal Gland   364
  Cushing's Syndrome   364
  Addison's Disease   365
  Cretenism   366
  Myxedema (Secondary Hypothyroidism)   366
  Grave's Disease   366
  Erectile Dysfunction   367
  Hypothalamus   368
  Pituitary Gland   368
Summary   371
Chapter Review Questions   372

18 **The Reproductive System**   **374**

Introduction   374
The Female Reproductive System   375
  Anatomy and Physiology   375
Contraceptives   377
  Topical Contraceptives   380
  Contraceptive Devices   380

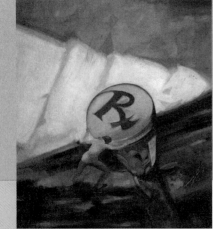

Diaphragms and Cervical Caps	381
Intrauterine Devices	382
STDs—Sexually Transmitted Diseases	382
Treatment and Prevention of STDs	383
Mammary Glands and Childbirth	383
Lactation	384
Infertility	384
Disease State, Causes, Symptoms, Outcome if Left Untreated	384
Causes of Infertility in Women	385
Pharmaceutical Treatment of Infertility in Women	386
The Male Reproductive System	386
Anatomy	386
Diseases of the Male Reproductive Tract	387
Summary	391
Chapter Review Questions	392

19   The Nervous System   395

Introduction	395
Anatomy of the Nervous System	396
Functions of the Nervous System	396
The Neuron	399
Neurotransmission and Receptors	400
The Central Nervous System	401
The Brain	402
Cerebellum	402
Cerebrum	402
Reticular Formation	404
The Limbic System	404
Blood Brain Barrier (BBB)	404
Diseases Affecting the Central Nervous System	405

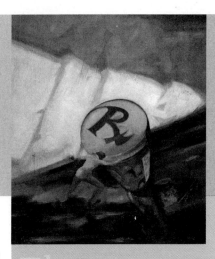

Anxiety 405
 Benzodiazepines 407
 Mechanism of Action of Buspirone 408
Mood Disorders 408
 Depression 408
Bipolar Disorder 412
 Mechanism of Action of Lithium 420
 Alcohol Withdrawal 420
 Treatment 421
Smoking Withdrawal and Cessation 422
 Antidepressants in Smoking Cessation 423
 Anti-anxiety Agents in Smoking Cessation 423
Psychosis 423
 Mechanism of Action of Antipsychotic Drugs 424
 Conventional, Traditional,
  or Typical Antipsychotic Drugs 425
Insomnia 425
 Prescription Hypnotics, Sedatives,
  and Barbiturate Medication 427
 Mechanism of Action for the Non-Benzodiazepines 428
Stimulants 431
 Adverse Actions of Stimulants 432
 Contraindications: Drug–Condition
  Interactions of Stimulants 432
 Withdrawal Treatment 432
ADD and ADHD 432
 Stimulants Used in the Treatment of ADHD
  and ADD 432
 Nonstimulants Used in the Treatment of ADHD
  and ADD 434
 Adverse Reactions of Strattera® (atomoxetine) 434
 Contraindications of Strattera® (atomoxetine) 434

The
Pharmacy
Technician
Series

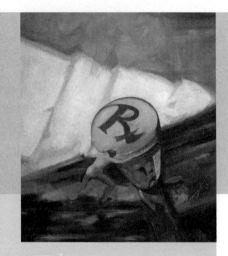

Convulsions, Seizures, and Epilepsy	434
Different Types and Classifications of Seizures	435
Status Epilepticus	436
Treatment of Seizures and Convulsions	437
Parkinson's Disease	437
Nonpharmaceutical Treatments of Parkinson's Disease, or PD	439
Future Treatments	439
Pharmaceutical Treatments of PD	439
Dementia and Alzheimer's Disease	442
Signs and Symptoms of Dementia	443
Treatment of Dementia	444
Migraine Headaches	446
Classic Migraine	447
Common Migraine	447
Pharmaceutical Treatment of Migraine Headache	448
Reye's Syndrome	448
Other drugs	450
Cancer Pain	453
Treatment of Cancer Pain	454
Nonpharmaceutical Pain Relief	455
Scheduled Narcotic Analgesics	455
The Peripheral Nervous System	458
Summary	459
Chapter Review Questions	460
APPENDIX A **Terminology**	465
APPENDIX B **Answers**	476
INDEX	485

Preface

Pharmacology is a key title in Prentice Hall's newest series for pharmacy technician education. *The Pharmacy Technician Series* is made up of six books that have been developed and designed together, ensuring greater success for the pharmacy technician student.

About the Book

Pharmacology is a detailed and complicated science; however, it is vital for the pharmacy technician to understand this subject. This book has been designed to guide the students through with ease, while building a solid foundation of knowledge for their careers.

The core features of this book include the following:

- Chapter Introductions and Summaries, which provide the student with a clearer understanding and rationale of the content being covered.
- Profiles of Practice boxes provide practical tips and quick statistics to engage the student in the learning process.
- Chapter Reviews provide a learning assessment for both the student and instructor to evaluate concept comprehension.
- Extensive illustrations—this book, while focused on pharmacology, is built on an anatomy and physiology approach to teaching. Students will treasure the quantity and detail of illustrations in this book.
- Terminology Appendix—students will appreciate the quick reference on pharmacology-related terminology found at the back of the book.

About the Series

While there have been a variety of textbooks and training manuals available for pharmacy technician education, none has met the true educational needs of the industry—until now.

We set out to develop the most comprehensive, accurate, and current texts ever published for pharmacy technicians. One method we used to achieve this goal was to involve pharmacy technician educators and trainers from across the country in every phase of the project. You will find that each title in this series has been developed, written, and reviewed exclusively by practicing pharmacy technician educators and practicing pharmacy professionals—a winning approach.

About the Authors

Jeanetta Mastron, **BS, CPhT**

Jeanetta has worked in pharmacy since 1989; for the past nine years she has served as a pharmacy technician educator. Currently, she works for the American Institute of Health Science in Long Beach, California, as Program Director and pharmacy technician educator.

Jeanetta earned her Bachelor of Science degree in Chemistry at Chapman College in 1977. In the past, she has served as the Contributing Editor for continuing education programs in *Today's Technician*™ magazine, and she is a regular presenter at pharmacy-related seminars across the United States. Jeanetta was awarded Technician Educator of the Year by NPTA in 2002.

Robin Luke, **CPhT**

Robin is a founding member of NPTA's Executive Advisory Board, the elected body of leaders for the National Pharmacy Technician Association. She has over ten years of experience in institutional pharmacy, sterile product preparation, compounding, bulk-manufacturing, and management, with a specialized knowledge of herbals and homeopathic treatments.

Robin has developed a variety of continuing education programs with a strong emphasis on reducing medication errors; she also speaks at meetings and conferences across the United States.

with

Mike Johnston, **CPhT**

Mike is known internationally as a respected author and speaker in the field of pharmacy. He published his first book, *Rx for Success—A Career Enhancement Guide for Pharmacy Technicians*, in 2002.

In 1999, Mike founded NPTA in Houston, Texas, and led the association from 3 members to over 20,000 in less than two years. Today, as Executive Director of the National Pharmacy Technician Association and publisher of *Today's Technician* magazine, he spends the majority of his time meeting with and speaking to employers, manufacturers, association leaders, and elected officials on issues related to pharmacy technicians.

About NPTA

NPTA, the National Pharmacy Technician Association, is the world's largest professional organization established specifically for pharmacy technicians. The association is dedicated to advancing the value of pharmacy technicians and the vital roles they play in pharmaceutical care. In a society of countless associations, we believe it takes much more than a mission statement to meet the professional needs and provide the needed leadership for the pharmacy technician profession—it takes action and results.

The organization is composed of pharmacy technicians practicing in a variety of practice settings, such as: retail, independent, hospital, mail-order, home care, long-term care, nuclear, military, correctional facility, formal education, training, management, sales, and many more. NPTA is a reflection of this diverse profession and provides unparallel support and resources to members.

NPTA is The Foundation of the Pharmacy Technician Profession; we have an unprecedented past, a strong presence, and a promising future. We are dedicated to improving our profession, while remaining focused on our members.

For more information on NPTA:
Call 888-247-8700
Visit www.pharmacytechnician.org

Acknowledgments

This book, which is part of a six title series, has been both an exhilarating and exhausting project. To say that this series is the result of a collaborative, team effort would be a gross understatement.

Mark — thank you for believing in my initial vision and concept for this series, which was anything but traditional. I will always remember the day we spent in New York City talking about cover concepts, and the like, at coffee shops and art galleries. More importantly, I am honored to have gotten to know you, Alex, and now little Sophie—and I consider each of you as friends.

Joan — you are truly gifted at what you do. I am amazed at your ability to join this project, at the point you did, and to literally guide each daunting task into a smooth and successful accomplishment. I feel that your leadership have created a better final product.

Julie — thank you for taking risks (plural) on this project, compared with standard policies and procedures. In the end, your support and belief in this project have allowed for a truly innovative product to be published.

Robin — your commitment to this project . . . to exceeding all expectations . . . to developing the best training series for pharmacy technicians available has been amazing. You are a wonderful, gifted individual—but most importantly I am thankful to call you "friend."

Andrew and Jenny — thank you for supporting this project, each in your own unique ways; thank you for supporting me and the entire organization. This project tested each of us . . . our character and our will . . . and I am honored to know you both.

Most important, I wish to thank my family. The past several years have been difficult and trying, but the strength, love, and support that you've given me has always pulled me through. *Thank you*.

Contributor

Mark Abell, PA
Lowell, FL

Reviewers

The reviewers of The Pharmacy Technician Series have provided many excellent suggestions and ideas for improving these texts. The quality of the reviews has been outstanding, and the reviews have been a major aid in the preparation of the manuscript. The assistance provided by these experts is deeply appreciated.

Lisa C. Barnes, B. Pharm., M.B.A.
ACPE Program Administrator, Adjunct Assistant Professor of Pharmacy Practice
University of Montana School of Pharmacy and Allied Health Sciences
Missoula, Montana

Kimberly Brown, CPhT
Associate Director and Instructor of Pharmacy Technology
Walters State Community College
Morristown, Tennessee

Ralph P. Casas, Pharm. D., Ph.D.
Associate Professor of Pharmacology
Cerritos Community College
Norwalk, California

Kristie Fitzgerald, BS, Pharm
Clinical Pharmacist, Department of Neonatology; Instructor
Salt Lake Community College
Salt Lake City, Utah

Madeline Jensen-Grauel, BS, Ed., M.Sc
Director, Pharmacy Technician Training Program
The University of Texas Medical Branch at Galveston
Galveston, Texas

Robert D. Kwiatkowski, BS, MA
Adjunct Instructor
PIMA Medical Institute
Colorado Springs, Colorado

Herminio Maldonado, Jr., MS, BS
Pharmacy Technician Instructor
PIMA Medical Institute
Colorado Springs, Colorado

Bradley Moore, MSN
Director of Health Science
Remington Administrative Services, Inc.
Little Rock, Arkansas

Hieu Nguyen, BS, CPhT
Pharmacy Technician Program Director
Western Career College
Sacramento, California

Introduction to Pharmacology

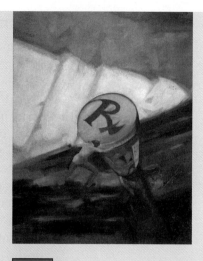

After completing this chapter, you should be able to:

- Define pharmacology and explain its importance as it relates to pharmacy technicians.
- Recognize and define the basic terms used in pharmacology.
- List and describe the major areas of pharmacology.

INTRODUCTION

Pharmacology is the medical science that deals with the discovery, chemistry, effects, uses, and manufacture of drugs. It builds on key concepts of physiology, biochemistry, microbiology, and pathology to help explain the mechanisms, uses, and adverse effects of pharmaceuticals used in clinical medicine. It is a very complex discipline, and it would take more than merely a few chapters or even this entire book to understand all of its components. But, by using this book, you will be introduced to a number of different aspects of the science of pharmacology. Primarily, the focus will be on the aspects of the science that will affect your work with patients—how pharmacology works clinically.

Studying Pharmacology

Due to its enormous, multifaceted complexity, pharmacology provides multiple challenges to various health care personnel. Each medical discipline may have different reasons for and concerns about understanding and using pharmacological information. Anyone who studies pharmacology will learn the basic principles, such as understanding drug actions and patient dosing (receptors, pharmacodynamics, pharmacokinetics, biotransformation, toxicology, and so on). A deeper understanding would incorporate the major therapeutics available and their uses. There are thousands of FDA-approved drugs that can be grouped into dozens of distinct categories on the bases on mechanism of action and therapeutic use. Furthermore, for any given mechanism or use, multiple agents generally exist, often with important differences among each other.

For the pharmacy technician, understanding the basic principles (at the very least) enhances the understanding of drugs and can be of great value in their chosen career. For example, during cart fill procedures, the patient drawer requires diphenhydramine with no particular amount stated for the fill. With basic knowledge of the drug diphenhydramine, a pharmacy technician understands enough to know how much to fill, what is a normal dose and frequency, and how much is too much. By knowing a little something about the patient, the pharmacy technician may also realize if the fill requires oral or intravenous (IV) form. Further study of pharmacology would provide integrative understanding of drug interactions with complex physiological and pathological processes. With this type of knowledge, a pharmacy technician could more fully understand drug–drug interactions. Realizing that there is so much more, a pharmacy technician is not limited and can only benefit from further learning. Also, can you just imagine with this knowledge how many medication errors are prevented?

There are any number of textbooks on the market to teach the subject of pharmacology. The material is presented in a way that is intended for a particular profession such as nursing. The same material may be presented in another textbook for another type of health-care related professional such as a microbiologist. Part of the confusion and frustration a student may experience is sometimes due to studying the right material with the wrong presentation. Other textbooks may oversimplify the complex material to a point where important concepts are neither understood nor retained. It is not only difficult to present the subject of pharmacology, but also challenging to present it in such a way that the student understands and retains the information. One way is to present the material with a particular health-care professional in mind. This book is written for the pharmacy technician.

By looking through this section, you will be exposed to many different aspects of how a drug or a chemical is permitted to enter the body and travel through the system and how it is handled by the body at the cellular level. Why? Because you, as a pharmacy technician, will not only be responsible for filling some prescription vials under the supervision of a pharmacist, but you will probably also be the first person and the last person the patient sees.

There are many different kinds of pharmaceuticals, from the ones patients will take through their mouths (orally, or PO) to the ones that they will apply to their skin, as in a patch or a paste. You will be exposed to different kinds of drugs and chemicals, and you will learn how they are absorbed. You will also be exposed to situations in which you might be able to detect whether a person is, perhaps, taking his medications the wrong way. (You will be surprised how many patients actually swallow a suppository!)

You will be taken through a course that will teach you not only what medications are called, but also the reasons behind the names. That's the realm of pharmacology—for a pharmacy technician.

Remember the following points:

- Drugs and the therapy by which they are being used to treat people are always changing, which means that you will also be required to change—you will always have to be willing to learn.
- All of the technological advancements over the last 50 years have developed a world in which patients are ever more demanding. They want their medications now. Be there for these people, as you will be one of them someday. "It remains the responsibility of every practitioner to evaluate the appropriateness of a particular opinion or therapy in the context of the actual clinical situation and with due consideration of any new developments in the field."

What does that last statement mean to you? It should indicate that, while you are not a practitioner in the same sense as a health care provider (such as a doctor) is, you should continue to aim high, keeping abreast of changes as they occur in medicine and applying them to the safety of your patients at all times. During such times throughout your career, patients will expect you to come through with answers to their questions. And if you don't have the answer, you will know how to find it.

Basic Terminology

As with any other profession, pharmacology has specific terms that you will be using throughout your career. You will hear these terms over and over again, so get used to reading them and understanding their meanings.

While the following terms do not nearly represent all of the terms applicable to the study of drugs, they do represent some of the key words that are most used in the functions of a pharmacy technician, and they will provide the foundation you will need when starting to understand pharmacology. As you continue with your studies, you will come across more terms and more definitions.

Adverse effect—a general term that applies to instances when there is an undesirable and potentially hazardous effect after the ingestion of a drug.

Agonist—a drug that binds to a specific receptor on a cell, typically called a target cell, and which produces a specific action within the cell and then within the body.

Antagonist—an inhibitor; a drug that counteracts, or provides the opposite effect of, an agonist.

Chemical name—the chemical composition of a specific drug. For example, the chemical name for ranitidine is quite foreign to most people and would have no meaning except to chemists.

Contraindications—a term denoting that a specific drug or combination of drugs should not be used by a person or a certain class of people because the use of the drug may have a dangerous and possibly fatal effect.

Dose—the exact amount of a drug that is to be administered to a specific person to produce a desirable effect.

Drug—any chemical substance that, when ingested, injected, applied to the skin, or administered in any other fashion will cause a specific change in the body.

Drug indication—the exact reason for the use of a drug.

ED50— a name that is applied to exactly one-half of the maximum dose of a drug, so that, when the maximum is used, the exact effects will be known.

Generic name—Drugs are released into market with two names: the generic name and the nongeneric name. The generic name is more appropriately used for the exact name of the drug, as it defines the class and something about the drug's use.

Mechanism of action—how a drug works or, after the drug is ingested, what effect it will have on the body (whether good or bad).

Over-the-counter (OTC) drugs—available to the public without a prescription. These drugs will change from time to time, as the FDA will commonly permit new drugs to be released to the public after the potential dangers have been eliminated.

Pharmacology—the study of drugs, how they work, and how they are metabolized and secreted from the body.

Receptor—the specific location on the cell membrane where, as with the agonist and the antagonist examples, a drug will become attached to the cell, enter the cell, and produce the desired effects.

Schedule I drug—the class of drugs that have the highest potential for abuse and, because of their actions, have no acceptable medical use.

Schedule II drug—the class of drugs that do have acceptable medical use, but are also extremely addictive. As a pharmacy technician, because of state and federal laws, you will probably not be exposed to these drugs unless you are under the direct supervision of the pharmacist. Schedule II drugs are highly regulated and monitored; if even one is missing, the federal or state government can actually revoke the license of the pharmacy.

Schedule III drugs—the class of drugs that are addictive, but the potential for abuse is considerably less than Schedule I and II drugs. There is a moderate potential for abuse, and, therefore, you will probably not be exposed to these drugs unless for exceptional purposes.

Schedule IV drugs—the class of drugs with a very limited degree of potential abuse. You will probably have some contact with them and will develop into a good adjunct to your pharmacist.

Schedule V drugs—the class of drugs that have the most limited degree of potential abuse. They are typically handled by both pharmacists and pharmacy technicians.

Side effect—an effect that a drug has on the body. While unexpected and undesirable, this effect is not necessarily deemed harmful. An example would be an upset stomach after taking a prescription antibiotic.

Site of action—the location where a drug will typically be expected to exert its effect—that is, at the cellular level.

Trade name—different from the generic name, this is the name that the pharmaceutical company uses, as a registered trademark, to promote the drug.

Major Areas of Pharmacology

There are a number of areas associated with the study of drugs, and you will be exposed to most of these in this book. While this is not an exhaustive list, it is a start and a basis on which other areas of pharmacology will build as you do your research.

Pharmacodynamics—the study of how drugs affect the body, including all of the different cells in the body (collectively called tissues).

Pharmacokinetics—the study of how drugs are introduced into the body and then absorbed, distributed, metabolized, and excreted out of the body.

Pharmacotherapeutics—a major study in the realm of pharmacology concerned with how drugs are used in the treatment of disease within the human body.

Pharmacy—an actual science, and not merely a place where people go to retrieve their medications. Pharmacy is the study of preparing and dispensing medications.

Posology—the study of the exact amount of a drug that is needed in order to produce a therapeutic effect.

Toxicology—the study of drugs that is concerned with harmful effects that any specific or any number of drugs have on living human tissue. For the pharmacy technician, it is important to understand that all drugs, to one extent or another, can have a toxic effect, just as water, as vital as it is to life, can cause one to drown.

SUMMARY

A thorough knowledge of pharmacology is essential to the pharmacy technician. Working under the supervision of a pharmacist, you will be responsible for filling prescriptions and interacting with patients. Keeping abreast of new technological advancements and new developments in the field of pharmacology will enable you to help minimize medication errors, and ensure the well-being and safety of the patients you serve.

Understanding the basic terms of pharmacology will provide you with a strong foundation to use throughout your career as a pharmacy technician. It is important to the safety of your patients that terms, such as adverse effect, contraindication, and mechanism of action, be fully understood. Familiarity with generic vs. trade names, dosage regimens, and drug interactions are important aspects of your knowledge base.

Finally, you will be exposed to a number of major areas of pharmacology, including how a drug works in the body (Pharmacodynamics), how the body affects the drug (Pharmacokinetics), and how drugs exert their therapeutic effect (Phamacotherapeutics). A solid understanding of these, and other, areas of pharmacology are necessary to enable you to assist the pharmacist in providing the best patient care.

CHAPTER REVIEW QUESTIONS

1. The study of how drugs have an effect on the body is known as:

   a. pharmacology

   b. pharmacotherapuetics

   c. pharmacokinetics

   d. pharmacodynamics

2. The cellular location where a drug will take effect is the receptor.

   a. true   b. false

3. Why is it important to study pharmacology on a continuous basis?

4. An agonist is a drug that binds to a specific receptor on a cell.

   a. true   b. false

5. _____ is the exact reason for the use of a drug.

Resources and References

1. Hitner, H. and Barbara Nagle. *Basic Pharmacology, 4th Ed.* New York and other cities: Glencoe/McGraw-Hill Publishers, Inc., 1999.

2. Koda-Kimble, Mary Anne. *Applied Therapeutics: The Clinical Use of Drugs, 4th Ed.* Vancouver, Washington: Applied Therapeutics, Inc., 1992.

3. Allen, Loyd V. Jr., Ph.D. *The Art, Science, and Technology of Pharmaceutical Compounding.* Washington, DC: American Pharmaceutical Association, 1998

4. Holland, Norman and Michael Patrick Adams. *Core Concepts in Pharmacology.* Upper Saddle River, NJ: Pearson Education, 2003.

5. Adams, Michael Patrick, Dianne L. Josephson, and Leland Norman Holland, Jr. *Pharmacology for Nurses—A Pathophysiologic Approach.* Upper Saddle River, NJ: Pearson Education, 2005.

The Realm of Pharmacology

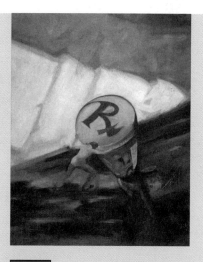

INTRODUCTION

Pharmacology is a very complex, diversified, and yet intriguing science. Those who leave high school and decide to take the road toward a degree in pharmacology spend countless hours with their eyes glued to textbooks.

By their own right, pharmacists are truly scientists. They take the responsibility for the health of others into their own hands, and a majority of them are now heavily involved in advancing their own degrees and taking their careers into the area of compounding medicines. This is far beyond what most people once thought about seeing the window with the Rx sign in the front.

Your responsibilities and how you view your job will depend very much on the pharmacist or pharmacists with whom you will be working. Although their knowledge might be advanced compared with yours, your ability to perform may be congruent with theirs. Knowing this can boost your confidence and improve your attitude as you continue with your studies as a pharmacy technician.

There remains so much to learn about pharmacology, even for those who practice the study of drugs and how they react to the human body each and every day. One issue that you should keep in mind is that all of the knowledge in the world will never be equal to experience, and that's where you, as an experienced pharmacy technician, will become a valuable tool to your pharmacist. Applying what you know toward the advancement of your career will help separate you from the rest. People will respect you not only for your knowledge, but also for how well you treat them. But, before we get there, we must know the basics about the science ofpharmacology.

Classification of Drugs

Why do you suppose drugs are listed in classes? What prompted the creation of such a classification? It's actually a good question, and it deserves a good answer. The answer is all in the history of pharmacy and the ways in which the *Federal Drug Administration* has, through the years, modified society's view of medications and addictions. How these medications can have adverse effects on a variety of different organs in the body is also a factor.

A category may be based on the following considerations:

- the chemical ingredients
- the method by which a drug is used (for example, by mouth, by injection, or applied to the skin)
- the organ in the body that is treated (such as the stomach, head, or eye)

Any one of these categories is called a class, and any drug fitting designated criteria belongs to that class of drugs. Putting drugs in the same class can provide effective treatment and cost savings.

Although there are numerous ways to classify drugs, for many reasons, drugs are often classified into groups according to two primary methods. Grouping drugs according to therapeutic classification as determined by their therapeutic usefulness is one way. Grouping drugs according to how they work pharmacologically, referred to as pharmacological classification, is the other. For example, a **diuretic** (an agent that promotes the excretion of urine) is an example of a pharmacological classification, as it describes an effect on the body, whereas a drug for vomiting (**emesis**) is an example of a therapeutic classification, as it describes a more straightforward clinical action of a drug.

Following are some of the universally accepted drug classifications, including either drug examples or subclassifications. (This is not a complete list.)

Analgesic (a drug that selectively suppresses pain)

narcotic

nonnarcotic

antirheumatic

Antiinfective

aminoglycosides

antifungals

antivirals
cephalosporins
florquinolones
macrolide antibiotics
peniciliins
tetracyclines

Antineoplastics (drug that is selectively toxic to rapidly dividing cells and is used to treat cancer)

Antiseptics (drug that inhibits bacterial growth, but does not destroy bacteria)

Antiviral (drug used to treat viral infections)
epivir
famvir
acyclovir

Cardiovascular
antihypertensive
antihyperlipidemic
beta blockers
calcium channel blockers
diuretics

Central Nervous System
antianxiety
antidepressants
antipsychotics
hypnotics
stimulants

Endocrine and Metabolic
androgen
anabolic
corticosteroids
estrogens
progestins
thyroid

Gastrointestinal
antidiarrheals
antimetics
laxatives
digestive aids

Hematological
anticoagulants
hemostatics

Neuromuscular

anticonvulsant

skeletal muscle relaxants

Nonsteroidal Anti-Inflammatory Drugs (NSAID)

ibuprofen

Nutritional

minerals

vitamins

electrolytes

Proton Pump Inhibitor

omeprazole

lansoprazole

Respiratory

antiasthmatics

antihistamines

decongestants

Topical

ophthalmic

otic

intrarectal steroids

Certain drugs, because of specific reasons, are classified into categories according to important factors. Two such categories are pregnancy and scheduled drugs or *controlled substances*.

Pregnancy categories are determined on the basis of the potential harm to the unborn. The five pregnancy categories of safety are A, B, C, D, and X, with A being the lowest risk and X being the highest. (See Table 2-1.)

TABLE 2-1 The Five Pregnancy Categories

Category	Description
A (lowest risk)	No known studies proving risk or harm to fetus have been performed.
B	No known animal studies show risk. If animal studies have shown risk, no studies in women confirm risk.
C	Animal studies show risk, but controlled studies in women have not been performed.
D	These drugs may cause harm, but also may provide benefit if no other drug is available or a life-threatening situation is present.
X (highest risk)	Studies show significant risk to women and fetus.

If you were to ask someone about the classification, for example, of an *antibiotic* that can be used for a female who is expecting to deliver a child, you could expect to hear any one of the following responses:

- These drugs are proven safe in pregnancies.

- These drugs are inadequate for those who are pregnant, mainly because they have not been tested in such a realm. (This is usually because there has been no reason to do so.)

- These drugs have been proven to be *teratogenic* (tending to produce anomalies of formation) in animals, which means that they have been proven not to be safe in gestating animals; but, again, because there has been no reason to test in female humans who are expecting, they are considered not to be safe in pregnant women at any point in their pregnancies.

- These are the types of drugs that have enough evidence to pose a fetal risk in humans; therefore, they should not be used at any cost or for any reason.

Controlled substances or scheduled medications require strict records to be kept of the amounts received by warehouses; these records can be compared with lists of the amounts prescribed.

Controlled substances are classified into scheduled class 1, 2, 3, 4, or 5 according to their potential for abuse. The classes and descriptions are as follows:

- **Class I**—There are no medical needs for these drugs, and they are not used in medicine for any reason; they are highly *addictive.* These are usually what we call street drugs.

- **Class II**—These drugs are highly addictive, but they do have a role in medicine. In most states, they cannot be released other than through a specific route; specifically, there must be a prescription with no refills. They must be counted and controlled by a licensed pharmacist and otherwise locked up. These drugs are exposed to the scrutiny of the FDA. For any reason, an agent can walk into a pharmacy, request to see the "Control II list," and then proceed to count the corresponding inventory, pill by pill, to ensure that no problems are indicated. At no time will these prescriptions be filled in response to a telephone call to a pharmacy. The pharmacy must keep strict records of all activity regarding these drugs.

- **Class III**—These drugs have less addictive value, and therefore, depending upon the state in which you will be employed and the company for which you will work, you may or may not be permitted to handle prescriptions for them. Generally, pharmacy technicians fill these prescriptions. Class III drugs may be kept in a separate locked area or vault.

- **Class IV**—These prescriptions have less addictive value. Usually, the pharmacist and company will permit the pharmacy technician to handle these drugs.

- **Class V**—Because of specific qualities, these drugs are addictive, but the potential for addiction is very rare.

The most important legislation that you should be aware of is the *Controlled Substances Act of 1970*, which was designed to regulate how pharmaceuticals are handled, how they are dispensed, and how they are directed by physicians. Remember, the physician–pharmacist relationship is one of trust, and that trust is controlled by many factors—not just laws, but also integrity and the realm of health care. The aforementioned schedule was designed as an offshoot of this enactment and has been a framework by which all controlled drugs have been handled since that time.

Drug Names

As you may already know, there are many different ways to describe one drug, but there are three basic types of name given to each drug: the chemical, *generic*, and *trade* names. Practicing pharmacy technicians will typically use and rely mostly on the brand and generic names during prescription filling and processing tasks.

There are a few things that you will need to know about the important differences between these two names. They can be very difficult to differentiate if you don't commit yourself to remembering them, but in time the distinctions will become second nature to you.

- *The generic name* describes the active ingredient(s) in the drug. Each drug has only one generic name given by the United States Adopted Name Council. (See Figure 2-1.)
- *The trade name* (also known as the brand or proprietary name) is the name that the pharmaceutical company develops to give the drug social and public significance. An example is the drug Zantac®, an *H2 blocker* which works by reducing the amount of acid in the stomach; ranitidine is the generic name. The trade name is given by the company that has researched, developed, and marketed the drug. (See Figure 2-2.)

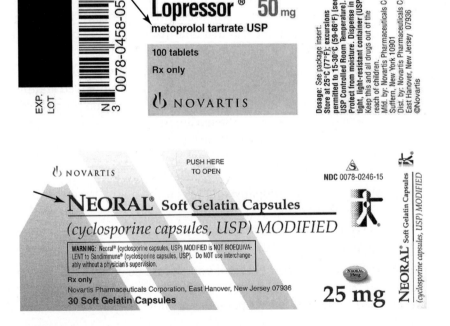

Figure 2-1 The generic name is metoprolol tartrate (*Lopressor is a registered trade mark of Novartis Corporation*)

Figure 2-2 The trade name is "Neoral" (*Neoral is a registered trademark of Novartis AG*)

When written, the trade name is generally capitalized, while the generic name is usually in lowercase letters. It is very important for the pharmacy technician to become familiar with the generic names. In efforts to contain escalating drug costs, increasingly, generic medications are the only allowable drugs that insurance plans will consider payment for to the pharmacy under many *health maintenance organizations* and *formularies*. Also, many pharmacy stock areas file their medications alphabetically according to generic names.

The chemical name of a drug is often complicated and generally refers to the chemical nature of the drug. These names can be extremely lengthy and difficult to remember and pronounce for many pharmacy technicians. Each drug is named by employing IUPAC's (International Union of Pure and Applied Chemistry) strict *nomenclature* guidelines. Each drug has only one chemical name.

If you ever had the opportunity to work with a physician or to review a patient's record, you would most likely see the trade names for most of the drugs. The reason for that is quite simple—physicians are inundated with visits from representatives of all of the major drug companies, who want the physicians to use their drugs. The representatives do not "push" their generic drugs, which are typically far beyond patent protection. The newer drugs are the ones that make the money, and once a physician, a physician assistant, or a nurse practitioner learns these trade names, they usually stick—it's a matter of memory and habit.

Routes of Administration

When most people think about pharmaceuticals, they think about the pill. But, in the real world of medicine, there are a number of different ways in which a health care provider can get a chemical compound—a drug—into a patient's body. These routes of administration are important to remember. Some drugs are packaged in a number of different forms, and this can be especially troublesome if the pharmacy in which you work deals with diverse patient populations. Getting a liquid mixed up with a solid is an easy mistake, but one that can produce some very dangerous consequences.

ORAL ADMINISTRATION

A tablet is a solid, whereas a capsule is an amount of liquid or solid granules contained in a "capsule" that is dissolved once it hits the acidic environment of the stomach. By far, this is the most common means by which a medication gets into a body. However, it's not quite as simple as merely swallowing the tablet or the capsule. There are many different chemical processes that must take place before the medication can become available to the body. (This will be discussed further in the sections on pharmacokinetics and pharmacodynamics).

Oral administration might be the most common form of administration (see Figure 2-3), but it is not always the best. Some people have specific problems, such as gastric emptying difficulties or a decreased intestinal transit time that will either inhibit the use of a pill or a capsule or delay the process of absorption.

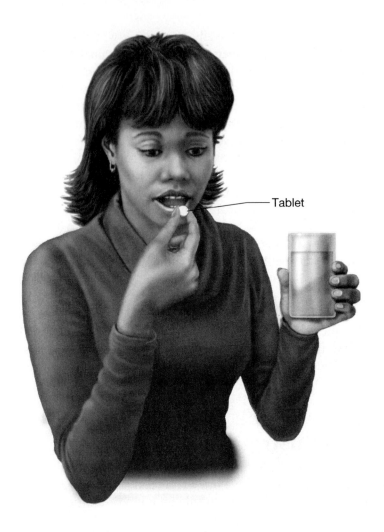

Tablet

Figure 2-3 The oral
route of administration

Oral tablets are available in various modified forms such as enteric coated, chewable, sustained release, and extended release forms. These products have been developed to aid in numerous types of patient situations—for example, when a drug should be released over a period of time (as in sustained release form) or when the action of the drug is to last for a period of time (as in extended release for optimum therapeutic effect).

Enteric coated medications can be used for patients who suffer from some sort of irritation to the medication's ingredients. The manufacturer may coat the tablet for ease of use to improve patient compliance. Another reason could be that the medication is coated to keep it binded, as it may otherwise break apart too easily. To accommodate different situations that may hinder absorption, when the medicine is to be released over a specific period of time, or to reduce stomach or other irritation, there are subforms of oral medication available in the tablet form.

Chewable forms of medications may be available especially for children. They may be beneficial in situations where it is difficult for the patient to swallow. A patient can chew the medication to a smaller form that may dissolve in his own saliva and thus be a lot easier to take. Often, they are flavored to make them more palatable to the patient.

There are a number of ways to administer a medication in oral form. Medications in capsule form sometimes work faster to dissolve in the body because they break down more quickly. There are two types of capsules. One capsule has a soft, gelatin-like shell, such as docusate sodium, and contains a liquid inside. The other has two harder shell pieces that fit together and contain a powder or granulated medication.

When a patient cannot or does not wish to take a tablet or capsule at all, a suspension can be made with some medications. For example, a child who is prescribed amoxicillin may require a liquid form. For many parents, it is difficult to get a young child to take tablets for various reasons. However, when given an amoxicillin suspension (referred to affectionately by many children as the "bubble gum" medicine), compliance is greatly increased. Each patient is different, and the provider has some options when attempting to increase compliance by choosing oral forms preferred by patients.

Sometimes, there is no apparent explanation at all, except that the patient just wants a capsule and not a tablet. You may notice this with some OTC (over the counter) medications on your store shelves, such as cold or *analgesic* remedies. They may be available as tablets, capsules, coated tablets, liqui-gels, or liquid. In addition to therapeutic reasons, there are also many consumer-driven reasons for the availability of various oral forms of medications.

Other oral forms may include troches, or lozenges designed to dissolve slowly in the mouth. Other preparations may be provided in a liquid form. These include solutions, emulsions, suspensions, syrups, elixirs, and tinctures.

Solutions include the elixirs, syrups, tinctures, and foams and contain medications in a water base. Some are rather sweet or thick, like syrups, and others that contain alcohol and are more watery are called elixirs.

Although the physician means no harm, there will be times when the route of administration of the medication prescribed will not be in the best interest of the patient. This may be especially true in pediatric cases and for those patients who suffer from cancer or some form of blood disease. You may hear the pharmacists talking with the health care providers (usually over the phone) when these issues arise.

Good relationships among all professionals, therefore, are paramount. In time, with the necessary experience, you may one day be able to alert the pharmacist to a dangerous situation, make an important difference in someone's life, or even stop a potentially harmful problem from occurring.

BUCCAL AND SUBLINGUAL ABSORPTION

These are means of getting drugs into the system via the mouth, but inside the cheek or under the tongue, respectively. (See Figure 2-4.) One advantage of these routes is that, because of the way in which the drug is manufactured, it does not need to go through the first-pass effect by way of the liver. (This will be discussed further in other parts of the text.) These means of getting the drug into the system work not only more easily, but also much faster than swallowing a pill.

Because of the structure of the tissue under the tongue and the way the saliva affects the medication (which is the first means by which anything

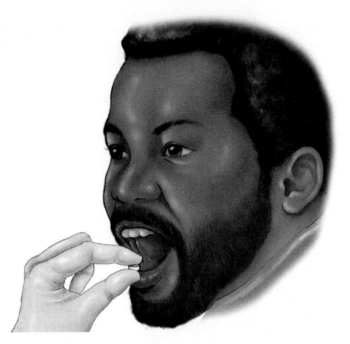

Figure 2-4 Sublingual route (*Holland, Norman; Adams, Michael Patrick, Core Concepts in Pharmacology, 1st Edition,* © 2003. Reprinted by permission of Pearson Education, Inc., Upper Saddle River, NJ)

becomes absorbed into the body), this method is excellent for situations when, for instance, a patient is complaining about chest pain—within minutes, the medication is available to the tissues around the heart muscle.

TOPICAL ADMINISTRATION

Medications applied to the skin or *mucous membranes* are known as being applied topically. Topical preparations may be administered to the skin, mouth, nose, oropharynx, cornea, ear, urethra, vagina, or rectum. These preparations may be available in a variety of forms, including the following:

- creams
- ointments
- gels
- lotions
- aerosols
- foams
- plasters
- powders
- patches
- suppositories
- sprays

Creams are a semisolid drug emulsion made of oil and water. An emulsifier is added so that the water and oil blend. The consistency is described as "creamy," and the product spreads easily. An example is hydrocortisone cream.

Ointments are much like creams, in terms of ingredients, but tend to be a little more "oily." Some patients prefer creams, which appear to "dissolve" more easily; others actually prefer a more oily consistency. Some medications come only in one form or the other.

Lotions differ, in that they come in a thicker water base. Many patients prefer them for their spreadability and familiarity, as many items they use every day come in this form (such as hand lotions). In gels, the medication or active ingredients are suspended in a thicker water base.

Medicinal advancements are just around the corner, but currently there are only a few medications that are designed to be administered by the placement of a patch on the skin for absorption into the body. (See Figure 2-5.) The skin is an organ like the liver or the heart; it has a *lipophillic* barrier, which means that it does not have an affinity for substances that contain fats. The patient can place a patch on the skin once a week, for example, and not worry about it until the following week.

RECTAL AND VAGINAL ADMINISTRATION

These methods use the rectum or vagina for administration, and while they bypass the first-pass system of the liver to some extent, they are not always the best means of getting a medication into the body. However, they are excellent for patients who are not cooperative with pills or other means of drug delivery.

Suppositories are usually made of medication and a solid base of glycerin or cocoa butter. They are made in adult and pediatric sizes and are meant to dissolve over a period of time after being inserted.

INHALATION ADMINISTRATION

This form involves inhaling medications (in gas, liquid, or powder form) that are then absorbed by the lung tissue for therapeutic effects. There are a host of medications—and more to come to the market—that are made in

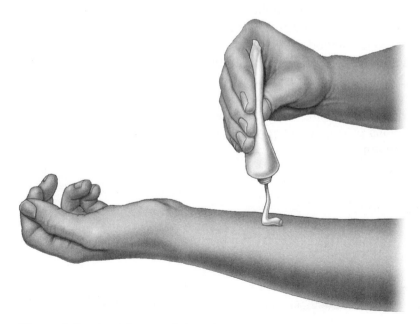

Figure 2-5 Applying an ointment

such a way that they can be administered through the lungs or the tissue within the pulmonary system. Because of certain characteristics of the pulmonary system (specifically, the high blood flow in combination with a relatively large surface area), many medications can be delivered directly to the bloodstream through the lungs, or the medication can be used to treat an ailment in the lungs themselves, such as asthma or some other problem. Nasal inhalation is used for medications in such products as nasal sprays, typically to relieve nasal congestion.

NASOGASTRAL ADMINISTRATION

This method bypasses oral administration and consists of pouring medication into a tube lowered through the mouth and throat into the stomach.

PARENTERAL ADMINISTRATION

Primarily, this method refers to the delivery of medication by way of an *intravenous* system (injection of liquid into the vein), *subcutaneous* injection (under the skin), or *intramuscular* (injection of liquid into a muscle). (See Figure 2-6.) Other less-used methods include intra-articular, intradermal, intrathecal, and intra-arterial.

The major benefit of IV (intravenous) administration is the rate at which the medication will be able to take effect. Since the medication is injected into the vein, the therapeutic effect can be much quicker than if another administration method is used. Many medications come readily available in IV form, while others have to be mixed with a combination of two or more ingredients, as is the case with IV fluids like antibiotics or maintenance IV bags often seen in hospitals. These products generally contain a base fluid, such as *normal saline* or *dextrose*, and have medications added to them in a certain concentration. The method of administration is referred to as an IV drip, and the drug is administered at a prescribed rate over a certain period of time, such as 100 mls per hour for 10 hours.

Numerous medications considered emergency drugs are available in injectable form, such as pain medications, sedation or anesthetics for surgery, and medications to stop an *anaphylactic* reaction (leading to damaging effects on the organism).

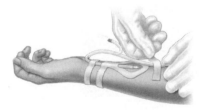

Figure 2-6   Parenteral administration

SUMMARY

Drugs are classified into three categories according to their chemical ingredients, the method by which the drug is used (by mouth, by injection, etc.), and by the organ in the body that is affected by the drug (heart, eye, stomach). They are further designated by separate classes and groups. Two of the most common classifications are therapeutic usefulness, i.e., analgesics (used to relieve pain), and pharmacological activity, i.e., diuretics (used to promote the excretion of urine). Two other important classifications of drugs are: Pregnancy Categories, which are used to determine the potential harm to the fetus if taken by a pregnant woman, and Controlled Substances, which are used to indicate the potential for abuse, or the addictive nature of the drug.

Drugs also have different names. The generic name of a drug describes the active ingredient, while the trade name (or proprietary name) of the drug is the name given to the drug by the pharmaceutical company that developed the drug. The chemical name of a drug is usually extremely long, and actually refers to the exact chemical structure of the drug. These chemical names are seldom used.

Drugs can also be classified according to their route of administration. While the most common method of administering a drug is orally (by mouth), drugs can also be administered parenterally (intravenously, intramuscularly, subcutaneously), topically (through the skin), and by inhalation, to name a few. Each route of administration has advantages and disadvantages which must be considered.

CHAPTER REVIEW QUESTIONS

1. Drugs are classified:
   a. according to the way they affect the body
   b. by cost savings
   c. because there are so many
   d. due to side effects

2. List the scheduled drug classes, and briefly explain their distinctions.

3. Which schedule class has the highest risk of addiction? The lowest?

4. Which agency determines the classification of drugs?
   a. DEA
   b. OSHA
   c. FDA
   d. JCAHO

5. What act was designed to regulate how pharmaceuticals are handled?
   a. the AMA act of 1974
   b. the DAA act of 1977
   c. the Controlled Substance Act of 1970
   d. HIPAA

6. Zantac is classified as:
   a. beta-adrenergic blocker
   b. H_2 blocker
   c. calcium channel blocker
   d. antibiotic

7. The skin is:
   a. an organ
   b. a disorder
   c. a skeletal muscle
   d. a heartbeat regulator

8. Name some alternative ways a patient could receive medications if he were not able to ingest orally.

9. Name a drug that is given through pulmonary administration.

10. List three drugs that can be applied topically.

Resources and References

1. Hitner, Henry and Barbara Nagle. *Basic Pharmacology, 4th Ed.* New York and other cities: Glencoe/McGraw-Hill Publishers, Inc., 1999.

2. Robert Berkow. *The Merck Manual, 16th Ed.* Rahway, N.J. Merck Research Laboratories, Inc., 1992.

3. Andreoli, Thomas, Charles Carpenter, Claude Bennett, and Fred Plum. *Essentials of Medicine, 4th Ed.* Philadelphia and other cities: Cecil W.B. Saunders, Inc., 1997.

4. Holland, Norman and Michael Patrick Adams. *Core Concepts in Pharmacology.* Upper Saddle River, NJ: Pearson Education, 2003.

5. Adams, Michael Patrick, Dianne L. Josephson, and Leland Norman Holland, Jr. *Pharmacology for Nurses—A Pathophysiologic Approach.* Upper Saddle River, NJ: Pearson Education, 2005.

The Body and Drugs

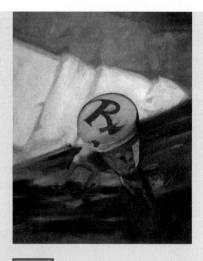

INTRODUCTION

If there were any two elements of medicine that require a
close, reliable relationship to be effective, they would be the
health care provider and the pharmacist. These two
individuals form a team that holds the keys to the processes of
diagnosis and medication that will, hopefully, bring an end to
the suffering of the patient.

There is an important reason to increase your knowledge
about medicine in its broadest sense. In order to understand
more about the medications that you will be handling on a
daily basis, you will require a sense of the inner workings of
the human body. Not knowing the basics would be like
getting a car without the keys. It just will not start.
So, let's begin.

Structure of the Human Body

A complete study of medicine, pathology, and physiology would certainly require more than this text can offer. We will focus on the basics, so that when a prescription (for example, for Atenolol©) is called into the pharmacy, you know what the drug is and what it is, theoretically, used for. Realize, however, that although this medication is designed to be used to treat *hypertension*, it can also be used to treat a number of other conditions, some of which you probably will not find in a textbook.

Presented next is a brief review of the systems in the body, followed by a discussion of the classes of drugs that are used to regulate these systems.

CARDIOVASCULAR SYSTEM

This is a nice term for the heart and all of the *vessels* that come into and out of the heart, including all of the smallest vessels in the foot. It's a very complicated and integrated system that contains numerous hormonal control systems. The smallest of muscles are actually responsible for the overall blood pressure. This network has complicated *neurological* and electrical systems that, when written about, fill volumes of information.

The heart is actually a muscle that contains four chambers. The left ventricle, the largest and most powerful chamber, is the one involved with most of the heart drugs used. (See Figure 3-1.)

The heart relies on the delivery of oxygen in order to survive. Without oxygen, the heart (or at least some parts of it) can die. The heart's reaction to a loss of oxygen is called a *myocardial infarction*, or a heart attack. You might think that the heart supplies its own blood, but it does not. It relies on a system wherein, during rest, blood rushes into the large vessels, thus providing the tissue with the needed oxygen and carrying away the dangerous chemicals, such as *carbon dioxide*, that can destroy the muscle.

The main function of the heart is to pump blood to the tissues of the body; while it does have other functions, they are insignificant in comparison. When the heart contracts, this action is called *systole*. It is represented by the top number when taking someone's blood pressure. When the heart is at rest, the action is called *diasystole*, which is represented by the bottom number on the blood pressure monitor.

Any problems with the heart, such as a lack of oxygen, an elevated heart rate, or an increased level of carbon dioxide, can have drastic and possibly fatal effects on the body. If a patient should approach you and tell you that he has chest pain, arm pain, or back pain, and he is short of breath, don't hesitate to either get your pharmacist or call your local emergency medical service. (And, indeed, patients will ask you questions rather than seek the advice of their health care provider—you are right there, and they think of you as the keeper of the keys.)

As alluded to previously, the body's blood pressure is not regulated only by the heart. In fact, the real pressure is regulated by the very small vessels in the body, called *capillaries*; and around some of them are small muscle systems controlled by proteins, hormones, and other compounds in the body.

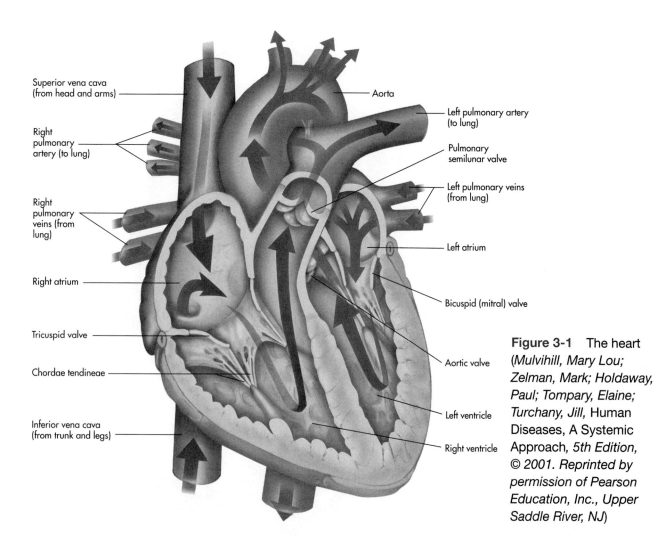

Superior vena cava
(from head and arms)

Right
pulmonary
artery (to lung)

Right
pulmonary
veins (from
lung)

Right atrium

Tricuspid valve

Chordae tendineae

Inferior vena cava
(from trunk and legs)

Aorta

Left pulmonary artery
(to lung)

Pulmonary
semilunar valve

Left pulmonary veins
(from lung)

Left atrium

Bicuspid (mitral) valve

Aortic valve

Left ventricle

Right ventricle

Figure 3-1 The heart (*Mulvihill, Mary Lou; Zelman, Mark; Holdaway, Paul; Tompary, Elaine; Turchany, Jill*, Human Diseases, A Systemic Approach, *5th Edition*, © 2001. Reprinted by permission of Pearson Education, Inc., Upper Saddle River, NJ)

So, when a chemist decides how to best control blood pressure, it is not always the heart that becomes the target, but also the small vessels in the body.

One of the key elements to remember about the cardiovascular system is that it is not all just mechanical. If it were not for the *electrolytes* in the body, such as *potassium* (K^+), sodium (Na^+), and *chloride* (Cl^-), to mention a few, the heart would not pump. In fact, just as an example, there is a sodium–potassium pump that regulates almost all of the electrical systems in the body, including the heart. By studying this system as well as a number of others, the pharmaceutical companies, through years of research, have been able to either block the action of the pump or cause it to work faster.

The remaining parts of the cardiovascular system are just as complex as the aforementioned. Through research on the many systems within the body that control blood pressure (not always directly related to the heart or the vessels), the pharmaceutical companies have designed drugs to ensure that blood pressure is better controlled. (See Figure 3-2.)

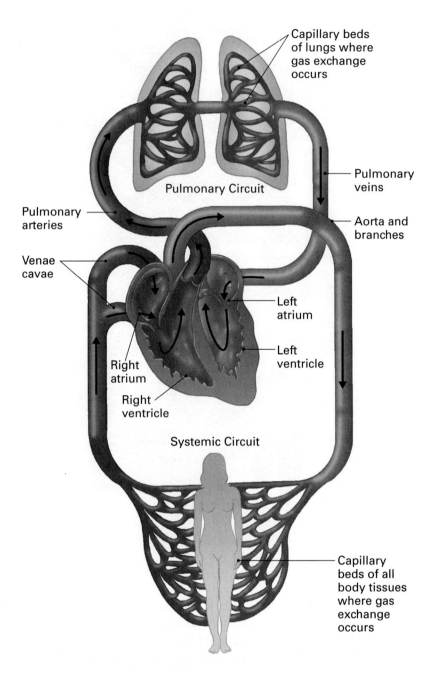

Figure 3-2   The cardiovascular system

There are specific diseases of the cardiovascular system that, were it not for the advancements made with respect to medications, would probably have kept the average age in the world in the 40–45 year range. The following is a short list of some of those diseases:

- congestive heart failure, or *CHF*
- heart/valve disease (a long list of diseases in this catagory)
- coronary artery disease, or *CAD*—from cholesterol, congenital reasons, and others

- *arrhythmias*—irregular heartbeats caused by a varied number of problems
- myocardial and pericardial disease (a long list of diseases in this category)
- cardiac tumors
- aortic disease (the aorta is the large artery through which the blood is pumped into the body)
- peripheral vascular disease (a long list of diseases in this category)

RESPIRATORY SYSTEM

The respiratory system is responsible for exchanging oxygen and carbon dioxide (Figure 3-3). This exchange is the definition of respiration. As the exchange continues from the lungs down to the individual cells, it is known as the Krebs cycle. At the cellular level, oxygen is actually the last component of the transformation that permits the cell to create energy. At the clinical level, where oxygen is taken in and carbon dioxide is taken out, oxygen is actually the last byproduct of the processes in the body that allows the body to continue to live, from the cellular level onward.

Clinically speaking, what you really need to know is that the lungs are important, and specific problems can develop that are able to cause greater problems. The heart is between the two lungs. If there is a problem with the

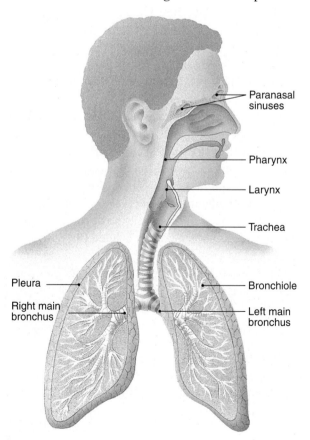

Paranasal sinuses

Pharynx

Larynx

Trachea

Pleura

Bronchiole

Right main bronchus

Left main bronchus

Figure 3-3 The respiratory system

system that permits blood to get through the lungs, there will also be a problem that will back up into the heart. Furthermore, the problems that affect breathing, such as asthma, while not totally preventable, are very well controlled if patients take their medications.

Typically, but not always, the asthmatics are children. Some parents are far too reluctant to show their children how to use their medications, such as the handheld mechanisms that deliver medication right to the lung tissue. It would be a proud moment for you, as a pharmacy technician, if you could demonstrate to a child or a parent the ways in which these canisters are properly used and why it might be important to use them before breathing becomes a real problem. However, you must be able to discuss these issues generally—how the medications work to alleviate the symptoms of asthma, for instance—without actually counseling patients about their medications, for that is the exclusive responsibility of the pharmacist.

A large array of problems can develop in the human lung. The more severe cases you will encounter will have already been through some of the other, less dangerous problems; therefore, these individuals will typically know how to use their medications, and they could probably teach you (and the pharmacist) a few things. However, realizing the functions of the lungs—that they are responsible for the final exchange of blood gases—is adequate.

Many other functions are interwoven with other organ systems, and specific medications are used to help treat problems when they occur. An excellent example of this would be the dreadful disease *cystic fibrosis*, which has a median age of about the late 20s. This disease currently has no cure, and for the majority of their lives, cystic fibrosis patients are on a wide array of drugs, including, at times, oxygen (which can be used as a drug).

A common form of lung disease, besides lung cancer, is chronic obstructive pulmonary disease, or *COPD*. In a clinical sense, you can identify a person who has this disease merely by observing them and taking a few notes about their appearance. For example, they usually take shorter, but a lot faster breaths than normal; they also (at late stages) have what is called "clubbing of the fingernails," which means that the nail beds are flat, no longer curved as normally seen. Some of these people have barrel chests, and, at the late stages, they usually carry the all-too-common sign of lung disease: oxygen.

At this stage, it is really important for you to know and understand the large array of medications that can be used to treat the many different types of lung diseases. When a specific medication is called in to your pharmacy, the dosage should be checked to ensure that the person making the phone call actually knows the prescription. This is vital because sometimes physicians permit non-medically-trained personnel to relay the calls to the pharmacies. That can be a hazardous error—and one that could be overlooked until it is too late.

There is nothing worse than seeing someone in respiratory distress. Upon occasion, patients will walk into the pharmacy with severe symptoms. Your job will be to send them to the emergency room or pick up the phone and call the local emergency medical service. The respiratory system can affect more than breathing; it can also raise or lower blood pressure, increase the heart rate, and, if the patient is in heart failure, it can exacerbate the problems. Don't wait, and don't try to treat these patients; get help.

Some of the more common diseases of the respiratory system include the following:

- COPD or chronic obstructive pulmonary disease
- chronic *bronchitis*
- *asthma*
- bronchiectasis (a viral infection in children)
- cystic fibrosis
- pulmonary hypertension
- emphysema (a component of COPD)
- lung cancer
- pneumonconioses—a set of diseases that are caused by the inhalation of dust and dust particles, as well as other substances
- pneumonitis
- sarcoidosis

RENAL SYSTEM

The renal system encompasses not only the two kidneys, but also a number of systems that control blood pressure. There are specific organs within the renal system that, when stimulated, will either produce a drastic increase in the blood pressure or just the opposite (Figure 3-4). The renal system is very

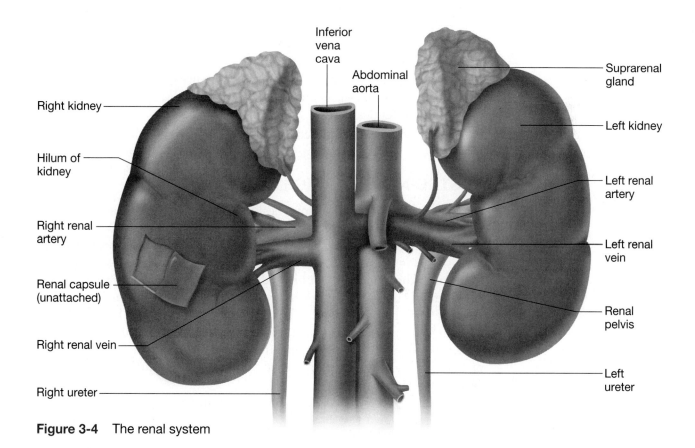

Figure 3-4 The renal system

much tied in with the other systems, such as the vessels in the body, the lungs, and the heart.

The renal system, in general terms, is responsible for the overall volume of the body. However, of more importance to the pharmacological realm of medicine, the kidneys are also responsible for the elimination or excretion of a large amount of the medications that people will take into their bodies. Of even more importance (but not so much of a clinical significance) are the specific sites within what are called the tubules of the kidneys that permit the elimination of such medications.

This is important particularly when specific medications are used alongside others. What is also important is that some medications, because of their characteristics, remain unchanged from intake to output. This is useful to know when treating, for example, bladder infections. An excellent example would be some of the sulfa medications, because they are used to treat the infections within the bladder and we want them to remain unchanged.

Understanding the normal kidney functions is important, especially if you are going to be expected to know what sort of medications will be used to treat specific diseases. New medications are coming upon the horizon every day, but the physiology of the human body will remain the same.

The following represents a relatively easy list to remember when studying the kidneys' normal functions:

- maintenance of the overall volume of the body and the electrolyte balance (referred to as *homeostasis*)
- the elimination of waste from the body, as well as unused portions of medications and other chemicals that, if left in the body, can become toxic
- regulation of blood pressure through the use of specific hormones, which will be important to remember when dealing with pharmaceuticals
- the overall control of red blood cells through hormones

GASTROINTESTINAL (GI) SYSTEM

Perhaps one of the chief reasons besides a headache, for a patient to seek medical attention, is abdominal pain. Realizing the host of reasons for abdominal pain and understanding the physiology of the gastrointestinal tract are essential to the pharmacy technician. This is not only because of the multitude of medications that can be used to treat the many symptoms related to the GI tract, but also because certain medications are transformed into their effective form before they are taken into molecules that can be used by the body to treat specific diseases. While some of these issues will be covered in pharmacodynamics and pharmacokinetics, this section will discuss the normal physiology of the gastrointestinal tract, from the mouth to the anus, in a very abbreviated manner.

The digestive process begins in the mouth, where proteins are used to start to break down starches and other items (Figure 3-5). Following this, the food (as well as medications) is sent to the stomach, where it is mixed

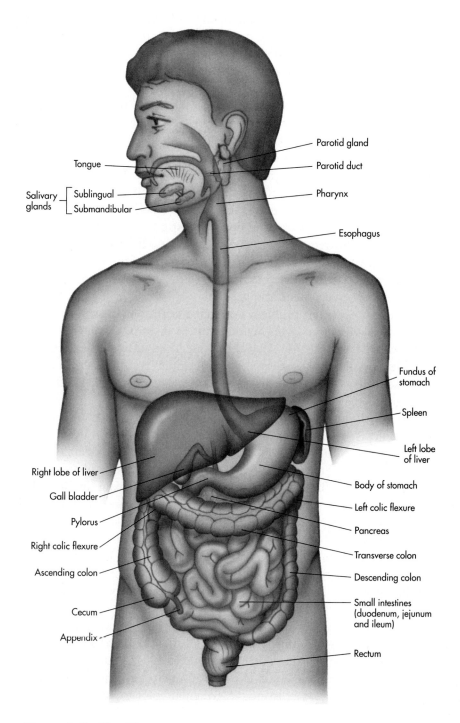

Figure 3-5 The GI system

with many different kinds of chemicals, chiefly acids. This is important to know because, in certain disease states, such as *peptic ulcer disease*, medications are used to help either reduce or almost totally eliminate the amount of acid in the stomach. Gastro and peptic acid disease states can cause severe pain as well as permanent damage to the lining of the stomach and the esophagus. Years ago, the only option was to remove a portion of the stomach. Now, the public has a totally new perspective on medicine in general, as new medications have put an end to a number of potentially life-altering surgeries.

After leaving the stomach, where most foods and medications are at least slightly altered with respect to their *molecular* structure, they enter the small intestines, which typically accept about 2 liters of ingested food and other items per day. If you follow this general rule with respect to the absorption of specific materials in the gut, then, usually, you won't go wrong.

Solutions are absorbed by specific mechanisms, which usually mimic the ways in which chemicals are permitted into a single cell of the body; water is generally transported from the intestines into the bloodstream passively. The mechanisms, however, that are used in the transport of nonwater substances employ "pumps" that require the use of electrolytes. If a patient appears dehydrated or has a known problem with absorption, or if the patient has been experiencing a great deal of diarrhea, there will most likely be a problem with the absorption of certain medications.

Diarrhea is a common problem associated with the absorption of some classes of medications; however, with regard to most of them, the diarrhea will soon pass. Therefore, you should be concerned only with patients who have problems with the absorption of medications because of chronic diseases. These problems can lead to other issues, such as a lack of efficacy of the medications themselves.

Because of the many problems associated with the gastrointestinal system as a whole, it would not be of much clinical benefit to list even some of the most common forms of diseases, mostly because they are usually associated with a number of other problems. The real issue, from a pharmacological standpoint, is deciding whether a patient is an appropriate candidate for a medication; and that issue is the domain of the health care provider and, at times, the pharmacist.

If a patient should ask you about his abdominal problems, you should have him seek medical attention as soon as possible. Your job is not to diagnose; to do so would be practicing medicine without a license. (This is also true of the pharmacist.) There should always be a correspondence with the health care provider, at all costs.

A word must be said, however, with respect to certain aspects of the patients' presentations—specifically, the color of their skin and eyes. This will be covered in more detail later, but as a general rule, ask your pharmacist before you hand over certain kinds of medications to any patient with a yellowish color in his eyes or a distinctive, irregular color to his skin.

ENDOCRINE SYSTEM

The endocrine system comprises a vast array of hormones and organs that help regulate many specific bodily functions (Figure 3-6), such as blood sugar and the thyroid gland. There are many more, most of which will not concern your everyday duties, as these patients are typically handled by

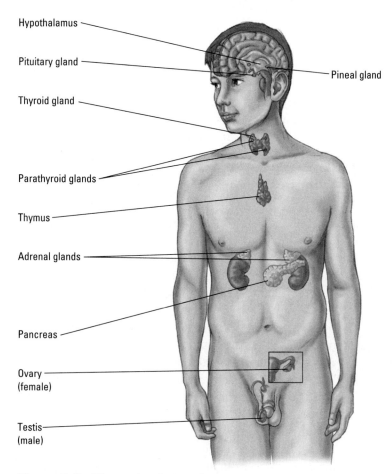

Figure 3-6   The endocrine system

highly trained specialists; the typical pharmacy is not involved with the treatment of these diseases. (You may encounter them, however, if you choose to work in a hospital or other closed facility where patients with severe disorders are sometimes stabilized.)

The endocrine system is regulated by what is referred to as the hypothalamic-pituitary axis. This axis is responsible for the overall regulation of such hormonal changes as the growth hormone, *ACTH* (or the adenocorticotropic hormone), prolactin (which is related to pregnancy and the delivery of breast milk), and *TSH* (or the thyroid-stimulating hormone). Other hormones, such as the luteinizing hormone and the follicular stimulating hormone, are related to both the female and the male reproductive systems.

The endocrine system also controls other functions, especially the body's blood sugar, but through a different organ, called the pancreas. A problem with one of the main hormonal systems can have an effect on the others, and therefore, the number of medications that can be associated with these systems is enormous. Because the names used for the various medications can be complex, your knowledge of the terminology will have to come from experience; but, a review of them appears in the next section of the text.

HEMATOLOGIC SYSTEM

The hematologic system contains all of the parts of blood, including the proteins, red blood cells, and other constituents of what makes up the fluid that carries oxygen to the cells and takes the many waste products away from the cells and eventually out of the body.

From a basic perspective, there are two main parts of this system that you ought to know to start with, while others will eventually follow with experience and time. One of the most important components of blood and blood products is the process of *coagulation*, which is the ability of the blood to clot. Most of the time, this system is very valuable to the life of an individual; however, in some situations, such as when a patient undergoes certain surgeries (for example, a heart valve replacement), there is a tendency of the blood to coagulate (clot) because of the presence of a foreign object in contact with the blood.

Within the blood, there are small cells called *platelets*. When platelets come in contact with an injury to the inside of a blood vessel or with a foreign object, they collect into small groups that become larger over time. Along with other substances in the blood, these platelets can cause the development of clots, which help the body by protecting a cut from bleeding. This system and another system, called the cascading effect of blood coagulation, can sometimes work together to form a barrier or a clot, (Figure 3-7). This is not necessarily a problem; but in the case of a patient with a heart valve transplant, the situation can cause a clot that can migrate from the heart to other parts of the body. If the clot reaches the brain, the result is usually a stroke.

A number of medications can help the blood in the prevention of coagulation; such drugs can range from simple aspirin to a drug by the name of Warfarin® (a type of rat poison, actually). Without these drugs, however, surgeries such as those which replace heart valves or arteries that are clogged due to cholesterol cannot be performed. There are potential risks to the use of these medications; these will be discussed in another section of this text.

With regard to other aspects of the blood and blood systems, it is important to know that the blood contains large proteins (discussed to some degree in other sections) that have a number of qualities. They help retain the blood in the vessels of the body, and they assist in the transportation of some drugs from the intestines to other parts of the body.

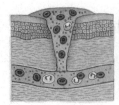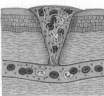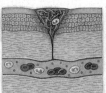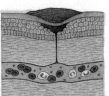

Figure 3-7 Blood clotting (© *Dorling Kindersley*)

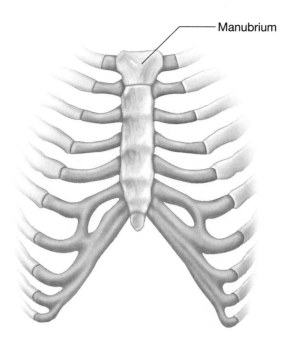

Figure 3-8 The manubrium

Blood is formed within the bone marrow of the body, mostly in the large bones, as well as in the *manubrium* (Figure 3-8), a bone situated in the center of the chest wall. Blood is a necessary part of the body due to its function in delivering oxygen and due to other qualities. Specific problems occur with diseases such as anemia or a low iron level in the blood. Low iron in blood can lead to a decreased affinity for oxygen, which, in turn, can cause a decrease in the energy level and other problems.

There are so many different kinds of anemia that to discuss them all is well beyond the scope of this text. There are a great many medications used to treat them as well; however, most of these medications will not usually be found in an ordinary pharmacy, but do often appear in a hospital setting, because some of the anemias are related to specific forms of cancer.

The normal red blood cell, which is responsible not only for the color of blood, but also for the transportation of oxygen, usually lives for about 120 days. Red blood cells that are over the age limit are usually destroyed through a variety of systems.

Specific kinds of tests are used to detect the level of coagulation of the blood; while these tests are typically done in the physician's office, you will grow accustomed to hearing about them because of the two types of drugs that are used to treat anemic patients: *PTT* (partial thromboplastin time), used to detect the primary means by which the body conducts homeostasis, and *PT* (prothrobin time), used to detect the secondary means of homeostasis.

PTT can be regulated through the use of aspirin, whereas PT requires warfarin or other types of drugs. Through the use of warfarin, a specific pathway of coagulation is actually interrupted. Warfarin interferes with the synthesis and availability of vitamin K, which is found abundantly in certain fruits (such as bananas) and many green leafy vegetables. It is very important for the patient to know these vitamin K rich foods so that they can limit their consumption while on warfarin therapy.

Through many different complex mechanisms, vitamin K becomes the one *catalyst* that will promote coagulation. Warfarin reduces the amount of vitamin K by inhibiting the way it is available. Conversely, the antidote to warfarin is vitamin K, which can be injected into the body through the muscle tissue, where it will alter the effects of warfarin.

SUMMARY

The structure of the body is divided into various systems, such as the Cardiovascular, respiratory, and renal systems. It is important to understand the functions of the different systems and how those functions are affected in a patient in a diseased state. Some abnormalities can have drastic, even fatal, effects on the body.

Pharmacotherapeutics plays a vital role in the overall treatment of dysfunction of the body. The significant advancements in the field of pharmacology enable many people to live longer, healthier lives.

A broad understanding of how abnormalities in the body affect the functioning of a body system, and how, in turn, dysfunction in one body system can affect other systems, is of utmost importance in optimizing the use of the vast array of pharmaceuticals available today.

The goal of pharmacotherapeutics is to work in conjunction with other medical interventions to return the body's function to as close to its normal state as possible.

CHAPTER REVIEW QUESTIONS

1. The heart contains how many chambers?
   a. 6
   b. 2
   c. 4
   d. 1

2. Myocardial infarction is another term for what condition?
   a. difficulty breathing
   b. heart attack
   c. severe rash
   d. cystic fibrosis

3. Real pressure in the body is regulated by very small vessels in the body called:
   a. capillaries
   b. platelets
   c. coagulants
   d. PTT indicators

4. What regulates almost all of the electrical systems in the body?
   a. fluid balance
   b. resistance
   c. central nervous system
   d. sodium-potassium pump

5. The respiratory system is responsible for exchanging what?
   a. red blood cells and white blood cells
   b. "bad" blood for "good" blood
   c. "bad" cholesterol for "good" cholesterol
   d. oxygen and carbon dioxide

6. The typical age that cystic fibrosis affects a person is what?

   a. mid 20s
   b. adolescence
   c. under 12 years of age
   d. after 40 years of age

7. Clubbing of the fingernails is a symptom of what disease?
   a. cystic fibrosis
   b. myocardial infarction
   c. COPD
   d. CHF

8. What organs are also responsible for the elimination or excretion of a large amount of the medications that people will take into their bodies?
   a. skin
   b. kidneys
   c. bowels
   d. liver

9. A deficiency in the kidneys is known as what?
   a. atopic dermatitis
   b. irritable bowel syndrome
   c. renal dysfunction
   d. hepatitis

10. The gastrointestinal system begins at what body part?
    a. the stomach
    b. the throat
    c. the esophagus
    d. the mouth

11. Explain how diarrhea can be a problem when a patient is taking medications.

Resources and References

1. Andreoli, T., Charles Carpenter, Claude Bennett, and Fred Plum. *Essentials of Medicine, 4th Ed.* Philadelphia and other cities: Cecil W.B. Saunders, Inc., 1997.

2. Wyngaarden, J., Lloyd Smith, and Claude Bennett. *Cecil Textbook of Medicine, 19th Ed.* Philadelphia and other cities: W.B. Saunders, Inc., 1992.

3. Robert Berkow. *The Merck Manual,* Rahway, *16th Ed.* NJ. Merck Research Laboratories, 1992.

4. Holland, Norman and Michael Patrick Adams. *Core Concepts in Pharmacology.* Upper Saddle River, NJ: Pearson Education, 2003.

5. Adams, Michael Patrick, Dianne L. Josephson, and Leland Norman Holland, Jr. *Pharmacology for Nurses—A Pathophysiologic Approach.* Upper Saddle River, NJ: Pearson Education, 2005.

Pharmacodynamics

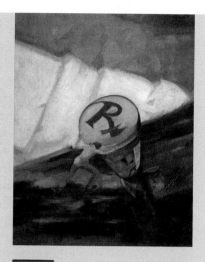

Learning Objectives

After completing this chapter,
you should be able to:

- Explain the importance of the effect of drugs to receptors.

- Describe mechanism of action and all it entails.

- Identify and understand key factors for mechanism of action.

- Explain how certain classes of drugs react in the body or cause reactions.

INTRODUCTION

Most manufactured drugs affect the cells in the body through a process that permits the drug to interact with specific drug receptors. Think about it as if each cell in the body has a specific key that can be locked or unlocked; and specific drugs are manufactured for specific receptors. The drug manufacturers have learned how to manipulate the cells, the different parts of the cells, and how they interact with yet other cells. The effect is a certain and expected response that can be measured.

Receptor Complex

A receptor (again, think of it as a key) on the cell interacts with a specific drug because the drug "fits" the specific structure of the receptor. The drug often has been designed to have the same or a similar structure as the cells. Once the key is "turned," so to speak, the chemical structure of the drug is permitted into the cell, where it performs most of its functions (Figure 4-1).

Let's look at, for example, the drug and the receptor responsible for controlling allergies. These drugs, called *antihistamines*, react in a specific manner called the drug-plus-the-receptor—or the drug–receptor—complex, which in turn has a specific effect. In this case, the antihistamine actually turns off the parts of certain cells in the body that cause the common symptoms of allergies, such as the burning, red eyes (the white part, the sclera of the eye, not the internal parts of the eye), and the runny nose. These and other symptoms are commonly seen, for example, in the patient who has hay fever, a term that describes the allergic reaction to most of the substances in the air during the spring and parts of the summer.

There is a vast array of drugs, and you will find that most clinicians use certain kinds all the time (as they get used to the way they work), with few exceptions, as when newer drugs emerge. Some drugs have specific shapes and structures that actually "match up" with the shape of the receptor on specific cells. As you will find through your own experience in listening as patients talk, certain drugs are better at matching the receptor–drug complex than others, even when they are in the same class. There are drugs that, because of their characteristics, interact with more than just one receptor. A classic example is the diphenhydramine class. These drugs react both with histamine receptors and with specific cells that make up the nervous system, such as the hormone called *acetylcholine*, which has properties that control certain neurotransmitters in the central and peripheral nervous system. Hence, these drugs can cause drowsiness as well as a number of other side effects.

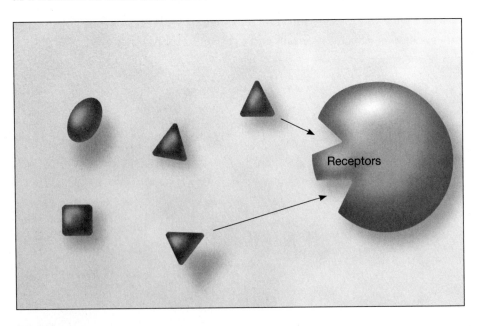

Figure 4-1   Receptor site

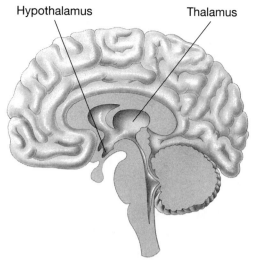

Hypothalamus   Thalamus

Figure 4-2 The hypothalamus (*Pearson Education/PH College*)

Site of Action

When a pharmaceutical agent is first developed, the scientists don't merely stumble upon a receptor (although that can happen). More often than not, they realize that there is a specific site of action for each drug class. It is equally true, however, that the specific site of action for some drugs is simply not known. The FDA requires the companies that manufacture these drugs to prove essentially two things: that the drug works (it does what the label says it will do), and that it is safe.

Chemistry is a science and sometimes an art. One of the most classic examples of knowing where a specific drug exerts its effects is the drug called aspirin. There are specific sites located in an area of the brain called the *hypothalamus* (Figure 4-2) which is called, among other things, the body's temperature regulator. By matching some of the sites on the cells of the hypothalamus, the body's temperature is reduced.

Mechanism of Action

Mechanism of action is a term that explains how a drug works and produces its desirable (and sometimes undesirable) effects. One of the more classic examples of this is when a patient undergoes anesthesia for surgery. The drugs used for the reduction of pain do their job by interrupting the pathway between the central nervous system and the peripheral nervous system; put another way, such a drug cuts the "cord" to the brain so that the person is no longer capable of sensing pain. Without this mechanism of action, patients who undergo massive surgical procedures would go into shock.

Receptor Site

The receptor site is the location where the drug (that is, the chemical) binds to the cell. Once the drug develops a bond, there are specific molecular changes that can occur (most of which are far beyond the scope of this text).

For example, when the opioids (narcotics) are used, they bind to cells, and the changes that occur within the cell itself are what cause a reduction in the amount of perceived pain. The pain remains there, as in surgery, where naturally there are areas where cells are damaged; but the brain does not perceive the pain, as specific qualities of the cells are turned off. (Recall the analogy of the key that turns a lock, which in turn, produces a specific response.) The known receptors are so numerous that it would be difficult to describe every one of them. New receptors are always being discovered; hence, the market for new, more powerful drugs is also enormous.

Agonists and Antagonists

Agonists and *antagonists* have been useful in studies of binding sites on receptors. In turn, such investigations are useful in drug design, with the goal of activating or inactivating certain classes of receptors. When these words are used, simply think about the terms, because they are defining their exact actions.

An *agonist* is a specific type of drug that, when it binds to the correct receptor for which it was designed, produces a certain, predicted action. In this case, the drug is doing exactly what it has been designed to do, although there may or may not be any predicted side effects. Agonists bind and produce cellular responses resulting in a therapeutic effect. Many hormones and neurotransmitters (such as acetylcholine, histamine, and norepinephrine) and many drugs (such as morphine, phenylephrine, and isoproterenol) act as agonists. For example, the agonist isoproterenol is used to treat asthma because it mimics the effects of catecholamines (hormones and neurotransmitters such as adrenaline, noradrenaline, and dopamine) in relaxing bronchial muscles in the lung. It does this by interacting with one specific class of adrenergic receptors.

On the other hand, an *antagonist* is a drug that, when it binds to a specific receptor on the cell, does not produce any noticeable or desirable effect; however, again, because it is a chemical, it may or may not have any predictable side effects. Antagonists interact selectively with receptors. They reduce the action of another substance (agonist) at the receptor site involved. For example, propranolol, a drug used to control blood pressure and pulse rate in cardiac patients, is an antagonist of another class of adrenergic receptors that control blood pressure and heartbeat rate.

It is helpful to know that agonists have two main properties; one of them is the *affinity*, or the ability of the agonist to actually bind to the cell receptor structure. (Again, if you think about this as a "lock and a key," it makes more sense.) The other property is the efficacy of the agonist, or the ability the drug imposes on the cell and its structure and how well it changes the way the cell behaves. In essence, if the drug is an agonist, and it does what it is designed to do, it is considered *efficacious*.

There are useful aspects for both kinds of these drugs; just because an antagonist does not produce a noticeable effect, it does not indicate that the drug is not useful. An antagonist has important uses; otherwise, such drugs would not exist.

While it is true that antagonists do bind to certain receptors and there is no noticeable action, the drug could become an advantage to the life of that cell as well as the life of the organism. Think about a person who has used the wrong drug, or, as in a more typical example, a patient who is brought into the emergency room because he has overdosed on some of the morphine-derivative drugs. A classic antagonist called naloxone, which binds to the exact sites where the illicit drug has attached itself, can be administered; the result is a prompt reversal of what would otherwise be a question of life and death.

There are literally thousands of other ways and reasons for which antagonists are used as pharmacological agents. As a pharmacy technician, will you be able to identify the agonists and the antagonists? Well, maybe if you are a chemistry buff; but knowing all of them is not a specific requirement. Knowing that they exist, how they work, and how to identify them is far more important.

Remember the *target cell*. When this term is used, it is actually referring to a large number of cells, all of which are quite similar. Target cells include the nerve cells and cells that are involved with the heart or with the vascular system, especially with respect to circulation and blood pressure. These and many others make up what the chemists and pharmacologists think of as the target cells—what cells and what receptors are becoming involved when a specific medication is being used.

The Dose–Response Curve

A relatively simple principle about pharmacology and pharmacodynamics is that the response of a drug is directly related to the amount of the drug taken or given. (See Figure 4-3.) As simple as this might seem, it is probably one of

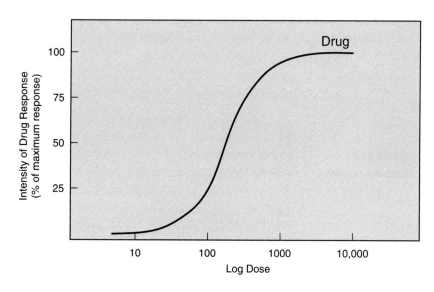

Figure 4-3 The dose–response curve

the most important aspects about pharmacology you may encounter as a technician. With respect to this dose–response curve, a dose is defined as the specific amount of the drug required to achieve a desired effect, which is referred to as the response to the drug. If the dose–response relationship were plotted on a chart, you could see a curve that would provide a picture of that relationship.

If you think about how a graph (a curve) might represent the way a drug reacts to a cell (and to all of the cells that are similar to the target cell), you can easily grasp the idea that, in time, a maximal response will be attained. After such a point, adding more of the same drug will be of no benefit. That does not mean, however, that adding more drugs will not cause harm, because in most cases, such harm does occur, especially when people abuse drugs.

The point on the graph that represents the maximal response is called the ceiling, and beyond that point drugs are often considered toxic, especially to the two systems that either change chemicals in the body or excrete other, nondesirable chemicals from the body: the liver and the kidneys. Knowing that there are drugs that do not have a ceiling is important in pharmacodynamics, as this is where your knowledge about what you do in the facility where you are employed counts the most. The position of the pharmacy technician is slowly and quite effectively moving from being just a cashier to being an expert about certain classes of drugs.

While it is true that you will probably not learn the mechanisms of the drugs at the chemical level, it is equally true that your knowing how they work and why specific chemicals can be a danger to a patient can become an asset to the pharmacist for whom you work. It is really that simple—well, not really. Because the science of medicine is becoming more fluid, your job will be ever changing and there always will be new things to learn.

POTENCY

The word *potency* in pharmacology means exactly what it does in general usage. It's a measurement of the strength of the drug that is required to have a specific effect on the body.

ED50

In medicine, there is a concept called the half-life of the drug. The ED50 is the measurement of the amount of a specific drug that will achieve one-half of the maximal response. This is an important concept because it is used to measure the potency of some drugs without having to actually achieve such a level.

Although this concept is used more in the experimental aspect of pharmacology, it is important to realize that not all drugs are tested by seeing what is needed in order to achieve the maximum effect, as this can become dangerous. In the laboratory setting, it is sometimes referred to as the

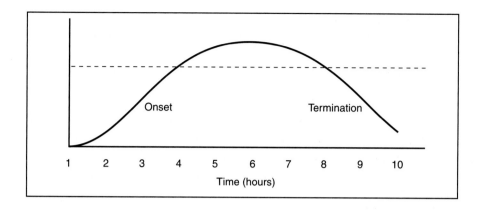

Figure 4-4 The time–response curve

quantal dose–response curve; and realizing that most medications work under the all-or-nothing principle will permit you to understand how medications perform the way they do. In other words, either the medication will work or it will not work—but if it does work, the effect will be in terms of the "all" concept.

The Time–Response Curve

This is simply a curve that gives the observer a means to determine the length of time in which a specific drug will continue to have the same degree of effect on a class of cells, an organ, or the entire body, depending upon the relationship between the body, the drug and, of course, what is being treated. (See Figure 4-4.) In the ideal world, when no other drugs (or foods) have an adverse effect on a drug, most curves will appear as a bell curve, showing a specific onset of action (which can be measured), the entire duration of action, and the termination of the action.

Pharmacodynamic Mechanisms

Much is known about the interactions between the many different drugs that can be taken into the human body. These interactions, sometimes referred to as the pharmacologic drug interactions, are an important aspect of pharmacology. For one reason or another, a lot of patients do not release information to their health care providers, and what happens next can become a dangerous problem to the health of the patient, to the integrity of the health care provider, and to the business of the pharmacy. Patients often do not think about these issues, and it's not your job to take the position of a health care provider. However, if you notice a problem, it would be foolish not to mention it.

Many of the problems related to drug–drug interactions occur because of the addition of a drug that is antagonistic in nature to one that is not, or adding an antagonistic drug to a number of drugs that are already designed to be antagonistic. This action, as you will learn later, creates a process by which a drug is either able to compete with specific sites on cells or prevent chemicals from competing on other cells.

As you will learn in the next section, specific sites on a cell, when turned on, will cause the cell to act in one way, while, on the contrary, a chemical can be used to turn off a mechanism. The chemicals connect to the cell and become the "key" that will lock or unlock a process of systems that then work together to make the cell react in a specific way. An excellent example of a problem that can occur with a drug–drug interaction is when a specific kind of medication, such as a tricyclic antidepressant, is used along with a specific kind of blood pressure medication, for instance, clonidine. These are two drugs that, when mixed, will tend to counteract each other, and the effect can be as severe as a drop in blood pressure.

Think, then, of the elderly patient who is being treated for neuropathic pain (the tricyclics are sometimes used to help control pain in certain conditions) and is also taking a patch called Catapress (which comes in a number of doses, 0.1, 0.2, and 0.3 mg). If the elderly patient were to stand up quickly in the morning, there could be a sudden problem with his blood pressure (because of the combination of medications) that causes what is called "postural *hypotension*." If, therefore, you notice that a patient's profile changes and a health care provider (such as a pain management physician) adds a tricyclic antidepressant without realizing that the patient is also on clonidine, your job could be to either tell the pharmacist or call the family physician to ensure that his patient's profile is changed accordingly.

Sometimes, a patient brings the common "brown paper bag" containing his medications into the clinic and then to the pharmacy. This is an opportunity for the clinician to make the appropriate adjustments, but typically what happens is that the patients bring one paper bag into the clinician's office and all the other paper bags into the pharmacy. In the better situation, the pharmacy has something that the clinician does not: the patient profile, which is automatically brought up on a computer screen. Most doctors don't have that sort of convenience, and they often resort to either the paper bag or the patient's words.

There are specific issues that are important to understand about the drug–drug interactions that you ought to keep in mind:

- The time it takes a drug to take an effect is important. Some drugs take an effect immediately, while other drugs take a much longer time, depending, of course, on the kind of drug, how it is absorbed, and how it is packaged (which also effects absorption). Some drugs, because of their constituency, take a long time—sometimes weeks to take a full effect, while others take even longer. So, just because a patient has recently received a new drug, it does not mean that the effect will be immediate. There is often little time to use immediate data to determine the way a body will react to a drug. Some drugs must first go through a process by way of the liver. Some drugs even build up *metabolites* that will not have an immediate effect on the body. Therefore, the patient is on his way home, on the way to a supermarket, or out of the area on vacation when the two drugs finally have a chance to create their individual effects to become one. The result can be very dangerous, particularly if the patient is the driver, not the passenger, driving down the highway.

- In many instances, the drug testing procedures performed on people to see if there are any complications are done on people who are not ill; these patients are usually well, and they offer themselves to science in an effort to help others. Suppose that a patient is taking an antibiotic, one of the drugs used to control acid secretion in the stomach (the H_2 blockers), and Warfarin, the chief drug used to keep blood from coagulating (clotting). Then the patient undergoes a heart valve transplant. If an antibiotic, such as Erythromycin®, is used along with Warfarin, the danger might not show up in specific studies; however, in the clinical world, there have been many instances when the combination of these two drugs has caused very severe problems, such as an increase in the levels of the prothrombin time, which measures the effect of how well the drug Warfarin works.

SUMMARY

Drugs available today have been designed to interact with specific receptors within the cells of the body. Drugs that have the same, or similar, chemical structure as the receptor cell can enter the cell to exert an expected response.

Once bound to the receptor cell, drugs can produce their effects in a variety of ways. Drugs can bind to cells to produce a desired effect, or they can work by either activating, or deactivating certain classes of receptors thereby either enhancing or blocking the activity of cell receptors. In some instances, the exact mechanism of action of a drug is not known.

The specific amount of drug needed to produce a desired effect will vary depending on how the body handles the drug once it is administered. This will be discussed in further detail in Chapter 5: Pharmacokinetics. The goal of pharmacotherapeutics is to determine the dose–response curve of a drug. If too little of the drug is available to the body (a sub-therapeutic level), the desired effect will not be produced. If too much of the drug (a toxic level) is available, undesired (or adverse) effects can result. Optimally, dosage regimens will result in blood levels sufficient to exert a therapeutic effect, while minimizing unwanted effects. Dose–response curves also give us valuable information that is of particular concern to your client, i.e., when to take the drug, how often to take the drug, when the drug will begin to exert its therapeutic effect.

Finally, it is important to recognize that drugs may bind to more than one receptor, and that multiple drugs can compete with one another for receptor sites. Familiarity with your client's concurrent medical problems and concomitant medications are essential for providing the best possible care.

CHAPTER REVIEW QUESTIONS

1. Structures on the cells that interact with a specific drug because they have a specific structure that permits the drug to fit are called:

    a. neurotransmitters

    b. receptors

    c. stimuli

    d. platelets

2. Define mechanism of action.

3. Antihistamines turn off the parts of certain cells in the body that cause the common symptoms of allergies, which are:

    a. red eyes, runny nose

    b. itchy skin, failing heart

    c. hepatitis, rapid hearbeat

    d. tears, difficulty hearing

4. Acetylcholine is a:

    a. nerve

    b. chromosome

    c. hormone

    d. capillary

5. Describe how an opiod helps a patient in pain. What happens in the body?

6. Describe the difference between an agonist and an antagonist, and give an example of each.

7. Agonists have two main properties. They are:

    a. affinity and efficacy

    b. bioavailability and dose–response time

    c. solubility and bioavailability

    d. efficacy and timeliness

8. Explain why, just because a drug does not produce a noticeable effect, it does not mean that the drug does not work.

9. The response of a drug that is directly related to the amount of the drug taken or given is referred to as:

    a. the first pass effect

    b. mechanism of action

    c. potency

    d. dose–response curve

10. Warfarin's active ingredient is the same ingredient found in what household product?

    a. Clorox

    b. laundry soap

    c. rat poison

    d. drain cleaner

Resources and References

1. Shlafer, M. "Pharmacodynamics—The Mechanisms of Drug Action," Pharm 210, 2003. Assessed October 30, 2003. Online at **http://wwwpersonal.umich.edu/~mshlafer/Lectures/Nursing/ nmechact.pdf**

2. Hitner, Henry and Barbara Nagle. *Basic Pharmacology*, 4th Ed. New York and other cities: Glencoe/McGraw-Hill Publishers, Inc., 1999.

3. Holland, Norman and Michael Patrick Adams. *Core Concepts in Pharmacology*. Upper Saddle River, NJ: Pearson Education, 2003.

4. Adams, Michael Patrick, Dianne L. Josephson, and Leland Norman Holland, Jr. *Pharmacology for Nurses—A Pathophysiologic Approach*. Upper Saddle River, NJ: Pearson Education, 2005.

Pharmacokinetics

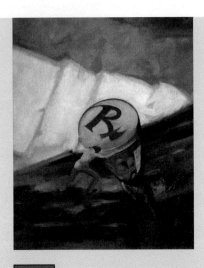

Learning Objectives

After completing this chapter, you should be able to:

- Explain how drugs travel through the body, depending on certain factors.
- List and identify the different absorption actions.
- Explain the difference between fat-soluble and water-soluble drugs, and give examples of each.
- Explain the concept of ionization and its importance.

INTRODUCTION

Pharmacology is a very broad topic, and there are many books that explain the ways in which drugs are absorbed, used, and secreted by the body. Many readers, however, get stuck when they are exposed to words such as *pharmacokinetics*. A broad definition of the term is "the study of the time course of a drug and its metabolites in the body following drug administration by any route."

In simple terms, pharmacokinetics is the study of how the body handles the drugs that are administered to it (whether they are administered orally, by way of IV, or any other means), how the drugs are changed from the original form into something that the body can use (typically by way of the liver or other organs), and then how they are secreted from the body and eliminated. In this chapter, we are more concerned about the medications once they are in the body than how they are presented to us before they are administered or what the dynamics of the administration are.

Throughout this chapter, you will be presented with terminology to which you may or may not have been exposed. The study of pharmacokinetics is one of the more difficult aspects of pharmacology, because it is pure science.

You may not think after reading the material that it will be important to know. As you proceed with your studies and with your career as a pharmacy technician, however, you will find yourself applying clinically a lot of what you understand about drugs and how they work.

This chapter will break down the ideas and the concepts about pharmacokinetics into smaller, more easily understood terms to ensure that the big picture will make sense. The most important thing to remember when learning about pharmacokinetics is not to become intimidated.

Plasma Concentration (Cp)

When a patient takes a pill or when a nurse injects a patient with a medication (which are two different methods of intake, which follow two different pathways, both of which end up in similar ways), the medication becomes absorbed into the body. The entire concept of plasma concentration is well beyond the scope of this text, and it has very little to do with the real clinical picture. After the absorption is complete, the level and concentration of a specific drug can be measured through certain tests in a laboratory setting. The test actually involves a combination of the measurement of the drug that is bound to the cells of the body and the amount of the drug that is not bound to cells in the body (in this case, blood cells).

One factor that determines the amount of the drug that is actually going to do any good for the body is the affinity of the drug to be bound to proteins that are available in the bloodstream. It is the bloodstream that will become the vehicle which will actually deliver the drug to the parts of the body where the drug will have an effect on whatever organ or organs (or systems, such as the cardiovascular system) need treatment.

Knowing that there is a way to measure the amount of a specific drug in a person's body has little to do with the overall clinical picture. So, let's get into only the "bare bones" of drug absorption, distribution, metabolism, and excretion, as well as how drugs are used to do the job for which they are designed.

Drug Absorption

This term refers to how a drug enters the body. In order for a drug such as a pill to enter the body, it must first, obviously, be swallowed. Then it begins the process by which it eventually enters the body's fluids, mainly, absorption into the bloodstream. For example, when you consider a drug contained in a pill, the medication passes into the bloodstream by getting through specific membranes, such as the membranes inside the stomach and the intestines. The absorption is largely dependent upon the type of the drug, how it is designed, and the reason the type of drug (e.g., a pill as opposed to a liquid) was used. Liquids are more readily absorbed than tablets or capsules, for they are already "broken down."

Cell membranes in the body are composed of special linings that make up the cell wall, each of which contains both lipids (fats) and proteins. This *semi-permeable* barrier is essentially a barrier that permits the entrance of some materials and the exit of others.

Some drugs actually bind to the stomach walls. One such drug is Metamucil©, which binds to the walls of the stomach to increase stool bulk. Thus, Metamucil is not absorbed by the body in any way.

With the exception of drugs that are administered by the use of an IV or intra-arterial method (injected into the bloodstream, bypassing some of the aspects of absorption), most drugs take a certain length of time before they start to act on the body.

Injections of numerous types of liquid drugs bypass the absorption process, as they are entered directly into the bloodstream. With this type of administration, observed results are often much quicker than with any other method.

Absorption of a drug does not always go by way of stomach to bloodstream. Inhaled medications are entered through the mouth to the lungs. The mucous membranes of the *alveoli* absorb the medication and send it into the capillaries to the bloodstream. Medications administered rectally or vaginally have a very slow release rate, as the medication dissolves and is actually considered to be applied topically.

Topical medications (with the exception of the transdermal "patch") are not necessarily absorbed through the skin into the bloodstream and display only a topical effect. An example is hydrocortisone cream used for inflammatory skin conditions. More and more medications are being made available in a "patch" form that allows penetration through the skin by reducing the size of the medication's particles.

Drug Distribution

Once a drug is absorbed, it then is distributed throughout the body by way of the circulatory system. Some of the drug binds to plasma proteins. Some of the drug that does not bind to plasma proteins "floats" through the bloodstream and may interact with receptors, producing a therapeutic effect. Plasma proteins, such as albumin, do not provide any therapeutic effect in and of themselves.

Membrane Transport Mechanisms

All cells in the human body have specialized transport mechanisms (recall the membrane concept mentioned earlier) through which all materials, including pharmaceuticals, must pass in order to perform their functions. There are special types of transport, including filtration, passive transport, and active transport.

This merely determines the ways in which most drugs get from outside of the cell into the cell. It is important, at least in the academic sense, for you to have some sort of idea as to how these mechanisms work. Following are more specific definitions of each of the mechanisms.

PASSIVE DIFFUSION

Passive diffusion is another term for passive transport, in this case across a cell membrane. The force that permits the substance to be transported from outside the cell into the cell depends largely on the concentration differences between the two environments (outside the cell and inside the cell). Due to equilibrium states that exist between the two environments, certain substances are permitted to pass through the membranes by using specific differences between these two *gradients*—that is, from a high concentration into a low concentration.

FACILITATED DIFFUSION

In facilitated diffusion, a carrier protein permits specific molecules, such as glucose (sugar), to pass through certain parts of the cells. This is far different from the preceding process, in that it does not require the expenditure of energy. In terms of some drugs, this is an important concept because of the rate at which the drug or the substance is permitted to pass through the membrane.

ACTIVE TRANSPORT

Active transport is a special kind of transportation system between the two environments—one that costs the cells energy; it uses the fact that certain substances are permitted to accumulate outside the cells. After a time, the accumulation of these substances will generate a special sort of concentration gradient that, in time, will permit the transportation of a substance from outside the cell into the cell.

PINOCYTOSIS

In this form of transportation, the cell actually engulfs the substance and, by doing so, permits the substance to enter the cell. This process also requires a degree of energy expenditure by the cell. Following absorption even at the point when someone takes a pill, there are specific mechanisms that must take place in order to cause the drug to become available to the body, as mentioned previously. However, there are other specific factors that determine how well or how fast a drug becomes available to the body, such as gastric emptying or the ability of the stomach to permit the passage of materials from the stomach to the small intestine. (Most drugs and foods are absorbed at a much faster rate in the small intestine than in the stomach.) Perhaps some of the exceptions to this rule are alcohol and other substances. Drugs use these mechanisms to become available to the body. Depending upon the reason for the drug and what it does, each drug has its own qualities that take advantage of how the body works to absorb it. So there is a great deal more involved in the transport of a drug into the body than just taking a pill and expecting it to work. For various specific reasons, there are time restrictions placed on the bioavailability of drugs—some drugs need an immediate access to the body's cells, whereas other drugs can afford to wait for the longer time it will take to become available to the body.

The Quality of Drugs—Solubility

Getting back to the cell membrane and its structure with respect to how drugs are absorbed into the cells themselves, recall that the cell membrane has already been defined as a protein and a lipid characteristic. That concept will depend largely on how fast a drug can become absorbed from outside a cell and make it into the cell to perform its designated function. In general terms, then, the more *lipid-soluble* the drug is, the faster the drug will be absorbed into a cell. As you continue with your studies as a pharmacy technician and start to really understand the makeup of different drugs (whether they are fat soluble or water soluble, for example), you will better understand how quickly different drugs are made available to the body. How does that help you clinically?

Suppose, for example, that a patient has a question about a specific drug. Even if you don't have a lot of chemistry knowledge, in time you will be able to tell which drugs are lipid soluble (meaning that they are composed of *buffers* that are lipids) compared with other drugs that, because of their chemical makeup, are more water soluble. The *Physician's Desk Reference* defines drugs in terms of their chemical structure, but some medical professionals describe the drug in terms of its makeup—for example, whether the drug is lipid soluble, water soluble, or both. Therefore, without giving it much thought, you will soon be able to tell a patient who asks you the question that a specific drug will take effect at a faster rate than, for example, a different kind of drug. This applies to most of the over-the-counter drugs as well; the labels will tell you about the basic chemical makeup, and you need not be a chemistry major to understand some of these concepts.

By and large, with the exception of most of the highly soluble general anesthetics used during surgery, drugs are water soluble and only partially soluble; and there are reasons for that. The human body is made up of mostly water, and, with the exception of most of the medications that are used in emergencies, drugs are not needed to work immediately. Because of the different mechanisms, specifically with respect to the cellular structure, there are specific reasons for the drugs being both water and lipid soluble medications. Because of the cell membrane, the drugs are manufactured to handle both the process of absorption into the body and the problems at the cellular level.

In order for a drug to be absorbed via the gastrointestinal (GI) tract, it must be both water and lipid soluble; if a drug is made of too much water, it cannot pass through the very fatty (lipid) layers of the GI tract. Drugs that have too much of a lipid makeup, on the other hand, will have a delayed absorption. (This is the very reason that some medications, such as Dilantin, sometimes do not work quite as effectively in some people as in others and why it can cause diarrhea.)

Drugs and Their Ionization

This is the concept of pharmacokinetics that will become your most likely friend, especially when you think about the *bioavailability* of drugs. Understanding electrolytes is not entirely essential; what you really need to understand is that drugs mainly exist in two basic forms, *ionized* and un-ionized. Think about two of the most common electrolytes, sodium and chloride, denoted by the symbols Na^+ and Cl^-, respectively. These symbols essentially mean that the molecules are either positively charged or negatively charged, or, in more chemical terms, these molecules have either lost or gained electrons. This concept is more important to understand than the lipid–nonlipid nature of drugs when thinking about chemicals (drugs or pharmaceuticals) crossing cell membranes so that they can perform their specific functions.

Generally speaking, chemicals that are ionized (positively or negatively charged) do not readily cross the cell membrane barrier; the un-ionized form of the chemical, or those chemicals that do not carry an electrical charge, negative or positive, are more readily absorbed into the cell.

The reason for this characteristic of drugs—that the electrically charged molecules cannot readily cross the barrier of a cell wall—is that most cell walls are composed of proteins and lipids (as well as other components) that are also electrically charged. Therefore, like two magnets, these components repel each other. This is an extremely limited review of the characteristics of cells and how chemicals are permitted to cross the barrier; but, again, you will want to know how it will help you clinically. The answer is simply that you will be better versed in the makeup of drugs, without having gone through an entire system of physiology and chemistry courses. Thus, you will function more effectively as a pharmacy technician, and you will be more valuable to yourself, your career, and your pharmacist.

SUMMARY

In order for drugs to produce their desired effects, they must be available to the cell receptor. There are many variables which influence how efficiently drugs are carried through the bloodstream to the target organ that they will affect.

The route of administration of a drug (liquid, tablet, parenteral administration) certainly plays an important role in determining the availability of the drug in the body. Other factors include: the affinity of the drug to be bound to proteins in the bloodstream and carried to the target organ, the transport mechanism of the target cell (filtration, passive or active transport) by which the drug enters the cell, and the solubility of the drug (cell membranes contain both lipids, or fats, and proteins).

But there are many other characteristics of cells, cell membranes, and drug molecules that will influence the outcome of drug therapy. Factors such as absorption, solubility, distribution, and ionization of the drug all contribute to how the body will handle a drug once it is taken.

CHAPTER REVIEW QUESTIONS

1. What are we looking for, physiologically speaking, when we medicate a patient?
   a. for the medication to become absorbed into the body
   b. to see if the patient has an allergic reaction
   c. to see if the medication will work
   d. a person with the right disease

2. What helps cells move a drug throughout the body?
   a. platelets
   b. specialized transport mechanisms
   c. bronchial tubes
   d. bloodstream

3. One of the chief concepts that determines the amount of the drug that is actually going to do any good for the body, in general terms, is the:
   a. bioavailability
   b. affinity
   c. processing
   d. solubility

4. Explain how alcohol consumption affects drug action in the body.

5. Explain why it matters to know if a drug is water or lipid soluble.

6. Which of the following is a common resource that defines drugs in terms of their chemical structure?
   a. *Trissel's*
   b. *Physician's Desk Reference*
   c. *The Handbook of Drugs*
   d. *The FDA Pharmaceutical Almanac*

7. Chemicals that are positively or negatively charged are known as what?
   a. receptors
   b. semipermeable
   c. lipid soluble
   d. ionized

8. Explain why ionization is important.

9. In order for a drug to be absorbed in the GI tract, it must be:
   a. water soluble
   b. lipid soluble
   c. semipermeable
   d. both a and b

10. The concept of solubility applies only to prescription drugs, not over-the-counter drugs.
    a. true
    b. false

Resources and References

1. Berkow, Robert. *The Merck Manual, 17th Ed.* Rahway, NJ: Merck Research Laboratories, 1992.

2. Winter, Michael. "Clinical Pharmacokinetics." *Applied Therapeutics: The Clinical Use of Drugs.* Vancouver, Washington: Applied Therapeutics, Inc., 1992.

3. Hitner, Henry and Barbara Nagle. *Basic Pharmacology, 4th Ed.* New York and other cities: Glencoe/McGraw-Hill Publishing Company, 1999.

4. Berkow, Robert. *The Merck Manual, 17th Ed.* Rahway, NJ: Merck Research Laboratories, 1992.

5. Hitner, Henry and Barbara Nagle. *Basic Pharmacology, 4th Ed.* New York and other cities: Glencoe/McGraw-Hill Publishing Company, 1999.

6. Holland, Norman and Michael Patrick Adams. *Core Concepts in Pharmacology.* Upper Saddle River, NJ: Pearson Education, 2003.

7. Adams, Michael Patrick, Dianne L. Josephson, and Leland Norman Holland, Jr. *Pharmacology for Nurses—A Pathophysiologic Approach.* Upper Saddle River, NJ: Pearson Education, 2005.

Drug Distribution and Metabolism

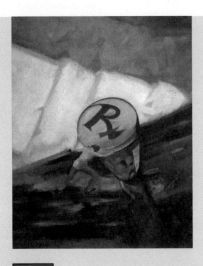

After completing this chapter, you should be able to:

- Describe protein binding and free-floating.
- Explain why solubility is important.
- Identify and explain the effect of bioavailability and its relationship to a drug's being effective.
- List and define the differences between the loading dose and the maintenance dose.
- Explain the importance of clearance of a drug and half life.

INTRODUCTION

Now that we have covered some of the basics with respect to drugs and the human body, it is time to talk about what happens to these medications when they are absorbed. With few exceptions, most medications undergo a number of different changes in the body in order to be effective. It's not quite as simple as most people think—their ability to take that pill this morning is the result of many, many years of research and development. The people who work behind the scenes in the pharmaceutical companies are responsible for ensuring that the medications work and are safe.

In this section, there will be more terms, presented as an overview of how medications work. Just the ideas, concepts, and theories regarding absorption can fill volumes of information—and this information is of no benefit to you, as you are concerned with only what you can apply to the practice of being a pharmacy technician.

The Path

In order for a medication to become absorbed into the body, it must first undergo what is called the first pass effect, which is completed in the liver. This process applies only to those medications taken orally, not the ones that are administered through other routes, which are manufactured in such a way that the body can more readily use them. (See Figure 6-1.)

However, patients cannot be expected to walk around with tubes sticking out everywhere, so, since the advent of the 20th century and with the advances made in physiology and pharmacology, medicine has made great strides in making a number of medications available in the tablet or capsule form.

Without going into much detail about the liver, how it functions, and other physiological concepts, what you will need to know is that specific medications are, indeed, passed through the liver first before they can be

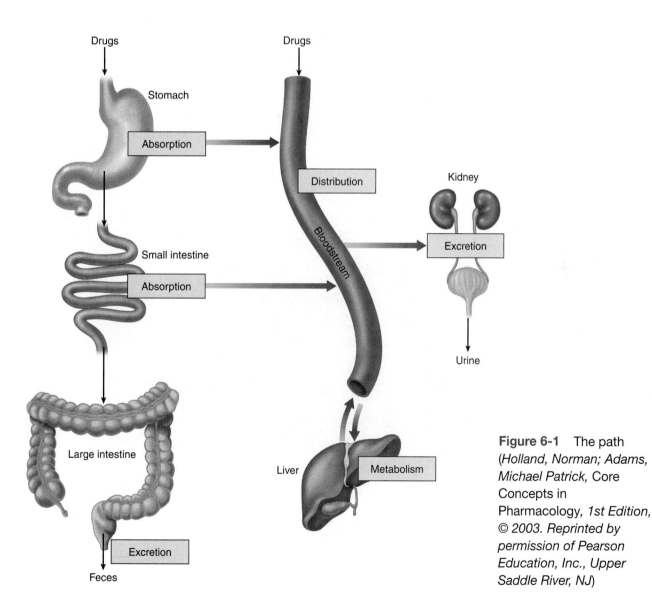

Figure 6-1 The path (*Holland, Norman; Adams, Michael Patrick,* Core Concepts in Pharmacology, *1st Edition,* © 2003. *Reprinted by permission of Pearson Education, Inc., Upper Saddle River, NJ*)

used by the body. Why is that important? Well, for instance, when people use alcohol in excess, their liver functions do not work as well as they should; therefore, some medications can become toxic to them. There are literally hundreds of other examples. When and if you see a patient come into the pharmacy who looks "bad," or has a great deal of yellow in the white part of their eyes (the sclera) (Figure 6-2), you will know that there is most probably a problem with the patient's liver. If the pharmacist doesn't see it, but you do, then your job is to alert the pharmacist. It would seem that this particular patient has not seen his health care provider in some time. The same is true if a patient has a sweet odor in his breath, which could mean that he is diabetic or has been drinking. Either way, your job is to be the eyes and the ears for your pharmacist; or you can call the physician yourself.

After someone takes a pill, it goes through the many different processes that ultimately lead to the bloodstream. It is from that point that the medication is delivered to the different organs in the body. There are several factors involved in the transportation of the drug from the blood to the tissues in the body, and these will be discussed next.

Plasma Binding Protein

This subject was addressed earlier, but in a different way. There are several large proteins responsible for delivering many substances from the intestines, through the blood, and then to the tissues of the body. These proteins are

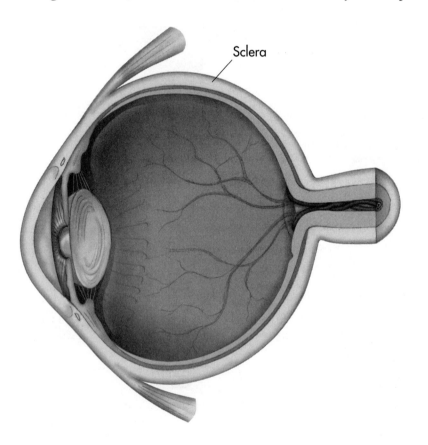

Sclera

Figure 6-2   The sclera

albumin and the several amounts of globulins. They have many different functions, including the ability to transport chemicals through the blood. Some drugs are transported by a means of attraction to these proteins by a process called protein binding, or they are freely floating through the blood.

The chemicals that are not bound to these proteins have their specific pharmacologic effect on the target organs—such as a sore throat treated by an antibiotic. Depending upon the molecule that was once a pill which the patient took this morning, some drugs are highly bound to the proteins, while a good majority of them are unbound. It is the free floating part of the drug that will make the difference.

WHAT DO YOU REALLY NEED TO KNOW ABOUT PHARMACOKINETICS?

The short answer is "a great deal." The long answer is "a lot." Why? Well, in order to have a basic understanding of the drugs that you are about to extend to a patient, you will need to know something about the drug, because the patient usually doesn't. And if you are going to rely on the pharmacist for the answer to every question of "How does this drug work," "How does this drug get into my system," or even "Why do I need this drug," then you will be really nothing more than a glorified cashier, and that's not what the pharmacist is looking for. He is looking for a person who can not only hand a bottle to a patient, but also explain some of the answers that patients might have.

No one is going to expect you to know all of the answers; all of the questions are not known yet. And the pharmacist, regardless of his educational degree and experience, is not a walking encyclopedia. When a question is posed, the educated person does not always know the answer; he knows where to get it; and that's what this review is all about, beyond the basics that you will need in order to operate as a technician.

Equilibrium

When all of the protein-bound sites are used up with respect to a specific drug, you can look for the unbound drug portion, measure it, and know how much chemical is really available for use. Two issues determine the degree to which a drug is bound to a protein site (as in cells in the bloodstream): (1) the binding affinity for the drug and (2) the number of available sites on the cells. As long as the volume of the drug is adequate, the amount of unbound drug will remain sufficient to get the job done.

Many equations and laws govern the pharmacokinetics of all of the drugs, and a chemist could tell you how all of this works. Although you don't need an extensive knowledge of these laws and equations, it would be helpful to understand why some drugs should be taken with food, some drugs should not be taken with milk, and some drugs should not be taken with anything, but on an empty stomach. The point is that you want as much of that drug unbound to proteins as is necessary to enable it to do the job. (There is a lot more to it than that, but you will learn more in time.)

Absorption

The absorption of a drug governs the *bioavailability* of the drug—that is, the amount of drug that is available for use. There are several factors that influence absorption.

As mentioned previously, a drug must be both lipid (fat) and water soluble in order to enter the body through the gastrointestinal tract. There is more to it than just what gets through the gut, however; how the drug is manufactured also plays a part. This could give you a clue as to why some patients (much to your chagrin) will demand the "real stuff," or the non-generic form of the drug—because, they claim, it works better. And, to some extent, they are right.

Some of the drugs that have lost their patent protection by their original manufacturer have been manufactured by other drug companies (as well as by warehouses that are owned by the original brand-name manufacturer). When these drugs are made, it's not always the chemical that effects absorption, but the buffer into which the drug has been instilled. Different buffers can completely change the degree to which these drugs will be able to reach the circulation.

When a drug enters the body via other routes, such as IV or IM (intermuscular) routes, whether it is brand name or generic, it is usually made almost completely available within minutes.

SALT FORMS

Consider the drug theophylline, which, by itself, has a bioavailability factor of 1.0 (meaning that it is completely available). However, this drug is often dispensed, not as theophylline, but as aminophylline, which is only 80 percent theophylline—the fraction of the drug salt, or *ester* that is the "parent" compound. The ratio between the two factors, the F (bioavailability) and the S (salt), will determine how well the drug is absorbed.

Rate of Administration

The rate by which a drug is administered to the body is not measured by the time it takes to swallow a pill, but by a formula that uses the two fractions identified previously with respect to the dosing interval. In other words, certain drugs are designed to be taken every four hours for many reasons, one of which is the half-life of the drug; another reason is the rate by which the drug can be absorbed over a given period. This helps the chemist (through the research and development process) as he determines the average rate of administration—to ensure that there is a certain amount of the drug in the system at all times.

Volume of Distribution

Theoretically, if you consider the body as one entity, you can assume that there is a specific amount of the drug in the body at any given time. This is not always true, however, because of many factors, including the different chemicals in the bloodstream, the bioavailability of the drug, the initial plasma concentration, and the amount of drug that is freely available at any given time. The actual volume of distribution, therefore, is determined by a number of factors, including the *loading dose*, which can sometimes be a higher dose than the patient will take on a regular basis. This is sometimes referred to as the difference between the loading dose and the maintenance dose. (This concept is more fully covered later.)

IMPORTANT NOTE ABOUT "TWO COMPARTMENTS"

As alluded to previously, most of the time a pharmacist considers a drug in terms of its being taken into the body—into one compartment, the entire body. However, the drug is actually in two compartments: Part of the drug is in the blood and in those organs which have a relatively high rate of blood flow, such as the heart; and part is in the different, minute tissues of the body. (At a certain point, whenever that is, there will be an equilibrium; but, clinically speaking, this concept is not relevant to you or the pharmacist unless you are working in an environment where there is compounding of drugs.)

Clearance

The clearance of a drug is determined by a number of factors, so when a manufacturer considers developing a new drug, one of the questions it must answer (for the company) is how it will be cleared and how fast. Ideally, drugs are eliminated from the body at the same rate at which they are absorbed, according to a "steady state" reading of the drug in the body at all times. However, due to the two-compartment model that was previously mentioned, such is not always the case.

The rate of distribution, the rate of absorption, and the rate of elimination will have to be determined to ensure that the body has enough of the drug at all times. This is particularly important with antibiotics, antihypertensives, or drugs that treat cancer. Through a calculation, a maintenance dose is determined, which tells the physician a number of things about the drug. The amount to be given over a period of time is important, as is your duty to tell the patient, for example, to "Make sure that you take these pills every six hours."

Half Life

This term is more useful for the chemist than for the clinician, unless you are in a hospital setting. Only applicable to those drugs that follow through with the first bypass of elimination (which means that it goes through the liver as well as the GI tract), it is the amount of time it would take for the drug to be reduced by one-half (a plasma level drug, not a protein bound drug).

There are all kinds of mathematical formulas that are used to help determine these values, but they mean little unless they can be applied clinically. However, suppose that you saw a patient walk into the pharmacy, obviously ill after you know that the patient just received two new medications not more than two days ago. The patient did not complain about a fever. Then you found out that the patient had inadvertently taken two more pills than he was supposed to take. What would you think? Would you think about the distribution, elimination, and excretion of that drug? Of course you would. And you would then alert the pharmacist, who would call the physician and, if warranted, the local emergency medical service.

Keep in mind that most patients do not think about how these medications work, nor do they consider how they work together. Likewise, some physicians, because of the size of their practice or the number of different doctors the patients are simultaneously consulting with, are not always aware of exactly what medications their patients are taking.

Information Resources

If you have a computer available at your facility, there are a number of websites you can access to find out more about medications. One of the more popular is **http://www.rxlist.com**. This site gives you a complete list of all medications as well as any side effects.

Another excellent Internet site, hosted by the Food and Drug Administration, is located at **http://www.fda.gov**. There you will find a variety of informative pages discussing drugs with respect to foods, cosmetics, and other issues.

Remember, all of this knowledge is of no use unless you can use it. Knowing the exact name for a drug is important; but knowing what it can do, especially with regard to other drugs, and how it is eliminated from the body and how fast is far more important.

SUMMARY

Most medications undergo a number of changes in the body in order to be effective. Medications taken orally pass through the liver in what is called, the first pass effect. It is especially important to remember that liver function can have a significant impact on the efficacy of a drug. Patients with impaired liver function may experience a lack of efficacy and, more importantly, toxic symptoms, that a patient with normal liver function will not. Also, we have learned (Chapter 5) that the solubility of a drug directly relates to the ability of chemicals to travel through the blood to the appropriate cell receptor site.

There are many other key components that affect drug distribution throughout the body, such as the bioavailability, rate of administration, half-life, and clearance of the drug.

The availability of receptor sites, the rate of clearance of a drug from the body, the rate of administration, the affinity of the drug for binding sites, and other factors all play a significant role in the outcome of pharmacotherapeutics: to ensure that, at any given time, there is a sufficient amount of drug in the body to produce the desired therapeutic effect.

CHAPTER 6

CHAPTER REVIEW QUESTIONS

1. Drugs either transported by means of attracting proteins are referred to as what?
   a. protein binding
   b. protein inhibiting
   c. protein synthesis
   d. none of the above

2. If a patient has a sweet odor in his breath, it could be an indication of what disease?
   a. COPD
   b. cystic fibrosis
   c. diabetes
   d. allergic rhinitus

3. Two issues that determine the degree to which a drug is bound to a protein site are:
   a. efficacy and bioavailability
   b. affinity and number of available sites on cells
   c. bioavailability and the number of T-cells
   d. absorption and evaporation

4. Aminophylline is what percent of actual theophylline?
   a. 20%
   b. 50%
   c. 60%
   d. 80%

5. Explain why a patient could be right in asserting that a generic drug does not work as well as a brand-name drug.

6. A dose that can sometimes be a higher dose than what the patient will take on a regular basis is called:
   a. an intermittent dose
   b. a STAT dose
   c. a loading dose
   d. a sub-therapeutic dose

7. Drugs are always eliminated from the body at the same rate that they were administered.
   a. true   b. false

Resources and References

1. Winter, Michael; Koda-Kimble, Mary Anne, Ed. "Clinical Pharmacokinetics." *Applied Therapeutics: The Clinical Use of Drugs, 4th Ed.* Vancouver, Washington: Applied Therapeutics, Inc., 1992.

2. Hitner, Henry and Barbara Nagle. *Basic Pharmacology, 4th Ed.* New York and other cities: Glencoe/McGraw-Hill Publishers, Inc., 1999.

3. Holland, Norman and Michael Patrick Adams. *Core Concepts in Pharmacology*. Upper Saddle River, NJ: Pearson Education, 2003.

4. Adams, Michael Patrick, Dianne L. Josephson, and Leland Norman Holland, Jr. *Pharmacology for Nurses—A Pathophysiologic Approach*. Upper Saddle River, NJ: Pearson Education, 2005.

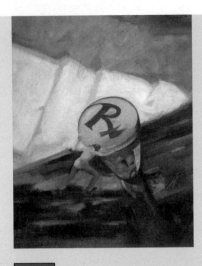

Addiction

Learning Objectives

Learning Objectives

After completing this chapter, you should be able to:

- Explain what happens physically and mentally during addictive behavior.
- List and define samples of drug and nondrug items that can be addictive.
- Explain the concept of the development of drug tolerance.
- Describe the role of the pharmacy technician in identifying drug abuse patients.
- List and identify some drugs that interact with alcohol.

INTRODUCTION

The term drug abuse is so broad as to have very little meaning outside of a specific context and is subject to a great deal of interpretation. Many negative societal connotations are applied to the term, however, whether referring to pharmaceutical medications or those agents commonly called street drugs.

Using Oxycontin®, for example, is quite different from using cocaine; but they might have the same potential power for abuse, depending upon the user and the person prescribing the narcotics.

There are specific reasons for the variety in the definitions, as the term *drug abuse* is actually a misnomer, applying to a large array of problems, including addiction, dependency, and even the occasional use of certain drugs. While all of these problems might present in the same way in terms of how the patient or user acts in public, it is important to understand the differences between dependency and addiction, as they carry two clearly different mechanisms and have different consequences.

For example, a patient who is taking narcotic medications for the treatment of an end-stage disease, such as cancer, may become chemically dependent upon that drug. For the patient and the practitioner, this is an acceptable evil connected with taking the medication, as the options are limited. In such cases, the issue of dependency has been well documented and understood by both parties.

Simultaneously, that same patient may become addicted to a prescribed medication. That, too, may be an acceptable risk, especially when the pain is associated with a type of cancer that cannot be treated and will result in death. The elimination of, or at least some control over, the pain warrants the addiction.

The Disease

Addiction is a disease. Chemical dependency is an associated risk and a result of taking a certain prescribed (or illegally obtained) drug for a specific period, but not to the point of addiction. These terms will be discussed in this section, along with the reasons for addiction, chemical dependency, and other terms associated with the use of certain narcotic medications.

There are important considerations for both the pharmacy technician and the pharmacist when releasing specific medications into the hands of patients who have had a clear history of problems with drugs, whether street drugs or pharmaceuticals, even when the person relinquishing the medication might simply have strong beliefs that the patient has had such problems in the past. This section will cover the question of when it is appropriate to hold a prescription until a physician or provider is consulted to ensure that problems do not arise due to the release of these chemicals.

Families and friends of a patient could very well become involved when addiction and dependency are problems, and this can create new issues. Such issues as these, and useful terms related to the world of the abuse of chemicals, will be examined in this section.

As a pharmacy technician, you will continue to learn more about the realm of drug and chemical misuse than what is presented here. While this section will be a valuable addition to your education, it is by no means meant to be comprehensive. Newer and more powerful chemicals are constantly introduced into the market; and, sad to say, stronger and more accessible forms of street drugs become available to users all the time.

The mixture of the two categories of chemicals (prescription and street drugs) can become a risk to a person's life. The essence of this section is that your pharmacy team can become an influential asset to the community concerning the use and misuse of specific chemicals, whether prescribed or obtained otherwise. The reasons people take controlled substances and how these substances react in the human brain are subjects well beyond the scope of this book. Identifying the symptoms of addiction or substance abuse can be an important function of your employment alongside a pharmacist; you and the pharmacist are a team, possibly representing the last element between the patient and a specific medication. Therefore, it will be important for you to remain alert to the symptoms and actions of those people who approach your facility for a specific drug.

Calling the physician or the health care provider can save a life or prevent problems such as damaged relationships—such serious matters can hinge on the dispensing of just one vial of medication. Read these sections, and you will begin to understand the concepts of addiction, substance abuse, and other aspects of using a medication inappropriately.

Characteristics

While the term *addiction* should not be used in the same context as *chemical dependency*, addiction is defined as both a psychological and physiological dependency. Dependency is defined as the feeling that something is needed in order to continue to exist in the same living situation and ways of thinking to which the person has become accustomed. For a drug or a chemical to be addictive, specific symptoms, called withdrawal symptoms, must be present following the abrupt change in the practice of use. Specific marks or signs of addiction are typically seen in people addicted to a specific substance, whether it is a prescribed drug or an illegally obtained substance. Some of these hallmarks are as follows:

- An absorbing focus—All addictions consume some time, thought, and energy.
- Increasing *tolerance*—In order to achieve the same effect as when the person first started using the agent, there must be more chemical ingested over time; later, there is a loss of control over the use of the agent.
- A growing denial—typically, the person becomes so sensitive to the thought of using the agent that he tends to deny any interest in the agent in order to sustain his previous pattern of life.
- Damaging consequences—There is no such thing as a harmless addiction, whether it is an addiction to a substance or to any other thing. All addicts eventually bring some form of destruction to themselves and their families. Typically, there is a loss of three things: employment, interest in self, and previous reputation. Addictions are enslaving and destructive dependencies on an agent, such as a drug or a pharmaceutical chemical.
- Painful withdrawal—Almost always, there is a painful withdrawal during the time the agent is abruptly stopped, for whatever reason. (This is sometimes also true with chemical dependency.) The addict has angry, uncontrollable outbursts, periods of anxiety, panic attacks, tremors, severe depression, and a sense of loss of life and all the good that life brings to the individual and the families involved.

Causes

Specific addictive street drugs such as cocaine, heroin, and morphine cause the release of *dopamine*, a neurotransmitting chemical in the brain. This is only one of the many different *neurotransmitters* in the brain that control such things as thought, actions, feelings, and other attributes. When these neurotransmitters are functioning normally, the person is also considered normal. Dopamine has been linked to some of the more common problems seen in those who are addicted. There is a proven link between dopamine and other *catecholamines* seen not only in the brain, but also in the adrenal system, leading to such problems as *hypertension* and other diseases.

Each higher dose of the drug causes higher dopamine levels, which is why people who are addicted to drugs are also *depressed*. In the addict's brain, the higher doses of dopamine activate a negative feedback system that, in time, causes the nervous system to be less sensitive to the neurotransmitter. The first high, therefore, is never duplicated by the second, the third, the fourth, and so on. Finally, the addict requires such high doses that the human body can no longer adapt. The results are sometimes fatal. Drug abusers increase the dose of a drug in an attempt to achieve the same effect as they achieved previously; this repeated effort causes the disease.

The Criteria for Addiction

In order to identify a person who is addicted to a specific chemical or a drug, you need to understand that there are specific criteria. Nine different items are sometimes all present and sometimes present but to a smaller degree, depending upon the level of addiction. It can be difficult to identify an addicted person; addicts have the time-tested strength of holding up a false front before others without being detected (that is, without blood or urine tests). However, in general, the following nine criteria are typically present in most people who are addicted, in one form or another, to one or more drugs:

The patient is noted taking the drug (or drugs) in larger amounts than are needed to achieve the expected results. Patients taking narcotics for pain relief reach this threshold when they take more than they need to achieve the pain relief and are seeking other effects of the medications. The patient develops what is called a high "tolerance" for the drug.

There have been many unsuccessful attempts to quit taking the medication, accompanied by a persistent period of craving and a desire to obtain the medication, sometimes at any cost to the patient or others involved, such as a ring of family members or friends.

Excessive time is used in seeking the medication; a patient, for example, uses many different health care providers and pharmacies to obtain a specific medication. There are periods when the patient feels *intoxicated* (or appears to you to be intoxicated or acting strange or unusual compared with previous encounters). The patient thinks about giving up other things in life for the purpose of drug seeking. He continues to use the drug or medication, even after he and his family have been told of the potential damages to his life or vital organs—or danger to others in his life.

The marked tolerance for the medication can leave a trail of information that can sometimes be determined by checking databases or talking with other providers or pharmacists. There are characteristic withdrawal symptoms manifested with any attempt to stop taking specific drugs, particularly during times when the pharmacies are closed, such as holidays, weekends, or any other periods when the drug is not available. There is a consistent use of the drug in order to prevent withdrawal symptoms.

The Roots of Drug Abuse

Drug abuse is not new; discoveries have been made indicating that approximately 5000 B.C. the cocoa plant was valued for its stimulant effects along with the nutritious properties of the plant. Even today, Peruvian Indians chew the plant leaves to achieve a gentle stimulation of their gums as well as a concomitant loss of appetite. City dwellers around the same area extract the more potent properties of the plant, called cocaine and distribute it as well as smoke it. Some continue to use the leaves as well as the extracted cocaine to fight off fatigue while they work in fields. If not for the substance, these people would remain exhausted because of the long hours of hard labor.

After long periods of use of the drug, these people undergo changes in their brains, which cause them to crave more and more of the extracted cocaine. This has been continuing for years.

Imagine this scenario: In California, a 19-year-old mother who has been marked with holes throughout her skin gives birth to a small, almost lifeless child. The child dies, but not before experiencing a long period of withdrawal. These events ignite the father into a murderous rage because his practice of injecting cocaine has been discovered. And the plot thickens from there: Many children who witness their parents high on cocaine or other substances eventually die from neglect because money that could have been used to purchase food is used to buy cocaine or heroin.

Getting high can be cheap, legal, and deadly. Children as young as nine years of age have died from intentional *Freon* inhalation. Every year, teenagers die from inhaling butane lighter fluid fumes. Others die from deliberately breathing typewriter correction fluid, fabric protector sprays, aerosol propellants, paints, paint thinners, and gasoline. While most people who use these sort of legal but dangerous elements found in our homes do not die, they can suffer consequences that are far beyond anything they gambled on—such as the death of a fetus, long-term brain damage, or a host of other problems. The highs that are associated with these sort of products are typically short-lived, and the substances are not detected by the most typical drug screens; but the effects can be devastating.

Alcohol

Alcohol, although legal in certain circumstances, is a depressant; other depressants include some of the oldest drugs known to mankind, such as the opiates. Despite the many programs that have been implemented to try to curb the use of alcohol, dangers still abound. One of the largest problems associated with the use of alcohol is its concomitant use with prescribed medications. Typically, a pharmaceutical label will have instructions on it which indicate that the medication should not be used along with alcohol. Because alcohol is a highly addictive substance, it is prudent and appropriate to discuss this drug and list some of the more commonly abused drugs associated with the consumption of alcohol.

A complete list of drugs that can have an adverse effect on any of the more important organs in the body, such as the heart, brain, kidneys, and others, is too long to list here. However, before you hand anyone a prescription for an addictive drug or any of the common pharmaceutical agents that pass through the liver for metabolism, you should be certain that the patient has been thoroughly counseled with respect to the use of alcohol along with the prescription.

There are times when the pharmacist deems it appropriate that certain patients who have been known to consume alcohol undergo more counseling than the typical patient who does not have a problem with alcohol. If the pharmacist is unaware of a patient's problem with alcohol, the pharmacy technician may take the initiative by performing the appropriate counseling as to the guidelines, as well as pointing out that the prescription bottle has a sticker on it that explains these same issues.

ALCOHOL, OTHER DRUGS, AND THE BRAIN

Alcohol and some of the more common drugs that are addictive or cause harm to the body have an immediate and altering effect on specific perceptions and emotions. After repeated use of these substances, there are reasons to consider that some form of dependence is being developed—symptoms are produced that are consistent with tolerance and withdrawal.

It is essential that you, as the pharmacy technician, realize that many of the commonly prescribed drugs can, when mixed with alcohol (ETOH), cause devastating effects. Not only should the sticker indicating such information be placed on the vial for that particular medication, but also it might be in your best interest to personally tell patients of the warning.

When asked, most alcoholics will deny that they even "touch that stuff." Syphilis was once called the "Great Impostor" because it mimicked a host of other problems; our society should use this term to define alcoholism. Over 20 percent of all patients who visit medical clinics or hospitals suffer from some sort of problem as a result of using alcohol in an excessive amount.

According to the American Society of Addiction Medicine, alcoholism is a "primary, *chronic* disease with genetic, psychosocial, and environmental factors influencing its development and manifestations."

As a representative of your company or institution, the pharmacist to whom you are responsible, the patient, and your own integrity, your challenge is to pick one of those 20 people out of a crowd of 100 people—and it is not easy.

Alcoholism is a disease, pure and simple. It refers to consuming ethanol in a potentially hazardous or harmful manner. Your responsibility cannot possibly be the patient's problem with this disease, but only the types of medications that are dispensed from your institution, because the list of medications that can cause problems when these alcoholics take them is long.

Table 7-1 contains a list of medications that are potentially problematic when mixed with other medications. This list should be posted somewhere in your pharmacy to ensure that patients can review what they have in their bag and what they have at home.

Like some of the drugs that are dispensed from any typical pharmacy, alcohol has the following effects:

Immediate effects: Alcohol (and some of the drugs that effect the neurotransmitters discussed previously) has specific mood-altering effects on the mind. Alcohol and some other drugs alter the levels of dopamine in the brain;

TABLE 7-1

Drug	Common Problems Associated with the Use of Alcohol
Isosorbide, NTG	Rapid heartbeat, sudden changes in blood pressure
Alprazalom, Diazepam	Drowsiness, dizziness, and an increased risk for overdose
Warfarin	Occasional drinking may lead to internal bleeding; heavier drinking may have the opposite effect, resulting in clots
Diphenhydramine	Drowsiness, dizziness, and an increased risk for overdose
Glyburide, Metformin,	Rapid heart rate, sudden changes in blood pressure, convulsions, and possibly coma
Cimetidine, Nizatidine	Rapid heart rate, sudden changes in blood pressure
Griseofulvin, Flagyl,	Rapid heart rate, sudden changes in blood pressure, liver damage
Aspirin, Advil, Tylenol	Stomach upset, bleeding ulcers, liver damage, increased heart rate
Chlonazepam, Phenytoin	Drowsiness, increased risk of seizures
Hydrocodone, Oxycodone	Drowsiness, dizziness, and risk for overdose
Temazepam, Diphenhydramine	Drowsiness, dizziness
Herbal Preparations	Increased drowsiness

this neurotransmitter effects the degree to which *synapses* (the connections between brain cells) can interact with each other. Alcohol causes the level of dopamine to elevate in the brain; and according to some recent research, even the anticipation of alcohol can have an effect on dopamine levels. Drugs such as the amphetamines increase the release of dopamine by blocking the molecule that would act to transport it away from specific centers of the brain where it has most of its activity. Another neurotransmitter, *serotonin*, is thought to have an even more immediate effect through the use of alcohol as well as some other drugs, particularly those currently used for the treatment of depression (the SSRIs, or the serotonin secretion re-uptake inhibitors).

Long-term effects: Cells in the brain, like cells in other parts of the body, are subject to change, given the right situation. Drugs and alcohol, over time, can impose such a change on the chemical composition of the brain with respect to how the cells react to each other. These changes can result in neuroadaptation; in other words, the brain learns other ways to function over time due to the damage imposed upon it by drugs and alcohol. For example, excessive consumption of alcohol can cause a sudden change in the amount of neurotransmitters, which can decrease the number of dopamine receptors in the brain. In time, this can have a long-term effect on the ways in which the abuser makes decisions and exercises judgment.

Neurotoxic effects: Over a longer period of time, chronic abuse of drugs or alcohol (or both) can have a long term effect on the brain to the point that a person develops dementia (loss of memory). Long-term use of such drugs as methamphetamine and cocaine can produce such long-term effects as an altered ability to see correctly and impaired hearing. One of the most commonly known problems associated with long-term use of alcohol is a disease called Weicke–Korsakoff's syndrome, which is a special type of dementia that is often accompanied by specific nutritional problems. This disease is often associated with an inability to learn new topics, recall people's names and addresses, or even remember a subject that was just recently mentioned.

TREATMENT FOR ALCOHOLISM

Excessive alcohol consumption is a great concern as it involves both damaging physical effects and psychological effects, including dependency. Alcohol is a central nervous system (CNS) depressant. This means that consumption can slow down normal thinking and impair judgment and motor skills. In addition, alcohol damages the liver and has been identified as the leading cause of cirrhosis (failure of the liver to function). Many medications taken while consuming alcohol may hinder absorption of the drug or interact, causing such effects as increased sedation.

As a pharmacy technician, you should alert the pharmacist if you suspect that a patient consumes an excessive amount of alcohol. Sometimes this may be easy to identify, while other times patients will deny such use, even with solid proof. Alcohol withdrawal can be quite devastating and painful for the patient. In some cases, it can also be life-threatening.

Treatment for alcoholism primarily involves counseling or entering a program such as Alcoholics Anonymous (AA). Joining a program such as AA is usually a time-sensitive matter, with intense counseling and support from other members and counselors. The format is that of a self-help group.

One type of medication used in the treatment of severe alcoholism is Disulfram© (Antabuse). It works by producing a violent reaction within the patient if he continues to consume alcohol. The patient will vomit and may experience other symptoms, including severe headaches, shortness of breath, and other ill effects.

SUMMARY

One of the purposes of this chapter (and Chapter 8) is to differentiate drug addiction and drug dependency.

Drug addiction is a disease. It is defined as the habitual use of a drug (including alcohol) that is beyond one's voluntary control. Addiction involves both psychological and physiological dependence on a substance to alter one's mood, emotion, or state of consciousness. Drug addiction can affect all aspects of the addict's life because it is enslaving in terms of time, thought, and energy. Loss of family, employment, reputation, and self-interest can be damaging results of drug addiction. In addition, drug addiction can have serious, long-term physiological effects. The causes, roots, and physiological consequences of drug addiction are covered in detail in this chapter.

Drug addiction is a disease that can cause tremendous suffering, pain, and devastating consequences. As a pharmacy technician, you may be in a position to identify problems of drug addiction. Recognizing the hallmarks of addiction that are discussed in this chapter can alert you to potential abuse problems. It is your duty as a pharmacy technician to be vigilant with regard to patients who take controlled substances, and to report your concerns to the pharmacist.

CHAPTER REVIEW QUESTIONS

1. Is addiction considered a disease or a disorder?
   a. disease
   b. disorder

2. What is the need for something or the feeling that something is needed in order to continue to exist called?
   a. addiction
   b. dependency
   c. coexistence
   d. craving

3. Drugs such as cocaine, heroin, and morphine cause the release of a chemical in the brain called:

   a. dopamine
   b. seratonin
   c. neurotransmitter
   d. adrenaline

4. Explain how, with higher doses of some drugs, a person may actually become depressed.

5. The connections between brain cells that interact with each other are known as:
   a. sedation
   b. synapses
   c. both a and b
   d. none of the above

Resources and References

1. Koda-Kimble, Mary Anne., Pharm. D. *Applied Therapeutics: The Clinical Use of Drugs, 5th Ed.* Vancouver, Washington: Applied Therapeutics, Inc., 1992.

2. "The Marks of Addiction." Accessed October 20, 2003.
http://www.gospelcom.net/rbc/ds/cb961/page2.html

3. Wyngaarden, James, Lloyd Smith, and J. W. B. Bennett. *Cecil's Textbook of Medicine, 19th Ed.* Philadelphia and other cities: Saunders Company, 1988. pp. 1390–1391.

4. "Nicotine and Cocaine Are Similar Types of Addictive Drugs." Accessed October 20, 2003.
http://stage.mhhe.com/sciencemath/biology/maderinquiry/aug5.html

5. "Addiction Criteria." Accessed October 20, 2003.
http://calyx.com/~schaffer/library/addcrit.html

6. Landry, Mim. *Understanding Drugs and Abuse: The Processes of Addiction, Treatment and Recovery.* Los Angeles, CA. American Psychiatric Press, 1994. pp. 41-89, 113–120.

7. "Alcohol, Drugs and the Brain." Accessed October 22, 2003.
http://www.open.org/tahana/ADA/twfadbr.htm

8. Baker, Ray. Rakel, Robert and Edward Bope, Eds. "Psychiatric Disorders: Alcoholism." *Conn's Current Therapy 2002.* Philadelphia and other cities: W. B. Saunders, Inc., 2002.

9. "Harmful Interactions: Mixing Alcohol with Medicines." National Institute on Alcohol Abuse and Alcoholism, Bethesda, MD. Publication Number 03-5329, Printed February 2003.

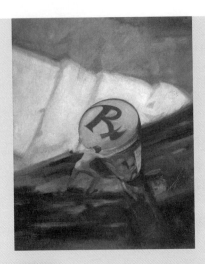

Drug Dependency

INTRODUCTION

Picture yourself as a pharmacy technician taking a call from a physician's office informing you that a patient has just left his office attempting to get some medication for his pain. The physician did not treat the patient, but you know the patient rather well.

While this patient might be looked upon as a drug seeker, you and the pharmacist realize through the patient's profile that he never engaged a physician in such a way in the past. Upon further investigation and discussion with your pharmacist, you realize that the physician who made the most recent phone call (which was ultimately referred to the pharmacist) is a new physician in town. Because the patient's own physician, a pain management physician, is not currently available, the patient chose to see a new physician for the time being.

After talking with your pharmacist and obtaining an approval to make a phone call, you call the patient and suggest that he go to the nearest emergency department or seek the attention of one of the pain management physicians with whom your pharmacy has developed a relationship.

The Problem

This is an important, but frequently overlooked issue in medicine that creates concern among primary care physicians. Because of the risk of abuse of specific narcotics, many physicians refuse to write prescriptions for them for fear of being not only "tagged" by the community as a physician who hands out pain prescriptions casually, but also of being charged for doing so by the legal authorities. There are legitimate cases, however, such as when a patient is being treated for an ailment like chronic pain that has been non-responsive to all other treatment. Sometimes there are very few options available, and when a patient such as the one discussed previously is a very responsible person with a clear understanding of the problems associated with taking the medication, he respects the dangers of dependency and addiction and uses only the amount allocated by the physician.

While this scenario might never happen in your entire career as a pharmacy technician, the probability for it to occur is greater now than it was yesterday, and it will become greater as the days go by. Therefore, while you are not the one who is ultimately responsible for a patient's physiological position, you need to be aware of the differences between what it means when your pharmacist tells you a patient is addicted and when the patient is chemically dependent. You also need to be aware of the consequences of other issues as they apply to the use of medications, and the list includes more than just the narcotics.

The term addiction applies to a person who is using a pharmacological agent compulsively; there is a psychological dependence; and the person continues to use the chemical in spite of all indications that, if the drug is continued, it will harm the body. The term addiction, however, has been used in the wrong context in all aspects of our society, including referring to patients of those who have licenses to practice medicine, such as physicians and other health care providers. Not all patients who ask for pain medications are addicts, clear and simple. Just because someone experiences a period of withdrawal following a halt to a medication does not mean that the person is an addict. Addiction is a psychological dependence, not just a physiological dependence.

Controlled Medications

According to the United States Controlled Substances Act of 1970, each medication that has a potential for abuse is identified by a number ranging from I through V, determined by the medication's ability to influence behavior and potential for abuse. The following considerations apply when, for example, a new medication for pain control is released into the market: the degree to which the medication has a potential for abuse, whether the substance has been determined to have a current and acceptable medical use, whether the use of the medication, under medical supervision, is safe.

Let's look at some medications that are generally classified for pain relief and their properties that can lead to abuse.

An *opiate* is a drug that has its origin in the opium poppy, from which such substances as cocaine and morphine are manufactured. An opioid is a scientific term that is used to describe a long list of medications and substances that includes the opiates, those made synthetically (such as methadone), and those medications having properties that interfere with specific receptors in the brain that "turn off" pain in the body.

The list also includes a number of other drugs that either compete with specific *receptors* or *antagonize* other receptors in the brain. The ultimate effect to the normal user is an eradication of the problem. The abuser is actually looking for some of the side effects, most of which, over time, can cause damage to the brain, the kidneys, and the liver, to mention a few of the important organs that keep the body alive. The federal government controls these substances for the safety and well being of society.

There is a point when a patient starts to abuse medications and becomes a drug abuser. This point is reached when a person knowingly continues to use a specific medication beyond its normal prescribed level. At this point, there is a noticeable psychological dependence on the drug that will lead to a large array of psychological problems if the drug is stopped. This person will do almost anything to achieve what is needed, including rob his own family, cheat his boss, or harm others to lay his claim to a specific drug. This is a vastly different from the patient who, because of pain that is unrelieved through all other measures, receives prescriptions for narcotics to achieve some relief.

For example, a patient may be taking a specific medication, such as one of the aforementioned opiates, for the relief of pain. Even if the condition is chronic and the patient continues to use the medication, addiction may not be a problem. Here, the patient understands that he should not take too much of the medication. When the pain is resolved, the physician will taper the medication off over time in order to prevent any withdrawal problems.

A great deal of confusion exists, even among clinicians, about the differences between physical dependence and addiction. The fundamental distinction between the two requires that clinicians never label patients who are presumed to be at risk for an *abstinence* syndrome (being physically dependent) as an addict.

Such a description misrepresents reality and essentially wrongfully identifies a patient as addicted when he is not. A clinician and a patient should have a conversation about the use of narcotics when other available drugs and alternative treatments are not effective. Having a profile on the patient gives you, as the pharmacy technician, the opportunity to further justify the distinction.

If a patient should present himself to your pharmacy with a prescription for a medication that has a clear indication for the potential for chemical dependence, or, in the worst case, addiction, and the patient is not known to the facility, the pharmacist has a legal and ethical responsibility to call the physician or access other means of identifying the patient. If there is no clear indication that the patient is addicted, then even the issue of dependency does not necessarily mean that the drug should not be dispensed.

In a case like this, if your pharmacist does not perform an adequate check, there could be an injustice brought upon the patient. Not only will withholding the medication leave him in continued pain, but also symptoms of withdrawal will appear eventually that could cause others to view the patient as addicted, because the proper, supervised, tapered withdrawal was not perfomed.

Without any doubt, the inconsistent use of the terms addiction, dependence, and tolerance leads to many misunderstandings among those who regulate the system of dispensing narcotics or other medications that have the potential of chemical dependence or addiction. Most of this misunderstanding, obviously, refers to those patients who are taking medications designed for pain and labeled as narcotics. Because of the many misunderstandings, there are a good number of patients who suffer with pain, untreated. Some patients have been identified as using such medications for issues other than pain relief, but there is no reason why a few should suffer because of this misunderstanding.

While it is not within your own jurisdiction to take these matters into your own hands, it is your responsibility to bring these and other situations to the attention of your pharmacist so that he can take the appropriate actions. Your pharmacist might know the patient in a different way; his license depends on what is dispensed, when it is dispensed, and for what reasons. Your position, however, does have its advantages, in that you may know something about the patient that the pharmacist does not know. A discussion between you and the pharmacist is therefore justified. The point is to be able to distinguish between the patient who might be chemically dependent, but legitimately needs the medication for the relief and adjustment of pain; the patient who, for whatever reason, may be using the medications for a recreational drug; and the patient who is actually psychologically addicted to the pharmaceutical agent.

Addiction Versus Dependence

For further reading on the differences between addiction and dependence— which has been a social issue since well before the 1940s—visit "The Definition of Addiction," by Steven L. Booker, Department of Psychology, the University of Sydney, at the following website: defofaddiction.html, at **www.pysch.su.oz.au**

SUMMARY

The purpose of this chapter is to further differentiate between drug addiction and drug dependency. The differences between addiction and dependency can sometimes be blurred, and you may find that, quite often, these terms are used interchangeably. However, the key difference between drug dependency and addiction is the absence of the psychological component. Drug dependency usually involves a physiological dependence.

It is your responsibility as a pharmacy technician to assist the pharmacist in identifying patients who may be having problems with drug dependency.

CHAPTER REVIEW QUESTIONS

1. Define the differences between drug addiction and dependency.

2. In your own opinion, why do some people become addicted or dependent physically? Why mentally?

Resources and References

1. Glossary of Terms. Accessed October 25, 2003.
   http://www.medsch.wisc.edu/painpolicy/glossary.htm

2. Carmichael, Blaine P. *Drug Abuse: Addiction vs. Dependency*. MPAS, A-C.

3. "Advocacy and Policy." Definitions Related to the Use of Opioids for the Treatment of Pain. A Consensus Document from the American Academy of Pain Medicine, the American Pain Society, and the American Society of Addiction Medicine. Accessed October 25, 2003.
   http://ampainsoc.org/cgi-bin/print/print.pl

CHAPTER 9

The Skin

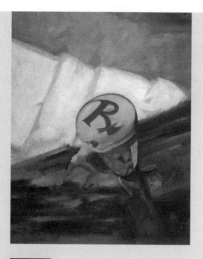

INTRODUCTION

There are many sense organs of the body. Immediately, the following senses come to mind: sight, hearing, smell, taste, and touch. All sensory receptors are microscopic-sized sense organs, which are the beginning of *dendrites* or sensory neurons (nerve cells). This chapter will explore the sense of touch, which utilizes the largest organ of the body—the skin. Chapter 10 will cover the senses of sight and hearing.

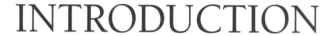

Learning Objectives

After completing this chapter, you should be able to:

- List, identify, and diagram the basic anatomical structure of the skin.

- Explain the function or physiology of the skin.

- List and define common diseases affecting the skin and comprehend the causes, symptoms, and pharmaceutical treatments associated with each disease.

- Explain the mechanisms of the following skin diseases and comprehend how each class of drugs works to mitigate the symptoms: chronic plaque psoriasis, eczema, impetigo, athlete's foot, acne, and lice.

- Describe and understand the significance of the development of the newest FDA approved drugs for the treatment of psoriasis.

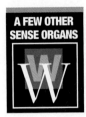
1. The olfactory nerve conducts impulses from the nose to the brain to create the sense of smell. Memory and smell play a big part in appetite. Smell plays a big part in the memory of events and people, as the olfactory nerve forms a direct link with the amygdala (emotion) and the hippocampus (memory). Odors can trigger memory, and memory can be evoked by odors. One can recall a person by the mere smell of a cologne, or an event by the smell of a fireplace. "It has been shown that patients of Korsakoff's syndrome, who suffer severe memory impairment, show less of an impairment for odor memory than for other kinds of memory. This suggests that there is in fact a mechanism for odor memory separate from other kinds of memory."[2]

2. The chemoreceptors for the gustatory sense organs are called the taste buds and are stimulated by chemicals. These taste sensations are sweet, sour, bitter, and salty. Any combination of tastes and odors makes tastes other than the four mentioned.

Anatomy

The skin is considered the largest organ of the body and performs several functions. The skin has three main layers: the epidermis, the dermis, and the subcutaneous layers. The epidermis is the outermost layer of the skin and contains *melanocytes*, where our pigment is stored. It is the thinnest part and known as the scarfskin or cuticle layer.

The dermis contains mostly fibroblasts that are responsible for secreting collagen, elastin, and ground substance. These substances provide the support and elasticity of the skin. In addition, immune cells involved in the defense against foreign invaders that may pass through the epidermis are found in the dermal layer. The dermal layer houses hair follicles, blood vessels, and sweat and oil glands. This is where the sensory receptors for touch, pain, heat, and cold are located.

The dermis is attached to an underlying subcutaneous layer, called the hypodermis, where the outmost part of the muscle is. The subcutaneous layer stores *adipose*, or fat tissue, and contains the connective tissue.

The dermis helps to keep the body at a normal temperature of 98.6 degrees Fahrenheit. The skin, or epidermis, provides protection from the heat, ultra violet radiation, and infection. Exposure of sunlight to the skin helps to produce Vitamin D, which is needed to help make cholesterol and to absorb calcium and phosphorus to make strong bones. The largest sensory organ provides the body with the ability to feel heat, cold, pain, and pleasure. (See Figure 9-1.)

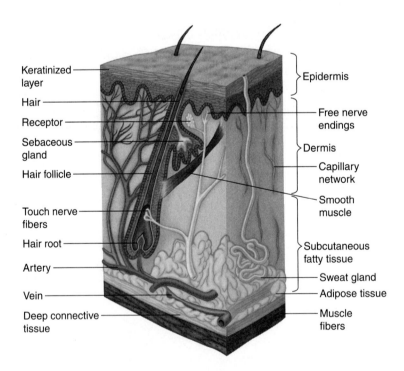

Figure 9-1 Structure of the skin (*Mulvihill, Mary Lou; Zelman, Mark; Holdaway, Paul; Tompary, Elaine; Turchany, Jill,* Human Diseases, A Systemic Approach, *5th Edition, © 2001. Reprinted by permission of Pearson Education, Inc., Upper Saddle River, NJ*)

Diseases and Conditions of the Skin

Over 1000 common skin problems fall into one of the following nine categories:

A *rash* is an area of red, inflamed skin, or a group of red spots, caused by irritation, allergy, infection, or defects to the skin's structure, such as blocked pores or malfunctioning oil glands. Examples of rashes are acne, contact dermatitis, eczema, hives, rosea, and psoriasis.

Eczema is an inflammation with pimple-like bumps characterized by itching, red, blistering, or oozing areas of the skin, progressing to scaly, brownish, or thickened skin. Some of the drugs that have recently been developed in new drug classifications for eczema are also used as new treatments for chronic plaque psoriasis. The following new immunomodulator creams and ointments were approved in 2003 and 2004: Elidel® (pimecrolimus)[3] cream is used for only mild to moderate atopic eczema. Protopic™ (tacrolimus)[4] tends to be used for severe atopic eczema. These creams and ointments are not steroids, but are used to treat the itch and inflammation associated with atopic eczema and psoriasis. Immunomodulators are agents that affect the body's immune system in some way.

Psoriasis is a chronic immune disorder in which specific immune cells become overactive and release excessive amounts of proteins called *cytokines*. One of the cytokines is called Tumor Necrosis Factor (TNF), which normally helps regulate the body's immune response to infection and inflammation. However, in patients with psoriasis, TNF causes inflammation instead of preventing it. This leads to the formation of painful, often disfiguring psoriasis plaques. Psoriasis is a noncontagious, chronic skin disease where the turnover of skin cells is rapid and the affected skin is thick, red, and scaly. Until recently, psoriasis had been treated in a manner that would only manage pain and inflammation. Some of the greatest discoveries known as "breakthrough drugs" in treating skin disorders and diseases have been drugs for chronic plaque psoriasis and psoriatic arthritis. Some of these drugs have recently been approved for use with rheumatoid arthritis. This chapter will review all of the newest types of drugs discovered in the last three years that have changed the way psoriasis is treated and managed. Discussion of these drugs in a textbook is also a first.

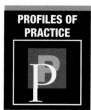

PROFILES OF PRACTICE

Psoriasis reportedly affects up to two percent of the U.S. population.

The FDA approved a new subcutaneous injectable drug for psoriasis on April 30, 2004. ENBREL® (etanercept),[5] an anti-TNF therapy agent, works by binding to the overproduced TNF. This attachment causes the TNF to be biologically inactive. This results in a significant reduction in inflammation. This SC injection can be self-administered. The previously available drugs are described as follows:

- Remicade® (infliximab)[6] is administered by intravenous infusion under the supervision of a specialist and in combination with MTX, a potent antineoplastic agent used for rheumatoid arthritis. MTX is given with infliximab to help prevent the formation of anti-infliximab antibodies.

- Amevive® (alefacept),[7] which is given by IM or infusion by a doctor, has the severe adverse reaction of lowering T-cell count. This lessens the ability of the immune system to fight cancer, infections, and other diseases. Amevive® works by binding to the specific lymphocyte antigen, CD2, and then inhibiting LFA-3/CD2 interaction, reducing lymphocyte counts (T-cells), and therefore treating the cause of psoriasis.

Raptiva® (efalizumab),[8] a newly approved drug (October 27, 2003) for plaque psoriasis, is an antibody that prevents activated T-cells from entering the skin. This drug is administered by subcutaneous injection once a week. Common side effects include H/A, chills, fever, nausea, muscle aches, and *thrombocytopenia*. The technical description of Raptiva®(efalizumab) is an "immunosuppressive recombinant humanized IgG1 kappa isotype monoclonal antibody."[8] This drug binds to CD11a receptor, part of the *antigen* that is expressed on all leukocytes. This attachment decreases cell surface expression of CD11a (number of receptors is decreased). This attachment allows Raptiva® to inhibit the binding of LFA-1 to the intercellular adhesion molecule-1 (ICAM-1). This action inhibits or blocks the adhesion of leukocytes to other cell types. The final result is that Raptiva® decreases the activation of T-lymphocytes and, therefore, the inflammation of psoriatic skin.

New research or "pipeline" information about ORAL Elidel® (pimecrolimus) made by Novartis, which selectively inhibits inflammatory cytokine release, has shown limited evidence suggesting the potential efficacy of 20 or 30 milligrams (mg) *orally* twice daily in chronic plaque psoriasis.[9] Another drug in the pipeline for psoriasis, Humirara® (adalimumab) by Abbott Labs, is in clinical trials administering 40 mg weekly or 40 mg every other week.[10] This drug was the first fully human monoclonal antibody DMARD, FDA approved on December 31, 2002, for rheumatoid arthritis. Older immunosupressant drugs, such as cyclosporine, attacked uninvolved organs and tissues. Newer drugs are target-specific, causing less damage.

Viral Infections—A virus penetrates the stratum corneum and infects the inner layers of the skin. Examples include herpes simplex, warts, and shingles (herpes zoster). Temporary viral infections, such as chicken pox and measles, also affect the skin. Antibiotics or antibacterial agents cannot cure viral infections. Antiviral medications and time are the only two treatments. A new drug for treating sexually transmitted external genital and anal warts is now available, an immunomodulator known as Aldara® (imiquimod) 5% cream.[11] The warts are caused by the human papilloma virus (HPV) and are not curable, but the drug can decrease the size and, therefore, the severity of pain. HPV is the most common sexually transmitted disease (STD).[12]

Bacterial skin infections are caused by many different bacteria, but the most common types are staphylococci, streptococci, and pseudomonas. Bacteria usually infect the topmost layers of skin, the follicles, or the deeper layers of skin. If left untreated, these infections may spread throughout the body, becoming more serious and possibly causing systemic infections. Examples include Lyme disease, impel folliculitis, and cellulitis. Cellulitis, impetigo, and folliculitis are the most common bacterial skin infections.[13] Antibiotics can be topically or orally administered, depending upon the microorganism and specific AB. Antibacterial agents are either bactericidal (kill the microorganism) or bacterostatic (stop the MO from reproducing and growing, allowing the immune system to take over). Chapter 15, on the immune system, will go into much more detail as to how antibiotics work. The main mechanism of action is to stop the production or function of the cell wall protein synthesis, which prevents the cell wall from growing. The inside of the cell continues to grow, bursting through the cell wall, leaking out the cytoplasm and nucleus. Thus, the microorganism cell collapses upon itself and dies.

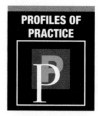

Acne is a special bacterial infection caused by Propioni bacterium and an overproduction of sebum, which causes an increase in hair follicles during puberty. Increased white blood cells to attack the hair follicles, causing inflammation that leads to papules, pustules, and nodules.

Cellulitis is an acute, deep infection of the connective tissue of the skin accompanied by inflammation. The culprit is staphylococcus, streptococcus, or other bacteria. The skin tissues of the infected area have all the cardinal signs of inflammation, becoming red (erythema), hot (warmth), swollen (inflammation), irritated, and painful. Those most prone to cellulites include those with a break in the skin due to an insect bite or injury; a history of PAD (peripheral vascular disease), diabetes, or ischemic ulcers; recent cardiovascular, pulmonary, or dental procedures or surgeries; and use of immunosuppressive or corticosteroid medications. Enzymes produced by the bacteria destroy skin cells.

Fungal skin infections, also known as "mycoses," occur when harmless fungi, which are usually present (parasites or saprophytes), gain entry into the skin rather than staying on the outer layer of the skin (epidermis). These infections are usually external, affecting the skin, hair, and nails. Yeasts form a subtype of fungus, characterized by clusters of round or oval cells. Fungal infections occur in damp, dark, and warm atmospheres, while yeasts must also have sugar. Examples include athlete's foot, jock itch, and ringworm. Fungal infections such as athlete's foot typically have itchy red areas that may crack or blister. They are common and generally mild; however, people with suppressed immune systems or who have been taking antibiotics for a long time are more susceptible to fungi spreading deep within the body, causing a more serious systemic disease. Patients with diabetes in particular are most at risk.

Parasitic infections are caused by insects or worms that burrow into the skin to live and/or lay their eggs. Some infections caused by parasites are scabies and lice. Parasites may enter and infect an injured or open wound caused by a blow, cut, or burn, which broke the surface of the skin. Scabies is characterized by small red bumps and intense itching caused by mites that burrow in the skin from bedding and mattresses. Lice are highly contagious and spread from person to person by close body contact, shared clothes, hats, hairbrushes, and combs. Lice are insects that look much like a crab under the microscope. There are three types of human lice: head lice, body lice, and pubic lice. The eggs and the adult must be killed and then removed from the hair. While lindane-containing products can kill head and body lice, these may cause severe damage to the nervous system. Lindane's use in adults is controversial, and it is no longer used in children. A better choice for children would be RID® (pyrethrins) gel or shampoo.

Tumors and *Cancerous growths* occur when skin cells multiply (reproduce) faster than normal. Some tumors or skin growths are harmless and will not spread. They are called benign (not cancer) if the cells are growing rapidly, but without mutation. On the other hand, skin cancer is characterized by the rapid reproduction and mutation of cells. Skin cancer affects 800,000 Americans each year, and more than 90 percent of all cases are caused by continuous or early-life sun exposure.[1] Avoidance of ultraviolet rays (the sun) and early detection with regular checkups can either prevent skin cancers or prevent benign conditions from advancing to malignancies. There are three types of skin cancer:[14]

Basal Cell Carcinoma (cancer) is the most curable, most common skin cancer. It commonly presents on the face and scalp and is mainly caused by sun exposure, often commencing in childhood. BCC accounts for 25 percent of all new cancers. It is located in the bottom layer of the outer skin layer or epidermis.

Squamous cell cancer is the second most common skin cancer. It can grow and spread rapidly, often appearing on the back of the hands, on the ears, or on the edges of the lips. This accounts for about 20 percent of all skin cancers. It usually arises in the outer layer of the epidermis. When this cancer spreads or *metastasizes*, it can invade distant organs and tissue and become fatal.

Malignant melanoma is the most deadly form of skin cancer; often, the signal is a mole that changes shape or color and may begin to bleed. However, it can be cured if caught when still thin and still in the outermost layer of the skin. It is usually localized (in situ) and spreads across the skin before it spreads deep into the skin.

Actinic keratosis (AK), also called a solar keratosis, is a scaly or crusty bump that originates on the skin surface. It may be light or dark and tan, pink, or red and is usually rough. While it may develop slowly, about 5 percent become squamous cell carcinoma and therefore are a *precurser* to cancer or a pre-cancer. It may also spread to other organs and tissues on its own.

Pigmentation Disorders—The color of the skin is determined by the amount of melanin produced by the body and, to some extent, genetics. Melanocytes produce this substance. Melanocyte malfunction or absence, exposure to cold or to other chemicals, infections, or severe skin burns can contribute to a loss of skin pigmentation (color), called hypopigmentation. An example of hypopigmentation is vitiligo. Hyperpigmentations can be caused by several factors, including hormonal changes (especially in women using systemic birth control), aging, and metabolic disorders. Examples are freckles and age spots (sometimes called liver spots).

Miscellaneous Skin Conditions and Diseases that do not fall under any of the preceding categories include hyperkeratosis, wrinkling, rosacea, spider veins, and varicose veins.

Hyperkeratosis is a condition of having too much keratin, which is a protein of the skin, hair, and nails. It causes the skin to harden into what is known as a callous. For example, a callous forms when the heel or ankle of the foot rubs against a hard surface like a shoe. Warts are small bumps on the skin surface that are caused by a human papilloma virus (HPV) infection; they are also a type of hyperkeratosis.

Wrinkles are caused by the combination of a breakdown of the collagen and elastin within the dermis and fat cells in the skin becoming smaller, which results in sagging skin. Less production of sebum causes the moisture barrier to become thinner, and more moisture is released, which results in dryer skin.

Rosacea is a chronic disorder of unknown cause, in which the skin of the face becomes red (erythema) and develops pimples, lesions, and possibly an enlargement of the nose. Oily, acne-prone areas (hyperplasia of the sebaceous glands) with deep-seated papules and pustules cause small blood vessels to enlarge (telangiectasia), resulting in a flushed appearance. It may last a very long time.

Spider veins are broken blood vessels, such as capillaries, which then enlarge. They become visible through the surface of the skin, varying in color from blue, purple, orchid, to bright red. The cause may be overweight, tight stockings, exposure to sun, or natural or drug-induced hormonal changes in women.

Burns are susceptible to infection due to the open lesions. The severity and depth of the burn are categorized as first degree, second degree, and third degree burns. The major cause of death among burn patients is not the burn itself, but the complication of infections caused by prolonged treatment and skin grafts. Silver sulfadiazine acts on the cell membrane wall to inhibit microbial activity and some yeasts. In addition, it allows oxygen to pass through the recommended $\frac{1}{16}$ of an inch thickness, to promote healing. It is applied once every 12 hours, along with a new dressing change.

Drugs versus Cosmetics for the Skin

The FDA defines cosmetics as "articles intended to be rubbed, poured, sprinkled, or sprayed on, introduced into, or otherwise applied to the human body or any part thereof for cleansing, beautifying, promoting attractiveness, or altering the appearance (excludes soap)."

The FDA defines the word "drug" in part as "articles intended for use in the diagnosis, cure, *mitigation*, treatment, or prevention of disease in man or other animals" and "articles (other than food) intended to affect the structure or any function of the body of man or other animals... ."[15]

Pharmaceutical Treatment of Various Skin Diseases

This book will focus on drugs for the skin, and not cosmetics, which are meant to enhance and beautify the skin (Table 9-1).

TABLE 9-1   Drugs Used to Treat Various Skin Diseases

Specific Disease	Type of Organism or Cause	Drug Classification	Name (Trade®/generic) and Dosage
Acne	Bacteria: *Propionibacterium acnes* Overproduction of sebum Clogged pores Infected hair follicles	Topical antiseptic: Rx anti-acne therapy: Topical preparation (Unblocks and prevents blockage of pores)	benzoyl peroxide solution 2-3x's/day Retin–A® (retinoic acid, tretinoin) cream. Apply as directed
		Oral/systemic acne	Accutane® (isotretinoin) PO 0.5-1 mg/kg/day × 20 weeks
		Antibiotic	TCN 250-500 mg TID × 10 d
Urticaria (hives)	Allergy or viral infection or can be idiopathic	Antihistamines	Claritin® (loratidine) 10 mg QD
		Anti-inflammatory Steroids PO	Prednisone PO as directed
		Immunomodulatory Agent PO	Sulfasalazine PO as directed
		Leukotriene inhibitors-PO	Accolate® (zafirlukast) 20 mg BID Singulair® (montelukast) 5 mg QD
Psoriasis	Poor immune system infections: HIV, *H. Pylori*, Streptococcal	Antibiotics, oral	PCN or TCN PO 250–500 mg TID
		Topical steroids:	Hydrocortisone, betamethasone, fluticasone, methylprednisolone apply as directed
		Immunosupressant: Topical	Cyclosporin NTE 5 mg/kg/day in two daily doses
		Immunomodulators:	Protopic® (tacrolimus) 0.03 or 0.1% ointment Apply BID Elidel® (pimecrolimus) cream, Apply BID
		Oral immunomodulators:	Elidel® (pimecrolimus) PO in clinical trials
		Humanized therapeutic antibody (monoclonal antibody)	Raptiva® (efalizumab) self administered SC injection 1/wk. Conditioning dose is 0.7 mg/kg, then 1 mg/kg (maximum single dose not to exceed a total of 200 mg).
		Biological drugs: biologic response modifiers or TNF blockers	Enbrel® (etanercept) SC injection, 50 mg twice–weekly × 3 months, then 50 mg/week.
		Immunosuppressive dimeric fusion protein	Amevive® (alefacept) 15 mg IM, once a week, for a total of 12 doses; administered by a doctor.

TABLE 9-1   Drugs Used to Treat Various Skin Diseases (*continued*)

Specific Disease	Type of Organism or Cause	Drug Classification	Name (Trade®/generic) and Dosage
		Drugs in the pipeline: TNF-blocking agents	Humira® (adalimumab) 40 mg SC injection QW or EOW
		Oral immunomodulator	Oral Fumarate for severe psoriasis[16]
Arthritic psoriasis	Poor immune system	Topical immunomodulators:	Protopic® (tacrolimus) 0.03 or 0.1% ointment. Apply BID
		Biological drugs: biologic response modifiers or TNF blockers	Remicaide (infliximab), IV infusion of 3–5 mg /kg Day 1, 2 and 6 weeks later (Given with MTX).
Eczema		Topical immunomodulators:	Protopic® (tacrolimus) 0.03 or 0.1% ointment. Apply BID Elidel® (pimecrolimus) cream. Apply BID
Lyme disease (early stages)	*Borrelia burgdorferi* (spirochete)	Oral antibiotics:	amoxicillin 250 to 500 mg TID doxycycline 250 to 500 mg BID
Cellulitis	*Staphylococcus, streptococcus*	Oral antibiotics OR	Ancef® (cefazolin) or Dynapen® (dicloxicillin) 250–500 mg TID × 10 days
		Intravenous (IV) antibiotics	IV cefazolin, oxacillin, or nafcillin Dosage varies
Impetigo (common in children 2 to 5 yrs old)	*Staphylococcus aureus,* streptococcus	Antibiotics: Erythromycin	Zithromax® (azithromycin) 500 mg on Day 1, then 250 mg qd × 5 days
		Cephalosporin	Keflex® (cephalexin) 250–500-mg × 10 days
Rosacea	Acne vulgaris, along with other causes	Topical antibiotics	sodium sulfacetamide Apply as directed
		Oral antibiotics	Oral tetracycline or metronidazole (also top) 500 mg PO TID
		*New oral AB Tx:	Periostat (R)® (doxycycline hyclate), PO 20 mg tablets[17]
Herpes cold sore	Herpes simplex labialis	Antiviral topical	Abreva® (docosanol) cream NPT 5 apps/day
External genital and anal warts (STD)	Human papilloma virus	Topical immunomodulator	Aldara 5% (imiquimod) cream. Apply once a day, 3 days a week, leave on 6 hrs.
Ringworm fungi or tinea	*Trichophyton rubrum*	Antifungal topical	Fulvicin® P/G (griseofulvin) Lotrimin® (clotrimazole)
Cuts	Infection prevention	Topical antibacterials	Neosporin®, Cortisporin®, Triple Antibiotic® ointment (Neomycin + Polymixin b, Bacitracin)

TABLE 9-1 Drugs Used to Treat Various Skin Diseases (*continued*)

Specific Disease	Type of Organism or Cause	Drug Classification	Name (Trade®/generic) and Dosage
Burns	Infection prevention and oxygen promoter	Topical anti-infective	Silvadene® (silver sulfadiazine), Sulfamylon® (mafenide Acetate) Apply as directed
Athlete's foot	*Tinea pedis, trichophyton rubrum epidermophyton floccosum*	Antifungal topical Cream, gel, spray and liquid forms	Miconazole 2%, Tolnaftate 1%, Clotrimazole 1%, and Naftifine 1% Fungizone® (amphotericin B) Apply as directed
Parasites	Lice or scabies	Antiparasitic topical agents	Kwell® (lindane) shampoo or solution [not for use in children] RID® gel (pyrethrins) Apply as directed
Hyperkeratosis	Excessive production of keratin	Keratolytics: Lactates for hardened dry skin	Alpha Keri Lotion®, Cetaphil® Apply as directed
	Warts are viral.	Warts, corns, and acne	Salicylic or beta hydroxy acids. benzoyl peroxide, creams, sol, gels Apply as directed
Pain	N/A	Topical analgesic	Solarcaine® (benzocaine), Nupercainal, Lidocaine®, xylocaine
Infection prevention	Various bacteria	Topical antiseptic	Alcohol, merthiolate, Zephiran® (benzalkonium chloride) Apply as directed
Anti itch	Allergic reactions, contact dermatitits, inflammation, dryness	Antihistamine, topical	Benadryl® gel, lotion, cream (diphenhydramine)
		Corticosteroid topical creams, ointments, solutions	Corticaine® (hydrocortisone), Valisone®, Celestone® (betamethas one) Kenalog®, Aristocort® (triamcinonide), Lidex® (fluocinonide) Synalar® (Fluocinolone) Cordan® (flurandrenolide) Apply as directed
Skin cancer	Exposure to sun, chemicals, genetic predisposition	Topical chemotherapeutic agent	5FU (fluorouraci) cream. Apply as directed
		Immunomodulator	Aldara® (imiquimod 5%) cream. Apply once a day for 2 days a week, 3 to 4 days apart.
		NSAID: Precancer treatment of actinic keratosis	Solaraze® (diclofenac sodium) 3% gel. Apply BID

No Pharmaceutical Treatment

There is no better preventive action for beautiful, healthy skin than to just do the basics. Outside of factors such as injury, aging, or true medical conditions, most skin conditions can be prevented with a simple daily routine. Keep skin clean and free from dirt with daily, gentle washing. Not only will this remove dirt, but it will prevent many skin conditions, such as pimples, from surfacing as you also remove residuals like oil and grease. This is not to say that you will never get a pimple, but that you greatly reduce the risk of developing a rash, acne, or other skin condition. If you are sensitive to a substance or have an allergy that produces a dermatological reaction, limit your exposure to that substance, whether it be animals, certain lotions, or cosmetics.

SUMMARY

The skin is considered to be the largest organ of the body, and consists of three main layers: the epidermis, the dermis, and the subcutaneous layers. The skin performs several important functions: it serves as a barrier to foreign organisms and debris, it is responsible for the regulation of temperature of the body, it excretes salts and excess water from the body, and it acts as a "shock absorber" to protect the underlying organs.

Diseases of the skin can range from simple rashes to deadly cancers (malignant melanoma). The most common skin disease, acne, affects approximately 17 million Americans.

Fortunately, a large armamentarium of pharmaceuticals is available to treat diseases of the skin. A special section of this chapter is devoted to recently-approved medications to treat psoriasis. This disfiguring, often painful, disease affects up to two percent of the U.S. population.

CHAPTER REVIEW QUESTIONS

1. Match the skin layer with the correct description:
   1. _____ scarfskin, has pigment
   2. _____ true skin, has nerves and blood vessels, sensory receptors for pain, heat, and cold
   3. _____ innermost layer, contains fat and connective tissue
   a. dermal layer
   b. subcutaneous layer
   c. epidermal layer

2. List the four main functions of the skin and explain what each does for the body.

   Answer:
   a. _____
   _____
   b. _____
   _____
   c. _____
   _____
   d. _____
   _____

3. Complete the following chart, matching each of the skin diseases with their respective symptoms and pharmaceutical treatments:

Symptoms:
   a. pimple-like bumps characterized by itching, red, blistering, or oozing areas of the skin
   b. red pimples and lesions on the face and neck with a possibility of enlargement of the nose
   c. itchy red areas that may crack or blister
   d. itchy, thick, red, and scaly patches
   e. highly contagious crab-like insects that burrow in the skin, feed on blood, and cause itching
   f. painful, red, deep skin infection, poorly marked perimeter or borders; may become serious if not treated immediately
   g. clogged sebaceous glands with possible folliculitis, causing red pimples, pustules, and nodules

Drugs Used to Treat:
   a. Antibiotics: Ancef®
   b. TNF blockers: Enbrel®, Corticosteroids: Hydrocortisone
   immunosuppressive dimeric fusion protein: Amevive® (alefacept) 15 mg IM, once a week, for a total of 12 doses; administered by a doctor
   c. Antifungal: Clotrimazole 1% cream or spray
   d. Keratolytic: salicylic acid
   e. Topical immunomodulators: Protopic® (tacrolimus) ung, Elidel® (pimecrolimus) cr
   f. Topical antibiotics: sodium sulfacetamide and oral antibiotics : TCN 500 mg PO TID
   g. RID® gel (pyrethrins)

Skin Disease	Symptoms	Drug Used to Treat
Chronic plaque psoriasis		
Eczema		
Cellulitis		
Athlete's foot		
Acne		
Lice		
Rosacea		

4. Match the drug with the correct mechanism of action:

1. _____ selectively inhibits inflammatory cytokine release

2. _____ binds to CD11a receptor, decreases the activation of T-lymphocytes and inflammation

3. _____ prevents the cell wall synthesis of protein, causing the cell to die

4. _____ soften and eliminate the hardened proteinized outer layer (epidermis)

a. topical immunomodulators
b. immunosuppressive monoclonal antibody
c. antibacterial/antibiotic
d. keratolytic

5. Describe the historical treatments, and explain the significance of the development of the newest FDA-approved drugs for chronic plaque psoriasis.

Resources and References

1. Kamel, Maged, N. M.D. Anatomy of the Skin
   http://www.telemedicine.org/anatomy.htm#functions

2. Healthepic Anatomy of Skin
   http://www.healthepic.com/hers/static/hers_beauty_skindeep_anotomy.htm

3. About Skin Anatomy and Physiology
   http://www.essentialdayspa.com/Skin_Anathomy_and_Physiology.htm

4. Holland, Norman and Michael Patrick Adams. *Core Concepts in Pharmacology*. Upper Saddle River, NJ: Prentice Hall, 2003.

Footnotes

1. About Skin Anatomy and Physiology
   http://www.essentialdayspa.com/Skin_Anatomy_and_Physiology.htm

2. Olfaction and Memory
   http://www.macalester.edu/~psych/whathap/UBNRP/Smell/memory.html

3. About Elidel® 1% (pimecrolimus) cream for eczema by National Eczema Society
   http://www.eczema.org/PIMECROLIMUSCREAM.pdf

4. About Tacrolimus for Eczema and Psoriasis: AAD: Tacrolimus Ointment Safe and Effective in All Ages for Mild to Moderate Eczema, by Bruce Sylvester
   http://www.docguide.com/news/content.nsf/news/8525697700573E18 85256E37006578F2?OpenDocument&id=48dde4a73e09a969852568 880078c249&c=Dermatitis&count=10

5. National Library of Medicine: Topical Tacrolimus: An Effective Therapy for Facial Psoriasis, by Yamamoto T, Nishioka K.
   http://www.ncbi.nlm.nih.gov/entrez/query.fcgi?cmd=Retrieve&db=Pub Med&list_uids=14693492&dopt=Abstract

6. About Enbrel® (etanercept) FDA approval of Enbrel (etanercept) for psoriasis on April 30, 2004
   http://www.amgen.com/news/viewPR.jsp?id=521767
   http://www.enbrel.com/news/pdf/Enbrel_Psoriasis_Approval.pdf
   http://my.webmd.com/content/article/86/99063.htm

7. About Remicade® (infliximab)
   http://www.dermnetnz.org/dna.psoriasis/infliximab.html

8. About Amevive® (alefacept) Doctor's Guide: Amevive (Alefacept), Treatment for Psoriasis, Approved in Israel, Receives "Positive Opinion" From Swiss Regulatory Authority, May 3, 2004
   http://www.pslgroup.com/dg/243fd2.htm
   http://www.rxlist.com/cgi/generic3/amevive.htm
   http://www.centerwatch.com/patient/drugs/dru820.html

9. About Raptiva® (efalizumab)
   http://www.thedrugdatabase.com/directory/R/Raptiva
   http://www.raptiva.com/about/faqs.jsp#Q7
   http://www.drugs.com/raptiva.html
   About Raptiva: Genetech Patient and Professional Information Website

10. About ORAL Elidel® AAD: Oral Pimecrolimus Effective in Treating Psoriasis, by Paula Moyer
    http://www.pslgroup.com/dg/22ebd2.htm

11. About Humirara (adalimumab) for psoriasis: Abbott Laboratories Announces Positive Results of Phase II HUMIRA(R) (adalimumab) Study in Psoriasis, February 9, 2004
    http://salesandmarketingnetwork.com/news_release.php?ID=14067& key=American%20Academy%20of%20Dermatology

12. About Aldara® (imiquimod)—Package Insert for both External Genital Warts and Actinic Keratoses:
http://www.3m.com/us/healthcare/pharma/aldara/AKPI.pdf

13. About Commonly Sexually Transmitted Diseases: HPV
http://www.princeton.edu/puhs/SECH/hpv.html

14. American Family Physician–Common Bacterial Skin Infections
http://www.aafp.org/afp/20020701/119.html

15. About Skin Cancer: The Skin Cancer Foundation
http://www.skincancer.org

16. FDA and Cosmetic ACT
http://www.fda.gov/opacom/laws/fdcact/fdcact1.htm

17. About Pipeline Oral Immunomodulator, Fumarate, for Psoriasis: Patients Show Improvement in Phase II Psoriasis Study of Novel Oral, April 29, 2004
http://salesandmarketingnetwork.com/news_release.php?ID=15454

18. Treatment of Rosacea CollaGenex Pharmaceuticals Initiates Multicenter Phase 3 Clinical Study to Evaluate Periostat as a Treatment for Rosacea
http://www.corporate-ir.net/ireye/ir_site.zhtml?ticker=CGPI&script=410&layout=-6&item_id=324979

19. Holland, Norman and Michael Patrick Adams. *Core Concepts in Pharmacology*. Upper Saddle River, NJ: Pearson Education, 2003.

20. Adams, Michael Patrick, Dianne L. Josephson, and Leland Norman Holland, Jr. *Pharmacology for Nurses—A Pathophysiologic Approach*. Upper Saddle River, NJ: Pearson Education, 2005.

Internet Sites to Visit

1. A look at photos of bacterial skin infections
http://matrix.ucdavis.edu/tumors/bacterial/bacterial.html

2. National Psoriasis Foundation: Research Pipeline
http://www.psoriasis.org/research/pipeline/chart.php

3. About Skin Cancer: The Skin Cancer Foundation
http://www.skincancer.org

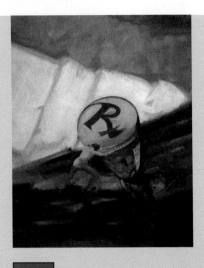

CHAPTER

10

Eyes and Ears

Learning Objectives

After completing this chapter,
you should be able to:

- List, identify, and diagram the basic anatomical structure and parts of the eye and ear.

- Describe the function or physiology of the ears and eyes (and the fluids within).

- List and define common diseases affecting the eyes and ears.

- Demonstrate a comprehension of the causes, symptoms, and pharmaceutical treatment associated with each disease.

- Understand the mechanisms of the following diseases and explain how each class of drugs works: glaucoma, cataracts, retinopathy, hearing loss, and otitis media.

- Describe and understand the indication for use and mechanism of action of anti-glaucoma agents.

- Define and utilize key terms.

INTRODUCTION

Previously, we discussed the largest sensory organ, the skin. In this chapter, we will explore the sense of sight, the sense of hearing, and the respective sensory organs, the eye and the ear.

Vision is the most basic and primary of all of our senses. We tend to value the sense of sight more than any other sense. Loss of sight usually means that a person will rely more acutely on the sense of hearing. Many parts of the eye contribute to the perception of a good image, but it is the retina, a piece of brain tissue, that is most vital for vision by getting direct stimulation from the world outside of ourselves in the form of lights and images.

Anatomy and Physiology of the Eye

Three pairs of extraocular muscles regulate the motion of each eye: the medial/lateral rectus muscles, the superior/inferior rectus muscles, and the superior/inferior oblique muscles. (See Figure 10-1.) The cranial nerve III innervates four of the six extraocular muscles: medial rectus, superior rectus, inferior rectus, and inferior oblique. The eye orbit is engulfed by layers of soft, fatty tissue, which protect and cushion the eye and enable it to turn easily. The most important structures of the eye are the cornea, conjunctiva, iris, lens, vitreous humor, retina, macula optic nerve, and the muscles. The vitreous humor, composed mostly of water, occupies about 80 percent of the eye's interior.

There are two types of photoreceptors, rods and cones. Cones are the most sensitive to bright light and color. The cornea is the primary and most powerful focusing structure of the eye, while the retina is comparable to the film of a camera because it senses light focused on it. The point of sharpest, most acute visual acuity within the eye is the macula.

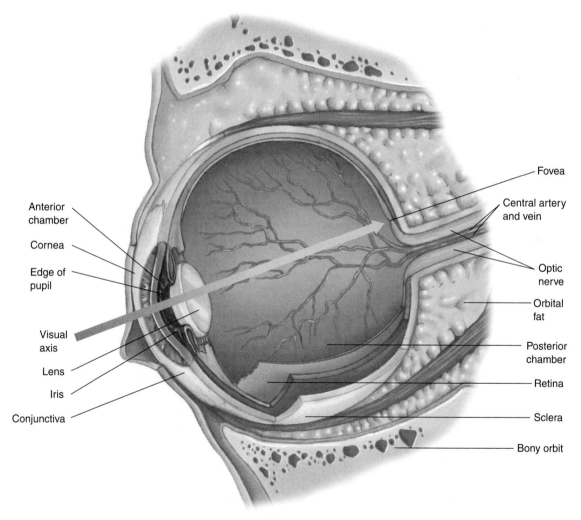

Figure 10-1 The eye (*Holland, Norman; Adams, Michael Patrick,* Core Concepts in Pharmacology, *1st Edition, © 2003. Reprinted by permission of Pearson Education, Inc., Upper Saddle River, NJ*)

Aqueous chamber filled with aqueous humor is the area bounded in front by the cornea and in back by the lens. Aqueous or aqueous humor is a clear, watery solution in the anterior and posterior chambers.

- Posterior chamber filled with aqueous humor is the area behind the iris, but in front of the lens.
- Vitreous humor is the transparent, colorless mass of soft, gelatinous material that fills the eyeball, behind the lens.
- Retina—often referred to as the "film" of the camera, located at the back of the eye and lining the innermost part of the eye, the retina is composed of light-sensitive nerve endings that take visual impulses to the optic nerve.
  - The optic nerve conducts visual impulses to the brain from the retina.
  - The macula is a small area in the retina that provides the most central, acute vision.
- Choroid, which carries blood vessels, is the inner coat between the sclera and the retina. The artery is the vessel supplying blood to the eye, and the vein is the vessel that carries blood away from the eye.

How the Eye Works

Understanding specific eye diseases begins with knowledge of how the eye works. The function of the eyes is to aid in sight. During the process of vision, light waves from an object, such as a building, enter the eye first through the clear cornea and then through the pupil, the circular aperture in the iris. The light waves are converged, or come together, first by the cornea, and then further by the crystalline lens, to a nodal point called "N," which is located immediately at the backside surface of the lens. This is the point where the image becomes inverted, or turned upside-down. In a young pair of eyes, the lens of the eye can modify its shape to change focus from distance to near.

The light progresses through the gelatinous vitreous humor and then, in perfect conditions, back to a clear focus on the retina, of which the most acute and central part is called the macula. If the eye is compared to a camera, the retina is then considered the film inside the camera, registering the tiny photons of light that interact with it. Inside of the retina, millions of tiny receptor cells, called photoreceptors, absorb the light energy.

This light energy, or light impulses, are sent along the optic nerve and turn it into electrical signals. These electrical impulses, or nerve impulses, are sent to the occipital lobe of the brain (posterior lobe). This part of the brain interprets these electrical signals as visual images. It is, therefore, our brain that "sees," as the eyes only aid in the visual process. (See Figure 10-2.)

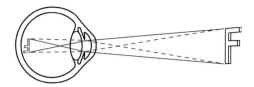

Figure 10-2 The eye as a camera

Diseases of the Eyes

While the eyes are prone to many diseases, only infection and vision problems will be addressed in this chapter. Common side effects of all of the ophthalmic products are minimal, with localized ocular toxicity and hypersensitivity, including eyelid itching and swelling, and conjunctival erythema as the most common. Eye products need to be sterile, pH balanced, clear, and particle free. Eye products can be used for dry eyes, infection, inflammation, and allergies. In this chapter, infections and vision disorders will be discussed, while treating allergic reactions involving the eyes with anti-allergenic agents, antihistamines, artificial tears, and anti-inflammatory products will be addressed in Chapter 13, The Respiratory System—Allergies.

Infections of the Eye and the Pharmaceutical Treatment

STYE

A stye, an infection of sebaceous gland also called a *hordeolum*, is a localized infection or inflammation of the eyelid margin involving hair follicles of the eyelashes. Visual acuity is unchanged. It is accompanied by redness, swelling, and pain in the eyelid, sometimes at the base of an eyelash. This type is an external hordeolum. If it is deep within the lid, it is called a meibomianitis or internal hordeolum, and is sometimes accompanied by conjunctivitis and a purulent drainage. Anti-infective eye drops are instilled into the lower conjunctival sac, and warm tap water or cold compresses can be applied for 10 minutes per hour, or 20 minutes four times a day, to control inflammation.

Treatment is with antibiotics; *Staphylococcus aureus* and *staphylococcus epidermidis* are the most likely culprits. Topical antibiotics are usually ineffective. Styes typically go away on their own, and therefore oral antibiotic therapy is usually not warranted. But in rare cases, oral antibiotic therapy could include a 10-day therapy of one of the following:

- dicloxacillin 250 mg PO Q6H
- erythromycin 250 mg PO QID
- tetracycline 250 mg PO QID
- amoxacillin 500 mg PO TID

BLEPHARITIS

This is inflammation of the eyelid margins, accompanied by redness, thickening, and possibly the formation of scales and crusts or shallow marginal ulcers. Ulcerative blepharitis is an acute bacterial, while seborrheic blepharitis and meibomian gland dysfunction (meibomitis) are chronic types of blepharitis. The latter is often associated with acne *rosacea*.

To treat ulcerative blepharitis, use one of the following antibiotic ointments for seven to ten days:

- bacitracin/polymyxin B
- gentamicin 0.3% qid

To treat seborrheic blepharitis, improve hygiene; use diluted baby shampoo to clean eyelid and remove greasy buildup.

To treat for meibomian gland dysfunction, use oral antibiotic: doxycycline 100 mg PO BID, over 3 to 4 months tapered down.

CONJUNCTIVITIS

Acute or chronic inflammation of the conjunctiva can be caused by viruses, bacteria, or allergy or may result from an irritation such as wind, smoke, or snow blindness. Conjunctivitis may also accompany the common cold and exanthems, such as the rubella measles, chicken pox, and mumps. Conjunctivitis, or pinkeye, is an inflammation of the thin lining (the conjunctiva) that covers the white of the eyeball and the inner surface of the eyelids. Pinkeye and redeye are terms that are used to refer to conjunctivitis. However, as a rule, pinkeye is a contagious infection, while redeye is a noncontagious inflammation due to an irritation.

Allergic conjunctivitis—allergy is fully discussed in Chapter 13, Respiratory System. "Redeye" is caused by hay fever, dust, mite dander, or animal dander. Specific treatment for allergy affecting the conjunctiva are presented as follows:

- Topical OTC combinations of antihistamine/vasoconstrictors such as naphazoline HCl/pheniramine maleate can be used for mild cases. Vasoconstrictors also known as decongestants may cause a rebound effect. (More details on rebound effect will be discussed later in this chapter.)
- Topical prescription antihistamines such as levocabastine, NSAIDs such as ketorolac, or topical mast cell inhibitors such as lodoxamide can be used separately or in combination if OTC preparations are not effective.
- Topical corticosteroids such as fluorometholone 0.1% or prednisolone acetate 0.12–1.0% drops tid can be useful in stubborn cases.

Bacterial conjunctivitis—The infection often starts in one eye, then soon spreads to the other. There is usually a thick, sticky *mucopurulent* discharge causing the eyelids and eyelashes to be matted or pasted shut upon awakening. There may be mild sensitivity to light (photophobia) with some discomfort, but usually no pain. Visual function is normal in most cases. The eye creates its own bacteriostatic lysozymes and immunoglobulins in the tear film, contributing to its strong immune system. The eye will fight to return to homeostasis, and bacteria will eventually be destroyed. However, an extra heavy load of external organisms can overpower the immune system, causing a conjunctival infection and setting the eye up for potential corneal infection. Therefore, antibiotics should be given to avoid such a possibility. Treatment with broad spectrum ophthalmics, treating both gram-positive and gram-negative organisms, and a anti-inflammatory will treat both the infection and inflammation (see table 10-1):

- Polytrim® (polymixin B sulfate and trimethoprim sulfate), gentamicin 0.3% tobramycin 0.3%.
- Resistant strains of pseudomonas call for fluoroquinolones such as Ciloxan, Ocuflox, and Chibroxin.

Viral conjunctivitis—The common cause adenovirus type 3 may also be caused by herpes simplex virus. "Pinkeye" has a short duration and is usually self-limiting, about one week in mild cases and up to three weeks in severe cases. It usually follows an upper respiratory infection or results from contact with someone who is infected. No treatment is available or needed for a viral eye infection. If it is suspected that a bacterial infection is also present, treat with topical antibiotics, such as sulfacetamide sodium 10% drops or trimethoprim/polymyxin B qid for seven to ten days. A matted-down, shut eyelid with a crust is indicative of viral conjunctivitis, while a wet, sticky, matted shut eyelid leads to a diagnosis of bacterial infection.

- Treatment for severe viral infection caused by HSV includes idozuridine solution or ointment, vidarabine ointment, or trifluridine solution.
- Treatment for VZV eye disease includes oral acyclovir, 600-800 mg, 5 times daily for 7–10 days, to terminate viral replication.

Conjunctivitis caused by Chlamydia and also known as neonatal inclusion conjunctivitis, is frequently acquired from birth canal infection due to *Chlamydia trachomatis* (serotypes *D* through *K*) or from swimming pools. Neonates are treated with systemic erythromycin 12.5 mg/kg PO or IV qid for 14 days, because pneumonia and other complications may result. Infected mothers and sexual partners are also treated to cure the conjunctivitis and concomitant genital infection with one of the following:

- azithromycin 1 g PO once
- doxycycline 100 mg PO bid for 1 week
- erythromycin 500 mg PO qid for 1 week, which will cure the conjunctivitis and concomitant genital infection.

TABLE 10-1 Various Topical Ophthalmics Used for Occular Infections

Trade	Generic	Indication and Classification	Sig
Antibacterials (AB's)			
Aminoglycosides - (AB's)			
Tobrex®	Tobramycin, 0.3% solution or ointment	Antibacterial, Aminoglycoside Tx Bacterial conjunctivitis, corneal infections	1 to 2 gtts q 4 hrs, severe infections: 2 gtts q1 hr until improvement, then the above regimen. Apply $\frac{1}{2}$ ribbon Ung q 3–4 hrs
Genoptic®, Garamycin Ophtalmic®	gentamycin Ophthalmic solution, 0.3%	Antibacterial, Aminoglycoside Tx Bacterial conjunctivitis, corneal ulcers, blepharitis	1 to 2 gtts q 4 hrs. Severe infections: 2 gtts q hr
Erythromycin (AB's)			
Ilotycin®	Erythromycin Ophthalmic Ointment, 0.5%	Tx neonatal inclusion or chlamydial, *Neisseria gonorrhea* or swimming pool conjunctivitis	Apply approx. 1 cm ribbon ung NTE 6 times/day
Sulfur Based Antibacterials			
Bleth—10®	Sulfacetamide sodium ophthalmic solution USP, 10%	Bacterial infections that may or may not accompany viral infection (secondary infections)	1 to 2 gtts q 2–3 hrs, tapered down for 7–10 days
Combination Antibiotics			
Maxitrol®	polymixin b sulfate, neomycin and bacitracin zinc ointment	Tx Blepharitis, Non-gonococcal bacterial and adult gonococcal conjunctivitis	Apply 1 cm ribbon ung, q 2 hrs - QID In addition: Tx single dose of ceftriaxone 1 g IM or ciprofloxacin 500 mg bid PO for 5 days
Polytrim®	polymixin B sulfate and trimethoprim sulfate, and gentamicin 0.3%	Bacterial infections blepharitis, non-gonococcal bacterial and adult gonococcal conjunctivitis	Apply 1 cm ribbon ung, q 2 hrs - QID
Fluoroquinalones (AB's)			
Ciloxan®		Tx bacterial infections caused by stubborn resistant pseudomonas	1–2 gtt - QID to Q1H for the first few days
Ocuflox®	Ofloxacin 0.3% solution	Same as above	1–2 gtts Q2-4 hrs $\times$ 2 day then, 1–2 q 4 hr $\times$ 7 day
Chibroxin®	Norfloxacin 0.3%	Same as above	1–2 gtts q 4 hr NTE 7 days

TABLE 10-1 Various Topical Ophthalmics Used for Occular Infections (*continued*)

Trade	Generic	Indication and Classification	Sig
Combination Drugs			
Tobradex®	Tobramycin and dexamethasone	Antibacterial and steroid combinations for infection and inflammation Tx bacterial Conjunctivitis, corneal ulcers	Apply approx. $\frac{1}{2}$ inch ribbon ung, NTE 4 times/day 1 to 2 gtts q 4–6 hrs
Antivirals			
Viroptic® {a pyrimidine (thymidine) analogue activated by cellular thymidine kinase}	trifluridine solution 1%	Tx epithelial keratitis caused by herpes simplex virus and keratoconjunctivitis, MOA—works by inhibition of DNA polymerase. DOC in U.S. for topical ophthalmic antiviral therapy as it is least vulnerable to resistant strains	To Cornea: 1gtt q 2 hrs NTE 9 gtts/day, then 1 gtt q 4 hr and tapered thereafter
Vira-A®	vidarabine ointment 3%,	Tx Acute keratoconjunctivitis epithelial keratitis caused by herpes simplex virus 1 & 2. MOA—interferes with early steps of viral DNA synthesis. Rapidly metabolizes to Ara - Hx	$\frac{1}{2}$ inch ribbon q 3hr, NTE 5 doses/day
Herplex® {halogenated pyrimidine derivatives}	idoxuridine solution 0.1% and ointment	Tx Acute keratoconjunctivitis epithelial keratitis caused by herpes simplex virus 1 & 2. MOA—slows growth of viruses by blocking reproduction of herpes simplex virus by producing incorrect DNA copies, preventing the virus from infecting or destroying tissue. IDU replaces thymidine (one of 4 building blocks of DNA) in an enzymatic step of viral replication	Oint. = $\frac{1}{3}$ inch ribbon q 4 hrs Sol. = 1 gtt q 1 hr during a.m. q 2 hr during p.m.
Antihistamines			
Emadine®	emedastine difumarate	Allergic conjunctivitis Rx antihistamine,	1 gtt in the affected eye, NTE 4 times daily

Trade	Generic	Indication and Classification	Sig
	ophthalmic solution) 0.05%	MOA—prevents H-1 binding on the eye cell, preventing itching, watering, and redness	
Livostin™ 0.05%®	levocabastine suspension, 0.05%	Allergic conjunctivitis Rx antihistamine for seasonal allergic conjunctivitis. MOA—same as above	1 gtt QID
Patanol®	olopatadine, 0.1%	Allergic conjunctivitis Rx antihistamine. MOA—same as above	1 drop, bid or q 6-8 hrs
Mast Cell Stabilizers Alomide ®	lodoxamide solution, 0.1%	Allergic conjunctivitis mast cell inhibitors for prevention of allergic reactions and for vernal keratoconjunctivitis, vernal conjunctivitis	1–2 gtts QID, NTE 3 months
Crolom®	Cromolyn Sodium, 4%	Allergic conjunctivitis same as above	1–2 drops, qid
Alamast®	Pemirolast potassium, 0.01%	Allergic conjunctivitis same as above	1–2 drops, qid
Anti-inflammatory Agents Acular®	ketorolac	Any conjunctivitis NSAID, Anti-inflammatory MOA—See Chapter 9 FIG08019 Musculoskeletal System—inflammation process and site of action of ASA, NSAID's, and Cox-2 Inhibitors	1 drop, qid
Eflone®, Forte Liquifilm®, FML Liquifilm®, FML S.O.P. 0.1% ointment®	fluorometholone 0.1% suspension or ointment	Any conjunctivitis Topical corticosteroids for inflammation in stubborn cases of conjunctivitis, keretitis, iritis MOA—inducing phospholipase A2 inhibitory proteins responsible for controlling the biosynthesis of prostaglandins and leukotrienes, thereby reducing or inhibiting the release of arachadonic	1–2 GTT BID, TID, and QID

Trade	Generic	Indication and Classification	Sig
		acid, interfereing with the inflammation cycle. See Chapter 9, The Skin	
Pred Forte®	prednisolone acetate 0.12 to 1.0%	Any conjunctivitis Topical corticosteroids for inflammation in stubborn cases, MOA—same as above	1 drop every 1–6 hr Careful—use may cause glaucoma
Decongestant/ Vasoconstrictors Naphcon ®, Allerest®, Clear Eyes®	Naphazoline HCl 0.1% solution	Allergic conjunctivitis Decongestant vasoconstrictor, returns blood to its origin, reducing redness. MOA—vasoconstrictor returns blood to its origin, reducing redness	1 drop, bid-qid, NTE 5 days
OcuClear®, Visine LR®	oxymetazolone 0.025% solution	Same as above	1–2 gtts qid
Visine®, Murine Plus®	tetrahydrozoline 0.05 % solution	Same as above	1–2 gtts bid-tid
Combination Drugs Naphcon-A®	naphazoline HCl/pheniramine maleate 0.1% solution	Allergic conjunctivitis Decongestant with an antihistamine MOA—Vasoconstriction, while antihistamine prevents H1 binding on eye cells	1 drop, bid-qid, NTE 5 days
Zaditor ®	Ketotifen fumarate, 0.025%	Allergic conjunctivitis Antihistamine-mast cell stabilizer with anti-inflammatory properties. MOA—1. Binds to H-1 receptors of the eyes, preventing allergic response 2. Mast cell stabilizer, prevents H-1 release, decreasing chemotaxis and activation of eosinophils 3. Inhibits pro-inflammatory mediators (IL-5, E-selectin, and ICAM-)	one drop q 8-12 hr (age > 3 yrs)

Eye Disorders that Affect Vision

While eye infections are usually self-limiting, and severe infections need treatment with antibiotics, only on a rare occasion does an infection contribute to vision problems. This section will address the diseases of the eye, that affect the function of the eye and contribute to irreversible vision problems. The pharmaceutical treatments available for each shall be explored.

GLAUCOMA

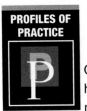
Glaucoma is one of the leading causes of permanent blindness, affecting more than two million Americans. Glaucoma is a slow, progressive disease that increases the intra optic pressure of the aqueous humor, in which there is also decreased outflow of aqueous humor. Visual impairment is irreversible and permanent. Blindness from glaucoma is inevitable. There is no cure for glaucoma; however, its progress can be slowed down with proper eye care. Glaucoma can affect anyone, but being over 50 years of age, of African descent, having diabetes, or a history of trauma to the eye are among the main risk factors. There are two types of glaucoma: closed angle glaucoma, or narrow angle; and open angle glaucoma, or wide angle. Inside the eye is a nourishing fluid called aqueous humor that circulates and feeds the eye. Patients with glaucoma should not take OTC drugs, especially ophthalmic decongestants and vasoconstrictors, as they may increase intraocular pressure (IOP).

In *closed angle glaucoma*, aka narrow angle, the anterior chamber is narrow, the outflow is impaired, and the iris thickens as a result of pupil dilation. This is the least common and most devastating form of the disease.

Symptoms include sudden intermittent changes in *intraocular* pressure due to extensive and prolonged pupil dilation, accompanied by ocular pain or inflammation, blurred vision, headache, pressure over the eye, cloudy cornea, extreme sensitivity to light or seeing halos around lights, nausea or vomiting, or a moderate pupil dilation that's nonreactive to light. If left untreated, blindness can occur within 3–5 days. Symptoms can come on rapidly, constituting an emergency in most cases.

Cause is usually an inherited anatomic deformity of the anterior chamber to be or to become narrow, in which aqueous humor cannot freely flow or drain out. Besides heredity, any one of the following may precipitate the closure of the anterior chamber:

- defect in the eye structure
- anything that causes the pupil to dilate—dim lighting, dilation drops for eye exams
- certain oral or injected medications
- blow to the eye
- diabetes-related growth of abnormal blood vessels over the angle
- most at risk are Asian, farsighted, or over the age of 60. These people should have their pressure checked every year or two.

Open angle glaucoma, aka wide angle, constitutes about 90 percent of all cases of glaucoma. It is an increase in intraocular pressure due to abnormality in the trabecular meshwork that impairs flow of aqueous humor between the anterior chamber and Canal of Schlemm. The canal is impaired and does not allow the fluid to return to the blood system. The fluid does not drain fast enough, and the IOP (intraocular pressure) builds up. This force or pressure hits the optic nerve, which causes blindness. There are basically three types of treatment: medicines, laser surgery, and filtration surgery. The goal of treatment is to lower the pressure in the eye.

Symptoms—open angle glaucoma is usually *asymptomatic* with a gradual, but progressive loss of field of vision, mild ache in the eyes, gradual loss of peripheral vision from all directions (the top, sides, and bottom areas of vision), seeing halos around lights, reduced visual acuity (especially at night) that is not correctable with glasses.

At risk are people with the following characteristics:

• African American
• family member with glaucoma
• diabetics
• very nearsighted
• over 35 years of age

Secondary Glaucoma occurs as the result of an eye injury, inflammation, a tumor, advanced cases of *cataracts*, diabetes or it can be drug induced (steroids). This form of glaucoma may be mild or severe, and may either be open angle or angle closure glaucoma. Treatment is the same as for primary.

Many cortisone-like drugs are widely used to treat a variety of conditions such as asthma, poison ivy, arthritis, and other inflammatory conditions. Such drugs as eye drops or ointments may cause secondary glaucoma; people with existing primary glaucoma must be sure not to use them. *Corticosteroids* that are injectable, oral, or topically applied to the skin are not a danger to most patients. However, after a surgery called "guarded filtration procedure," in which a new drain is made, post-surgical use of such corticosteroids will be required for about one month or so to reduce inflammation and prevent scarring that could close the new drain.

Oral medications taken for high blood pressure can cause problems for people with glaucoma. Therefore, it is advisable for glaucoma patients to try to control their blood pressure by nonmedicinal means, such as weight reduction and exercise. When lifestyle changes are not effective, antihypertensive medications will be indicated, but the glaucoma will need to be monitored and can worsen.

Oral cold remedies may contain drugs that enlarge or dilate the pupil by causing the iris to constrict. The dilated pupil places pressure on the drain, preventing the release of aqueous humor, because outflow channels are being blocked by the iris when the pupil is enlarged. These prescription drugs are atropine or atropine-like products. The same compound can be found in Lomotil® for diarrhea. Psychotropic agents and "tranquilizers" also dilate the pupil. Recall that fluid is constantly flowing into and out of the eye. If the flow out of the eye is blocked, the pressure inside the eye rises. Therefore, people with narrow anterior chamber angles are at risk for developing elevated IOP when their pupils are dilated (as in the dark or from the use of eye drops or oral medications that dilate the pupil). The FDA requires labels on these agents to warn consumers that the medications may cause glaucoma and should not be used by persons with existing glaucoma. (Those who have had iridotomy are not at risk of new closure by such drugs.)

Drugs for glaucoma either decrease the formation of aqueous humor, increase the outflow of aqueous humor, or both (see Table 10-2). The newest type of anti-glaucoma agent, a prostanoid selective FP receptor agonist, works by increasing the outflow of aqueous humor by two routes: the Canal of Schlem and trabecular meshwork, and the uveoscleral route.

CATARACT

A cataract is a condition in which the lens becomes opaque and interferes with the transmission of light to the retina and the vision is less sharp, less colorful, and less intense.

It is a myth that a film grows on the eyes; rather, the cataract grows within the eye. The cataract causes double or blurred images. The lens becomes opaque when old cells of the lens die and become trapped within the capsule that contains the lens. The cells accumulate over time, causing the lens to cloud, which makes images look blurred. Cataracts are usually a natural result of aging; however, eye injuries, diseases (diabetes and alcoholism), and certain medications can also cause them. At this time, cataracts can be treated only with surgery, in which the clouded lens is replaced with a clear, plastic lens. There are four classifications of cataracts:

- Congenital—hereditary or due to measles infection in mother during first trimester
- Trauma—injury to the lens
- Age—85 percent of all people over 80 years old have some clouding of lens
- Metabolic and toxic agents
  - Disorders of carbohydrate metabolism (diabetics)
  - Smoking
  - Drug induced (digoxin, alcohol)

VASCULAR RETINOPATHIES RETINOPATHY

Vascular retinopathies retinopathy is a noninflammatory disease in which the retina has become damaged. There is no pharmaceutical treatment for any of the many types of retinopathies. However, it is important that you understand that there are many causes, and some retinopathies are drug-induced. Some retinopathies may respond to laser treatment. A technician should pay attention and listen to a patient who mentions visual disturbances while taking specific medications. Report all discussions to the pharmacist, who better understands

TABLE 10-2   Drugs for Glaucoma with Various Mechanisms of Action

Trade	Generic	MOA	Indications	Side Effects	Sig
Beta blocking agents		MOA unknown, but may reduce aqueous humor formation and increase drainage	Chronic open-angle glaucoma and ocular hypertension	Stinging, oral dryness, ocular pruritus, drowsiness, conjunctival follicles, blurring of the eyes	1. Stinging or irritation of eye when medicine applied 2. Redness of eye or inside of eyelid 3. Decreased night vision 4. Blurred vision
Timolol®, Betimol®, OcuDose®, Timoptic-XE®	timolol maleate Ophthalmic Solutions 0.25% and 0.5%		Nonselective (Beta 1 and 2)		1 gtt 0.25% BID, NTE 1 gtt 0.5% BID
Betoptic®	betaxolol HCl solution 0.5% and 0.25% suspension		Beta 1 selective		1–2 gtts BID
Betoptic-S®	betaxolol HCl 0.25% suspension		Beta 1 selective		1–2 gtts BID
Betagan®	levobunolol HCl solution 0.25%, 0.5%		Nonselective (Beta 1 and 2)		1–2 gtts 0.5% sol. QD 1–2 gtts 0.25% sol. BID, NTE 2 gtts 0.5% sol. BID
Ocupress®	carteolol HCl solution, 1%		Nonselective (Beta 1 and 2)		1 gtt q 12 hr (or BID)
OptiPranolol®	metipranololet axolol HCl solution, 0.3%		Nonselective (Beta 1 and 2)		1 gtt q 12 hr or BID
Adrenergic agonists		Reduces the aqueous humor production and increases aqueous humor outflow	Selective Alpha-2 adrenergic agonist	Stinging, oral dryness, ocular pruritus, drowsiness, conjunctival follicles, blurring of the eyes	
Alphagan®	brimonidine 0.2%			The pressure lowering effects of brimonidine may decrease over time, must monitor Pt	1 gtt BID or TID
Iopidine®	apraclonidine, 0.5% and 1%				1–2 gtts q 8 hrs

Trade	Generic	MOA	Indications	Side Effects	Sig
Miotics		Pull on the ciliary muscle, which pulls the spaces between the meshwork to open more and increases the flow of fluid out of the eye. Decrease the size of the pupil, relaxing the iris, increasing fluid outflow through the trabecular meshwork only. Constrict the pupil.	Various purposes	Small pupil, headache, blurred vision, change in refraction, decreased visual field, retinal detachment	
Miostat®, Carbastat®	carbachol solution, 0.01%	cholinergic (parasympatho-mimetic) agent, constricts the iris and ciliary body, results in reduction of IOP. The exact MOA is not precisely known.	To obtain miosis during surgery		No more than one-half milliliter instilled into the anterior chamber for miosis
Cholinergic Agents Isoptocarpine®, Pilocar®	pilocarpine $\frac{1}{4}$, $\frac{1}{2}$, 1%, 2%, 3%, 4%, 5%, 6%, 8% Ophthalmic gel, 4%	Direct-acting cholinergic agent	Chronic simple open glaucoma, Chronic angle-closure glaucoma	Painful contraction of ciliary muscle, painful eye or brow, blurred vision, spasms, twitching, darkened vision, headaches	Open glaucoma. 1 gtt 0.5%–4% sol. QID Acute angle-closure. 1 gtt 1%–2% sol. q 5–10 min × 3–6 doses; then, 1 gtt q 1–3 hr until IOP is decreased $\frac{1}{2}$-in. ribbon QHS only
Phospholine Iodide®	echothiophate iodide ophthalmic solution 0.03%, 0.06%, 0.125%, and 0.25%	Long-acting cholinesterase inhibitor of endogenous ACH in iris, ciliary muscle, decreases Aq. Hmr outflow	Chronic angle-closure glaucoma		Lowest dose possible with least potent, qd or BID, NTE BID as it is long acting

TABLE 10-2 Drugs for Glaucoma with Various Mechanisms of Action (*continued*)

Trade	Generic	MOA	Indications	Side Effects	Sig
Carbopnic anhydrase inhibitors		Carbonic anhydrase inhibitors reduce the aqueous humor production, thus lowering the pressure in the eye	Open angle glaucoma or Ocular hypertension	1. Blurred vision 2. Bitter, sour, or unusual taste 3. Dermatitis 4. Chest pain 5. Conjunctivitis 6. Diarrhea 7. Dizziness 8. Double vision 9. Dry eye 10. Dry mouth	
Azopt®	Brinzolamide solution 1%			1. Chest pain 2. Jaundice	1 gtt q 8 hr
Truspot®	dorzolamide HCl 2% solution			Allergic reactions in patients who are also allergic to sulfonamides	1 gtt q 8 hr
Diamox®	acetazolamide 125 mg, 250 mg, 500 mg (sustained release)		DO NOT GIVE TO THOSE ALLERGIC TO SULFA DRUGS	1. Loss of appetite 2. Metallic taste 3. Diarrhea 4. Weakness 5. Tingling sensation in hands or feet or mouth area 6. Hearing impairment or ringing in the ears 7. Convulsions 8. Shortness of breath or difficulty breathing	125 mg or 250 mg, 1 to 4 times per day U.D. Diamox Sequels, 500 mg 1 cap Bid
Combination Product		Dual action of beta blocker and Carbonic Anhydrase Inhibitor		eye pain, tearing, itching, blurred or cloudy vision, ocular burning	
Cosopt®	dorzolamide hydrochloride and timolol maleate	Dorzolamide, a CAI and timolol, beta blocker, both decrease		Same as preceding, and keratitis, blepharitis, conjunctival	1 gtt BID

Trade	Generic	MOA	Indications	Side Effects	Sig
		aqueous humor production; timolol also increases drainage.		edema, discharge or follicles, corneal erosion, corneal cataracts, dizziness, bronchitis, dyspepsia, abdominal pain, back pain, bitter, sour, or unusual taste	
Osmodic Diuretics			For head or eye injury, before or after surgery acute closed angle glaucoma		
Ophthalagen	glycerin anhydrous	Clears the edema and enables outflow	Eye surgery in cases of head or eye injury	Adverse effects include diarrhea, back pain, confusion, and hyperosmolar coma	PO 1–1.8 gm/kg 1–1.5 hr before surgery, Q5 min
Osmitrol	mannitol	Increases glomerular filtration with minimal reabsorption of water in the tubules, enhances secretion of Na^+ and Cl^- ions.	Lowers IOP when other means and agents have failed	Rebound urinary retention, H/A, back/chest pain, chills/rigors, N&V, confusion, pulmonary edema, hypokalemia, and hyponatremia	IV Infusion: 1.5–2 mg/kg (15–20% sol) 30-50 min/hr, over 30 to 60 min. NTE 50 to 200 g in a 24-hour period
Prostamides and Prostaglandins		Exact MOA unknown, but believed to increase uveoscleral outflow of aqueous humor	For open angle glaucoma	Change of iris color, red eye, eye irritation or inflammation, flu-like syndrome, and arthritis	

TABLE 10-2   Drugs for Glaucoma with Various Mechanisms of Action (*continued*)

Trade	Generic	MOA	Indications	Side Effects	Sig
Lumigan®	bimatoprost ophthalmic solution, 0.03%	Dual action improve natural flow of fluid through both the trabecular meshwork and uveoscleral routes	Open angle glaucoma, Dual action improve natural flow of fluid through both the trabecular meshwork and uveoscleral routes	In addition to the preceding: may increase growth of eyelashes and increased pigmentation of the iris and periorbital tissue (eyelid)	1 gtt QD dosing only
Rescula®	Unoprostone isopropyl solution 0.15%	Inactive biosynthetic cyclic derivative of arachidonic acid, MOA is unknown, but does increase outflow of aqueous humor	For open angle glaucoma	May gradually change eye color, increasing the amount of brown pigment in the iris	1 gtt BID
Travatan®	trovoprost solution, 0.004%	Selective FP prostanoid receptor agonist, causing release of MMP (metalloproteini-ases) that degrade the cellular matrix that increases outflow; exact MOA unknown, believed to decrease IOP by increasing uveoscleral outflow of aqueous humor	Prostaglandin F2 alpha analogue (synthetic)	1. May gradually change eye color, increasing the amount of brown pigment in the iris. 2. May increase growth of eyelashes	1 gtt q p.m. ONLY, NTE 1 gtt qd Approved 3-2001
Xalatan®	0.005% latanaprost solution	Prostanoid selective FP receptor agonist MOA same as Travatan®		1. May gradually change eye color, increasing the amount of pigment in the iris. 2. May increase growth of eyelashes	1 gtt q p.m. only, NTE 1 gtt qd Approved 3-2001

the side effects and interactions of the drugs and may report to the attending physician for further observation and testing.

There are two major types of retinopathies:

- *Simple or nonproliferative retinopathies* are characterized by defective bulging in vessel walls, which causes bleeding into the eye. The bulging is caused by small clumps of dead retinal cells called cotton wool exudates and by closed vessels. This form of retinopathy is considered mild.
- *Proliferative retinopathies* are severe forms characterized by newly grown blood vessels and scar tissue formed within the eye, by closed-off blood vessels that are badly damaged, and by the retina breaking away or detaching from its mesh of blood vessels that nourish it.

A general sequence of events for many of the retinopathies is outlined as follows:

Blood flow to the retina is disrupted, either by blockage or breakdown of the various vessels. Bleeding or hemorrhage occurs, along with fluid, cells, and proteins known as exudates leaking into the area. A lack of oxygen to surrounding tissues and hypoxia or decreased blood flow results; *ischemia* may lead to necrotic retina or other ocular tissue. This causes chemicals to be produced by the body, which, in turn, cause new blood vessels to grow. This new growth is called neovascularization. However, these new vessels generally leak blood, causing more problems. The retina may swell, and vision will be affected. The retina may detach.

The following are some of the causes of retinopathies:

- Drug induced—chloroquine, thioridazine, and large doses of tamoxifen can cause the arteries and veins to become blocked, thus resulting in a retinal artery or vein occlusion. These are just some of the causes of the various retinopathies.
- Microaneurysms cause bleeding into the vitreous humor (fluid inside of the eyeball).
- Solar retinopathy—exposure to the sun or looking at the sun during an eclipse can cause damage.
- Neovascularizations is the formation of new blood vessels, which tend to be fragile, leak protein, and bleed.
- Central vein occlusion causes a rapid deterioration of visual acuity. This is often secondary to HTN, diabetes mellitus, or sickle cell anemia.
- Diabetic retinopathies are confined to the retina and involve thickening of capillary walls and microaneurysm formation, followed by rupture and bleeding into the retina. In proliferative diabetic retinopathies, the retina bleeds into the vitreous humor.
- Atherosclerosis—a hardening or thickening of the retinal arteries is called arteriosclerotic retinopathy.
- Retinal artery occlusion—complete blockage of an artery to the retina results in sudden unilateral blindness (one eye/sided anopsia).

- HTN—high blood pressure in the arteries of the body can damage the retinal arteries and is called hypertensive retinopathy.
- Syphilis infection causes infection of the retina, or syphilitic retinopathy.

Cycloplegic, Mydriatic Drugs, Lubricants

Certain drugs help the ophthalmologist to examine the patient's eyes. Drugs that will relax the ciliary muscle are cycloplegic drugs; and mydriatic drugs dilate the pupils. People with dilated pupils may experience blurred vision for a variable amount of time, usually 2–4 hours. While having your pupils dilated, brilliant lights may be bothersome. You should wear dark glasses until the dilation subsides.

Lubricants restore moisture to the dry eye. Dry eyes may result from exposure to the elements (sun, wind), chemicals such as chlorine, allergens, or certain drugs. Originally responding to possible injury or infection, the immune system sends white blood cells and other mediators in the blood to the eye. Since more blood is traveling to the eye, the whites of the eye get redder as blood vessels dilate (open up) to accommodate the blood.

Vasoconstrictors, also called decongestants, will return blood back to where it came from when the mediators are no longer needed. While short-term use may be warranted, unfortunately, a rebound effect will occur in long-term use. The rebound effect happens when the swelling goes down; the redness goes away, only to return again because the medication causes the dilation of the vessels. (What actually happens is that the blood vessels become dilated again to counter the vasoconstrictive effect of the medication.)

This paradoxical over-compensation, or "self-correcting" action, causes the blood vessels to dilate even more, resulting in a tolerance in 2–5 days. Because the blood vessels have dilated so much, they become tired. The patient then uses more drug to counter this dilation. This rebound effect goes on and on. Long-term use of vasoconstrictors should be avoided. There is some research that connects long-term use of vasoconstrictors with glaucoma.

Basics of Using an Ophthalmic Product

The following basic precautions and standard procedures must be followed when placing eye drops or ointment into the eye:

1. Wash hands thoroughly with soap and water.

2. Remove contact lenses before putting in ophthalmic medication, and wait 15 minutes after administering the medication before putting them back in.

3. Never touch the tip of the tube against the eye or to anything else— keep the medication and container sterile.

4. Wipe any excess ointment or gel from the eyelids and lashes by using a tissue. Wipe off the tip of the tube by using a second (clean) tissue. Recap right away. Store in a proper location and at the correct temperature.

5. Wash hands immediately to remove any medication.

6. If more than one type of eye drop is used, always wait 5–10 minutes between putting in each different type of drop.

7. Sometimes eye drops can cause a few moments of blurry vision; wait until the vision completely clears before resuming activities such as driving.

How to Apply an Ophthalmic Ointment

The stream of oil based ointment is measured in the length of the "ribbon" that comes out of the tube. Sometimes the measurement is stated in centimeters, or cm, while other times the manufacturers state it in terms of the English inch. For this reason, it is good to know that 1 inch is equivalent to 2.5 cm. (See Figure 10-3.) Some specific instructions for applying ointment to the eye are as follows, and are in addition to the basic instructions listed previously:

1. Hold the tube between your thumb and forefinger. Place it near the eye, but not touching any part of the eye or the eyelid. Tilt your head forward slightly.

2. With the index finger of your other hand, pull the lower eyelid down to form a "V" pocket. Squeeze the tube and place a ribbon of ointment or gel into the "V" pocket made by the opened lower eyelid. Do not let the tip of the tube touch the eye.

3. Blink the eye gently. Close the eye for 1–2 minutes.

How to Instill an Ophthalmic Solution

Solution or liquid that is to be placed into the eye must be "instilled"; otherwise, the liquid will immediately drain from the tear duct area, and the eye will not receive the medication. (See Figure 10-4.) Some specific instructions for instilling solution and suspensions into the eye are as follows and are in addition to the basic precautions and standard procedures listed previously:

1. Shake the bottle gently or roll it in your hand to be sure the medicine is well mixed, when directed by the instructions, and especially if the product is a suspension.

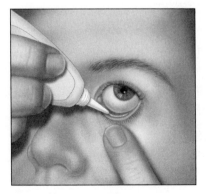

Figure 10-3 Applying an ophthalmic ointment

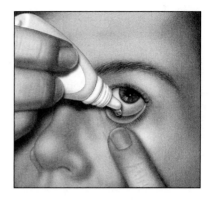

Figure 10-4 Instilling eye drops

2. Tilt your head back slightly; look at the ceiling.

3. Use your index finger to gently pull down on your lower eyelid to form a pocket.

4. Position the dropper above your eye. Look up and away from the dropper.

5. Squeeze out the prescribed number of drops, and gently close your eye.

6. Apply gentle pressure to the inside corner of your closed eye (near your nose) for about one minute to prevent the liquid from draining down your tear duct.

7. If you are using drops in both eyes, repeat the process in the other eye.

The Ear

Hearing starts with the outer ear, or pinna or auracle. Sound waves or vibrations travel from the outer ear down the external auditory canal and strike the eardrum, known as the tympanic membrane. The eardrum vibrates, and these vibrations are then passed to three tiny bones in the middle ear called the ossicles. The *ossicles* amplify the sound and send the sound waves to the inner ear and into the fluid-filled hearing organ, the cochlea. The *cochlea* is lined with cells that have thousands of tiny hairs (cilia) on their surfaces. The sound vibrations make the tiny hairs move. The hairs then change the sound vibrations into nerve signals, so your brain can interpret the sound. The signals travel to the brain along special nerves. After the sound waves reach the inner ear, they are converted into electrical impulses, which the auditory nerve sends to the brain. The brain then recognizes these electrical impulses as sound.

Anatomy and Physiology of the Ear

The ear has three major areas, the outer, middle, and inner ear. The outer ear structures, commonly called the flaps and ear lobes, are the cartilaginous portion known technically as the pinna or auricle. The pinna acts as a pre-amplifier that enhances the sensitivity of hearing.

The tympanic membrane, or "eardrum," receives the vibrations that travel up through the auditory canal. These vibrations are transferred first to the three tiny ossicles, and then to the oval opening into the inner ear. The ossicles are the three smallest bones in the body. They form the "coupling" between the vibration of the eardrum and the forces exerted on the oval opening of the inner ear. The eardrum provides amplification of about 15 times more than the oval opening. The auditory canal acts as a closed tube resonator, which boosts and improves sounds in the 2–5 kilohertz range. At the eardrum, sound energy or air pressure changes are converted into mechanical energy of eardrum movement. Sound travels through the three ossicles (bones)—the malleus (hammer), incus (anvil), and stapes (stirrup)—of the middle ear.

EUSTACHIAN TUBE

The eustachian tube connects the middle ear with the nasopharynx of the throat. When a person swallows or coughs, this tube "opens" to equalize the pressure between the middle ear and the outer ear. Proper transfer of sound waves occurs when the pressure is the same. The eustachian tube is shorter in children, often presenting a more horizontal orientation. It is therefore less likely to open and more likely to become blocked by enlarged adenoids. Fluid will collect more often within the middle ear area of young children, causing temporary hearing loss and/or a feeling of fullness and pain. This condition is called "serous otitis media," or SOM. SOM may occur shortly after or during an upper respiratory infection when the child produces more congestion. Allergy-induced congestion or SOM may require antihistamines to dry out the congestion and to stop the allergic response that is causing it. SOM is most common among children younger than five years old.

Sometimes surgical insertion of ventilation tubes into the middle ear needs to be performed; this operation is known as a myringotomy. Swimming with these tubes may cause a potentially serious infection, and should be avoided.

The middle ear serves as an equalizer, matching the impedance of air in the ear canal to the impedance of the perilymph of the inner ear. Perilymph is the same as cerebrospinal fluid (CSF), having a low potassium $-K^+-$ concentration and a high sodium $-Na^+-$ concentration. The scala tympani also contains perilymph. (See Figure 10-5.)

COCHLEA

This snail-shaped structure is the sensory organ of hearing, containing the nerves for hearing. The vibrational, wavelike patterns, initiated by vibration of the stapes footplate, causes a shearing of the cilia of the outer and inner hair cells. This process causes hair cell depolarization, which occurs in the Organ of Corti within the scala media of the cochlea. This results in the vibrational energy that changes into neural energy, or impulses, that the brain interprets as sound, as they are transmitted along the eighth nerve.

VESTIBULAR LABYRINTH

The vestibular labyrinth is composed of the sense organs of balance, the saccule and utricle, which notify the brain about an individual's linear and rotational movement in space. This vestibule contains the receptors for balance.

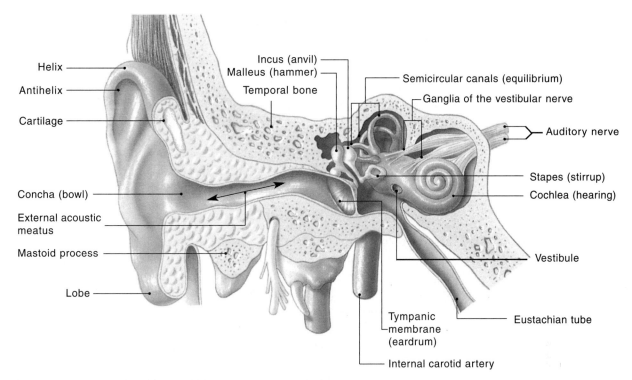

Figure 10-5 The ear (*Holland, Norman; Adams, Michael Patrick,* Core Concepts in Pharmacology, *1st Edition, © 2003. Reprinted by permission of Pearson Education, Inc., Upper Saddle River, NJ)*

Complications of Earwax Buildup

The skin of the outer part of the ear canal contains the ceruminous and sebaceous gland that produce earwax. The purposes of earwax are to trap dust, dirt, insects, and sand, preventing them from getting into the eardrum; keep the eardrum moist; and to inhibit the formation of bacteria in the eardrum. Usually, the wax will accumulate for a short period and in a small quantity and then dry up, before it comes out of the ear, carrying the offensive particles along with it.

Sometimes earwax will migrate to the outside (pinna) where it is easily wiped off. Wax does not form in the deep part of the ear canal near the tympanic membrane (eardrum). Normal amounts of earwax are healthy and also serve as a water repellent. Dry, itchy ears may be a result of wax deficiency. The homeostasis of self-cleaning—making more earwax, then drying, flaking, and falling out of the ear canal—is slow and constant.

Sometimes homeostasis is interrupted when the wax builds up against the eardrum. Using objects such as pens or cotton swabs serves only to push the earwax farther inside. Continuous scratching of the ear canal, which has very thin skin and is easily injured, can lead to pain and infection. Hearing aids can prevent the migration of the earwax out of the canal. Annual ear exams can prevent some temporary hearing loss. The audiologist may wash the ear out, vacuum it, or physically remove the wax with special instruments. OTC ear drops may be used to pre-soften the earwax before the "wash" or vacuum. A precautionary note—if the eardrum is punctured or perforated, infection may result from the use of water or presoftening ear drops. Examples of ear wax softeners are Debrox® and Murine Ear Drops® (carbamide peroxide).

Types of Hearing Loss

CONDUCTIVE HEARING LOSS

This type of loss happens when there is a problem with a part of the outer or middle ear. Usually this is a mild hearing loss, and it is usually temporary because, in most cases, medical treatment can help. Sometimes a blow to the head or ear will cause this. Birth defects of malformed parts of the outer or middle ear, a tiny hole or perforation in the eardrum, wax buildup in the ear canal, and middle ear infections can all be responsible.

SENSORY HEARING LOSS

This type of loss happens when the cochlea is not working correctly because the tiny hair cells or cilia are damaged or destroyed. It can affect one ear or both ears. Depending on the loss, sound may be muffled (mild loss), some sounds might be slightly inaudible (moderate loss), or no sounds at all may be heard (severe profound loss). Speech may also be affected. Sensory hearing impairment is almost always permanent. It may be due to heredity or may occur during the developmental stages of the fetus when a pregnant woman gets certain kinds of diseases, such as Rubella (German measles). Other possible causes are certain medications, severe injury to the head, listening to extremely loud music, exposure to other loud noises (factory machinery, race cars). (Tinnitus is ringing or buzzing in the ear that does not come from an external source and may also be caused by infections or drugs.)

DRUG INDUCED

Some drugs cause ototoxicity in which hearing and balance are impaired. Hearing loss can be reversible (temporary) or irreversible (permanent). Drugs that cause hearing loss belong to several classifications, such as the strong antibiotics known as aminoglycosides, which are given intraveneously; loop diuretics; antineoplastic agents; anti-cancer drugs; and antimalarial and antiarrhythmic drugs that contain quinine. Aspirin can contribute to ringing in the ear, or tinnitus. (See Table 10–3.)

NEURAL HEARING LOSS

This type of loss happens when there is a problem with the connection from the cochlea to the brain, such as when the nerve that carries the messages from the cochlea to the brain is damaged.

PRESBYCUSIS

This permanent loss is due to damaged hearing nerves. When hearing deteriorates with age, sensitivity for high-pitched sounds fades first. This is why people often say they can hear sounds, but they cannot understand. Presbycusis

TABLE 10-3 Drugs that Cause Sensory Hearing Loss	
Trade	Generic
Antibiotics	
Amickin®	amikacin IV
Garamycin®	gentamicin IV
Nebcin®	tobramycin IV
Loop Diuretics	
Bumex®	bumetanide
Edecrin ®	ethacrynic acid
Lasix®	furosemide
Demadex®	torsemide
Antineoplastic Agents—anti-cancer drugs	
Paraplatin®	carboplatin
Platinol®	cisplatin
Quinine products (selected)	
Tonic water	
Aralen®—chloroquine	
Quinaglute Dura-tabs®, Quinidex Extentab®	quinidine
Quinine	quinine sulfate

develops slowly and gradually. Recruitment, a progression of presbycusis, is a loss of sensitivity to soft sounds and decreased ability to tolerate loud sounds.

Otitis Media

One of the most common causes of conductive hearing loss is otitis media, an inflammation and infection of the middle ear that usually presents in one out of three children. Acute otitis media is an infection that produces pus, fluid, and inflammation within the middle ear. Older children may complain about ear pain, fullness, or hearing loss. Younger children may present irritability, fussiness, or difficulty in sleeping, feeding, or hearing. Fever is usually present.

These symptoms are frequently associated with signs of upper respiratory infection, such as a runny or stuffy nose or a cough. Otitis media, the most common childhood illness, usually appears four to seven days after the respiratory infection. Severe ear infections may cause the eardrum to rupture. Immediate medical treatment is then necessary. More than 80 percent of all children will have at least one middle-ear infection before they are three years old. Usually, otitis is easily treatable; however, a temporary hearing loss may result. This conductive hearing loss may cause delays in speech and language development and lead to learning difficulties. If left untreated, permanent hearing loss, rupture of the tympanic membrane, and/or meningitis may develop (see Table 10-4).

TABLE 10-4	Antibiotic Treatment of Otitis Media in Children

Prophylaxis

| Amoxil®, Trimox®, Wymox® | amoxicillin |
| | sulfisoxazole (DOC) |

First-line Therapy

Bactrim®,	
Septra®—Use for PCN allergy	trimethoprim-sulfamethoxazole (SMX TMP)
Amoxil®, Trimox®, Wymox®	amoxicillin

Second-line Therapy

Augmentin®	amoxicillin and clavulanate potassium
Zithromax®	azithromycin
Cefzil®	cefprozil
Vantin®	cefpodoxime proxetil
Cedax ®	ceftibuten
Ceftin®	cefuroxime axetil
Biaxin®	clarithromycin
Lorabid®	loracarbef

Third-line Therapy

Cleocin®	
(Use for resistant pneumococci)	Clindamycin
Rocephin	ceftriaxone sodium

SUMMARY

The most basic of all of our senses is sight. The anatomy and physiology of the eye are discussed extensively in this chapter.

The eyes are prone to many diseases, but eye infections are usually self-limiting and treatable and, only on rare occasions, lead to vision problems. More serious diseases of the eye can contribute to irreversible vision problems.

There are a wide variety of treatment modalities available to treat eye disorders. However, it is important that ophthalmic products be used safely and properly. One of your most important responsibilities as a pharmacy technician is to thoroughly understand the basics of safely using ophthalmic remedies.

The ear consists of three major areas, the outer, middle, and the inner ear. The functions of the ear include hearing and the maintenance of equilibrium or balance. Like the eye, the ear is susceptible to a variety of disorders, but these can normally be prevented, controlled, or reversed with treatment. While easily treatable, common problems such as otitis media, a middle ear infection, can lead to permanent hearing loss, if untreated. It is estimated that more than 80 percent of children will be affected with this disorder before reaching the age of three.

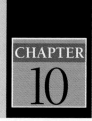
CHAPTER REVIEW QUESTIONS

1. The most common eye disease that results from a complication of diabetes is:
   a. conjuctivitis
   b. glaucoma
   c. retinopathy
   d. pinkeye

2. The treatment for glaucoma includes:
   a. medicines
   b. laser surgery
   c. both a and b
   d. none of the above

3. Patients with glaucoma should not:
   a. keep a patch over the eye
   b. use ointments directly in the eye
   c. use OTC drugs without consulting their doctor
   d. expose the eye to more than two hours of sunlight per day

4. The most common ear disease in children is:
   a. otitis media
   b. myringotomy
   c. glaucoma
   d. conjuctivitis

5. Otitis media is:
   a. a blockage in the tear ducts
   b. an inflammation and infection of the middle ear

   c. the first sign of the onset of diabetes
   d. not curable

6. Which part of the eye is the most sensitive for acute vision?
   a. lens
   b. cornea
   c. retina
   d. optic nerve

7. Explain the rebound effect.

8. Which part of the ear is where the brain interprets sound from electrical impulses?
   a. the Organ of Corti within the scala media of the cochlea
   b. the tympanic region
   c. the eustachian tubes extending into the eardrum
   d. both b and c

9. The reaction to a drug, which causes permanent damage to hearing and balance, is called:
   a. neurological detriment
   b. otitis media
   c. diabetes mellitus
   d. ototoxicity

10. Explain which sense, eyesight or hearing, is more important to you and why you would not want to lose it compared with losing the other sense.

Resources and References

1. *The Merck Manual of Diagnosis and Therapy*
   http://www.merck.com/mrkshared/mmanual/section8/chapter94/94c.jsp
2. Timolol® http://www.rxlist.com/cgi/generic/timolol_cp.htm
3. Lumigan® Package Insert http://www.lumigan.com/pdfs/PI.pdf
4. *Review of Anatomy: The Ear and Temporal Bone*
   http://www.bcm.tmc.edu/oto/studs/anat/tbone.html#EAR
5. Visit a website that simulates various eye conditions:
   www.visionsimulator.com. The site was reviewed by Philips Eye
   Institute Physicians for accuracy on November 13, 2002.
6. Beltone interactive Internet site for the Anatomy of the Ear
   http://www.beltone.com/ear_anatomy/ear_anatomy.asp#
7. Holland, Norman and Michael Patrick Adams. *Core Concepts in
   Pharmacology*. Upper Saddle River, NJ: Pearson Education, 2003.
8. Adams, Michael Patrick, Dianne L. Josephson, and Leland Norman
   Holland, Jr. *Pharmacology for Nurses—A Pathophysiologic Approach*.
   Upper Saddle River, NJ: Pearson Education, 2005.

The Gastrointestinal System

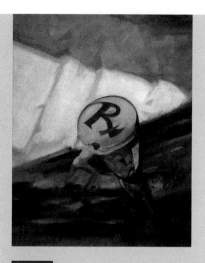

INTRODUCTION

Without digestion, the body would not get nourished or rehydrated. The cells of the body would die and, eventually, the body itself would die. The main purpose of the digestive system is to fuel the body so that it can continue to survive and function properly. A lack of proper nutrition and digestion can lead to numerous disease states. Therefore, the digestive system aids in the prevention of some diseases.

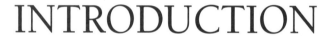

Learning Objectives

After completing this chapter, you should be able to:

- Identify and list the basic, anatomical, structural parts of the digestive system.
- Describe the physiology of the digestive system and each part's function.
- List vital amino acids, vitamins, and minerals needed for the body to function.
- Define the necessity, function, and disease state resulting from the depletion of each.
- List vital ingredients used in the TPN formula and describe how they are added.

Anatomy and Physiology of the Digestive System

The digestive system is a series of hollow organs connected in a long tube that twists and turns. It extends from the mouth to the anus (Figure 11-1). A protective lining of this tube, called the mucosa, prevents acid from causing sores known as ulcers. In the mouth, stomach, and small intestine, the mucosa contains tiny glands that produce the liquid digestive juices that help digest food. These liquids contain enzymes and acids.

Two organs produce digestive juices that are sent to the intestine through small vessels. The liver produces bile, which it stores in the gallbladder, and the pancreas produces enzymes. In addition, accessory organs, nerves, and blood play a major role in the digestive system.

Rings of muscles, called smooth muscle, help to produce a wave of synchronized contractions, or *peristalsis*, to help propel the food down the digestive tract. The six main parts or organs of the digestive system are as follows:

- mouth
- esophagus
- pharynx

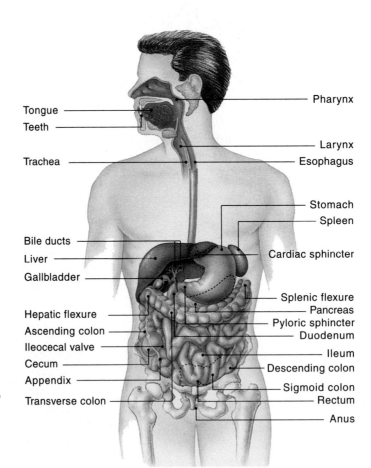

Figure 11-1 The digestive system (*Holland, Norman; Adams, Michael Patrick,* Core Concepts in Pharmacology, *1st Edition,* © 2003. Reprinted by permission of Pearson Education, Inc., Upper Saddle River, NJ)

- stomach
- small intestines
- large intestines

The six accessory organs are as follows:

- teeth
- tongue
- salivary glands
- liver
- gallbladder
- pancreas

Function of Digestion

Digestion is the process that the body uses to accomplish the following functions:

- break up food particles into smaller pieces
- break down food substances into nutrients that the body can use for body processes as energy
- transfer what it cannot use as "waste" out of the body; this elimination process is known as excretion
- reabsorb water into the body's tissue in order to prevent dehydration

The Digestive Process

THE MOUTH

Digestion first begins in the opening of the alimentary tract, the mouth, where accessory organs aid in physical digestion (Figure 11-2). The teeth assist in breaking up the food pieces into smaller particles; this is known as mastication. Saliva moistens the food to ease swallowing. The tongue moves the ball of food, known as a bolus, to the uvula, and both assist in swallowing, along with the epiglottis. Food then passes through the throat or pharynx into the esophagus, as the "windpipe," or trachea, is closed off. Before the food is swallowed, the carbohydrate content of the food is chemically broken down by an enzyme into simple sugars, or *monosaccharides*. This enzyme is an amylase known as ptyalin.

Monosaccharides are the building blocks of carbohydrates. Because food is usually swallowed before being completely chewed or moistened with the enzymes, physical and chemical digestion is not yet completed. The food mixture or bolus passes through the lower esophageal sphincter into the stomach. The "LES" is another name for the cardiac sphincter, as the esophagus, approximately 10 inches long, runs behind the heart before it curves to meet the stomach. (More details on the "LES" will be presented in the section on GERD.)

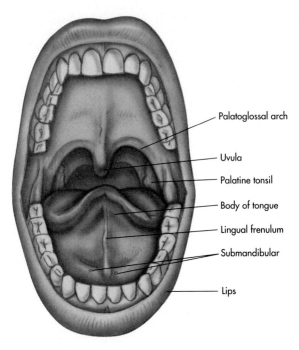

Figure 11-2   The mouth

THE STOMACH

There are three parts of the stomach: fundus, body, and pylorus. The smooth muscles of the stomach continue the peristalsis, which will continue to move the foodstuff—now called chyme and consisting of thick soupy liquid—along the digestive tract and break up the food into smaller pieces. (See Figure 11-3.) The chemical digestion in the stomach occurs when the walls of the stomach sense the weight or presence of the food or get stretched out.

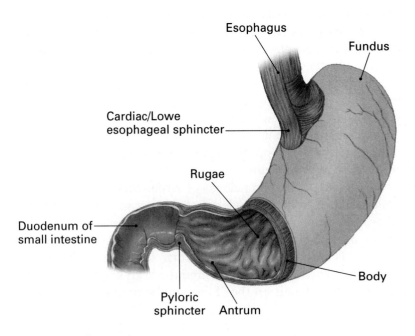

Figure 11-3   The stomach

In response, the parietal cells make and secrete HCL acid, which converts pepsinogen into the enzyme pepsin. The proteolytic enzyme pepsin chemically breaks down protein into amino acids. Amino acids are the building blocks of the protein. About four hours later, peristalsis will continue to move the chyme, consisting of carbohydrates, monosaccharides, protein, and amino acids, through the pyloric sphincter. (More details will be presented on gastric ulcers later in this chapter.)

THE SMALL INTESTINE

There are three parts of the small intestine: the duodenum, jejunum, and the ileum. The duodenum is the first part of the small intestine, where about 80 percent of all food is chemically digested. Also, 80 percent of all ulcers are found in the duodenum. As the highly acidic chyme enters the duodenum, it must be neutralized by an alkaline substance, bicarbonate; otherwise, a duodenal ulcer will result. The strong acidity of the chyme signals the pancreas to secrete bicarbonate along with its starch, protein, and fat digesting enzymes. Secreted bicarbonate neutralizes the stomach acids and raises the pH in the small intestine to just slightly acidic (about 5.5), which is the chemical environment in which the pancreatic enzymes work best. (See Figure 11-4.)

The small intestine will call upon the liver to make and secrete bile to help in digesting the fats. Stored bile from the gallbladder will be sent to the small intestine to break up the large molecules of fats into smaller ones—a process called emulsification—so they can be well absorbed from the intestine after enzymes break down the smaller globules of fat into absorbable nutrients.

Then the pancreas will send all three enzymes in a juice or secretion. Trypsin, a protease, will further break down any remaining proteins or amino acids into the simplest of amino acids. Amylopsin, an amylase, will further break down any remaining carbohydrates and simple sugars into the simplest of sugars or monosaccharides. Finally, and for the first time, a lipase called steapsin will break down the smaller molecules of fat into fatty acids

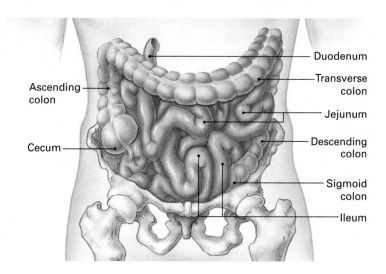

Figure 11-4 The small intestine

and glycerol, the building blocks of fats. Now that all food sources, carbohydrates, proteins, and fats (lipids) are broken down into their simple substances as nutrients so that they can enter the bloodstream, the body can use them as energy and to continue other body processes. The four nutrients, monosaccharides, amino acids, fatty acids, and glycerol, then are absorbed into the capilliaries of the blood system by the finger-like projections called *villi* and the micro villi in the small intestine. Whatever is not absorbable is then passed out of the small intestine into the large intestine (or the colon) and out of the large intestine and the body as waste.

The small intestine is where the majority of absorption takes place. The nutrients are absorbed into tiny lymph vessels called lacteals and are passed through a larger vein, the *portal vein*, to the liver. The liver breaks down any toxins that may be present and prepares the nutrients for release into the bloodstream. The bloodstream carries the nutrients to every cell in the body, where they are used for energy and for tissue building and repair.

Table 11-1 shows the chemical breakdown of specific foods in a typical sandwich and the function of the building blocks produced during the digestion.

THE LARGE INTESTINE OR COLON

The large intestine has seven parts: cecum, ascending colon, transverse colon, descending colon, sigmoid colon, rectum, and anus. The material or residue that is not absorbed, or waste, is moved through the ileocecal valve that connects the lower ileum of the small intestine to the cecum, the first part of the large intestine. The large intestine utilizes smooth muscle to mix the waste and allows the water to be re-absorbed through the large intestine. The contractions of the colon are unsynchronized (non-peristaltic) and constitute the "motility." A second and very important type of motility that occurs in the large intestine is the high amplitude propagating contraction (*HAPC*). These extremely strong contractions occur about six to eight times

TABLE 11-1 Comparison of Nutrient Functions within the Body			
Food Source	Chemical Base of of Food Source	Building Block (nutrient present at the end of digestion or hydrolysis)	Function of the Building Block or Nutrient
Bread or Bun	Complex Carbohydrates	Simple Sugars or Monosaccharides	Quick Energy
Hamburger Patty	Protein	Amino Acids	Growth repair of all cells, tissue, organs structure esp. muscle
Mayonnaise	Lipids (Fats)	Fatty Acids and Glycerol	Stored energy, lubrication, protection/padding, and insulation.

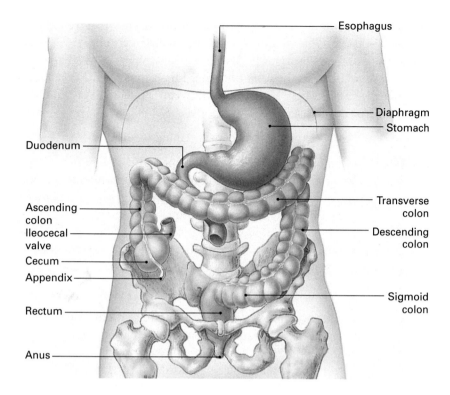

Figure 11-5 The large intestine

per day in healthy people. They are longitudinal and sweep from the cecum, stopping just above the rectum. They move the waste down the large intestine and may trigger a bowel movement. Food waste remains in the large intestine for about 30 hours, along with bacteria. (See Figure 11-5.)

The second phase of digestion begins when food passes from the stomach into the small intestine. As the partially digested food enters here, its strong acidity signals the pancreas to secrete bicarbonate along with its starch, protein, and fat digesting enzymes. Secreted bicarbonate neutralizes the stomach acids and raises the pH in the small intestine to just slightly acidic (about 5.5), which is the chemical environment in which the pancreatic enzymes work best. The gallbladder simultaneously secretes bile into the small intestine, which helps to emulsify dietary fats and fat-soluble vitamins so that they can be well absorbed from the intestine.

Disorders of the Digestive System

GERD OR GASTRIC ESOPHAGEAL REFLUX DISEASE

Commonly known as heartburn, GERD occurs because the lower esophageal sphincter relaxes when it should be contracting, and an excess amount of acid made in the stomach then rises up from the stomach into the esophagus.

The primary goal in treatment is to reduce the over-production of acid (these drugs will be discussed later in the Ulcer section) and to contract the LES. The LES connects the stomach and the esophagus. Relaxing the pyloric

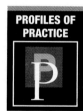

PROFILES OF PRACTICE

An estimated 70 million Americans are said to have one or more digestive disorders, which accounts for 13 percent of all hospitalizations.

sphincter will allow more food to continue to pass through the GI tract. Reglan® is an example of a drug used for this indication.

Reglan®—metoclopramide 5 and 10 mg tablets PO–10 to 15 mg qid 30 min ac and qhs—is the drug of choice for serious GERD that cannot be allieviated by OTC drugs. Metoclopramide can act as a GI stimulant or as an antiemetic or antinauseant.

a) GI Stimulant—Dopamine Receptor Antagonist

MOA 1—Stimulates peristalsis of the upper GI tract without causing more acid production, causes a relaxation of the pyloric sphincter and increasing resting tone of the LES. Increasing the resting tone means it allows the muscle of the LES to tighten more during its relaxed state, which increases contraction of the LES. Relaxing the pyloric sphincter and contracting the LES allow a quicker elimination process, also known as increased emptying time, whereby food goes through the stomach faster.

b) Antiemetic or Antinauseant

MOA 2—The antiemetic properties of metoclopramide are unknown, but are believed to be a result of its antagonism of central and peripheral dopamine receptors. Dopamine causes nausea and vomiting by stimulation of the medullary chemoreceptor trigger zone (CTZ). It promotes proper sphincter function by blocking stimulation of the CTZ by agents like L-dopa or apomorphine, which are known to increase dopamine levels and to have dopamine-like effects.

Side effects include drowsiness and urinary incontinence. Drug interactions to be alert for include anticholinergic drugs such as atropine and scopolamine, and narcotic analgesics such as Tylenol #3 and Vicodin. Additive sedative effects can occur when metoclopramide is given with alcohol, sedatives, hypnotics, narcotics, or tranquilizers such as Valium, Dalmane, Percocet, or Tofranil.

NAUSEA AND/OR VOMITING

Nausea precedes vomiting. It is a feeling of awareness that something is stimulating the vomit center and that vomiting is going to occur. Vomiting is produced by involuntary contraction of the abdominal musculature when the fundus and lower esophageal sphincter are relaxed, which causes a strong ejection of gastric contents. Nausea and vomiting occur when the vomiting center in the brain is activated by any of the following causes:

- migraines
- gallstones
- intestinal obstructions
- irritation of the stomach
- psychological—anxiety, depression, stress, fear, bulimia
- overeating
- eating foods that are spoiled

- drinking too much alcohol
- food allergies
- medication—NSAIDS, chemotherapy
- illness
- motion sickness
- various conditions of the body or disease states
- Projectile vomiting in infants can be a sign of pyloric stenosis, a blockage at the stomach outlet that must be treated immediately.
- Post-operative vomiting is caused by a lessened amount of narcotic or opium derivative in the body as it is excreted over time after the surgery. If left untreated, chronic vomiting can cause malnutrition, dehydration, KCl electrolyte deficiency, heart problems, and arrhythmias.

Other indications to use Antinauseants and Antiemetics include the following:

- *Pregnancy*—No drugs have been approved, but Vitamin B6 may help to reduce emotional stress. There is no deficiency associated with nauseau and vomiting of pregnancy.
- *Bacterial* or *Viral Gastroenteritis*—Acute onset is the most common cause of some type of bacteria or virus. This could be food contamination or *influenza* transmission. This is usually a sudden projectile vomiting that occurs in a one-time attack and does not require medication. The patient generally feels much better after the attack.
- *Psychogenic Vomiting*—Some nausea and vomiting are due to depression, anxiety, and emotional stress.
- *Motion sickness* or *vertigo*. Motion sickness occurs when the body is subjected to accelerations of movement in different directions or under conditions where visual contact with the actual outside horizon is lost. The balance center of the inner ear then sends information to the brain that conflicts with the visual clues of apparently standing still in the interior cabin of a ship or airplane.

Treatment for nausea and vomiting is typically through the relief of medications. Which medication is decided upon depends on certain factors, such as are shown in Table 11-2.

TABLE 11-2 Antihistamines Used as Antiemetics		
Antihistamines		
Dramamine®	Dimenhydrinate	50 mg tabs, 1–2 tablets q 4–6 hours, NTE 300 mg, 6 tablets in 24 hours
Transderm Scop® Anitvert®	Scoplamine meclizine {for vestibular disturbances (inner ear)}	one patch q 3 days

TABLE 11-3   Post-Operative Vomiting Drugs

Centrally acting non-phenothiazines		
Tigan®	trimethobenzamide	250 mg capsules t.i.d.-q.i.d.
Phenothiazines		
Compazine®	prochlorperazine	5–10 mg t.i.d.-q.i.d. tablets and capsules NTE 40 mg/day
Phenergan®	promethazine	12.5 mg, 25 mg, 50 mg tablet, 12.5–25 mg q 4–6 hr as needed

Antihistamines work by competitive inhibition or by blocking H1 receptor sites, slowing the response to the stimuli causing the nausea and vomiting. They are thought to block excitatory labyrinthine impulses at cholinergic synapses in the region of the vestibular nuclei. Side effects include drowsiness and dry mouth. Warnings listed advise to not take antihistamines if you have glaucoma or urinary disturbances.

Post-operative vomiting is generally caused by the decreased amount of narcotic or opium derivative in the body after surgery the drugs used for anesthesia are excreted and the half-lives are accrued (see Table 11-3).

Post-emetogenic is nausea and/or vomiting that occurs during or after chemotherapy administration and is caused by a side effect of the drugs. Serotonin receptors of the 5-HT$_3$ type are located peripherally on vagal nerve terminals and centrally in the chemoreceptor trigger zone of the area postrema. During chemotherapy that induces vomiting, mucosal enterochromaffin cells release serotonin, which stimulates 5-HT$_3$ receptors. This evokes vagal afferent discharge, or firing, inducing vomiting.

Drugs used for post-emetogenic nausea are called 5-HT$_3$ antagonists. These drugs block serotonin receptors from binding with the 5-HT$_3$, which prevents the stimulation of the receptors preventing N/V. Side effects are none to minimal—headache, diarrhea, or constipation. Drug interactions listed are none (see Table 11-4).

Ginger root is an herb that has been known to aid in combating nausea and vomiting. Ginger root lists as a minor side effect a burning stomach.

Ulcers

Ulcers are sores on the inside "flesh" wall of the stomach or intestines, caused by over-production and secretion of the parietal cell. A peptic ulcer is a sore that forms in the lining of the stomach or the duodenum. Symptoms of an ulcer can include burning pain in the upper abdomen, nausea, vomiting, loss of appetite, weight loss, fatigue, deep recurring ache relieved with food or antacids, gastric pain aggravated by general irritants, and nocturnal or nighttime pain.

TABLE 11-4 Drugs Used for Post-emetogenic Nausea

5-HT₃ Antagonists

Zofran®	ondansetron	1. Oral Sol: 4 mg/5 ml–50 ml bottle, 4 mg and 8 mg tablets, 2 mg/ml injectable 2. **Premixed**, 32 mg/50 mL, Oral - 8 mg 30 minutes prior to emetogenic chemotherapy, then BID to TID Infusion - 32 mg over 15 minutes 30 minutes before chemotherapy
Kytril®	granisetron HCl	1 mg tabs BID or infusion 1 mg/ml 10 mcg/Kg over 5 minutes within 30 minutes of administration of chemotherapy
Anzemet®	dolasetron mesylate	50 mg and 100 mg tablets Oral - 100 mg up to 1 hr before chemotherapy

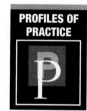

Over 400,000 new cases of peptic ulcers are diagnosed each year, and ulcers are the cause for nearly 40,000 surgeries annually.

Peptic ulcer disease affects all age groups, but is rare in children. Men have twice the risk for ulcers as women do. The risk for duodenal ulcers tends to occur first at around age 25 and continues until age 75; gastric ulcers peak in people between the ages of 55 and 65. There is an 80 percent incidence of duodenal ulcers. (See Figure 11-6.)

A major cause of peptic ulcers is infection with the bacterium *Helicobacter pylori* (*H. pylori*). It is estimated that approximately two-thirds of all ulcers are caused by *H. pylori*. Many people have *H. pylori* infections, but not everyone who has an infection develops a peptic ulcer.

NSAIDs

Some peptic ulcers are caused by the extended use of Nonsteroidal anti-inflammatory drugs (NSAIDs) such as aspirin, ibuprofen, and naproxen sodium.

As you know, NSAID medications such as ibuprofen can be found in most stores and are available without a prescription. Other NSAIDs, such as Celebrex©, require a prescription. NSAIDs are very effective at pain relief (analgesia) and are often prescribed to reduce inflammation.

NSAIDs work to block the effect of an enzyme called cyclooxygenase (Cox), which is critical for producing prostaglandins that protect the lining of the stomach from the damaging effects of acid.

Prostaglandins are produced within the body's cells by the enzyme cyclooxygenase. There actually are two Cox enzymes, Cox-1 and Cox-2. Both enzymes produce prostaglandins that promote inflammation, pain, and fever. However, only Cox-1 produces prostaglandins that support platelets and protect the stomach. Nonsteroidal anti-inflammatory drugs (NSAIDs) block the Cox enzymes and reduce prostaglandins throughout the body. As a consequence, ongoing inflammation, pain, and fever are reduced.

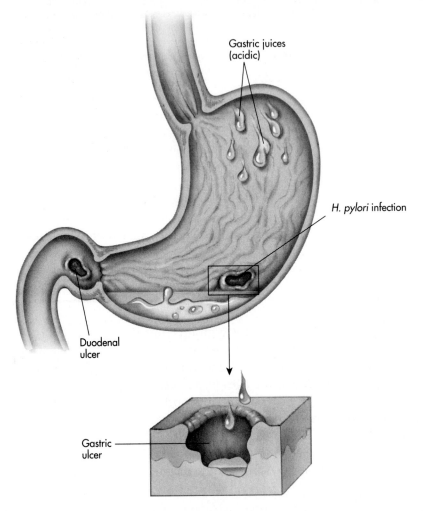

Figure 11-6 An ulcer (*Mulvihill, Mary Lou; Zelman, Mark; Holdaway, Paul; Tompary, Elaine; Turchany, Jill,* Human Diseases, A Systemic Approach, *5th Edition, © 2001. Reprinted by permission of Pearson Education, Inc., Upper Saddle River, NJ*)

One type of prostaglandin (there are many varieties) helps line the stomach with a protective fluid (called gastric mucosa). When the production of this protective fluid is diminished, there is an increased risk for stomach ulcers developing.

This group of drugs is now thought to increase the risk of heart attack and stroke. Studies show an increased risk of cardiovascular events (including heart attack and stroke) in patients on Vioxx® compared with placebo, particularly those who had been taking the drug for longer than 18 months. Vioxx® was pulled from the market in 2004 by its manufacturer because studies indicated that long-term use greatly increased the likelihood of these cardiovascular events, and similar results have been coming out regarding other NSAIDs, such as Celebrex®.

CAUSES AND TREATMENTS

Factors that can induce the over-production of acid include the following:

Smoking   In 1989, the U.S. Surgeon General's report stated that ulcers are more likely to occur, less likely to heal, and more likely to cause death in smokers than in nonsmokers. Some studies show that smoking reduces the bicarbonate produced by the pancreas, interfering with the neutralization of acid in the duodenum. Some research shows that smoking lessens the power of the immune system to fight the *H. pylori* bacteria. The advice is to discontinue smoking habits.

Alcohol   Reports are mixed, but include prevention of *H. pylori* and causing more bleeding. The advice is to decrease alcohol consumption or discontinue in severe cases.

NSAIDs   NSAIDs work by inhibiting prostaglandins, the hormone-like compounds that can cause inflammation. Because prostaglandins also protect the stomach lining, NSAIDs can promote GI distress such as mild upset stomach and bleeding ulcers. NSAIDs do not cause bleeding, but they make bleeding worse.

NSAIDs hinder protective mechanisms, such as the mucosal lining of the stomach, by prostaglandin depletion, causing less protection of the stomach and intestinal wall. Nearly four percent of regular NSAID users develop serious gastrointestinal conditions. Patients are advised to always take NSAID medications with food to help prevent stomach problems. NSAID induced ulcers usually heal once the person stops taking the medication.

Excessive peristalsis   Motility leads to stimulation of the parietal cells to secrete more acid. It is believed by some that the peristalsis that accompanies stress can lead to this. Since diarrhea may be caused by an increase in motility and peristalsis, or "spasms of the colon," antidiarrheals may help in alleviating the acid caused by the increased motility, by reducing motility. Antispasmodics, also known as muscarinic receptor antagonists, are usually prescribed. Antispasmodics cause a direct antispasmodic effect on smooth muscle. An example of this type of medication is Donnatal®–Belladonna alkaloids.

Anticholinergics   These medications inhibit the actions of acetylcholine at the postganglionic parasympathetic neuroeffector sites. Large doses block nicotinic sites, inhibit gastric acid secretion, and decrease GI and urinary tract motility. Moderate doses dilate the pupil and increase heart rate and small doses inhibit salivary and bronchial secretions. A high protein diet causes more HCL to be required for digestion. Drugs prescribed for this include prostaglandin replacement. An example would be Cytotec®–misoprostol. Take misoprostol along with NSAIDs to prevent the thinning of the mucosal lining by increasing the prostaglandin that increases the viscosity of the mucosal lining—100 mg tablets 100 to 200 mcg q.i.d. with food. Dose can be reduced to 100 mcg if the larger dose cannot be tolerated. Available in 100 and 200 mg tablets, as a prostaglandin-like substance or agonist, it stimulates the production of the mucosal lining. By increasing its viscosity, it offers greater protection from the acid when the patient takes the NSAID. Adverse reactions include diarrhea, cramping, miscarriage, premature labor, and birth defects.

> **Note:** This is now one of the ingredients in the Cervical ripening agent PGE and one of the ingredients of the RU486 abortion pill known as Mifeprex®.

Certain foods cause the mast cells to release histamine 2. H2 binds to the H2 receptor site of the parietal cells that line the stomach wall, which triggers the acid to be made and released. This follows the lock and key theory. H2 antagonists enter the H2 receptor in the parietal cell, preventing H2 from binding, by getting to the binding site first. This prevents the lock and key from working, blocking acid production and secretion. This is called competitive inhibition.

Drugs prescribed for this situation include H2 receptor antagonists. Examples are as follows:

- Aciphex® = nizatidine 150 mg tablet 1 tab BID or Qhs and 300 mg 1 tablet Qhs
- Pepcid® = famotidine 20 mg and 40 mg tablets and *RPD Orally*. Disintegrating Tablets, Oral suspension: 40 mg of famotidine per 5 ml, 20 or 40 mg Qhs or BID, intermittent infusion—premixed is 20 mg every 12 hours.
- Tagamet® = cimetidine tablets 200 mg qid, 300 BID, 400 BID and 800 mg BID tablets and 300 mg/2 ml vials for intermittent infusion Q 6–8 hrs
- Zantac® = ranitidine 150 mg and 300 mg tablets, one tablet Qhs or BID, intermittent infusion

Adverse reactions include fatigue, hypertension, muscle pain, bronchiospasm, grand mal seizures, impotence, and gynecomastia.

H. pylori This is a spiral shaped bacterium found in the gut, more specifically, the gastric mucous layer or adherent to the epithelial lining of the stomach. It can over-produce, or multiply. A byproduct of its cell division is an acid production that leads to more acid in the stomach and intestines. *H. pylori* mainly causes about 90 percent of duodenal ulcers and 80 percent of gastric ulcers. Therapy for *H. pylori* infection consists of ten days to two weeks of one or two effective antibiotics, such as amoxicillin, tetracycline (not to be used for children under 12 years old), metronidazole, clarithromycin, plus ranitidine bismuth citrate or bismuth subsalicylate, or a proton pump inhibitor. Acid suppression by the H2 blocker or proton pump inhibitor, in conjunction with the antibiotics, helps alleviate ulcer-related symptoms, helps heal gastric mucosal inflammation, and may enhance efficacy of the antibiotics against *H. pylori* (see Table 11–5 and Table 11-6).

Proton Pump Inhibitors block the enzyme that turns on the H^+–ATPase Enzyme System. By blocking this enzyme, the parietal cell will not secrete hydrogen, which is the last step in making the HCl. Side effects include headache, nausea, and vomiting. Drug interactions—digoxin causes an ↑ in plasma levels of digoxin, while ketoconazole decreases ↓ plasma levels of ketoconazole.

TABLE 11-5   Drugs Used against *H. pylori*

Drug Regimens

Non-PPI Drug Regimen	Bismuth subsalicylate (Pepto Bismol®) 525 mg QID + metronidazole (Flagyl®) 250 mg QID + tetracycline 500 mg QID* × 2 wks + H2 receptor antagonist therapy as directed × 4 wks
Double Drug Theory	Lansoprazole 30 mg TID + amoxicillin 1 g TID × 2 weeks
Triple Drug Theory	1. omeprazole 20 mg BID + clarithromycin 500 mg BID + amoxicillin 1 g BID × 10 days 2. Lansoprazole 30 mg BID + clarithromycin 500 mg BID + amoxicillin 1 g BID × 10 days

TABLE 11-6   Drugs Used against *H. pylori*

PPI	Availability	Dosage
Aciphex®	20 mg tablets	20 to 40 mg qd
Prilosec®	10 and 20 mg capsules	20 or 40 mg Qd
Nexium®	20 and 40 mg capsules	20 or 40 mg Qd
Prevacid®	15 and 30 mg enteric coated delayed release capsule	15 or 30 mg qd ac
Protonix®	40 mg delayed release tablet	1 tablet qd

Nutrition

Modern daily food intake recommendations are based upon the *Nutrition and Your Health: Dietary Guidelines for Americans*. This publication was first developed in 1980 by the U.S. Department of Agriculture (USDA) and the Department of Health and Human Services (DHHS) for use in consumer nutrition education efforts with healthy Americans aged two years and older. The fifth edition, issued in 2000, contains ten guidelines. Its message, built around three actions, "Aim, Build, and Choose," strives to motivate Americans with the following advice:

- Aim for fitness.
- Aim for a healthy weight.
- Be physically active each day.
- Build a healthy base.
- Let the Pyramid guide your food choices.
- Choose a variety of grains daily, especially whole grains.

- Choose a variety of fruits and vegetables daily.
- Keep food safe to eat.
- Choose sensibly.
- Choose a diet that is low in saturated fat and cholesterol and moderate in total fat.
- Choose beverages and foods to moderate your intake of sugars.
- Choose and prepare foods with less salt.
- If you drink alcoholic beverages, do so in moderation.

The Recommended Dietary Allowances (RDA) were established to cover the nutritional needs of all normal, healthy persons living in the United States. The Food and Nutrition Board of the National Academy of Sciences set the values for the RDAs on the bases of human and animal research. They usually meet every five years to review current research on nutrients.

Note: RDA stands for the Recommended Dietary Allowance, although many refer to it as the Recommended Daily Allowance. The RDA is being revised and will be called the Dietary Reference Intake (DRI). The revision is a collaborative effort between the United States and Canada. Until publication of the new DRI, the information reported herein refers to the old RDA schedule.

Basic Nutrition

There are six categories of nutrition described as follows:

MACRONUTRIENTS

There are three types of macronutrients: carbohydrates, proteins, and fats. Kilocalories (kcal) are the units by which energy is measured when referring to the energy taken in by food and expended with exercise. Fats are the most concentrated source of food energy. One gram of fat supplies about 9 kcal, compared to the 4 kcal supplied by carbohydrates and protein. The three micronutrients—vitamins, minerals, and water—provide no calories or energy.

CARBOHYDRATES

Sources of carbohydrates include fruit, vegetables, whole grains, and legumes, which all contain fiber, starch, and some vitamins and minerals. The two types of carbohydrates are simple and complex. Simple carbohydrates are known as sugars and contain no energy-yielding calories. They are "empty calories," for example, candy. Complex carbohydrates are known as starches. They take longer to be broken down in the digestive tract and have more nutritional value than sugars. An example is whole grain bread.

Carbohydrates such as starch and sugar provide immediate energy and are the most readily available sources of food energy. During digestion and metabolism, all carbohydrates are broken down to a simple sugar called glucose for use as the body's principal energy source. Glucose is stored in the liver and muscle tissue as glycogen. A carbohydrate-rich diet is necessary to maintain muscle glycogen, the preferred fuel for most types of exercise. Dietary recommendations state that 55 percent of daily calories should be complex carbohydrates. Simple carbohydrates should be limited to 10 percent or less of daily calories.

FATS

Dietary fats are the body's only source of the fatty acid linoleic acid that is essential for growth and skin maintenance. Fat insulates and protects the body's organs against trauma and exposure to cold and is involved in the absorption and transport of the fat-soluble vitamins.

Fats are the source of fatty acids, which are divided into two categories: saturated and unsaturated (including monounsaturated and polyunsaturated fatty acids). These fatty acids differ from each other chemically, based on the nature of the bond between carbon and hydrogen atoms.

As a general rule, saturated fat is solid at room temperature and is derived mainly from animal sources. Unsaturated fat is liquid at room temperature and is found mainly in plants. Monounsaturated and polyunsaturated fats should be emphasized, since they tend to lower the blood cholesterol level. Saturated fats tend to raise the level of blood cholesterol, and high blood cholesterol levels are associated with an increased risk of coronary heart disease. Of the two types of fat, saturated is considered bad fat because the entire chain of fat has hydrogens covering it, which leads to increased LDL and cholesterol. Saturated fats contain more cholesterol and are derived from animal sources such as meat (pork and beef), dairy, and dairy products. They are known as hydrogenated fats and are solid at room temperature. Butter, skin of the animal, and mayonnaise are saturated fats, along with steak and pork chops. Oils such as palm and coconut oil actually cause the body to manufacture cholesterol.

Unsaturated fat is considered good or better fat to eat because it has double bonds-monounsaturated fat. Examples are olive oil, canola oil. While polyunsaturated fats are found in most other vegetable oils and nuts, deep cold water fish such as salmon, mackerel, tuna or bluefish are all sources of the "good" fat.

Note: Current studies show diets that contain a certain type of polyunsaturated fatty acid are associated with a decreased risk for heart disease in certain people.

Hydrogenated fats are created when an oil that is largely unsaturated, such as corn oil, has hydrogen added to it. Taking the unsaturated fat and chemically making it saturated by adding hydrogens produces trans-fatty acid. Trans-fatty acids act like saturated fats in the body. Hydrogenated fat is solid or semi-solid at room temperature. The best example of this is margarine. Hydrogenated fats are found in almost every processed food in the supermarket. Hydrogenated oils are fats with *trans-fatty acids* that have the same capacity to do harm as saturated fats. Research has shown that trans-fatty acids increase the LDL cholesterol, decrease the HDL cholesterol, and thus increase the risk of coronary heart disease.

Worse yet are the trans-fatty acids also found in most packaged foods and listed on the label as partially hydrogenated or hydrogenated oil. They are chemically altered (processed) fats. The more solid and hydrogenated the fat is, the more trans-fatty acids there are in the product. Commercial peanut butter is an example.

Palm and coconut oils are high in saturated fats, even though they stay liquid at room temperature. They will raise blood levels of bad cholesterol or LDL and VLDL and lower good cholesterol of HDL.

Essential fatty acids, Omega-3 and Omega-6, are fats that are needed by the body, but the body does not make them. Omega-3 is found in fish and helps prevent heart disease, arthritis, and cancer growth and development.

The functions of fats or lipids in the body are as follows:

- Helps to provide lubrication
- Stored fat used for
  - Energy reserve
  - Insulation—provides warmth
  - As cushion or protection, acts as shock absorbers to protect vital organs
- Helps metabolize carbohydrates and proteins more efficiently
- Carrier for fat soluble Vitamins A, D, E, K

These fats should be avoided: saturated (animal), hydrogenated or partially hydrogenated fats or oils (made more semisolid at room temperature), trans fats (chemically altered), palm and coconut oils that raise blood bad cholesterol (LDL and VLDL), fats hidden in animal skin and meat, cookies, crackers, bread, peanut butter, margarine, and frozen foods. More olive oil and canola oil should be eaten.

No more that 30 percent of food intake calories should be from fat, and then preferably from monosaturated fat. The new proposed food pyramid may require more fat that is monosaturated.

PROTEIN

The nine essential proteins have all essential amino acids. Essential proteins are found in the muscle of the animal such as: Meat, dairy, fish, beef, chicken, and pork. Incomplete proteins come from plant-based foods such as soy, tofu, beans, and peanuts. Building blocks for the body are enzymes, hormones, and antibodies. Proteins are also necessary components of hormones, enzymes, and blood-plasma transport systems. Protein is not a significant energy source during rest or exercise. However, the body will use protein for energy when calorie or carbohydrate intake is inadequate (during fasting or a low carbohydrate diet). Protein is necessary to make and repair body cells, tissue, and muscle.

Protein breaks down into amino acids. There are 20 amino acids that the body needs. The nine essential amino acids the body must take in through food are as follows:

- valine
- leucine
- isoleucine
- threonine
- lysine
- histidine
- phenylalanine
- tryptophan
- methionine

The 11 amino acids that the body makes are as follows:

- glycine
- alanine
- serine
- aspartic acid
- glutamic acid
- asparagine
- glutamine
- arginine
- tyrosine
- cysteine
- proline

Following are some adverse reactions to certain nutrients:

- Excessive protein intake causes urinary calcium loss.
- Restriction of protein results in decreased iron intake.
- Lipoproteins carry fatty substances.

The requirement for dietary fats is 15 percent of total calories, 0.8 g per kg of body weight. When someone eats a lot of extra protein, a lot of extra nitrogen must be excreted, so a lot of urine needs to be made, which requires a lot of extra fluid. This places many athletes, particularly those less than amply hydrated, at risk for dehydration. In extreme cases, excess protein or amino acid intake can lead to kidney damage.

VITAMINS

Consuming the RDA requirements of vitamins may help to prevent diseases and to maintain good health. Good food instead of vitamin supplements is preferred, because food has fiber. The following are for the average adult male and female 25 to 50 years old.

Fat-soluble vitamins are found in the fat and oily parts of foods. They tend to be stored in the liver and adipose tissue and remain there, rather than being excreted like most water-soluble vitamins. The storage of fat-soluble vitamins in the body makes it possible to survive long periods of time without having to supplement them in the diet. Because they are stored in the body, there is a risk of toxicity with fat-soluble vitamins.

Vitamin A—Betacarotene is found in orange, yellow-orange, and green leafy vegetable foods such as carrots, pumpkin, apricot, squash, peaches, and spinach. Vitamin A is found in animals also, but only in beef liver and fish liver oil.

Most of the body's vitamin A is stored in the liver as retinyl palmitate, then released into the blood circulation as retinal. It binds to *retinol* binding protein and prealbumin (transthyretin). It helps with eyesight and epithelial cells and tissues (skin cells).

Deficiencies in vitamin A may cause night blindness; xerosis (dryness) of the conjunctiva and cornea; xerophthalmia and keratomalacia; keratinization of lung, GI tract, and urinary tract; and increased susceptibility to infections. Follicular hyperkeratosis of the skin is common (raised pink bumps where hair exits).

Acute toxicity occurs in children from taking large doses ($> 100,000 \mu$g or 300,000 IU), resulting in increased intracranial pressure and vomiting. Death may ensue, unless ingestion is discontinued. Chronic toxicity in adult women may cause birth defects in infants of women receiving 13-*cis*-retinoic acid (isotretinoin) for skin conditions during pregnancy. Adults may also exhibit *carotenosis*, in which the skin (not including the sclera) becomes deep yellow or orange-yellow, especially on the palms and soles. Early warning signs may include sparse or coarse hair, eyebrows thinning, dry rough skin, and cracked lips. RDA requirements suggest a daily intake of males-5000 IU and females-4000 IU of this vitamin.

Vitamin D—Sunshine allows the skin to make vitamin D with cholesterol. Milk is fortified with vitamin D; canned salmon and tuna also contain it. The main function of vitamin D is to help the absorption of calcium from the intestine to make stronger bones and teeth. Deficiency causes a metabolic bone disease called *rickets* in children and *osteomalacia* in adults. A softening of the bones can lead to bowed legs. RDA recommendations are 400 IU for both males and females.

Vitamin E—Found in wheat germ oil, sunflower seeds, and nuts, vitamin E helps to make the reproductive hormones. It manufactures RBCs (red blood counts) and WBCs (white blood counts) and helps convert energy.

This vitamin deficiency is generally caused by *malabsorption*, not by lack of ingestion, and may cause disorders of the reproductive system; abnormalities of muscle, liver, and bone marrow; hemolysis of RBCs; defective embryogenesis; brain dysfunction; and a disorder of capillary permeability. RDA recommendations for vitamin E are males 15 IU and females 12 IU.

Vitamin K is primarily found in dark green leafy vegetables. Vitamin K is necessary for forming clots. It is used as an antidote for too much coumadin (hemorrhaging). Vitamin K controls the formation of coagulation factors II (prothrombin), VII (proconvertin), IX (Christmas factor, plasma thromboplastin component), and X (Stuart factor) in the liver. Vitamin K is necessary for coagulation and for the calcium uptake in bones.

Deficiency is rare in adults due to microbiologic flora of the normal gut, which synthesizes menaquinones (from Vitamin K). However, the following can contribute to an increased need for Vitamin K: trauma, extensive surgery, long-term parenteral nutrition with or without treatment with broad-spectrum antibiotics, and overdose of coumadin. Drugs that contribute to vitamin K-related hemorrhagic disease are anticonvulsants, anticoagulants, certain antibiotics (particularly cephalosporins), salicylates, and megadoses of vitamin A or E.

Note: In infants, the livers, where vitamin K is stored, are not fully developed. So Vitamin K deficiency in breastfed infants remains a major worldwide cause of infant morbidity and mortality. One to seven days postpartum, the infant may have skin, GI, or chest hemorrhage. RDA requirements state that males receive 80 mcg and females 65 mcg.

Water-soluble vitamins, for the most part, are carried in the bloodstream and excreted in the urine. They are needed in small doses, are unlikely to be toxic, and have to be replaced on a regular daily basis. Vitamins B-1, B-2, B-6, B-12, and C are known as water-soluble vitamins. Excess of Vitamin C and B6 may have serious side effects. Vitamins are destroyed by high heat or overcooking. Vitamin Bs are from animal products and enriched breads and cereals.

Vitamin B1—Known as thiamin and found in fortified bread and cereals, sunflower seeds, peanuts, wheat bran, beef liver, pork, seafood, egg-yolk, and beans, vitamin B1 is necessary for carbohydrate metabolism, possibly in nerve conduction, essential for the synthesis of acetylcholine and muscle movement and gamma-aminobutyric acid (GABA). It is used in the manufacture of hydrochloric acid, and therefore plays a part in digestion.

Deficiency causes *beriberi*, affecting peripheral neurologic, cerebral, cardiovascular, and GI systems. Those most at risk are breastfeeding infants whose mothers are thiamin-deficient, adults with high consumption of polished rice, alcoholics, patients on renal dialysis, patients on total parenteral nutrition (TPN) (high concentrations of dextrose infusions or frequent or long-term infusions can lead to increased need for B1, especially if vitamin B1 is not administered), and patients with hypermetabolic states in which more carbohydrate is needed or metabolized (for example, fever, infection, pregnancy, and strenuous exercise). RDA recommendations for Vitamin B1 are males 1.4 mg and females 1 mg.

Vitamin B2, also know as riboflavin, can be found in organ meats, nuts, cheese, eggs, milk, lean meat, green leafy vegetables, fish, legumes, whole grains, and yogurt. The body requires B2 to use oxygen and metabolize amino acids, fatty acids, and carbohydrates.

Riboflavin activates vitamin B6 (pyridoxine), which helps to create niacin and assists the adrenal gland. B6 is used for red blood cell formation, antibody production, cell respiration, and growth. Vitamin B2 is needed for the health of the mucous membranes in the digestive tract and aids absorption of iron and vitamin B6.

Deficiency of vitamin B2 leads to oral, eye, skin, and genital lesions; dizziness; hair loss; insomnia; light sensitivity; poor digestion; retarded growth; slow mental responses; and burning feet. RDA recommendations are for males 1.6 mg and for females 1.2 mg.

Vitamin B3—Also known as Niacin, vitamin B3 is found in meat and amino acids. Vitamin B3 is very important in oxidation-reduction reactions, and is vital in cell metabolism.

Deficiencies of niacin and tryptophan, a precursor that allows the body to synthesize niacin, are the main causes of *pellagra*. Pellegra affects the skin, mucous *membrane*, GI and brain/cns systems, with photosensitive rash, scarlet stomatitis, glossitis, diarrhea, and mental aberrations. Deficiency is found in diets high in corn (maize), common in India and Central and South America. RDA requirements for males are 18 mg and females 13 mg.

Vitamin B5—Pantothenic acid is found in beef, brewer's yeast, eggs, fresh vegetables, kidney, legumes, liver, mushrooms, nuts, pork, fish, torula yeast, whole rye flour, and whole wheat. Vitamin B5 is important for the secretion of hormones (cortisone), which assist metabolism and help to fight allergies, and for maintenance of healthy skin, muscles, and nerves. Pantothenic acid is used in the release of energy as well as the metabolism of fat, protein, and carbohydrates. It is used in the manufacture of lipids (fats), neurotransmitters, steroid hormones, and hemoglobin.

> **Note:** Some are of the opinion that pantothenic acid is also helpful in fighting wrinkles and graying of the hair. Deficiency is extremely rare. Adult volunteers on a deficient diet experienced malaise, abdominal discomfort, and burning feet associated with paresthesias, which responded to pantothenic acid. No RDA guidelines here, but 10 to 100 mg is suggested.

Vitamin B6, also known as pyridoxine, can be found in fortified cereals, beans, meat, poultry, fish, and some fruits and vegetables. When caloric intake is low, the body needs vitamin B6 to help convert stored carbohydrate or other nutrients to glucose to maintain normal blood sugar levels. Important in blood, CNS, skin metabolism, and erythropoiesis. It is also essential for red blood cell metabolism, manufacture of hemoglobin to carry oxygen, function of nervous and immune systems due to its protein metabolism and cellular growth, and for the conversion of tryptophan to niacin. B6 helps maintain the normal range of blood glucose, and the health of lymphoid organs (thymus, spleen, and lymph nodes) that make white blood cells. Vitamin B6 is needed for the synthesis of neurotransmitters such as serotonin and dopamine, required for normal nerve cell communication.

> **Note:** While a shortage of vitamin B6 will limit these functions, supplements of this vitamin do not enhance them in well-nourished individuals.

Vitamin B6 deficiency can result in a form of anemia that is similar to iron deficiency anemia. B6 deficiency can decrease antibody production and suppress the immune response. Signs and symptoms include dermatitis, glossitis (a sore tongue), depression, confusion, and convulsions.

Toxicity of vitamin B6 may cause sensory ataxia, profound lower limb impairment of position and vibration sense, and nerve damage to the arms and legs. This neuropathy is usually related to high intake of vitamin B6 from supplements and is reversible when supplementation is stopped. Senses of touch, temperature, and pain are only somewhat affected. RDA requirements for vitamin B6 in both males and females is 2 mg.

Vitamin B9, more commonly known as folic acid, is found in barley, beef, bran, brewer's yeast, brown rice, cheese, chicken, dates, green leafy vegetables, lamb, legumes, lentils, liver, milk, mushrooms, oranges, split peas, pork, root vegetables, salmon, tuna, wheat germ, whole grains, and whole wheat. Vitamin B9 is important for energy production and the formation of red blood cells. It strengthens immunity, healthy cell division and replication, protein metabolism, and prevents depression and anxiety.

Deficiency in folic acid can be serious and may result in sore, red tongue, anemia, apathy, digestive disturbances, fatigue, graying hair, growth impairment, insomnia, labored breathing, memory problems, paranoia, weakness, and the birth defect spina bifida if a pregnant mother does not intake this vitamin, especially in the first trimester. RDA requirements suggest a daily dose of folic acid of 400 mcg.

Vitamin B12, also known as cyanocobalamin, needs to be supplemented in vegetarians because it is only found in animal products. Vitamin B12 is not found in plants, but in the microorganisms found on plants. Therefore, sources for vegetarians are nutritional yeast supplement, fortified cereals, soy milk, and taking a vitamin supplement. Vitamin B12 is needed for cell division, to make DNA, and blood formation (RBC's). Vitamin B12 is bound to the protein in food. Hydrochloric acid in the stomach releases B12 from protein during digestion. Once released, B12 combines with a substance called intrinsic factor (IF) before it is absorbed into the bloodstream.

Deficiency is a very serious problem leading ultimately to irreversible nerve damage signified by numbness and tingling in the hands and feet. Signs and symptoms include fatigue, weakness, nausea, constipation, flatulence, loss of appetite, weight loss, difficulty in maintaining balance, depression, confusion, poor memory, and soreness of the mouth or tongue.

Note: Pernicious anemia is an anemia that occurs in the absence of intrinsic factor, normally present in the stomach. Vitamin B12 binds with IF before it is absorbed and used by the body. An absence of intrinsic factor prevents normal absorption of B12 and results in pernicious anemia. Patients with pernicious anemia need IM injections of B12, as it is a chronic condition requiring monitoring by a physician and lifelong supplementation of vitamin B12. RDA recommendations are 2 to 3 mcg for both males and females.

Vitamin C, or ascorbic acid, is found in citrus fruits, oranges, lemons, limes, and grapefruits. Vitamin C is an *antioxidant*, which prevents free radicals from causing cancer. Citric acid or ascorbic acid is essential for collagen formation and helps maintain the integrity of connective tissue, bone or osteoid tissue, and teeth or dentin. Important for wound healing and recovery from burns, vitamin C helps the absorption of iron. Vitamin C functions as a redox system in the cells of the body. It activates enzymes that hydroxylate procollagen proline and lysine to procollagen hydroxyproline and hydroxylysine.

Severe deficiency results in *scurvy*, an acute or chronic disease of bleeding gums, with poor dentin formation, weakened and leaking capillaries, defects in bone and related structures, wounds that heal poorly and break open easily, and a poor immune system. RDA recommendations for both males and females is 60 mg. Many nutritionists suggest 100 mg per day.

MINERALS

Minerals are inorganic compounds much smaller than vitamins that occur in much simpler forms; but like vitamins, minerals do not provide energy. There are dozens of minerals found in nature and of them, 21 are essential for human nutrition. Minerals also act as helpers in delivering nutrients and aiding in certain functions in the body. They are different, however, from vitamins due to the fact that they are indestructible. Minerals are not made by the body; therefore, *exogenous* sources must be used.

Some minerals, such as calcium and phosphorus, are used to build bones and teeth. Others are important components of hormones, such as iodine in thyroxine. Iron is essential for the formation of hemoglobin, the oxygen carrier within red blood cells. Certain minerals called electrolytes help regulate muscle contraction, conduction of nerve impulses, and regulation of normal heart rhythm.

Minerals are classified into two groups, based on the body's need. Major minerals are needed in amounts greater than 100 mg per day. Calcium, phosphorus, magnesium, sodium, and chloride fall into this category. Minor minerals, or trace elements, are needed in amounts less than 100 mg per day. Iron, zinc, selenium, copper, and iodine are minor minerals. Minerals have no calories and do not provide energy.

Minerals are very important for numerous regulations of body functions. Certain minerals and their purposes are listed as follows:

- Calcium—important to bones, muscles, nerves, and blood development
- Iron—necessary to keep oxygen in the carried blood; RDA males 8 mg females 18 mg
- Phosphorus—helps builds bones and teeth, along with calcium
- Sodium—regulates body fluids
- Zinc—aids in the healing process
- Potassium—proper muscle memory function
- Selenium—helps make efficient immune system, supports thyroid, and helps make antioxidants; RDA 55 mcg
- Magnesium—aids in energy metabolism and protein synthesis, needed for more than 300 biochemical reactions in the body, aids in maintaining normal muscle and nerve function and steady heart rhythm, and keeps bones strong; RDA 300 to 400 mg

WATER

Found as 60 percent of adult's body weight, the average adult needs about six to eight 8 oz. glasses of water a day. Most water should come from liquids and foods. Water is indispensable and abundant in the body. It actually forms the major part of every tissue within the body and provides the medium for which most of the body's activities are conducted. It also facilitates many of the metabolic reactions that occur in the body and helps transport vital materials to the cells. One function of great importance is that water serves as the vehicle in which glycogen is transported into muscle cells. Glycogen is often referred to as muscle fuel, because it powers muscle contractions.

Determining Your Water Requirements

Body Weight $\times$ 0.6 $\div$ 12

Example:

200(lbs.) $\times$ 0.6 $\div$ 12 = 10 (8 oz. glasses of water a day)

Regular intake helps maintain normal functions of the body. Thirst is a weak signal to drink water. Lack of water can lead to dehydration.

Food Guide Pyramid

The food guide pyramid was developed by the USDA and supported by the Department of Health and Human Services (1984) and is currently being revised to reflect more individual dietary needs. The Pyramid is a food guide for people to make healthy food choices. Pay close attention to the serving sizes in each category. (See Figure 11-7.)

FOOD ALLERGIES

Some people develop food allergies to all kinds of foods. Food allergies involve the immune system and can be quite troublesome for those who experience such symptoms as swelling, hives, rashes, nasal congestion, asthma, nausea, diarrhea, and gas. Symptoms can be immediate or delayed up to 48 hours after eating the food. They can be severe and life threatening, causing anaphylactic shock.

While food allergies can sometimes cause a life-threatening event, food intolerance will have the same symptoms as food allergies but without involving the immune system. For example, a lactose deficiency can cause symptoms similar to mild allergy—gas and diarrhea. These symptoms need an expert to evaluate. Lactose intolerance also includes mucous lining thinning, cramping, and bleeding during defecation, whereas allergy to milk would not produce these effects.

Total Parenteral Nutrition

A TPN is all the food and calories that the body needs given intravenously. It is used for patients with long-term requirements for intravenous feeding, who cannot receive adequate oral intake of nutrients to meet physiologic

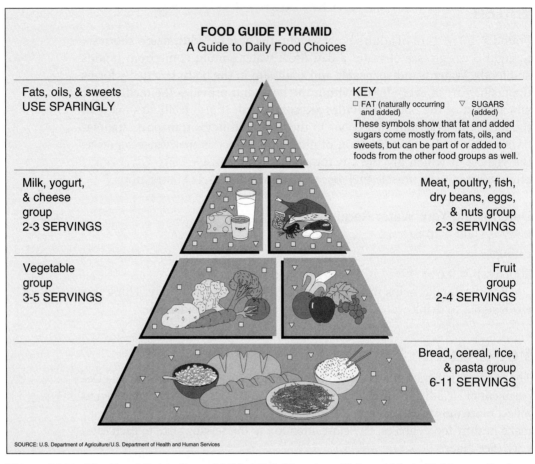

FOOD GUIDE PYRAMID
A Guide to Daily Food Choices

Fats, oils, & sweets
USE SPARINGLY

KEY
□ FAT (naturally occurring and added)   ▽ SUGARS (added)
These symbols show that fat and added sugars come mostly from fats, oils, and sweets, but can be part of or added to foods from the other food groups as well.

Milk, yogurt, & cheese group
2-3 SERVINGS

Meat, poultry, fish, dry beans, eggs, & nuts group
2-3 SERVINGS

Vegetable group
3-5 SERVINGS

Fruit group
2-4 SERVINGS

Bread, cereal, rice, & pasta group
6-11 SERVINGS

SOURCE: U.S. Department of Agriculture/U.S. Department of Health and Human Services

Figure 11-7 The Food Guide Pyramid (*Mulvihill, Mary Lou; Zelman, Mark; Holdaway, Paul; Tompary, Elaine; Turchany, Jill,* Human Diseases, A Systemic Approach*, 5th Edition, © 2001. Reprinted by permission of Pearson Education, Inc., Upper Saddle River, NJ*)

needs through the gastrointestinal system. The conditions that may require a TPN would include hypercatabolic states such as patients with burns, sepsis, trauma, various gastrointestinal diseases, renal failure, and pancreatitis. Some patients who refuse to eat or cannot eat will also benefit from a TPN.

INDICATIONS

A TPN is required when a patient is in one of the following situations:

- chooses not to eat, such as in a case of anorexia or depression
- is unable to eat after a mouth surgery or injury to the mouth, or is in a coma
- should not eat—pre-operative or post-operative patient
- requires more nutrition than the average person can eat to provide adequate calories and protein, such as in the case of the burn patient
- is unable to absorb or digest nutrients properly via the alimentary tract, for example, with malabsorption or malnutrition, such as in short bowel syndrome

- has a disease state that is causing a bowel obstruction or needs prolonged bowel rest due to pancreatitis
- has severe weight loss, gastrointestinal fistula

Providing good nutrition for the patient's well being and progress toward good health and recovery is a team effort by the physician, nurse, pharmacist, dietitian, and social worker.

Physician will decide if the patient needs to have TPN. If so, the patient will be assessed and appropriate nutrition and electrolytes ordered, after evaluation of lab values for potential TPN line infections.

Nurse will hold all key information during the TPN therapy for all health care workers. The nurse will monitor quality care for parenteral nutrition therapy and central venous catheters, inspecting for infection. The nurse will be involved in the discharge planning and patient education of home TPN infusion therapy. The nurse may also follow up with the home TPN therapy patients post-discharge from the hospital.

Pharmacist will assess many factors of total *parenteral* nutrition for each patient and evaluate the physical, chemical, and therapeutic compatibility of the parenteral nutrition solution with other drugs that the patient is on. The pharmacist will also evaluate the stability of the TPN products. The pharmacist will assist the physician in initiating, maintaining, and monitoring the TPN therapy's effect on the patient's disease state and metabolic condition. The pharmacist will be a resource and reference for provision of educational programs on important parenteral nutrition subject matter and assist in the planning and coordination of home TPN therapy orders.

Dietitian will determine the nutritional status and TPN needs of the specific patient, and then develop and initiate a plan of nutritional care accordingly. The dietician will usually watch and evaluate the nutritional status continually and recommend changes as needed. The dietician may be involved in educating patients, physicians, and other health professionals on the various types and methods of nutritional support and delivery systems for both hospital and home use.

Social Worker assesses and evaluates the patient's environment and abilities, family's ability and level of understanding of TPN, and any psychosocial issues that may affect the caretaker's or the patient's ability to cope with TPN therapy. The social worker may assist and work closely with the nurses in regards to the discharge planning of the home TPN therapy patients to facilitate a smooth transition from institution to home.

A TPN contains carbohydrates in the form of dextrose, lipids in a fat emulsion of fatty acids and glycerol, protein in the form of amino acids, vitamins, minerals, and water.

A TPN is a solution that has dextrose and amino acids as its base, plus vitamins, minerals, electrolytes, and water. It is commonly called a 2 in 1, or 2:1. Another type of a TPN is a TNA, or Total Nutrient Admixture, also known as a 3 in 1, or a 3:1. This is made up of the preceding ingredients, plus a fat emulsion, or lipid. A TNA is a TPN, but not all TPNs are TNAs. A 3:1 is a TPN, but a 2:1 is not a TNA. Because many times a mixture of fat, dextrose, and amino acids can clog the vein or heart, many protocols call for the fat emulsion to be administered separately.

TWO TYPES OF TPN LINES

There are two kinds of TPN lines for infusion. The central line is attached via the superior vena cava to the heart, and the peripheral line is attached to an extremity, usually in the arm at the wrist or the back of the knee (see Table 11-7).

In the central line infusion, the amino acids and dextrose solution with additives are mixed in a one-bag-per-day system at many hospitals, while at other hospitals a 24-hour supply of one-liter TPN bags is made. The fat emulsions are a separate solution, which are added to the intravenous tubing at a specific connection port at some hospitals.

At other hospitals, the fat emulsions or lipids are added to the TPN mixture. Starting and stopping the TPN should be done gradually. The administration of the TPN is to be weaned. The starting rate should be no more than 50 cc/hour for 4–6 hours. The rate can be increased 25 percent every 4–6 hours. Weaning is accomplished by decreasing the rate by 25 percent every 4–6 hours.

Blood glucose monitoring is recommended 4–6 hours after TPN initiation. Because the patient is on dextrose intravenously, a diabetic state can be induced, and therefore insulin may be needed.

Peripheral venous nutrition (PVN)—A peripheral TPN is used when a patient is unable to ingest adequate calories orally or enterally or when central venous nutrition is not feasible. Perhaps the patient has nausea or is a central line risk patient. The TPN solution can be caustic to the peripheral veins. Solution is commonly made with 4.25 percent amino acid concentration and 10 percent dextrose. The IV fat emulsion should be run simultaneously with the PVN to minimize thrombophlebitis (unless contraindicated).

Formulas for TPNs can be made from a predetermined "basic" replenishment standard or custom. A standard TPN solution is often the answer to the pharmacoeconomics of total parenteral nutritional therapy, as it can be cost effective and meet most patients' nutritional needs.

Electrolytes are substances that dissociate into positively and negatively charged ions in aqueous solution (see Table 11-8). Electrolytes help to conduct electrical current in the body in order for muscle and nerves to work together for normal contractibility and messaging. Electrolytes are included when ordering the standard TPN solution. Sometimes an electrolyte-free solution is used, and then the physician orders the more appropriate specific electrolytes for that patient (see Table 11-9).

Note: Vitamin K is not included in the MVI-12 vial, and 10 mg needs to be added each week. Sometimes an older doctor will order "1 amp,"

TABLE 11-7   The Use of a Central Line versus a Peripheral Line Can Be Distinguished by the Following Criteria

Peripheral TPN Line	Central TPN Line
Less than 2 weeks of therapy	Greater than 3 weeks of therapy
Central catheter risk	Collapsed or rolling veins
Less than or equal to 2000 daily calories	Greater than or equal to 3000 daily calories
Less than or equal to 10% dextrose	Greater than 10% dextrose
Less than or equal to 10% lipid	Greater than 10% lipid
Limited NPO (short period of time)	

meaning one vial of 10 cc. If the patient is on anticoagulant therapy, such as with warfarin/Coumadin®, the doctor, pharmacist, and dietitian must be consulted on the lab results. They must be in agreement before Vitamin K can be added. Vitamin K helps in clotting, but may exacerbate a condition of stroke or MI.

Some patients may require selenium and zinc supplementation. Zinc is good for healing. Too much zinc may throw off the copper, and too much copper will lower zinc.

Insulin can be added to the TPN bag if needed to offset hyperglycemia. Sometimes insulin is added "on the floor" by the nurse. If the patient is a "brittle diabetic," it is possible that the patient's most immediate blood glucose reading must be taken by the nurse and the appropriate amount of insulin adjusted.

Note: Only regular insulin can be added to a TPN, as it is clear, or particle free.

Lipids are fats that are in an emulsion form. They are used as a calorie source, especially for burn victims. Lipids are used to prevent fatty acid deficiency. Fat emulsions are available as a 10 percent product (which is 1.1 Kcal/cc) and as a 20 percent product (which is 2.0 Kcal/cc). There are also 5 and 30 percent formulas available, all in 250 or 500 ml containers.

A three-in-one (3-in-1) mixture is a TPN in which the fat emulsion is mixed in with the TPN dextrose and amino acids. This is not done at many hospitals because the mixture is hard to keep "homogenized." It is an emulsion that must stay an emulsion, or else the "oiling out" can cause problems in the administration, clogging of the line, or even clotting.

TABLE 11-8 Suggested Daily Electrolytes	
Potassium	50–80 mEq/day
Sodium	60–120 mEq/day
Calcium	8–20 mEq/day (160–400 mg)
Magnesium	10–30 mEq/day (120–360 mg)
Chloride	100–120 mEq/day
Phosphate	12–30 mmol/day (463–927 mg)
Acetate	no defined daily need

TABLE 11-9 Suggested Electrolytes versus Electrolyte-free TPN Solutions		
	Standard Electrolyte	Electrolyte Free
Sodium (mEq/L)	35	0
Potassium	30	0
Calcium	5	0
Magnesium	5	0
Chloride	47–50	17–20
Phosphate	14.3	0
Acetate	67–74	37–44

Medications that are extremely necessary and compatible with the TPN may be needed at some time, and could be added to the admixture (see Table 11-10 and Table 11-11). These include H2 antagonists, Pepcid® or Zantac®; antidiarrheal for some cancer patients, Sandostatin® (decreases growth hormone); or anti-emetics, Reglan®.

TPN SOLUTIONS FOR SPECIAL DISEASE STATE DIETARY NEEDS

Patients with *renal failure* need a balance of both essential and nonessential amino acids. Renamine® contains only essential amino acids. Close monitoring of blood serum ammonia levels is important in kidney patients. Careful attention must be paid to the fluid restricted patient, by increasing the concentration of dextrose and fat emulsion in order to reduce volume.

Patients with chronic liver disease, such as drug induced hepatic cirrhosis or cirrhosis of the liver, are usually malnourished. TPN complications such as an infection can compromise any patient's nutritional status. Hepatamine can be used with patients with hepatic encephalopathy. It is a liver-specific amino acid mixture.

The *catabolic* patient has a metabolic response to injury, burn, or sepsis that generates a neuroendocrine response which induces hypermetabolism, proteolysis, insulin resistance with hyperglycemia, and a depletion of lean body mass. The bottom line is that the patient needs more calories than

TABLE 11-10	Standard Multivitamin Additive Is MVI-12 and Should Be Added Every Day
Vitamin C (ascorbic acid)	100 mg
Vitamin A (retinol)	3300 IU
Vitamin D (ergocalciferol)	200 IU
Vitamin B1 (thiamine)	3.0 mg
Vitamin B2 (riboflavin)	3.6 mg
Vitamin B6 (pyridozine HCl)	4.0 mg
Niacinamide	40.0 mg
Pantothenic acid	15.0 mg
Vitamin E	10 IU
Biotin	60 mcg
Folic Acid	400 mcg
Vitamin B12	5 mcg

TABLE 11-11	Trace Elements
Zinc	5 mg
Copper	1 mg
Manganese	0.5 mg
Chromium	10 mcg

Note: The container will read MTE −4, MTE −5, or MTE −6, also known as Mineral Trace Elements, Minerals, or Metals.

usual. Novamine is a high concentration amino acid, and it is used for the catabolic patient with a fluid restriction. The use of IV fat emulsion as the main calorie source is encouraged in catabolic patients.

The patient who has or who develops poor glucose metabolism may become critically ill. Metabolism of glucose can increase CO_2 production and O_2 consumption. Insulin may be required.

COMPATIBILITY

There are some components of a TPN that are not compatible, yet are required in the same solution and by the body. If the pharmacy uses an automated pump to make the TPN, the technician will not have to be concerned with the order in which additives are added. The pumps have been preprogrammed to use the correct order to avoid precipitation of calcium and phosphate. However, if you are making a TPN by the gravity method, you will have to ensure that the order of the addition of calcium and phosphorous-containing solutions is correct. There must be at least two additives between the addition of these two items, sometimes referred to as "flushers." Additional calcium is usually added last, and phosphate is usually added first. If the two come in contact with each other, the complex calcium phosphate will be made. This precipitate will cause a clogging of the line, and worse yet, clot the patient's vein, causing an ischemia, which may lead to death.

Inside the body, calcium and phosphate both help to form the bone matrix and dentin. Compatibility can be a problem when adding certain electrolytes together. A pharmacy technician should contact the pharmacist before preparing a TPN.

If there are not enough electrolytes to separate the phosphates from the calcium, another method can be employed in which the calcium is added to the dextrose, the other additives to the amino acids, and then the admixtures are added to an empty bottle one after another. After each additive, the contents of the container are mixed.

STABILITY

The TPN bag is protected against light. If the TPN contains vitamin B12, the color of the TPN will be yellow. TPN is to be changed a minimum of once a day to avoid deterioration or expiration of the TPN components. To avoid infection, the lines are to be changed daily also.

Strict aseptic technique must be used while preparing TPN admixtures, using a filtered-air, laminar flow hood to avoid bacterial contamination. In addition, the high sugar content of these products supports prolific bacterial growth. Sepsis is a potentially severe patient problem. To avoid infection, the IV lines are to be changed at least once a day, and the nurse will monitor the patient's temperature, Q 4 to Q 8 hours If the temperature is over 38 degrees Celsius, the doctor will be notified immediately.

When TPN nutrition infusion is being cycled, a heparin flush is needed to maintain *patency* of the central venous catheter when the solution is not being infused. The sodium or heparin flush is done at least every shift.

Thrombosis should be suspected if the patient complains of pain or swelling in the extremity or surrounding area on the side where the catheter is located. The catheter may leak at the insertion site. A venogram should be ordered to confirm a thrombosis. The nurse must assess for thrombosis with each patient check.

Hyperglycemia may set in due to the high amount of dextrose the patient is infused with. Blood sugars should be obtained to assess the patient for hypo/hyperglycemia. It is also thought that the higher the blood glucose is, the more likely infection may occur. It can occur when the TPN is infused too fast or if the body cannot tolerate the sugar. Sometimes having an infection or taking a medication, such as a steroid, will make the body less tolerant of large amounts of sugar. Stopping a TPN infusion abruptly without a "taper down" or too much insulin in the TPN bag may cause hypoglycemia. When the body is receiving a large amount of sugar, it produces more insulin. When the TPN infusion is suddenly halted, the insulin takes longer to stop being produced. This will result in a drop in the blood sugar below normal.

Catheter insertion avoids a *tamonade*. This would be the filling of the outer cardiac sac or pericardium of TPN solution, resulting in death. A correctly placed TPN central catheter is essential to avoid this complication during infusion into the patient. An X-ray should be taken as a precaution and studied to avoid infusing into the pericardium.

There are three types of catheters: non-tunneled catheters, tunneled catheters, and the implanted ports.

Non-tunneled catheters are usually placed in the subclavian, jugular, or femoral for a short-term therapy of less than eight weeks. Generally they are not used for home TPN. These catheters should be inserted with sterile technique in a surgical setting, but can be done at the patient's bedside. Immediately after insertion, a stat portable chest X-ray is taken. This ensures correct placement, avoiding insertion complications. The tip of the catheter must be in the superior or inferior vena cava to infuse TPN through the catheter. Single lumen catheters are recommended because of the decreased risk of infection.

Tunneled catheters, commonly known as Hickmans®, Groshongs®, and Broviac®, are used in patients who need more of a long-term therapy. Placed either in the clinic procedure room or in the hospital operation room and made of silicone, they are inserted most commonly in the chest area. The catheter is tunneled under the skin, enters a large vein, and then is "threaded" into the superior vena cava.

Implanted ports, commonly known as Infusaport® or Port-A-Cath®, are placed in the patient in a clinic procedure room or in the hospital operating room. These are used for more intermittent therapies, but can be used for TPN infusion both in the hospital and in the home setting. The catheter is sutured under the skin in the subcutaneous tissue. The silicone catheter that attaches to the septum is then threaded into a major vein.

Contraindications of TPN therapy—Some studies have demonstrated TPN's ability to stimulate tumor growth (Brennan, 1981; Torosian, 1992) leading some researchers to suggest that anorexia and semi-starvation are associated with a slowing of tumor growth. These can result from opportunistic infection and poor wound healing leading to a high morbidity and mortality. TPN in cancer patients is controversial because the patient's specific micronutrient deficiencies of Ca, Fe, Mg, or Vitamin B12 can be present even in the absence of weight loss (Blackburn *et al.*, 1977).

The following are adverse reactions, usually related to TPN's components or additives:

- Water may cause fluid overload or retention.
- Insulin and dextrose may lead to hypoglycemia or hyperglycemia.
- Heparin may lead to hemorrhage.
- Electrolytes may cause abnormal levels of sodium, chloride, potassium, or magnesium.
- Vitamins may lead to a deficiency in Vitamin D or an excess of Vitamin A.
- Dextrose may lead to respiratory distress or liver dysfunction, since TPN is a customized mixture of dextrose ranging from 10 percent to 35 percent.

Symptoms may include the following: body swelling, respiratory distress, high or low blood glucose, bleeding, changes in level of consciousness, cardiac arrhythmias, diaphoresis, confusion, lethargy, headache, hunger, tremors, fever, and sepsis.

SUMMARY

The gastrointestinal system is the system in which food travels through the body. Food is broken down, absorbed, or chemically modified into substances that are required by the cells to survive and function properly. Waste products that the body cannot use are eliminated. The gastrointestinal system extends from the mouth to the anus. Its six main parts are the mouth, esophagus, pharynx, stomach, and small and large intestines. Various supportive structures, accessory glands, and accessory organs also help to make up the complete digestive system. The main purpose of the digestive system is to fuel the body. A thorough review of the gastrointestinal system is presented in this chapter.

An estimated 70 million Americans suffer from one or more digestive disorders; this accounts for 13 percent of all hospitalizations. Over 400,000 new cases of peptic ulcer are diagnosed each year, resulting in nearly 40,000 surgeries annually. As a pharmacy technician, you should be aware of the important digestive disorders discussed throughout the chapter.

There are many over-the-counter remedies available to treat the "milder" forms of digestive disease with which you should be familiar. Of course, the more serious gastrointestinal diseases often require more aggressive therapies, including surgery. Total Parenteral Nutrition (TPN) is used for patients who cannot receive adequate oral intake of the nutrients necessary to meet the body's physiological needs. TPN is administered intravenously, and is not a treatment modality that you would normally encounter.

Of course, as with any disease, the primary goal is prevention. As a pharmacy technician, you need to be prepared to assist the pharmacist in providing information to clients about proper nutrition. You should have a firm grasp of the approved recommendations for daily food intake, and the Recommended Dietary Allowances (RDA) that have been established.

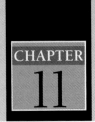

CHAPTER 11

CHAPTER REVIEW QUESTIONS

1. What are the six accessory organs of the digestive system?

2. What two organs produce digestive juices, which are sent to the intestine through small vessels, and what are the juices?

3. The process of breaking up large molecules of fats into smaller ones in the gallbladder is known as:
   a. anticholinergic effect
   b. emulsification
   c. hydrogenation
   d. delipidization

4. What percentage of daily calories recommended by the RDA should be complex carbohydrates?
   a. 14%
   b. 22%
   c. 55%
   d. 35%

5. During digestion and metabolism, all carbohydrates are broken down to glucose.
   a. true
   b. false

6. Name 5 reasons a TPN may be required for a patient.

7. What is the maximum starting rate of a TPN?
   a. 50 cc/hour for 4–6 hours
   b. 25 cc/hour for 4–6 hours
   c. 10 cc/hour for 4–6 hours
   d. 75 cc/hour for 4–6 hours

8. What two products precipitate in the TPN if not added in the correct order?

9. What are the six categories of nutrition?

10. The three parts of the small intestine are:
    a. jejunum, duodenum, ileum
    b. esophagus, stomach, duodenum
    c. duodenum, diaphragm, ileum
    d. stomach, esophagus, jejunum

11. Name seven parts of the large intestine.

12. An important motility that takes place in the large intestine to help eliminate waste is known as:
    a. cecum contraction
    b. high amplitude propagating contraction
    c. synchonized contraction
    d. peristalitic contraction

13. How long is it estimated that food remains in the large intestine along with bacteria?
    a. 24 hours
    b. 18 hours
    c. 30 hours
    d. 4 hours

Resources and References

1. MOA of APAP News on APAP
   http://www.pharmweb.net/pwmirror/pwy/paracetamol/pharmwebpicm echs.html
2. Arthritis Today 2004 Drug Guide DMARDs
   http://www.arthritis.org/conditions/DrugGuide/about_dmards.asp
3. *Merck Manual of Diagnosis and Therapy*
   http://www.merck.com/mrkshared/mmanual/section5/chapter57/57a.jsp
4. National Library of Medicine: A Review of SERM's and National Surgical Adjuvant Breast and Bowel Project Clinical Trials.
   http://www.ncbi.nlm.nih.gov/entrez/query.fcgi?cmd=Retrieve&db=Pub Med&listuids=14613021&dopt=Abstract
5. Holland, Norman and Michael Patrick Adams. *Core Concepts in Pharmacology*. Upper Saddle River, NJ: Pearson Education, 2003.
6. Adams, Michael Patrick, Dianne L. Josephson, and Leland Norman Holland, Jr. *Pharmacology for Nurses—A Pathophysiologic Approach*. Upper Saddle River, NJ: Pearson Education, 2005.

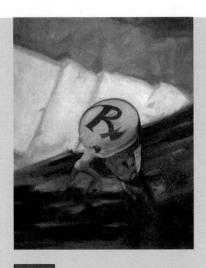

The Musculoskeletal System

After completing this chapter, you should be able to:

- List, identify, and diagram the basic anatomical structure and parts of the muscles and bones.

- Describe the function or physiology of the muscles and bones and their inter-workings and independent contributions to the human body.

- List and define common diseases affecting the muscles and bones and comprehend the causes, symptoms, and pharmaceutical treatment associated with each disease.

- Describe the mechanisms and the complications of the following musculoskeletal diseases and comprehend how each class of drugs work: osteomyelitis, osteoarthritis, gout, inflammation, multiple sclerosis, and cerebral palsy.

- List the indications for use and mechanisms of action of ASA, NSAIDs, Cox-2 inhibitors, antigout agents, calcitonin, bisphosphonates, SERMs, and skeletal muscle relaxants.

- Define and utilize key terms.

INTRODUCTION

Without muscles, you would not be able to move. Muscles work very hard during exercise or simple movement. The energy that provides work has to come from somewhere. The energy comes from food and is carried as nutrients to the muscles by the blood. To release the energy and do work, the muscles also need oxygen, which is likewise carried to the muscle by the blood. The energy, now called ATP (adenosine triphosphate), carries out the work of the contractions of the muscles.

The musculoskeletal system is extremely important, as it provides the framework of the human body for both support and movement. More importantly, not even one body function can take place without at least a part of this system contributing to its action. All body movement is coordinated between the nervous system and the bones, joints, muscles, ligaments, cartilage, and tendons. Whether you are eating, riding a bike, eliminating waste, or simply breathing, the musculoskeletal system is underlying that action. The largest system in the body synchronizes movement at both the cellular level and at the gross muscular tissue level. Failure of any one of the components of this system will bring a somatic complaint or disaster to the body.

Anatomy of the Muscles

Skeletal muscles are attached to bones and provide body movement, or kinetics. These muscles are voluntary, striated in shape, and contain multiple peripheral nuclei (Figure 12-1).

Cardiac muscle is attached to the heart and is known as the myocardium. The myocardium is discussed in another chapter. This muscle helps with the transmission of electrical impulses from nerve to muscle fibers. The *cadence* and rhythm of the heart, as well as the force of contraction, are dependent upon this muscle. This muscle is involuntary and striated with a single central nucleus.

Smooth muscle is attached to, or lines, other organs such as the stomach, intestines, lungs, and blood vessels. This type of muscle, referred to as visceral muscle, is discussed in the chapters on the circulatory (vasculature), digestive, respiratory, and nervous systems. Visceral muscle is involuntary and nonstriated and has a single central nucleus.

Muscle Action

The thick and thin filaments of the muscles do the actual work of a muscle. The thick filaments are made of a protein called myosin. A thick filament is a shaft of myosin molecules arranged in the shape of a cylinder. Thin filaments are also made of a protein called actin. It has been said that thin filaments look like two strands of pearls twisted around each other.

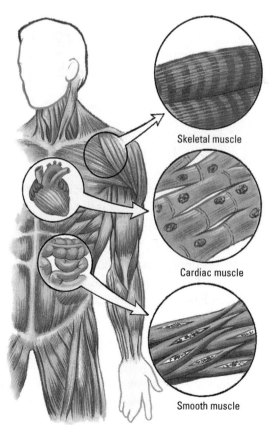

Skeletal muscle

Cardiac muscle

Smooth muscle

Figure 12-1 Skeletal muscle - Cardiac muscle - Smooth muscle

The thick myosin filaments grab onto the thin actin filaments by forming cross bridges during a contraction of a muscle. The thick filaments grab and pull the thin filaments past them, which shortens the *sarcomere*. The signal for contraction in a muscle fiber is synchronized over the entire fiber so that all of the myofibrils that make up the sarcomere shorten at the same time. Two substances in the grooves of each thin filament enable the thin filaments to slide along the thick ones. These proteins are tropomyosin, a long rod-like protein, and troponin, a shorter bead-like protein complex. Troponin and tropomyosin are the molecular chemicals, or "switches," that control the interaction of actin and myosin during contraction.

Chemical and physical interactions between the actin and myosin cause the sarcomere length to shorten, and therefore the myocyte to contract, during the process of excitation coupling contraction.

There are about 300 molecules of *myosin* per thick filament. An enzyme (ATPase) hydrolyzes ATP, which is required for actin and myosin cross bridge formation.

The thin filaments are composed of three different types of protein: actin, tropomyosin, and troponin. Together these are termed the regulatory protein complex. The *actin* is a globular protein.

The Bones

A baby has about 300 "soft" bones, which eventually grow together, or fuse, to form the 206 bones that adults have. Some of a baby's bones are made of a special material called cartilage. Cartilage is a soft and flexible cushion. During childhood, the cartilage grows and slowly hardens into bone, with help from calcium. At about the age of 25, the cartilage will have finished hardening into bone. After cartilage has hardened, there can be no more growth—the bones are as big as they will ever get.

There are five classes of bones:

- **Long**—for example, the femur of the leg
- **Short**—bones that are roughly cube-shaped; for example: the carpals of the hand
- **Flat**—bones that are generally more flat than round; for example, the cranial bones and the ribs
- **Irregular**—bones that have no defined shape; for example, the scapula and the 26 vertebrae
- **Sesamoid**—bones that often have cartilage and fibrous tissue mixed in. These bones are found in the joints and help to lower friction and enhance joint movement; for example, the patella or kneecap.

LONG BONES

The most common bone is long bone, which this chapter will concentrate on. Let's look inside a long bone, which is divided into two areas: the epiphysis (the rounded end of the bone) and the *diaphysis* (the main shaft or central part of the bone).

The epiphysis is covered with articular cartilage, which is smooth and slippery, and helps bones move against each other within joints. The inside of the epiphysis is made up of spongy or cancellous bone, which is made from criss-crossed strands of bone, and the spaces between the strands are filled with bone marrow.

The diaphysis has a hollow core called the medullary cavity and is filled with red marrow in children and yellow marrow in adults. The walls of the diaphysis is made of a second type of bone called compact bone, which is much harder and more solid than spongy bone. The outermost layer of the long bone is the periosteum, which covers the diaphysis and part of the epiphysis, but it does not cover the articular cartilage. This layer contains cells, or osteoblasts, which make new bone to replace the older bone cells, osteoclasts, and also provide nourishment for the bone. (See Figures 12-2 and 12-3.)

Bone Marrow

Bone marrow is the gelatinous substance inside bones. Red bone marrow functions to produce red blood cells, white blood cells, and blood platelets. In infants, red marrow is found in the bone cavities. With age, it is replaced by yellow marrow for fat storage. In adults, red marrow is found mainly in the spongy bone in the clavicles, pelvis, ribs, skull, sternum, and vertebrae.

There are two types of bone marrow:

Red Marrow—a red, jelly-like substance that contains blood cells and is usually found only in the sternum, vertebrae, ribs, hips, clavicles, and cranial bones. As you age, red converts to yellow, has less fat, and is high in erythrocytes (red blood cells).

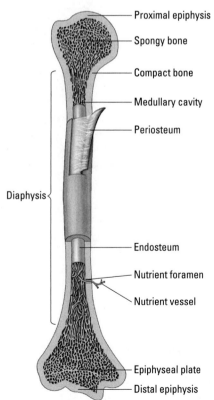

Figure 12-2 The long bone (*Mulvihill, Mary Lou; Zelman, Mark; Holdaway, Paul; Tompary, Elaine; Turchany, Jill,* Human Diseases, A Systemic Approach, *5th Edition,* © *2001. Reprinted by permission of Pearson Education, Inc., Upper Saddle River, NJ)*

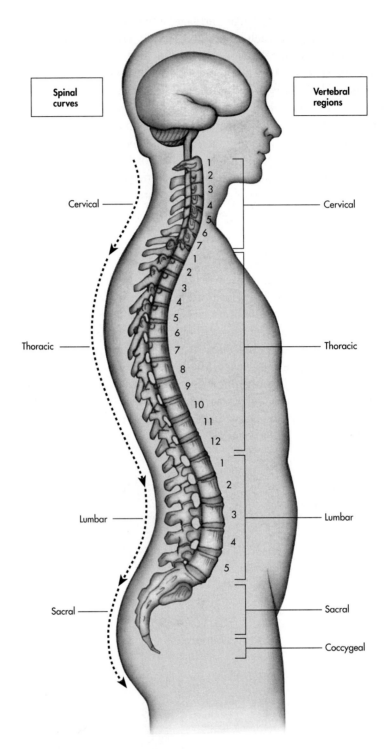

Figure 12-3   The spine

Yellow Marrow—a fatty yellow substance that replaces red marrow in long bones in adults and does not produce blood cells. Yellow bone marrow has less pluripotential hematopoietic (fewer stem cells) and what stem cells are there are inactive. Yellow marrow has more fat in muscles to the bones.

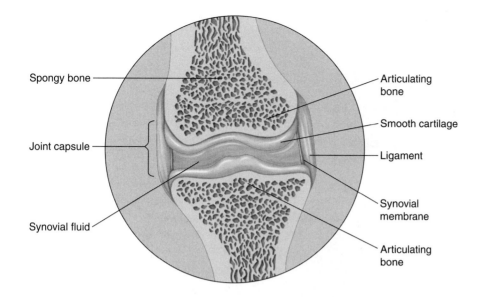

Spongy bone

Joint capsule

Synovial fluid

Articulating bone

Smooth cartilage

Ligament

Synovial membrane

Articulating bone

Figure 12-4 The joint (*Mulvihill, Mary Lou; Zelman, Mark; Holdaway, Paul; Tompary, Elaine; Turchany, Jill,* Human Diseases, A Systemic Approach, *5th Edition,* © *2001. Reprinted by permission of Pearson Education, Inc., Upper Saddle River, NJ*)

Anatomical Vocabulary

- **Bones:** Specialized form of dense connective tissue consisting of calcified intercellular substance that provides the shape and support for the body. Bones are made of calcium and phosphate. Injuries can result in fractures.
- **Joints:** The location or position where bones are connected to each other. A joint contains synovial fluid and cartilage.
- **Cartilage:** Soft bones that line every joint and give shape to the ears and nose. Injuries can result in tears or degeneration of the cartilage and arthritis.
- **Synovial Fluid:** Fills the space between the cartilage of each bone to provide smooth movement by lubricating the cartilage.
- **Ligaments:** Strong fibrous bands of connective tissue that hold bones together. Injuries can result in sprains.
- **Tendons:** Cords of connective tissue that attach muscle to bone. Injuries can result in strains, ruptures, or inflammation.
- **Bone Marrow:** Spongy type of tissue found inside most bones and responsible for the manufacture of red blood cells, some white blood cells, and platelets. Also acts as storage area for fat. (See Figures 12-4, 12-5, and 12-6.)

The Functions of Bones

The bones serve the body in many ways. If any one of these functions is endangered or compromised, the body would suffer immensely.

- The bones provide the framework or foundation of the body.
- Bones lend to the support of the body to keep it in an upright position. The skeleton supports the body against the pull of gravity with the weight of the bones.
- The bones protect the internal organs—heart, lungs, brain, liver—by enveloping them in a "cage."

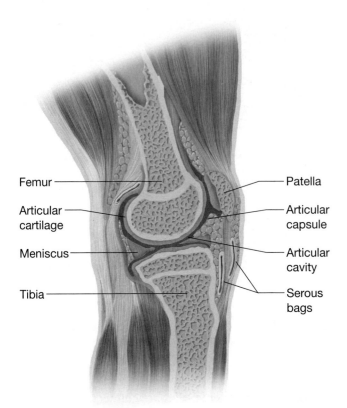

Femur

Articular
cartilage

Meniscus

Tibia

Patella

Articular
capsule

Articular
cavity

Serous
bags

Figure 12-5 The knee
joint

- The tunnels within the bone's living tissue allow for the exchange of nutrients and waste products.
- Bones help the muscular system to allow the body to move. Muscles are attached to the bones and pull them, causing the bones to move. Bones act as simple mechanical lever systems.
- *Hematopoiesis*, the formation of blood cells, mostly takes place in the red marrow of the bones. Bone marrow produces red blood cells to transport oxygen, white blood cells to fight disease-causing bacteria, and platelets to stop bleeding and makes new cells to replace worn out cells.
- Bone marrow stores nutrients such as calcium and phosphorus. When the calcium levels in the blood decrease below normal, the bones release calcium so that there will be an adequate supply for metabolic needs. When blood calcium levels are increased, the excess calcium is stored in the bone matrix (marrow). The dynamic process of releasing and storing calcium goes on almost continuously, lending to homeostasis. (See Figure 12-7.)

Musculoskeletal Disorders

There are many diseases of the muscles and bones. Here are only a few that will be explored in this chapter.

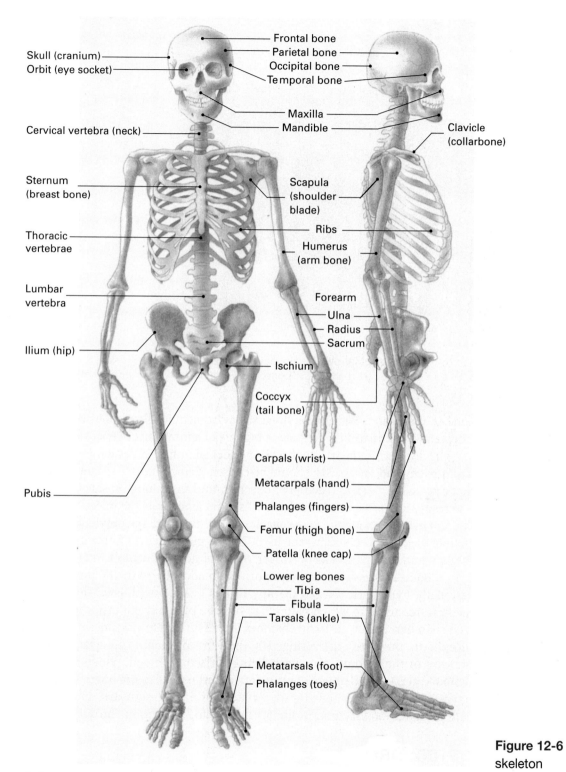

Figure 12-6   The skeleton

OSTEOMYELITIS

This is an infection inside the bone that destroys bone tissue that occurs usually after multiple fractures or trauma in patients with diabetes or tuberculosis. Often, the original site of infection was other than the bone, and infection spread to the

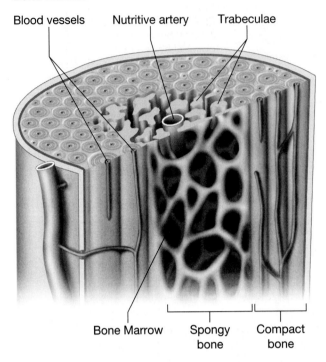

Bone Marrow

Blood vessels   Nutritive artery   Trabeculae

Bone Marrow   Spongy bone   Compact bone

Figure 12-7 Bone marrow

bone by the blood. Bacteria or fungus may sometimes be responsible for osteomyelitis. Pharmacokinetics plays a big role in anitinfective agent selection.

The drug exhibiting the highest bacteriocidal or fungicidal activity with the least toxicity and lowest cost should be chosen. Penicillinase-resistant semisynthetic penicillin, such as nafcillin or oxacillin, and an aminoglycoside (until culture results and sensitivities are known) should ameliorate the infection.

Staphylococcus aureus is the usual culprit of spinal osteomyelitis and responds well to IV clindamycin in PCN allergic patients. Antimicrobial IV therapy may last six weeks or longer. Surgical debridement of infected devitalized bone and tissue must be performed in addition to the IV therapy. Occasionally, hyperbaric oxygen therapy, or HBO, is required. HBO therapy is a medical treatment in which patients to breathe pure oxygen inside a pressurized chamber. The hyperbaric chamber is pressurized to 2.5 times normal atmospheric pressure, delivering 100 percent oxygen. This produces an increase in the amount of oxygen being carried by blood, which results in more oxygen being delivered to the organs and tissues in the body. This extra oxygen improves the benefits of certain antibiotics, activates white blood cells to fight infection, and promotes the healing process in chronic wounds.

OSTEOPOROSIS

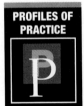

PROFILES OF PRACTICE

Osteoporosis, which is the most prevelant bone disorder in the United States, is 400 percent more prevalent in women than in men.

Brittleness of the bones due to lack of calcium is called osteoporosis. Estrogen keeps calcium in the bone, while PTH and calcitonin contribute to the homeostasis of calcium in the bone and blood and vitamin D is required for absorption of calcium. Menopause is a major cause of osteoporosis. (See Treatment of Weak, Fragile, or Soft Bones.) (See Figures 12-8 and 12-9.)

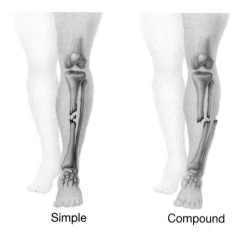

Simple Compound

Bone Fractures

Complete Incomplete

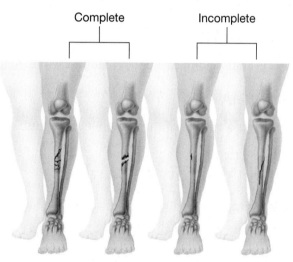

Comminuted Simple Greenstick Fissured

Figure 12-8 Bone fractures

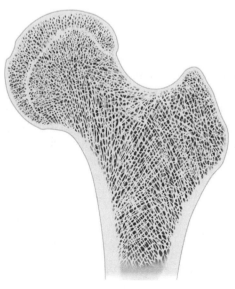

Normal Bone Tissue

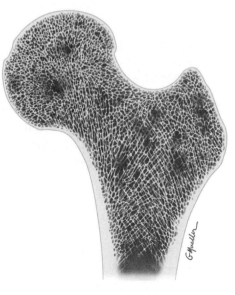

Bone Tissue with Osteoporosis

Figure 12-9 Bone density (*Mulvihill, Mary Lou; Zelman, Mark; Holdaway, Paul; Tompary, Elaine; Turchany, Jill,* Human Diseases, A Systemic Approach, *5th Edition,* © 2001. Reprinted by permission of Pearson Education, Inc., Upper Saddle River, NJ)

PAGET'S DISEASE

Pronounced paj-ets, in this disease, the normal process of bone growth is changed—it breaks down more quickly and then grows softer than normal bone. Normally, bone is continually breaking down and rebuilding. Paget's disease causes a malfunction in the normal process of bone remodeling. This process of bone destruction and growth, which is usually slow, is somehow altered in Paget's disease. Soft bones can bend or break more easily and can also grow larger than before. It can affect any bone, but usually affects the skull, the hip and pelvis bones, and bones in the legs and back. (See Treatment of Weak, Fragile, or Soft Bones.)

BURSITIS

This is an inflammation of the bursa, the small, fluid-filled pouch located between bones and ligaments or between bones and muscles (serves as a cushion).

TENDONITIS

This is an inflammation of the tendons, which hold muscles to bone.

MYALGIA

Myalgia is a term used that simply means muscle pain.

Bone Marrow Disorders

ANEMIA

Anemia is failure of the bone marrow to produce the components of the red blood cells. A lack of iron that causes a lack of oxygen inside the erythrocyte and leads to fatigue is a common cause. However, blood loss or hemolysis (red blood cell destruction) can also cause a variety of anemias.

LEUKEMIA

Leukemia begins when one or more white blood cells experience DNA loss or damage. The results are copied and passed on to subsequent generations of cells. They do not die off like normal cells, but instead multiply and accumulate within the body. No one really knows why such changes occur. There are some factors that increase risk, such as genetics or age. Other factors that may play a part are environmental or lifestyle-related variables. All cancers, including leukemia, begin as a mutation in the genetic material—the DNA (deoxyribonucleic acid)—within certain cells.

Arthritis

There are many types of arthritis, which begins with an inflammation of the joint.

RHEUMATOID ARTHRITIS

Rheumatoid arthritis (RA) is a progressive form of arthritis that has devastating effects on the joints, body organs, and health in general. It is classified as an *autoimmune* disease because the disease is caused by the body's immune system attacking the body itself. Symptoms include painful, stiff, swollen joints, fever, and fatigue. RA is an inflammation of the cartilage around the joints that leads to a thickening and hardening of the synovial fluid. Eventually, the visceral organs are attacked.

OSTEOARTHRITIS

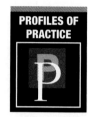

Osteoarthritis is a progressive disease. The breakdown of cartilage that is seen with this condition occurs in several phases. Knee joint pain is the most common musculoskeletal complaint that brings people to their doctor. With today's increasingly active society, the number of knee problems is increasing.

Reports indicate that as many as 40 million Americans are affected by osteoarthritis.

The cause of the breakdown is a wear and tear of the joint due to weight bearing activities such as marching, running, and jogging. The erosion of the joint may allow particles of the worn bone to be considered as foreign material in the joint, summoning phagocytes to come to the aid. This begins some irritation and swelling known as inflammation.

GOUT

Gouty arthritis is a painful joint inflammatory disease that was first described in the days of *Hippocrates*, 400 to 300 B.C. This special inflammatory disease is associated with the deposition of uric acid in the joint synovial fluid of the big toes, knees, and elbows, as well as in soft tissue. Therefore, this is a systemic disease, not just localized in the joints. The uric acid and the synovial joint fluid interact to form precipitates in the form of needle-like crystals, which cause tremendous pain. The irritation leads to the bone and cartilage meeting against the solid foreign particles, which imitates osteoarthritis. An increase in the amount of uric acid in the blood leads to uric acid crystals in the joints, which act as an irritant and cause an arthritis-like pain, along with inflammation. It is sometimes confused with pseudoarthritis or false gout. Calcium pyrophosphate deposits, rather than uric acid crystals, cause pseudoarthritis. When uric acid in the blood is high, not filtered, and cleared via the glomerulus of the nephrons in the kidneys, the acid is deposited in the joint. (See Chapter 16, Renal System.) The uric acid and the synovial fluid combine to make uric acid crystals. This precipitation leads to the disease often referred to as gouty arthritis.

Gout is caused by an excess (overproduction) of uric acid in the body or by the inability of the kidneys to adequately clear uric acid from the body (inadequate excretion). Uric acid is formed every day from the metabolism of nucleic acids. Humans cannot use uric acid. It is normally secreted into the urine by renal tubules. The condition of having too much uric acid in the blood is called *hyperuricemia*.

An excess of certain fermented alcoholic beverages (wine and beer) and certain foods (such as legumes—peas, lentils, beans—cheeses, anchovies, sardines, scallops, muscles, shellfish, organ meats—liver, kidneys, heart—and red meats) that are aged and contain a high purine content which increases the uric acid level of the blood may increase uric acid levels and precipitate gout attacks.

Medications, including hydrochlorothiazide, a diuretic, and some transplant immunosupressant medications, such as cyclosporine and tacrolimus, can also increase uric acid levels.

Certain disease states and genetic factors can predispose to gout: A high incidence has been noted in New Zealanders, Pacific Islanders, and postmenopausal women; but it affects men more than women by a ratio of 20:1. Obesity, high blood pressure, kidney disease, and genetics are risk factors for gout.

With time, elevated levels of uric acid in the blood may lead to deposits around joints. Eventually, with hyperuricemia, the uric acid may form needle-like crystals in joints, leading to acute gout attacks. Uric acid may also collect under the skin, which is known as tophi, or in the urinary tract as kidney stones.

While uric acid crystals accumulate in the joint fluid, phagocytes (leukocytes) enter the same area and attack the uric acid crystals. This phagic activity leads to a decrease in the pH (acid) of the joint fluid, causing more uric acid to accumulate in the joint.

Acute gout is the vicious cycle of inflammation producing edema, redness, and severe pain characteristic of acute gout. In chronic gout, uric acid slowly deposits in soft tissues causing tophi, or the bulging, deformed joints that were characteristic of King Henry VIII, who was known to have suffered from gout. This may also happen in the kidney and is known as kidney stones.

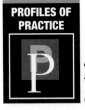

PROFILES OF PRACTICE

As much as three percent of the United States population is affected by gout.

Treatment of Arthritis

DISEASE MODIFYING ANTI-RHEUMATIC DRUGS (DMARDs)

Taken early in the disease, these drugs can help prevent the progression of the disease. DMARDs usually take up to six to eight months to evoke a response; they are considered slow-acting drugs (remittive). DMARDs are now regarded as a long-term solution to controlling symptoms. Generally, DMARDs are used for RA, but some can also be used for juvenile RA, ankylosing spondylitis, psoriatic arthritis, and lupus. To date, only Arava (leflunomide) has been developed for RA, while the others have been used to treat different disease states. A major adverse reaction is an acquired illness due to the mechanism of action that lowers the immune system response, which is called immunosuppression. DMARDs are immunosppressants. Therefore, the patient must watch for such signs of infection as sore throat, cough, fever, or chills. Vaccinations may pose a problem for those taking DMARDs as they suppress or lower the immune system.

GOLD (RIDAURA®)

Ridaura® was discovered accidentally by a French physician, Jacques Forrestier. Gold salts have been used for the treatment of RA for over 50 years. After he injected gold salts into a tuberculosis (TB) patient, who coincidentally had arthritis, the arthritis improved. Gold has been used to treat arthritis ever since. The mechanism of action is not exactly known, but it is believed that the gold interferes with functions of white blood cells responsible for joint damage and inflammation. Gold slows destruction, but it cannot cure existing joint deformities. Side effects include an itchy rash on the lower extremities and mouth ulcers, which disappear when the medicine is discontinued; and transitory diarrhea or loose bowel movements. Fifty percent of users discontinue this medication due to the side effects.

PENICILLAMINE

This is a cousin of PCN, also a known *chelator* because it binds to heavy metals in the body. However, patients who are allergic to PCN can take penicillamine. It may become more active or potent if combined with copper, which is present naturally in the body. Used since the 1970s for RA, the exact MOA is unknown, but believed to act like gold, interfering with functions of white blood cells responsible for joint damage and inflammation. Side effects include skin rashes, mouth sores, loss of taste, and GI upset. Kidney damage may also occur; therefore, the patient must be monitored for protein in the urine.

SULFASALAZINEIS

A combination of salicylate and an antibiotic and originally used to treat inflammatory bowel disease, it has been on the scene since the 1940s. Since it is not as toxic as gold or penicillinamine, a renewed interest in usage of this drug for RA has developed. Side effects include loss of appetite, N/V/D. The toxic effects include renal problems and blood dyscrasias. In addition, because it is a sulfur based drug, it may cause severe allergic reactions or anaphylactic shock.

HYDROXYCHLOROQUINE (PLAQUENIL®)

Originally used to treat malaria and recently SLE (lupus), this medication has been around for many years. Plaquenil is indicated for patients with RA who have not responded well to NSAIDs. It has few side effects, and blood test monitoring is not required. Once a day dosing is usual, with one rare toxic effect. The drug may deposit in the retina and cause visual impairment. Therefore, an ophthalmology exam is recommended every six months.

LEFLUNOMIDE (ARAVA®)

Arava helps to slow the progression of joint damage caused by RA. While there is no cure for RA, Arava may help prevent RA from getting worse. It has been shown to inhibit structural damage (as evidenced by X-ray erosions and joint space narrowing) and improve physical function. Leflunomide is an isoxazole immunomodulatory agent that inhibits dihydroorotate dehydrogenase and has antiproliferative activity. DHODHase is an enzyme involved in *de novo* pyrimidine synthesis. By blocking this enzyme, Arava® prevents T-cell actions and proliferation that lead to the disabling inflammation of RA. Arava also has demonstrated an anti-inflammatory effect. The drug is available in tablets containing 10 mg, 20 mg, or a loading dose of 100 mg of active drug. Side effects include dry mouth, insomnia, hair loss, nausea, diarrhea, tiredness, and acne. Toxic effects include dark yellow urine, difficulty breathing or shortness of breath, increases in blood pressure, and yellowing of the skin or eyes. Leflunomide has the potential to cause liver damage; therefore, patients must be monitored. Rash, swelling, and difficulty breathing may be signs of a possible allergic reaction and should be reported immediately.

SECOND LINE OF THERAPY

NSAIDs or nonsteroidal anti-inflammatory drugs and other steroidal anti-inflammatory drugs are commonly used for the symptoms of rheumatoid arthritis, but they do not prevent the progression of the disease. There is also some research that shows NSAIDs interfere with the bone rebuilding process.

Inflammation

Inflammation is a symptom common with bursitis, tendonitis, muscle pain, dysmenorrhea, arthritis, and gout. Inflammation, along with pain, is the most common symptom associated with the previous inflammatory diseases. The inflammatory process is a normal response to injury. When tissues are damaged, substances such as histamine, prostaglandins, and serotonin are released. These substances produce vasodilation and increased permeability of the capillary walls. As more inflammation is made, the inflamed tissue hits nerves, which causes pain because the pain receptors are stimulated. This occurs while proteins and fluid leak out of the injured cells. As blood flow to the damaged area increases, leukocytes migrate to the area to destroy harmful substances introduced by the injury. All of this results in the development of the cardinal signs of inflammation:

- redness
- swelling
- edema
- warmth
- pain
- loss of function (immobilization)

Note: In some instances, the inflammatory process becomes chronic and repeats over a long period of time. Exaggerated or prolonged, it results in further tissue damage. The inflammation becomes a disease in itself.

Treatment for Inflammatory Diseases

There are basically three choices of anti-inflammatory agents used to treat the aforementioned conditions: salicylates, NSAIDs, and corticosteroids.

SALICYLATES

Salicylates relieve inflammation by inhibiting the synthesis of prostaglandin. Salicylates are also used as anti-inflammatory drugs to reduce swelling and further tissue damage, analgesics to relieve pain or lower the threshold of pain without affecting consciousness, and antipyretics to reduce fever or body temperature. Salicylates are older products made by various manufacturers.

Examples of salicylates are as follows:

- aspirin—various manufacturers such as St. Joseph and Bayer
- salicylamide—various manufacturers
- sodium salicylates—various manufacturers

Side effects of salicylates include the following:

Nausea and *vomiting*—Salicylates directly irritate the stomach mucosal lining and stimulate the chemoreceptor trigger zone (CTZ) in the medulla oblongata located in the brain stem, which directly excites the vomiting center.

Hemorrhagic effect—Inhibition of the aggregation of platelets—Platelets are the sticky substance in the blood necessary for clot formation. The anti-coagulation effect of ASA thins out the blood, increasing the risk of hemorrhage and GI ulcer. Therefore, patients can bleed excessively if cut, undergo surgery, or have dental work while taking ASA and salicylamides. This is called the antiplatelet effect of the drug.

Tinnitus—Salicylates relieve pain, aches, and fever in low doses. Unfortunately, to relieve the pain of arthritis, gout, and rheumatoid arthritis, they must be used in large doses for extensive periods of time. Megadose therapy is frequently associated with toxic effects. Megadoses of ASA or NSAIDs may also cause tinnitus, by their effect on the hearing organ of the inner ear, the cochlea, and specifically the spiral ganglion. Tinnitus is a ringing in the ear.

The dangerous and often fatal reactions of acute salicylate poisoning are respiratory depression and acidosis.

Very good documentation supports the fact that ASA blocks the enzyme Cox-2, thereby blocking the first step in the inflammatory process and further blocking of prostaglandins from being made. In addition, platelet-aggregating substance thromboxane A2, preventing further stroke or MI, is also blocked when ASA blocks the production of prostaglandin.

Other indications of salicylates include antiplatelet or anticoagulant effect. If ulcers are not present, continual administration of aspirin may be beneficial to prevent the formation of thromboemboli. Usually, a child's dose of 81 mg is given. In layman's terms, this "thins out" the blood. While too much aspirin or other salicylates may cause hemorrhage, a small amount on a daily basis for the patient with a potential for stroke or MI will be a benefit. (Read more about this in Chapter 14, Circulatory System, "Antiplatelet Agents.")

Reye's Syndrome, a fatal disease affecting the brain and liver in children who have taken aspirin after or during a viral infection, has been the main reason for the decrease in the use of ASA. (Learn more about this in Chapter 13, Respiratory System, "Treating the Common Cold with Drugs." A comparison chart of the properties of ASA, APAP, and NSAIDs is also presented in Chapter 13.)

NONSTEROIDAL ANTI-INFLAMMATORY DRUGS (NSAIDs)

NSAIDs, or nonsteroidal anti-inflammatory drugs, relieve inflammation and pain (see Table 12-1). Some of the many types of arthritis are associated with infection. An NSAID will reduce the fever as well as relieve pain associated with fever, but not affect the infection. Antibiotics would be needed for the infection.

Adverse reaction of NSAIDs with long-term use of NSAIDs may have a damaging effect on chondrocyte (cartilage) function, which leads to more arthritic symptoms and disease. With chronic use, all anti-inflammatory and salicylate drugs may produce nausea, GI distress, and ulceration. However, ibuprofen has been reported to produce less gastric distress. Toxic effects of NSAIDs include bone marrow suppression leading to dyscrasias. (Blood disorders have been reported in patients who received nonsteroidal anti-inflammatory drugs.) Therefore, these drugs (NSAIDs) are strictly used for their anti-inflammatory effect and are not used as often for their analgesic (pain relieving) or antipyretic (fever reducing) effects. If another pain reliever or fever reducer with less harmful adverse reactions can be used, it may be the preferred drug over an NSAID.

A possible benefit of NSAIDs may exist. At the time of this writing, recent research indicates that NSAIDs may contribute to the brain redeveloping neurons disease states that involve brain inflammation or amyloid-beta, such as Alzheimers and other dementias. Lowered amyloid-beta occurs as NSAIDs, including ASA, inhibit the RHO-ROCK interaction (G-protein and rock). The future neurogenesis may help in head trauma patients or stroke. More studies are underway, and others are needed.

While it has been accepted in the past that the brain does not replace neurons, this is no longer considered true. There are small areas of the brain wherein stem cells make neurons throughout life, and this may help the learning and memory processes.

The MOA of NSAIDs is to inhibit or block the enzyme that starts the reaction of inflammation by making prostaglandin. The enzyme that it blocks is cycoloxygenase II, which catalyzes arachidonic acid to prostaglandins and leukotrienes. Further NSAIDs block the action of the synthesis of prostaglandin that promotes inflammation.

COX-2 INHIBITORS

Cycoloxygenase I is the enzyme that produces prostaglandins that cause the building and thickening of the mucosal lining of the stomach, which would

TABLE 12-1　Examples of NSAIDs

Trade	Generic	Usual Adult Dose
Motrin® Motrin IB® (OTC)	ibuprofen	1200 mg–3200 mg daily 100 mg qid, 300 mg qid, 400 mg, 600 mg or 800 mg tid or qid NTE 3200 mg/d
Feldene®	piroxicam	10 mg (qd or bid)–20 mg qd, NTE 20 mg qd
Ansaid®	flurbiprophen	100 to 300 mg total/day BID, TID, or QID NTE 400 mg/d
Voltaren® Voltaren-XR®	diclofenac	100 mg–200 mg/day NTE 225 mg/day
Indocin®	indomethacin	25 mg or 50 mg bid, tid NTE 200 mg/d
Dolobid®	diflunisal	500 or 1000 mg LD, 250 or 500 mg q8 to q12hr NTE 1500 mg/day
Nalfon®	fenoprofen	200, 300, 600 mg dose q8–6 hr NTE 3200 mg
Orudis® Oruvail® capsules	ketoprofen ketoprofen extended– release	50 mg qid, 75 mg tid, NTE 300 mg/d, 200 mg Ext. Rel./day
Meclomen®	meclofenamate	50–100 mg q4–6hrs, NTE 400 mg/day
Naprosyn®	naproxen	250 mg, 375 mg, or 500 mg tabs bid 125 mg/5 ml 10 to 40 ml suspension bid NTE 1500 mg/day
Anaprox® Naprelan® Controlled Release	naproxen sodium	375 mg tablets bid or 750 mg qa or two Naprelan 500 mg tabs (1000 mg once/day) NTE 1500 mg/d
Clinoril®	sulindac	100 mg, 200 mg tabs qd to bid NTE 400 mg qd
Tolectin®	tolmetin	200 mg, 400 mg, 600 mg tabs tid NTE 1800 mg/day
Daypro®	oxaprozin	1–2 600 mg caplets/day NTE 1800 mg (or 26 mg/kg, whichever is *lower*) in divided doses
Relafen®	nabumetone	2–4 500 mg tablets/day NTE 2000 mg/day

protect the stomach against acid. Cycoloxygenase II is the enzyme that produces the prostaglandins that contribute to inflammation.

When NSAIDs block *all* prostaglandin synthesis by blocking both Cox-1 and Cox-2, which can thin out the mucosal lining of the GI tract and reduce inflammation, a patient can then get a GI ulcer while successfully treating inflammation. Therefore, Cox-2 inhibitors, which block only the Cycoloxygenase II that makes PGE-2, but not C-1 (PGE-1), contribute less to ulcers while treating inflammation. Only the inflammation process is inhibited, not the viscosity of the mucosal lining.

The Cox-2 inhibitors have successfully been marketed on the basis of the belief that the main mechanism by which nonselective NSAIDs cause gastrointestinal ulcers is inhibition of Cox-1. According to this hypothesis, selective Cox-2 inhibitors will have similar anti-inflammatory activity with less GI toxicity. Short-term clinical studies (CLASS and VIGOR), in which all patients underwent endoscopy, showed fewer cumulative gastroduodenal erosions and ulcers with the Cox-2 inhibitors (9–15 percent) than with non-selective NSAIDs (41–46 percent). The FDA authorities judged this outcome as insufficient to prove that Cox-2 selective inhibitors were better than nonselective NSAIDs in terms of the life-threatening complications of NSAIDs, ulcers complicated by GI bleeds, perforations, and obstructions. Therefore, the monographs and package inserts of celecoxib (Celecoxib®) and meloxicam (Mobicox®) include the same warnings and patient precautions of GI toxicity as all other NSAIDs.

Current studies—according to the VIGOR and CLASS studies, Cox-2 selective inhibitors are associated with an increased incidence of serious adverse events as compared with nonselective NSAIDs. Therefore, more studies are underway to prove or disprove this hypothesis.

Current study—at the time of this writing, a study in Germany shows that the benefit of using leeches in knee arthritis is a great reduction in swelling and pain. Acetaminophen (trade name, Tylenol®), also known as paracetamol, N-Acetyl P-Aminophenol, is now thought to selectively block the newly discovered enzyme Cox-3 in the brain and spinal cord, which reduces pain and fever without unwanted gastrointestinal side effects. Still, there is no or very little anti-inflammatory effect with this drug.[1]

It is important to emphasize the adverse reactions of NSAIDs. Long-term use of NSAIDs may have a damaging effect on chondrocyte (or cartilage) function, which leads to more arthritic symptoms and disease. Therefore, in the long run, use of NSAIDs may play an important role in exacerbating any arthritis-related disease. Yet, the immediate relief that they bring many patients cannot be denied.

Skeletal Muscle Relaxants

Skeletal muscle relaxants (SMRs) are used to relax specific muscles in the body and relieve the pain, stiffness, and discomfort associated with strains, sprains, or other injury to muscles. SMRs may also be used in spastic diseases such as multiple sclerosis and cerebral palsy and to help relax the patient or a specific part of the body prior to surgery. Drug therapy does not take the place of recommended rest, exercise, or muscle problems caused by tetanus. Skeletal muscle relaxants act either in the central nervous system (CNS) or directly on the muscle to produce their muscle relaxant effects (see Table 12-2).

Surgical and orthopedic procedures and intubations can be facilitated by the use of skeletal muscle relaxants. SMRs can be used for over exertion of the muscles and injuries accompanied by aches and pain of sore, stiff, and swollen joints. Other drugs used to alleviate the sore aches and pains associated with overworked muscles are analgesics and anti-inflammatory agents.

There are two actions of skeletal muscle relaxants that inhibit neuromuscular function: peripheral acting and central acting. Direct acting skeletal muscle relaxants are a subtype of peripheral acting skeletal muscle relaxants. The peripheral acting skeletal muscle relaxants block muscle contraction at the neuromuscular junction within the contractile process. The contractile process begins with the electrical impulse originating in the CNS conducted via the spinal cord to the somatic, or voluntary, motor neurons. These motor neurons connect to skeletal muscle fibers, creating the NMJ or neuromuscular junction. ACH (acetylcholine) forms the endings of the somatic motor fiber endings, which then travel to the neuromuscular synapse, an area between two neurons. When the ACH attaches to the Nicotinic–II receptors, depolarization occurs, causing the contractile substances of myosin and actin to produce a muscle contraction. Therefore, the peripheral acting skeletal muscle relaxants inhibit contraction in two ways: as nondepolarizing agents and depolarizing agents.

Nondepolarizing skeletal muscle relaxants block NII receptors, thereby inhibiting depolarization or contraction, which stops nerve transmission. Depolarizing skeletal muscle relaxants attach to the NII receptors, stimulating them to cause depolarization or contraction, which then changes the NII receptors so that they do not respond to the natural ACH neurotransmitter in

TABLE 12-2 Skeletal Muscle Relaxants	
Trade®	Generic
Peripheral—Direct Acting Skeletal Muscle Relaxant	
Dantrium®	dantrolene
Central Acting Skeletal Muscle Relaxants	
Librium®	chlordiazepoxide (primarily anti-anxiety)
Valium®	diazepam
Parafon Forte DSC®	chlorzoxazone
Flexeril®	cyclobenzaprine
Soma®	carisoprodol
Robaxin®	methocarbamol
Norflex®	orphenadrine

the future. This one–two punch is considered the neuromuscular blockade (see Table 12-3).

ADVERSE ACTIONS

The adverse actions of skeletal muscle relaxants vary from mild to major. An overdose will produce toxic effects in which possible paralysis of the respiratory muscles causing respiratory failure and death may result. It is well documented that, in order to fall asleep, you must relax the body and muscles as well as the brain's thoughts and impulses. When you relax the muscles, you may also become sleepy, drowsy, or asleep. Therefore, you can expect the following side effects: drowsiness, dizziness, nausea, vomiting, fatigue, and weakness (see Table 12-4).

The main problem is the potentiation of the neuromuscular blocker by any CNS depressant or other muscle relaxant, which would lead to an increased and faster approach to death by respiratory depression (when respiratory muscles are depressed).

Treatment of Weak, Fragile, or Soft Bones

Osteoporosis, the thinning of bones in postmenopausal women and elderly men, is a major cause of bone fractures, affecting 20 million Americans. Women over age 45 commonly suffer fractures of the hip, wrist, or spine due to loss of bone mass from osteoporosis. Think of bone remodeling as a ditch digger digging a ditch and another person right beside him filling up the ditch. As old bone is worn away or removed, new bone is made. As calcium

TABLE 12-3 Agents for Surgical Procedures that Provide Temporary Muscle Paralysis	
Trade	Generic
Nonpolarizing Agents	
Curare—no trade name, available in nature	from South American plants such as *Strychnos toxifera, Strychnos castelnaei*, originally *used as an arrow poison*. When prepared and used properly, curare may assist in temporary muscle paralysis for surgery.
Flaxedil®	gallamine
Mivacron®	mivacurium
Pavalon®	pancuronium
Norcuron®	vecuronium
Tracrium®	atracurium
Zemuron®	rocuronium
Depolarizing Agents	
Quelicin®, Anectine®, or Sucostrin®	succinylcholine

TABLE 12-4 Examples of Drugs that Interact with Muscle Relaxants

Classification	Trade	Generic
Alchohol		
	Various	Various (even if in another medication preparation)
Antibiotics		
	Cleocin®	clindamycin
	Pipracil®	piperacillin
		neomycin
	Achromycin V®, Tetracyn®, Sumycin®	tetracycline - TCN
Benzodiazepines and other tranquilizers or sedatives		
	Halcion®	triazolam
	Valium®	diazepam
	Dalmane®	flurazepam
	Xanax®	alprazolam
Antiarrhythmics		
	Lidocaine®	xylocaine
General Anesthetics		
	Amidate®	etomidate
	Brevital®	methohexital
	Diprivan®	propofol
	Ethrane®	enflurane
	Fluothane®	halothane
	Forane®	isoflurane
	Ketalar®	ketamine
	Penthrane®	methoxyflurane
	Pentothal®	thiopental sodium

removal leaves a hole in the bone, new calcium is laid to fill in the holes, making new bone. PTH and calcitonin hormones from the parathyroid gland and thyroid gland, respectively, contribute to this homeostasis.

If there is too much calcium in the blood, the condition is called hypercalcemia. Hypercalcemia causes a decrease of sodium permeability across the cell membrane, decreasing nerve conduction. Since muscles such as the heart depend upon the influx of sodium, hypercalcemia will result in poor muscle function. If this muscle happens to be the heart, it will have less contractility and stop beating. The opposite is true with hypocalcemia, which would increase sodium influx, causing excitability to the nerve and increased conduction. Again, if this were the myocardium, increased excitability would increase contractility, and therefore tachycardia would result with possible myocardial infarction. Prolonged muscle spasms resulting from increased calcium in the blood are called tetany. Hypocalcemia causes increased spasms and convulsions.

In addition to vitamin D and mineral calcium replacement therapy, weak, fragile, and soft bones may respond to hormonal therapy (estrogen, calcitonin) and bisphosphonates. ERT (estrogen hormonal therapy) is used for osteoporosis, while bisphosphonates and HRT of calcitonin are used for both Paget's disease and osteoporosis.

Cholesterol in the skin, along with sunlight, generates the inactive form of vitamin D to become choecalciferol. Then it is sent to the blood system, where it becomes calcifediol, and finally to the kidneys, where it is changed by enzymes to active vitamin D called calcitriol.

The parathyroid gland and the thyroid gland work in a homeostatic way to ensure the bone building and bone demineralization (dissolution). Osteoclasts, bone cells that arise from marrow stroma cells and found on the surfaces where bone is being formed, are generally regarded as bone forming cells (the "good guys"). Osteoclasts, enriched with identifier acid phospatase, are large, multinucleated cells that play an active role in bone resorption or breakdown (the "bad guys"). PTH (parathyroid hormone) from the parathyroid gland and calcitonin from the thyroid gland work in tandem to accomplish this. When PTU is released, it stimulates bone demineralization or breaking down of bone. This is the process called bone resorption (not to be confused with term absorption, or reabsorption) in which the smaller minerals enter the bloodstream. One of the minerals that enters the blood system is calcium. Calcium is necessary for proper nerve and muscle function. PTH allows the kidneys to change the calcifediol to calcitriol.

When calcitriol is released from the kidneys back into the blood system, if there is too much in the blood, you would have hypercalemia. When this happens, the normal functioning thyroid gland will secrete calcitonin to counter the increase of Ca^{++} in the blood. While calcium is coming out of the bone into the blood, the bone is left with "holes" in it that may contribute to osteoporosis if the calcium is not put back—if the bone is not rebuilt.

BISPHOSPHONATES

Bisphosphonates are a very common treatment for osteoporosis. Bisphosphonates work by mimicking the natural organic bisphosphonate salts found in the body, inhibiting bone resorption and osteoclast activity. Bone mass and density are actually restored. There are two types of bisphosphonates: non-nitrogen side chain and nitrogen side chain bisphosphonates. The nitrogen side chains are preferred because they are more potent. Bisphosphonates irreversibly bind and inactivate osteoclasts and induce apoptosis of the osteoclast. In addition, they decrease osteoclast action. Bisphosphonates work by inhibition of the mevolonate pathway, the pathway responsible for cholesterol synthesis. The inactivated osteoclast is then incorporated into the bone matrix.

CALCITONIN

Calcitonin inhibits bone resorption and decreases the number of bone fractures from low bone density, increasing bone growth, or osteoblasts. Calcitonin blocks the bone-mineral-absorbing activity of the osteoclasts (bone cells), increases calcium excretion by the kidneys, and slows bone resorption—the speed at which bone is broken down before it is replaced. It acts directly on osteoclasts (via receptors on the cell surface for calcitonin). Often, calcitonin from eel or salmon is used, as it is many times stronger and longer lasting than the human form. Calcitonin is a polypeptide hormone that is a potent inhibitor of osteoclastic bone resorption, but its effects are only transient (temporary and come-and-go). The calcitonin receptor is specific for osteoclasts and causes rapid shrinkage of the osteoclasts with initial exposure. Osteoclasts avoid the inhibitory effects of calcitonin following continued exposure. It is available in a nasal spray or injection. Calcitonin produces small increments in the bone mass of the spine, with a modest reduction of bone turnover in women with osteoporosis (see Table 12-5).

While calcitonin reduces the risk of vertebral fracture in postmenopausal women with osteoporosis, it does not show much sign of helping nonvertebral (hip, wrist) fractures. Calcitonin may have an analgesic benefit. Miacalcin Nasal Spray® has a new delivery system via the nose, as opposed to injection. Inhalation of 200 units/day may exhibit the minor side effect of nasal irritation.

SELECTIVE ESTROGEN RECEPTOR MODULATORS

Another option for postmenopausal women is the class of drugs called SERMs (selective estrogen receptor modulators). SERMs, such as raloxifene used to prevent and treat osteoporosis, have a protective effect on the bones and heart; however, they do not control the hot flashes associated with menopause. Early studies report a significant reduction in the number of cases of breast cancer detected in women using SERMs.[4] Due to the lack of uterine stimulation with SERMs, there is no increased risk for endometrial cancer and no vaginal bleeding. The most common side effects are leg cramps and hot flashes that are worse than without the drug. Contraindictions include a history of breast cancer, liver problems, or blood clots; or if the patient is on HRT (see Table 12-6).

Ormeloxifene, a SERM being used in India and considered the "perfect SERM," may be approved by FDA soon. At this time, Ormeloxifene has not been approved in the United States.

NONPHARMACOLOGIC TREATMENTS OF OSTEOPOROSIS

These include weight-bearing exercise such as daily walking. Lifestyle changes include quitting smoking and reducing intake of caffeinated and alcoholic beverages. Calcium intake from diet and supplement needs to be

TABLE 12-5	Bone Resorption Inhibitors	
Bone Resorption Inhibitor	**Trade and Generic Names**	**Notes**
Nonnitrogen Side Bisphosphonates	1. Didronel® - etidronate 2. Skelid® - tiludronate	First and second generation Tx: Paget's Disease
Nitrogen Side Bisphosphonates	1. Fosamax® - alendronate 2. Actonel® - risedronate 3. Zomig® - zolendronate 4. Boniva® - ibandronate 5. Aredia® - pamidronate	The newer, more potent bisphosphonates, also called third generation bisphoshonates, Tx: hypercalcemia with metastases, menopausal osteoporosis
Calcitonin—polypeptide hormone	Miacalcin Nasal Spray®	Reduces the risk of vertebral fracture, but not hip or wrist, in postmenopausal women with osteoporosis

TABLE 12-6	Comparison Chart of Health Benefits and Risks of Drugs Used for Osteoporosis in Menopause			
	Parathyroid Hormone	**Hormone Replacement Therapy**	**SERMs**	**Bisphosphonates**
Selected Examples	Forteo® - teriparatide FDA approved	Premarin®, Climara®	Evista® - raloxifene, the only SERM approved for osteoporosis. Others in the investigational pipeline as of 2004.	**Oral agents:** Fosamax® - alendronate, Actonel®, risedronate. **Injected agents:** Aredia® - pamidronate Zometa® - zoledronic acid
Osteoporosis and Fracture	↑ bone mineral density ↓ risk for fracture	↑ bone density. ↓ fracture, although not significantly in women over 60. Not currently recommended for prevention of osteoporosis in most women (2004)	↑ bone density ↓ spinal fractures. Does not appear to prevent hip fractures as bisphosphonates do.	**DOC**—for most women. Only agents as of 2004 proven in large studies to **prevent** fractures, including hip and spine.

TABLE 12-6 Comparison Chart of Health Benefits and Risks of Drugs Used for Osteoporosis in Menopause (*continued*)

	Parathyroid Hormone	Hormone Replacement Therapy	SERMs	Bisphosphonates
Heart Disease	Unknown	No overall benefit, as there is an increased risk for MI and stroke within the first two years in women with existing heart disease	Possible protection, according to a 2002 study, in women with existing heart disease	No known effects
Cancer	Animal studies report higher risk for bone tumors. Human cancer risk unknown	Increased risk for breast cancer. Estrogen without progesterone increases risk for uterine cancer. Possible protection against colon cancer.	Tamoxifen and raloxifene reduce breast cancer risk. Tamoxifen, only, increases risk for uterine cancer.	May have anti-tumor properties. May slow metastasis to the bone in cancer patients.
Other Positive Effects	Unknown	Possible protection for urinary tract infections with vaginal application **only**, incontinence, glaucoma, macular degeneration	No vaginal bleeding. ↓ side effects more than HRT or bisphosphonates.	Unknown.
Other Negative Effects	Injectable only (pain)	↑ Risk for blood clots, vaginal bleeding, breast pain, asthma, endometriosis, fibroids, TMJ, varicose veins, gallstones. Mixed studies on Alzheimer's, osteoarthritis, migraines, and cataracts.	↑ Risk for blood clots. Side effects include menopausal symptoms of hot flashes, leg cramps. Swelling in the legs	Increased risk for GERD. Possible long-term risk for ulcers, especially in combination with NSAIDs or ASA. Administration of some requires empty stomach and 30 minutes of sitting up.

1500 mg per day for a postmenopausal woman or 1000 mg per day if she is receiving hormone replacement. U.S. RDA for men aged 25–65 is 1000 mg per day, and for men over 65, 1500 mg per day.

Treatment of Gout

DRUGS OF CHOICE

Colchicine is mainly used during the first 48 hours of an acute attack, because it will cause nausea and vomiting when given longer than that. Colchicine will alter the ability of the phagocytes to attack the uric acid crystals, which prevents the fall of the pH of the joint or synovial fluid. The cycle of the depositing of uric acid crystals and acid is broken. The gouty attack subsides. If a patient is taking "blood thinners," such as aspirin, persantine, or warfarin or is prone to ulcers with an NSAID or ASA, colchicines may be the drug of choice.

Anti-inflammatory analgesics such as aspirin and ibuprofen can be used to reduce the pain and inflammation of acute gouty attacks. Indomethacin is most often prescribed for gout inflammation.

PREVENTATIVE TREATMENT

Prophylactic therapy is the long-term use of drugs to prevent the reoccurrence of gouty attacks and tophi. There are two major types of drugs used: hypouricemic agents and uricosuric agents. Hypouricemic agents affect the amount of uric acid in the blood, whereas the uricosuric agents affect the elimination of uric acid from the kidneys via urination.

- **Hypouricemic agents** decrease production of uric acid in the blood. The enzyme xanthine oxidase is necessary to convert hypoxanthine into uric acid. The MOA is inhibition of the enzyme xanthine oxidase so that hypoxanthine is not made. Therefore, uric acid is *not* formed, and hypoxanthine is then excreted into the urine. Over a period of time, the uric acid in the blood decreases, preventing the future formation of tophi and urate stones in the kidney.
- **Uricosuric agents** increase the excretion of uric acid. Uricosuric drugs promote the excretion of uric acid via the kidney, without altering the formation of uric acid, which leads to a rapid clearance of uric acid from the blood. These drugs block the renal re-absorption (in the renal tubules) of uric acid so that uric acid passes into the urine.

Uricosuric drugs frequently cause GI distress. It is recommended that these drugs be taken with meals, milk, or antacids.

Combination drugs for gout are prophylactic and other drugs used as maintenance drugs. This type of drug would be Colbenemid® = probenecid + colchicine, which reduces urate blood levels and prevents further gouty attacks. Often, probenecid is administered in combination with colchicine as a preparation called Colbenemid®. To reduce the likelihood of developing renal urate stones, it is also recommended to drink plenty of water daily (see Table 12-7).

TABLE 12-7	Comparative Chart of Drugs Used to Treat Gout				
Indication	Classification	Trade	Generic	Purpose	MOA
Acute Gout Attack	Anti-Gout Agent	No trade name	colchicine	To stop the cycle of the depositing UA crystals and lowering the pH, during an immediate acute attack, within the first 48 hours	Alters phagocytes' ability to attack uric acid crystals, prevents the fall of the pH of the joint or synovial fluid. Stops the cycle of the uric acid crystals and low pH acid
Acute or Chronic	NSAID	Indocin®	indomethicine	Anti-inflammatory analgesics, reduce pain and swelling	Inhibits/blocks the enzyme Cox-2, starts the reaction of inflammation, preventing prostaglandin synthesis
Chronic	Hypouricemic agent	Zyloprim®	allopurinol	Prophylactic therapy—decreases production of uric acid in the blood	Inhibition of the enzyme xanthine oxidase, stopping production of hypoxanthine preventing formation of UA
Chronic	Uricosuric agent	Benemid®	probenecid	Prophylactic therapy—increases the excretion of uric acid	Blocks the tubule renal re-absorption of uric acid, so that uric acid passes into the urine
Chronic	Uricosuric agent	Anturane®	sulfinpyrazone	Prophylactic therapy—increases the excretion of uric acid	Blocks the tubule renal re-absorption of uric acid, so that uric acid passes into the urine
Chronic	Combination drug	Colbenemid®	probenecid + colchicine	Reduces urate blood levels and prevents further gouty attacks	MOA is same for the individual drugs (see the preceding)

Spastic Diseases

MULTIPLE SCLEROSIS

More commonly known as MS, this disease is signified by more than one (multiple) area of inflammation and scarring of the myelin in the brain and spinal cord. MS is an "autoimmune" disease in which, for unknown reasons, the body's immune system begins to attack normal body tissue. In the case of MS, the body attacks the cells that make myelin. Myelin is the tissue that covers and protects the nerve fibers. Nerve "communication" is disrupted. A person with MS experiences varying degrees of neurological impairment, depending on the location and extent of the scarring. Although there is no known cure for MS at this time, there is much that can be done to make the patient's life easier.

Symptoms of MS may include fatigue, weakness, spasticity, balance problems, bladder and bowel problems, numbness, vision loss, tremor, and vertigo. Not all symptoms affect all MS patients, and symptoms and signs may be persistent or may cease from time to time.

Treatment of MS includes steroidal anti-inflammatory agents, aka synthetic adrenal glucocorticoids, and corticosteroids such as betamethasone, dexamethasone, methylprednisolone, prednisone, and prednisolone.

CEREBRAL PALSY

Cerebral palsy refers to poor control of the brain, muscles, and joints. Cerebral palsy is caused by an injury to the brain before, during, or shortly after birth affecting body movements and muscle coordination. Affected children may not be able to walk, talk, eat, or play in the same ways as most other children.

CP is characterized by an inability to fully control motor function, particularly muscle control and coordination, and manifested by the following symptoms:

- muscle tightness or spasm
- involuntary movement
- disturbance in gait and mobility
- abnormal sensation and perception
- impairment of sight, hearing, or speech
- seizures

It is caused by damage to one or more specific areas of the brain, usually occurring during fetal development or infancy. It can also occur before, during, or shortly following birth.

Depending on the individual child's needs, physical therapy, occupational therapy, and a speech–language therapy are employed to improve posture and movement of the child. Pharmaceutical therapy includes drugs to prevent seizures and spasticity (see Tables 12-8 and 12-9).

TABLE 12-8   Drugs to Treat Seizures Associated with Cerebral Palsy

Trade®	Generic
Dilantin®	phenytoin
Tegretol®	carbamazepine
Luminal®, generic manufactures	phenobarbital

TABLE 12-9   Drugs to Treat Spasticity Associated with Cerebral Palsy

Trade®	Generic
Lioresal®	baclofen—muscle relaxant, MOA acts like GABA and decreases activity of nerves, blocking nerves within the reticular formation
Dantrium®—Peripheral Direct Acting SMA	dantrolene
Valium®— Benzodiazepine SMA	diazepam

SUMMARY

The musculoskeletal system provides the body with both form and movement and consists of bones and skeletal muscles. The musculoskeletal system has four main functions: to provide a framework or shape for the body, to protect the internal organs, to allow for body movement, and to provide storage for essential minerals. There are 206 bones in the human body. The five classes of bones are long, short, flat, irregular, and sesamoid. Skeletal muscles are classified as skeletal (voluntary muscles attached to the bone to provide body movement), cardiac (involuntary muscle attached to the heart), or smooth muscle (involuntary muscles attached to, or lining, the internal organs).

There are many disorders of the musculoskeletal system, some of which cause only discomfort and pain, and some of which can completely disable an individual. Osteoporosis, the most prevalent bone disorder in the U.S. affects approximately 20 million Americans, and is a major cause of bone fractures. Osteoarthritis, a progressive disease of the joints, affects up to 40 million Americans. A discussion of many, but not all, of the disorders affecting the musculoskeletal system is contained in this chapter.

There is a wide range of pharmaceuticals used for the treatment of diseases of the musculoskeletal system; many of them provide only symptomatic relief. However, as a result of intensive research, new products aimed at the prevention or retardation of disease, particularly in the areas of osteoporosis and osteoarthritis, may provide hope for the millions of Americans afflicted with these debilitating diseases.

CHAPTER REVIEW QUESTIONS

1. Identify the parts of this long bone:

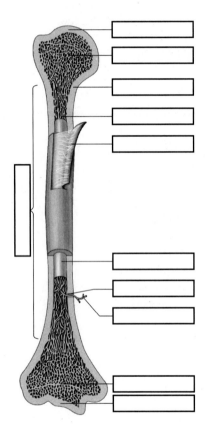

2. The purpose of bone marrow is to:
   a. produce red, purple, and yellow blood cells for oxygen production
   b. produce red blood cells, some white blood cells, and platelets, as well as acting as storage area for fat
   c. produce immune cells only
   d. separate the yellow fat cells from the red heme, or oxygen, cells.

3. The osteoclasts attach to the bone and dig up the bone matrix, leaving holes contributing to weak bones.
   a. true
   b. false

4. Osteoarthritis is a disease that results from infection in the spine.
   a. true
   b. false

5. Osteomyelitis can be treated with:
   a. HBO
   b. Clindamycin and PCN
   c. debrasion
   d. all of the above

6. Osteoarthritis can be treated with:
   a. nonsteroidal anti-inflammatories
   b. ibuprofen and fenoprofen
   c. ASA and gold
   d. a and b only

7. Gout is a condition of edema of the foot and toe.
   a. true
   b. false

8. Gout is caused by:
   a. too much uric acid in the blood
   b. too much uric acid combining at the joint with synovial fluid
   c. crystals of uric acid in the joint
   d. high purine diet
   e. all of the above

9. Rheumatoid arthritis is treated with:
   a. MTX and gold
   b. antimalarial drugs such as hydroxychloroquine
   c. penicillamine and sulfasalazines

d. dihydroorotate dehydrogenase inhibitors such as leflunomide

e. all of the above

10. Gout is treated with:

a. cochicine during an acute attack

b. hyporuricemics and uricosurics during chronic phases

c. hypercalcemics during chronic phases

d. a and b only

e. b and c only

11. How do hyporuricemics decrease production of uric acid in the blood?

a. by inhibition of the enzyme "xanthine oxidase" so that hypoxanthine is not made

b. increase the excretion of uric acid

c. cause a rapid clearance of uric acid from the blood

d. are prophylactic only

e. a and d only

f. b and c only

12. Uricosuric agents:

a. increase the excretion of uric acid

b. promote the excretion of uric acid via the kidney, without altering the formation of uric acid

c. cause a rapid clearance of uric acid from the blood

d. block the renal re-absorption (in the renal tubules) of uric acid so that uric acid passes into the urine

e. promote inhibition of the enzyme "xanthine oxidase"

f. a, b, c, and d only

g. b, c, d, and f only

13. Cox-2 inhibitors:

a. produce prostaglandins that contribute to inflammation

b. block Cycoloxygenase II, the enzyme that produces the prostaglandins that contribute to inflammation

c. block the NSAID effect

d. increase the viscosity of the mucosal lining of the GI tract, reducing ulcers

14. The DOC for osteoporosis in menopausal women is:

a. calcitonin, which inhibits bone resorption

b. bisphosphonates, which inhibit bone resorption and osteoclast activity

c. calcium and vitamin D supplements

d. SERMs

15. PTH and calcitonin produce a homeostasis for bone remodeling.

a. true

b. false

16. Alcohol, benzodiazepines, and general anesthetics produce an adverse reaction that will promote respiratory depression and possible death.

a. true

b. false

17. Which of the following treats seizures associated with cerebral palsy?

a. Dilantin®

b. Tegretol®

c. phenobarbitol

d. all of the above

18. The MOA of acting like GABA, blocking the nerves within the reticular formation of the brain that control the muscles, thus inhibiting muscular function, belongs to which drug?

a. Dilantin®

b. Cleocin®

c. Lioresal®

d. bisphosphonates

19. The direct acting skeletal muscle relaxants act by:
    a. interfering with the actin and myosin biochemical pathways on the muscle itself, preventing contraction
    b. interfering with the calcium release from the sarcoplasmic reticulum, thereby dissociating the excitation coupling
    c. blocking descending reticular formation and spinal cord neuronal activity
    d. stimulating GABA-b receptors, causing relaxation
    e. a and d
    f. a and c

Resources and References

1. MOA of APAP News on APAP:
   http://www.pharmweb.net/pwmirror/pwy/paracetamol/pharmwebpicmechs.html
2. Arthritis Today, 2004 Drug Guide, DMARDs:
   http://www.arthritis.org/conditions/DrugGuide/about_dmards.asp
3. *Merck Manual of Diagnosis and Therapy*:
   http://www.merck.com/mrkshared/mmanual/section5/chapter57/57a.jsp
4. National Library of Medicine: A review of SERM's and National Surgical Adjuvant Breast and Bowel Project Clinical Trials:
   http://www.ncbi.nlm.nih.gov/entrez/query.fcgi?cmd=Retrieve&db=PubMed&listuids=14613021&dopt=Abstract
5. Chart 8–1 Comparison Chart of Health Benefits and Risks of Drugs Used for Osteoporosis in Menopause: information gathered from
   http://www.hosppract.com/cc/1999/cc9908
   http://www.ubcpharmacy.org/cpe/resources/highlights/fall2000.pdf
   Facts and Comparisons 200
6. Cerebral Palsy—A multimedia tutorial for children and parents
   http://www.people.virginia.edu/~smb4v/tutorials/cp/cp.htm
7. *The Virtual Anaesthesia Textbook Non-Opioid Analgesics*
   http://www.virtual-anaesthesia-textbook.com/vat/non_narcotics.html#intro
8. *Cerebral Palsy: A Guide for Care*, by Miller, Bachrach
   http://gait.aidi.udel.edu/res695/homepage/pd ortho/clinic.cpalsy/cpweb.htm#RTFT
9. Watch a Video on Arava for Rheumatoid Arthritis:
   http://www.arava.com/professional/about_arava/works.do
10. Holland, Norman and Michael Patrick Adams. *Core Concepts in Pharmacology*. Upper Saddle River, NJ: Pearson Education, 2003.
11. Adams, Michael Patrick, Dianne L. Josephson, and Leland Norman Holland, Jr. *Pharmacology for Nurses—A Pathophysiologic Approach*. Upper Saddle River, NJ: Pearson Education, 2005.

The Respiratory System

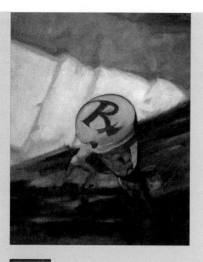

INTRODUCTION

Children commonly hold their breath to find out what it feels like. Adult do so while swimming or to prevent inhalation of an offending odor. This act cannot be performed very long without giving up, not only to the desire for air, but to the need for it. Oxygen and the action of getting it into the body and to the various parts of the body (known as respiration) are crucial to sustain life.

Most people can survive for weeks (probably 50–80 days) without food, for several days (3–14) without water, and a few hours without adequate warmth in cold weather. After several minutes without air, however, the brain begins to suffer serious consequences, major organs shut down, and eventually the person dies. The longer the body goes without air, the more damage is done. It is the respiratory system that performs the essential action of receiving and exchanging air through the lungs, known as breathing.

After completing this chapter, you should be able to:

- Identify and list the basic anatomical structural parts of the respiratory tract.

- Describe the function or physiology of the individual parts of the respiratory system and the external exchange of oxygen and waste.

- List and define common diseases affecting the respiratory tract and comprehend the causes, symptoms, and pharmaceutical treatment associated with each disease.

- Explain the mechanisms of the following respiratory diseases and comprehend how each class of drugs works in order to mitigate the symptoms: colds, allergies, asthma, emphysema, rhinitis, nasal congestion, bronchoconstriction, and COPD.

- Describe and understand the indication for use and mechanism of action of mucolytics for CF and their antidotal use for APAP overdose.

- List the trade and generic names for the various classifications of drugs for the respiratory tract.

- Define and utilize key terms.

Anatomy of the Respiratory System

The one respiratory system is divided into two parts. The upper respiratory tract consists of the nasal cavity (nose), paranasal sinuses, and pharynx (throat) and ends at the larynx. (See Figure 13-1.) The larynx acts in conjunction with the epiglottis to guard the entrance to the trachea and lower airways. It also functions as the voice box. The lower respiratory tract consists of the trachea (which enters the thoracic cavity), two lungs, two main bronchi (one to each lung), secondary and tertiary bronchi, bronchioles ending with the terminal respiratory bronchioles, alveolar ducts, and alveoli. (See Figure 13-2.)

The upper respiratory tract gets afflicted with diseases such as sinusitis, colds with either rhinitis or nasal congestion, and allergies: while the lower respiratory tract is affected by bronchial infections, bronchoconstriction, and chronic obstructive diseases such as asthma and emphysema.

Function of the Respiratory System

The primary function of the respiratory system is to supply oxygen to the blood, which carries it to all parts of the body. The blood carries oxygen via the "freeways" of the circulatory system, or the blood vessels known as the veins, arteries, and capillaries. The heart is the pump that propels the blood to and from the lungs. The purpose of the respiratory system is twofold in that it (1) transports air to and from the lungs and (2) exchanges gases within the blood vessels—oxygen for carbon dioxide. During its journey, air is *humidified*, warmed, and purified (suspended particles removed).

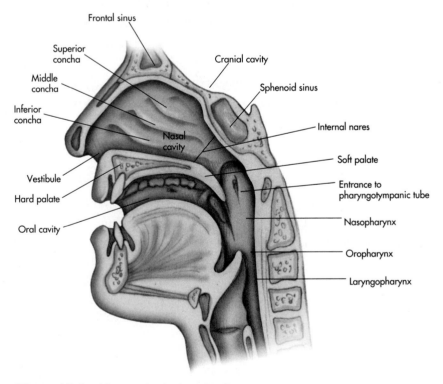

Figure 13-1 Upper respiratory tract

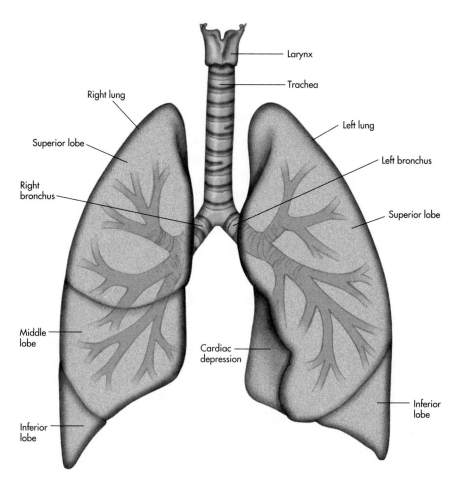

Figure 13-2   Lower respiratory tract

Respiration or breathing is the mechanism through which gas exchange is accomplished. When we breathe, we inhale air, which has oxygen in it, and when we exhale we release carbon dioxide, a byproduct of the usage of oxygen that plants utilize. This exchange of gases, called the external exchange, is the way in which the respiratory system gets oxygen to the blood. If oxygen does not get to a specific part of the body, that part would die. Without oxygen, for even a few seconds, the whole body would die. When blood stops moving, oxygen does not get to the tissue that it needs to "feed." This is called *ischemia*. (The "internal exchange" will be discussed in Chapter 14, The Circulatory System.)

The supportive functions of the lymphatic system of the lungs are three-fold: (1) maintains fluids, (2) provides respiratory immunity defenses, and (3) removes inhaled solid material and microorganisms. The sizable flow of lymph from the lung tissue interstitial spaces into the blood help to eliminate excess fluid, and the lymphoid tissue of the tonsils protect against infection at the entrance to the respiratory tract. (More discussion of the lymphatic system can be found in Chapter 14, The Circulatory System, and Chapter 15, The Immune System.)

In essence, there are two ways to get oxygen to the body: (1) via the respiratory system, which brings oxygen into the body and blood, and (2) the

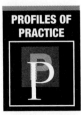
What is a hiccup? A hiccup is technically known as a singultus and diaphragmatic spasm. The diaphragm usually works without a hitch. But sometimes the diaphragm can become irritated and jerk, causing the breath to be exhaled differently. An irritation or stimulation of the glossopharyngeal area causes this irregular breath. During the jerking motion, the diaphragm contracts involuntarily. The person takes in a quick breath of air into the lungs. Then this irregular breath of air hits the voice box, and the sound it makes is called the hiccup. Things that can irritate the diaphragm are eating or swallowing too quickly, eating too much, an irritation in the stomach or the throat, or a feeling of being nervous or excited. Most cases of hiccups last only for a few minutes.

However, some cases of hiccups can last beyond a few days, which usually indicates that there is another medical problem. "The longest hiccup ever known was experienced by an American pig farmer whose hiccups persisted from 1922 to 1987."

circulatory system, which takes the oxygen in the blood to various parts of the body. The respiratory and circulatory systems work in tandem to accomplish their mutual goal of keeping the body alive.

A DIFFERENCE BETWEEN AIR AND OXYGEN

Air is a mixture of gases, not one pure element. The normal composition of air by volume is approximately 78 percent nitrogen, 21 percent oxygen, and 0.03 percent carbon dioxide. The balance is made up of other gases, like argon, helium, krypton, neon, and xenon, which occur in trace (small) amounts. In addition, air contains water vapor, traces of ammonia, and suspended matter such as bacteria, dust, spores, and plant debris. Oxygen is a gas that is one pure element. Oxygen is just one of the components of air.

ACTUAL RESPIRATION AND THE EXTERNAL EXCHANGE

Respiration is achieved through the mouth, nose, trachea, lungs, and diaphragm. Inspiration of air occurs when the pressure inside the lung, known as intrapulmonary pressure, becomes lower than the outside (atmospheric) pressure. This change in pressure allows the air to flow into the alveoli (tiny air sacs) of the lungs. During inspiration the intrapulmonary pressure would be less than the atmospheric pressure of 760 mm Hg. During inspiration, oxygen enters the upper respiratory system through the mouth and the nose, where it is warmed and filtered by *cilia*, the tiny hair-like organelles found in the nose and bronchial passageways.

Cilia provide another important function by adhering to inhaled dust, smoke and other pollutants and then moving in a specific manner to eliminate the irritants. The oxygen then passes through the larynx (the voice box) and the *trachea* (wind pipe). The trachea is a tube that enters the chest cavity, where it splits into two smaller tubes called the bronchi. Each bronchus then splits off into the bronchial tubes. The bronchial tubes lead into the lungs, where they split off into many smaller tubes, which connect to tiny air sacs called alveoli. This upside-down tree may look like broccoli. The small buds of the broccoli are the tiny air sacs known as alveoli.

The average adult human lungs contain about 600 million spongy alveoli, which are surrounded by capillaries. These alveoli are often referred to as grape-like clusters of air sacs. Inhaled air with oxygen passes into the alveoli and then diffuses oxygen through the capillaries. The oxygen then travels into the arterial blood (oxygen rich blood). During this same time, the blood that is full of waste, from the veins and capillaries, releases its carbon dioxide into the alveoli. The carbon dioxide leaves the lungs by the same capillaries during exhalation.

In review, alveoli bring new oxygen from the breathed-in air to the bloodstream. These alveoli, or "air sacs," exchange oxygen for waste products, like carbon dioxide, which the cells in the body have made and cannot use. In fact, if the waste does not leave the body, it will accumulate in the blood and cause suffocation to all body parts due to the lack of external exchange. There must be an external exchange of carbon dioxide for air, from which oxygen can be extracted. This external exchange that keeps the human body alive is directed by the brain, which does it automatically. (Read more about this and other autonomic functions in Chapter 19, The Nervous System.)

The Diaphragm

The diaphragm is a layer or sheet of muscles that lies across the bottom of the chest cavity. The shape of the diaphragm is often times referred to as a dome. The function of the diaphragm is to pump or push the carbon dioxide out of the lungs and take in or pull the oxygen into the lungs. Breathing occurs as the diaphragm contracts and relaxes. Contraction of the diaphragm causes oxygen to be pulled or taken into the lungs; the chest expands. Relaxation of the diaphragm causes carbon dioxide to be pumped out or pushed out of the lungs; as the abdomen pushes up against the diaphragm, the chest contracts or shrinks.

The Lung and the Conducting Airways

Only about 10 percent of the lung is occupied by solid tissue. The remainder is filled with air and blood. The functional structure of the lung can be divided into two parts: the conducting airways (aka dead air space) for ventilation and the gas exchange portions for perfusion, which utilizes the circulatory system. The conducting airways are tubes lined by cilia and respiratory *mucosa* and contain differing amounts of muscle or hyaline cartilage in their walls. Airways are for conducting air, which means passing it through the pathways to the destination for clearance and filtering foreign particles. The conducting airways move approximately 10,000 liters of inspired air per day. The main differences between the bronchi and the bronchioles are the presence or lack of cartilage. (See Figure 13-3.)

Cartilage is a form of protection and cushioning for the bronchi. The bronchioles contain little cartilage in their walls and instead have a thick layer of smooth muscle, which controls the size of the lumen. The lumen is the opening or inner diameter in which air passes—like a tunnel. The bronchi contain hyaline cartilage rings in their walls to keep the airways open.

How We Breathe

We inspire, or breathe in, about 20 times a minute. During inhalation, air passes through the nasal passages where it is filtered, heated, and moistened and enters the back of the throat. We breathe with the help of the diaphragm and other muscles in the chest and abdomen. These muscles physically change the space and pressure inside the body to assist breathing and to create a capacity for air. When the diaphragm pulls down or contracts, it leaves more space for the lungs to expand and also lowers the internal air pressure. The air then expands the lungs like a pair of balloons. Shortly thereafter, the diaphragm relaxes, and the cavity inside the body gets smaller again. These

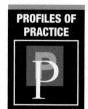

PROFILES OF PRACTICE

What is a yawn? Medical school teaches that a yawn, although not completely understood, is caused by a lack of oxygen in the alveoli, which makes the lungs stiffen and react to get more oxygen into the lungs.

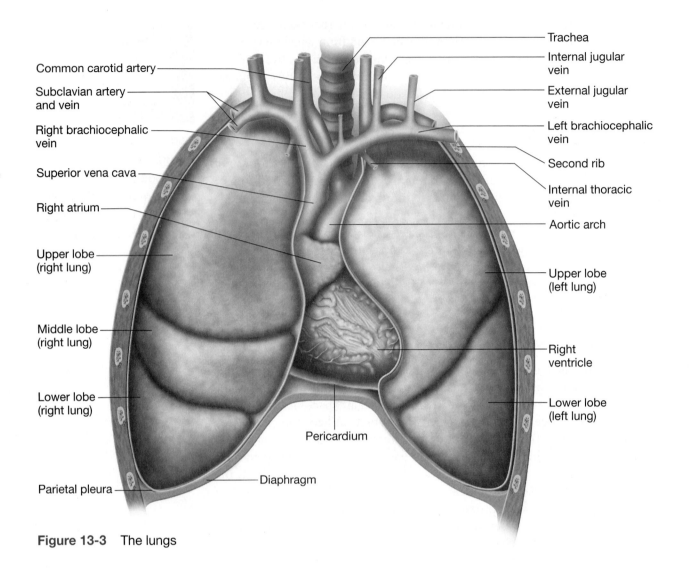

Common carotid artery

Subclavian artery and vein

Right brachiocephalic vein

Superior vena cava

Right atrium

Upper lobe (right lung)

Middle lobe (right lung)

Lower lobe (right lung)

Parietal pleura

Trachea

Internal jugular vein

External jugular vein

Left brachiocephalic vein

Second rib

Internal thoracic vein

Aortic arch

Upper lobe (left lung)

Right ventricle

Lower lobe (left lung)

Pericardium

Diaphragm

Figure 13-3   The lungs

muscles squeeze the rib cage, collapsing the lungs, and push air up and out of the body as an exhale. Inspiration is taking in air (to get oxygen), while expiration is letting out waste (carbon dioxide).

Note: **Do we breathe when we swallow?** The esophagus, or food pipe, is located at the back of the throat and the windpipe for air is located at the front. This prevents food from getting into the windpipe and causing us to choke. When we swallow during ingestion, a flap called the epiglottis swings down to cover the windpipe, so that food doesn't go down the windpipe ("wrong pipe"). This flap blocks the air coming in just for a second, so for that moment in time we are not breathing. Therefore, we do not breathe when we are swallowing. In addition, since smell and breathing help in tasting food, we are not tasting our food as we swallow—that has been done by our taste buds prior to swallowing!

Disease States of the Respiratory Tract

There are many diseases and conditions of the respiratory tract that can be treated with over the counter medications. However, infections and cancer must be treated with specific anti-infectives, antibiotics, and chemotherapeutic drugs. (Chapter 15, The Immune System, will address the issues regarding these disease states.) In this chapter, the common cold, allergies, anaphylactic shock, and chronic obstructive diseases such as emphysema and asthma will be explored. With COPD, the normal flow of air is blocked by excess mucus and inflammation such as with chronic bronchitis, by collapsed airways such as with emphysema, or by tightening of the muscles around the airways such as with chronic asthma. As a result, the patient will exhibit and feel a shortness of breath. The patient will also cough or wheeze or feel weak. Emphysema, asthma, or bronchitis may exist alone or co-exist.

Cough and Colds

Colds, caused by a viral infection, lead to more absences at work or school each year than any other medical reason. The cold inflames the membranes in the lining of the nose and throat, this inflammation is called rhinitis. Over 200 different viruses are responsible for the common cold. Among the most common are rhinoviruses, which thrive in the nasal mucosa, and corona viruses that cause respiratory, neurological, and *enteric* infections.

One of the reasons for the increased incidence of colds during the fall and winter months, or "cold season," is considered to be the fact that people are more often indoors, in closer proximity to each other, and often with a heater on. Many cold viruses flourish in low humidity during colder months, making the nasal passages drier and more vulnerable to infection. This susceptibility is especially intensified when the heater is on in indoors. Colds usually start two to three days after the virus enters the body, and symptoms last from several days to several weeks. The symptoms of the common cold may include the following:

- stuffy nose or congestion, swelling of the sinus membranes
- difficulty breathing
- runny nose, rhinitis
- sneezing
- sore or scratchy throat, mild hacking cough
- headache
- low-grade fever or chills
- achy muscles and bones or mild fatigue
- watery discharge from nose
- a discharge from the nose that thickens and turns yellow or green

Corona viruses are named for their corona-like or halo-like appearance in electron spectrographs, caused by various projections on the surface of the viral envelope, one of which is the E2 glycoprotein. E2 glyocprotein is the viral attachment protein and target of neutralizing antibodies. These viruses affect adults and are difficult to culture in a laboratory.

Colds can best be prevented by not being in contact with others with a cold and by washing your hands, which come in contact with the virus. Avoid touching your eyes, nose, or mouth when in contact with others who are contaminated with the virus. Lower the thermostat of the indoor heater; use more blankets as an alternative.

HOW A COLD VIRUS BECOMES A DISEASE

The exact mechanism of the cold virus is not fully known or understood, but the following is the most probable explanation of the sequence of events that cause a cold *virus* to become a disease. Viruses cause infection by overpowering the immune system. The first line of immunity defense is mucus, which is produced by the mucus membranes in the nose and throat. Mucus captures inhaled material such as pollen, dust, pollution, bacteria, and viruses. After a virus enters the mucus membrane, it then enters a nose, ear, eye, or skin cell, and overtakes protein synthesis to manufacture new viruses, which, in turn, attack surrounding body cells (see Table 13-1).

Cold symptoms are most likely a result of the immune response to the viral attack. Virus-infected nose cells emit (send out) signals that command white blood cells to the site of the infection. In turn, these cells send out immune system chemicals such as kinins. Kinins lead to the symptoms of the common cold by causing swelling and inflammation of the nasal membranes, leakage of proteins, fluid from capillaries and lymph vessels, and the increased production of mucus. Researchers are examining whether drugs to block kinins and other immune system substances, or the receptors on cells to which they bind, might benefit people with colds.

COUGH AS A SYMPTOM AND A COMPLICATION OF THE COMMON COLD

A cough may be a symptom of a cold, flu, other respiratory problems, or even non-respiratory tract diseases. There are many ways to look at a cough as a symptom:

TABLE 13-1   Comparison of the Cold and Flu Virus Symptoms

Cold Symptoms	Flu Symptoms
Low or no fever	High fever
Sometimes a headache	Usually a headache
Stuffy or a runny nose	Clear nose
Sneezing	Sometimes sneezing
Mild, hacking cough	Productive cough, may become severe
Slight aches and pains	Often severe aches and pains
Mild fatigue	Severe fatigue, may last for weeks
Sore throat	Usually a sore throat
Normal energy level	Extreme exhaustion
Colds occasionally can lead to secondary bacterial infections of the middle ear or sinuses, requiring treatment with antibiotics.	Influenzas occasionally can lead to secondary bacterial infections of the lungs/bronchi and bronchioles, or to pneumonia.

- Cough helps us to clear mucus and foreign material from our airways. In this respect, we can remove irritants and microorganisms, which means cough is purposeful and needs to be as effective as possible.
- Cough can be a sign of a problem, such as a chicken bone in the airway. Many times coughs have alerted others that the person coughing is choking and needs the Heimlich maneuver. Again, the cough is purposeful.
- Patients with heart problems such as CHF, with an acute stage of abnormal beating or rhythm of the heart, can be in need of restoring normal cadence or heartbeat. A cough can be a lifesaving effort to restore the normal heartbeat.

Patients seek treatment for cough due to complications of infectious cough such as the following:

- hoarseness or inability to speak clearly or be heard
- symptoms of insomnia due to coughing during the night
- musculoskeletal pain, especially in the respiratory muscles and diaphragm
- urinary incontinence—When the PC muscle weakens, the continence mechanism in the urethra does not work well, and small increases in abdominal pressure can cause urine to leak. Urine loss occurs with activities that increase intra-abdominal pressure—such as sneezing, coughing, laughing, standing, and lifting—when the PC muscle that helps to hold the urethra, bladder, vagina, and rectum in place weaken. This stress incontinence occurs more often, especially when the PC muscle is already weakened.
- subjective perceptions of exhaustion
- subjective perceptions of self-consciousness (being heard coughing)

There are many causes of cough, but it is agreed by most that a cough probably begins with an irritation of nerves in the respiratory tract. The irritation may come from a clump of mucus in the airway from exposure to an airborne offender such as a chemical aerosol (hair spray, room freshener, perfume, pesticides, paint fumes), or from postnasal drip.

There are many other causes. Postnasal drip, or PND, usually results in the patient who has recently had a cold or flu or suffers from *allergic rhinitis* or acute or chronic sinusitis. Disease states such as asthma, bronchitis, CHF, and GERD as well as side effects of certain drugs such as ACE inhibitors can also contribute to cough.

Psychogenic cough, which is emotional or psychological in origin, also known as "habit" or "nervous" cough, and sounds like a person clearing his throat, has other causes. Cystic fibrosis, an idiopathic pulmonary fibrosis disease, can cause thick mucus to build that needs to be expelled or expectorated. Asthma, sinusitis, and GERD are the most frequent causes of chronic cough in children. Serious respiratory complications of GERD include cough, chronic bronchitis, progressively worsening bronchial asthma, and other pulmonary diseases.

Post-infectious cough persists for three or more weeks, usually as the only remaining symptom after a viral upper respiratory tract infection such as flu. This condition is due to persistent inflammation after infection. It goes away in time. A persistent acute cough that lasts for three weeks or less is usually caused by the common cold, but can be a symptom of a more serious illness such as pneumonia or congestive heart failure.

A recurring cough that lasts for three or more weeks at a time is considered to be a chronic cough. It is sometimes caused by more than one condition and is most common among tobacco smokers, but also in nonsmokers with postnasal drip syndrome (PNDS), gastroesophageal asthma, or reflux disease (GERD). "Smokers' cough" can mask a more serious cause of cough, such as pneumonia or congestive heart failure.

If a pertussis such as whooping cough exists, antibiotic treatment is warranted to fight the bacterial infection in the patient and possibly in all persons who were exposed to pertussis. Children usually get pertussis. It is difficult for the child to stop coughing and to get air. There are coughing spasms with a typical "whooping" sound that follows the cough. This sound indicates that the child is trying to catch his breath before the next bout of whooping or coughing. Complications that may set in for children are pneumonia, seizures, brain damage, and death. Children under seven years of age need to be vaccinated against pertussis.

A series of five injections of DTaP (for Diphtheria/Tetanus/Pertussis) has prevented many deaths since its requirement in the United States. An effective, purposeful cough requires normal nerve pathways in the respiratory tract, so that cough can occur when needed. Normal muscle tone of the diaphragm and abdomen, the respiratory muscles, are required to create a strong push to the lungs for expiration to expel the air and normal mucus stickiness and viscosity. Excessive coughing can affect the normal muscle tone, hindering the dislodging of mucus or phlegm to be expelled from bronchial airways by the cough.

Mucus occurs in a productive cough, while a nonproductive cough is a dry, hacking cough. A productive cough is purposeful, requires drugs to promote the removal of the mucus, and may help some patients cough up and expel abnormally thick mucus by thinning it out. It is important to keep the airways free of mucus in order to prevent invasion by bacteria that can cause serious disease to the respiratory tract.

A nonproductive cough is usually not purposeful and may persist, becoming as problematic as it is annoying. A nonproductive cough can be exhausting, depending on the duration and forcefulness of the cough. Intercostal tissue of the rib cage may tear if the cough persists. Drugs can be given to stop the nonproductive cough. Some nonproductive coughs result as a side effect of a medication that is being taken for a different condition or disease.

TREATING THE COMMON COLD WITH DRUGS

Treatment of colds can only be considered as symptomatic treatment. OTC drugs and common-sense therapies are available for uncomplicated cases of the common cold. Among them, bed rest, keeping warm, drinking plenty of fluids, gargling with warm salt water, and using petroleum jelly for a raw nose are the most accepted. Treatments of colds with drugs, whether over the counter or prescription, include the following classifications:

- antihistamines, which allow one to get sleep and dry up mucus membranes
- decongestants, which thin mucus and allow easier passage of mucus
- cough suppressants, expectorants, and mucolytics
- analgesics, which relieve pain or body aches
- antipyretics, which reduce body temperature
- anti-inflammatory agents, which reduce inflammation

Note: Antibiotics will not cure the cold or any other viral infection. However, it is possible to develop a secondary bacterial infection, for which antibiotics will most likely be prescribed.

ANTIHISTAMINES FOR THE COMMON COLD

When used in cough or cold products, these agents dry the wet mucus lining due to their anti-cholinergic effects. They help the body to go to sleep to get the much-needed rest and to repair itself, due to their effects on the CNS. (Antihistamines, also used for allergic reactions, are discussed separately.) For symptoms of the common cold, antihistamines can be used to dry up mucus membranes in cold formulas, antihistamines for seasonal allergies, and as a sleep aid when repackaged and marketed for insomnia. Many drugs have many different uses, based upon what they do as a desired effect and what they do as a side effect. Can you name other drugs that are used for many different reasons?

Side effects of antihistamines are drowsiness, sleepiness, and dry mucus membranes, such as the mouth, nose, or eyes. Some antihistamines also stop nausea, vomiting, and motion sickness.

Antihistamines have two mechanisms of action (MOAs) to combat colds and one more MOA to combat allergies. First generation antihistamines cause the anti-cholinergic effects of drying of mucus membranes of the nose, mouth, and eyes—by attaching to muscarinic or cholinergic receptors, which blocks the effect of acetylcholine (ACH).

Note: Only first generation antihistamines work on cholinergic receptors. This MOA helps to combat both the common cold and allergies.

First generation antihistamines are lipophilic; therefore, they cross the blood brain barrier and enter the CNS, causing sedation as a side effect. This side effect can be desirable for those with a cold who may need to rest and sleep; but for the average person with allergies who wants to function normally on the job or at school this may be an unwanted side effect.

Antihistamines also are used to combat allergies and work by blocking the Histamine-1 or H-1, from entering the H-1 receptor site of a given body part such as the nose, eye, skin ear, or throat. If the H-1 cannot enter the H-1 receptor site, then no allergic reaction will occur (see Tables 13-2, 13-3, 13-4 and 13-5).

TABLE 13-2 Examples of OTC Antihistamines Used for Cold and Allergy Symptoms

Generic Name	Trade Name®
Antihistamines, H-1 Antagonists	
chlorpheniramine	Chlor-Trimeton® (CTM)®, Drowsy
clemastine	Tavist-1, Drowsy
cyproheptadine	Periactin, Drowsy
brompheniramine	Dimetapp®, Drowsy
brompheniramine	Nasahist B®, Drowsy
brompheniramine	Oraminic II®, Drowsy
diphenhydramine	Bendryl®, Drowsy
diphenhydramine	Banophen®, Drowsy
diphenhydramine	Diphedryl®, Drowsy
loratadine	Alavert®, Non-Drowsy
loratadine	Claritin, Non-Drowsy
loratadine/psuedoephedrine	Claritin-D®, Non-Drowsy

TABLE 13-3 Examples of Prescription (Rx) Antihistamines for Allergy

Generic Name	Trade Name®	Formula
Antihistamines, H-1 Antagonists		
azelastine	Astelin NS®	Possible Drowsy, nasal spray
cetirizne	Zyrtec®	Non-Drowsy, PO
fexofenadine	Allegra®	Non-Drowsy, PO
hydroxyzine	Atarax®	Drowsy, PO
hydroxyzine	Vistaril®	Drowsy, IV, IM
hydroxyzine	Vistazine®	Drowsy, PO
promethazine	Phenergan®	Drowsy, PO, IM, PR

TABLE 13-4 Examples of Prescription Antihistamines for Unusual Indications or Dosage Forms

Generic Name	Trade Name®	Indication
Antihistamines, H-1 Antagonists		
emedastine	Emadine®	Rx ophthalmic, allergic conjunctivitis
hydroxyzine	Atarax® (PO), Vistraril® (Inj.)	pre-op anxiety pruitus, nausea/vomiting
ketotifen fumarate	Zaditen®	Rx–Combination ophthalmic antihistamine and a mast cell stabilizer. Has a distinct inhibitory effect on eosinophil infiltration, activation, and degranulation
meclizine	Antivert® (PO)	OTC for motion sickness

TABLE 13-5 Table of Comparison of Degree of Sedation of Various Types of Antihistamines

Ethanolamines		Ethylenediamines		Alkylamines
1. clemastine 2. diphenhydramine 3. doxylamine	**Greater sedation than →**	1. pyrilamine 2. thonzylamine	**Greater sedation than →**	1. pheniramine 2. brompheniramine 3. chlropheniramine 4. triprolidine

DECONGESTANTS

Decongestants thin out the mucus in the inflamed, stuffy nose and clear the nasal passages, allowing for easier breathing. Indications for use are for nasal and bronchial congestion.

Examples of OTC decongestants are generic pseudoephedrine = Sudafed®, Allermed®, and Genaphed® Actifed®, Drixoral®. All that is mentioned for pseudoephedrine also applies to Nature's Way® and other "health store" products that contain naturally derived pseudoephedrine from the Chinese herb ephedra, or ma huang. Side effects apply to these products as well.

Only one oral decongestant, pseudoephedrine, is currently approved by the FDA. Pseudoephedrine is an alpha-adrenergic agonist, which acts on alpha-adrenergic receptors in the blood vessels of the nasal mucosa to produce vasoconstriction, resulting in decreased blood flow and shrinkage of tissue in the nasal passages, thus reducing vascular inflammation and edema that is associated with congestion. This drug is a sympathomimetic agent that mimics stimulation of the sympathetic nervous system and "acts like" Norepinephrine. It acts predominantly on the alpha–adrenergic receptors, but has a little effect on beta-2 receptors. By constricting or shrinking blood vessels (veins and arteries) in the nose, lungs, and other mucus membranes, it provides relief of nasal congestion known more commonly as "stuffy nose."

While pseudoephedrine, like ephedra, has an indirect effect by releasing norepinephrine from the storage sites in the neuronal terminals (nerve endings), it also can relax the bronchial smooth muscles by acting directly on Beta-2 adrenergic receptors in the mucosa of the respiratory tract. This stimulation produces vasoconstriction, which shrinks swollen nasal mucus membranes; reduces tissue hyperemia (excessive blood), edema, and nasal congestion; and increases the patency (openness) of the nasal airway passages. In addition, it promotes an increase in the drainage of sinus secretions. Obstructed eustachian tubes may also be opened. It has very little effect on the CNS, which is why this over the counter agent has been used successfully by so many for such a very long time. Some OTC diet aids also include pseudoephedrine as a mild stimulant.

Side effects of oral pseudoephedrine include irregular heartbeat, palpitations, hypertension, and shortness of breath. CNS toxic effects include convulsions, hallucinations, and stimulation. This drug may also cause asthmatic attacks.

Benefits and disadvantages of oral pseudoephedrine compared with topical nasal inhalation are as follows:

- PO—Prolonged decongestant effects, but has a delayed onset; topical usually works quickly within five minutes.

- PO—No rebound congestion; topical has a rebound effect. Rebound effect occurs with topical decongestants only when more and more product is needed to produce the same effect. This will increase side effects as well. This happens with prolonged use (more than three to five days) when nasal decongestants lose effectiveness and even cause swelling in the nasal passages. The patient then increases the frequency of the dose. Congestion worsens, and the patient responds by increasing the doses or frequency of doses to as often as every hour. Patients can become dependent upon use. This effect may occur with ophthalmic decongestants as well. PO is less potent than topical; topical has a direct effect and has less systemic effects.

Note: Pseudoephedrine is an essential chemical used in methamphetamine production, and therefore a sought-after ingredient. "Meth" is an illegal, highly addictive street stimulant. Because many pharmacies have had raids on this drug, some states have placed purchase restrictions of 9 grams of pseudoephedrine, with no more than three 3-gram packages in one purchase. Legitimate consumers stocking up on cold products will have to divide their purchases into more than one visit to a specific store.

Topical nasal decongestants act as *vasoconstrictors*, sending edema and blood back to the blood vessels from which they originally leaked out, thereby shrinking the dilated blood vessels. They are used for the temporary relief of nasal (nose) congestion or stuffiness caused by hay fever or other allergies, colds, or sinusitus.

Side effects of topical decongestants include burning, dryness, or stinging inside of nose; increase in nasal discharge; and sneezing. Toxic effects of topical decongestants include blurred vision; fast, irregular, or pounding heartbeat; headache, dizziness, drowsiness, or lightheadedness; high blood pressure, nervousness, trembling, trouble in sleeping, and weakness. Thinking that a topical agent is safe for all patients fools many people. But there is a long contraindication list for this simple dosage form of topical (and) nasal sprays and drops. Do not use on patients with the following conditions:

- diabetes mellitus (commonly called "sugar diabetes")
- excessively dry membranes in nose
- enlarged prostate—difficulty urinating may worsen
- glaucoma—mydriasis may worsen
- heart or blood vessel disease such as CHF or CAD
- high blood pressure—especially oxymetazoline may make the condition worse.
- overactive thyroid gland may cause the heart to speed up; decongestants may increase tachycardia.
- topical decongestants that are applied to the nasal membrane or sprayed into the nasal cavity are outlined in Table 13-6.

TABLE 13-6 Topical Nasal Decongestants	
Trade® Nasal Decongestants	Generic Nasal Decongestants
Afrin Topical Decongestant®, Dristan 12-Hr Nasal Spray®	oxymetazoline
Neo-Synephrine 4-Hr®, 4-Way Fast Acting®, Afrin Children's®	phenylephrine
Benzedrex Inhaler®	propylhexedrine

Note: After much debate and public hearings that began in 1985 and a controlled case study that began in 1994, phenylpropanolamine, aka PPA, was removed from the market in November 2000 due to its increased risk of intracranial bleeding associated with hemorrhagic stroke. PPA was used as in OTC cough and cold remedies as a decongestant, as well as an appetite suppressant in weight loss formulas. This risk was found to be higher in women than in men, mainly because the incidence of stroke occurred more with diet aids, which are used more by women than men, than cold medications.

COUGH MEDICATIONS

There are two types of coughs and two types of treatments. Nonproductive cough is treated with a cough suppressant or antitussive to quiet the cough; these allow the upper respiratory tract to stay moistened, since coughing dries it out, irritating the respiratory tract. Expectorants are used to increase the moisture and decrease the viscosity (thin out) of the mucus to ease the removal of the mucus during the coughing (see Table 13-7).

NONDRUG TREATMENT OF THE COMMON COLD

Throughout the centuries man has sought a cure for the common cold to no avail. There is no treatment to cure the common cold. It has been said that time and a good immune system are the only cures for the common cold. However, many treatments for the symptoms have been documented and used. Among them, the one with the most positive result is breathing in steam. Eating hot, steamy, homemade chicken soup can have the same effect, according to some researchers. The steam is believed to open up congested airway and nasal passages, allowing for easier breathing. Another treatment that may be employed is the administration of a 23 mg zinc lozenge within the first 24 hours of the onset of the symptoms of the common cold, and every two hours thereafter for the duration.

In 1992, studies proved that the duration of colds could be shortened by three days, from seven to four days, with the proper use of zinc. It is believed that zinc indications "interfere with the replication of cold viruses in the throat," according to George Eby, who conducted the initial study on zinc.

TABLE 13-7   Comparison of Cough Formula for Nonproductive versus Productive Coughs

Indications—Nonproductive Cough	Indications—Productive Cough
Symptoms—Dry, hacking cough does not produce mucus or phlegm.	**Symptoms**—A cough in which there is a production and removal of phlegm or mucus. Sometimes called a "wet" cough.
Purpose—Suppressants, aka antitussives, are drugs used to suppress cough centers in the brain and to moisten and lubricate the throat to relieve irritation and **quiet the cough**.	**Purpose**—Expectorants are drugs that **loosen and clear mucus and phlegm from the respiratory tract** and also moisten and lubricate the throat to relieve irritation.
Generic Ingredient— **(1) Non-narcotic Cough Suppressants**—dextromethorphan for nonproductive coughs **(2) Narcotic Cough Suppressants**—Codeine and hydrocodone usually added to guaifenesin	**Generic Ingredient**— **Non-narcotic Expectorant**—guaifenesin
(1) Trade Names of Non-narcotic Antitussives: Found in Dimetapp®, Robitussin-DM®, Delsym®, Pertussin®, Drixoral®, Vicks Formula 44®, Triaminic®, Coricidin®	**Trade Names of Non-narcotic Expectorants**: Robitussin®, Humibid®, Humibid LA®, Robitussin, Organidin NR®, Fenesin®
(2) Trade Names of Narcotic Antitussives: Hycodan®, Tussigon®, and Mycodone®	
(1) Mechanism of Action of Suppressants-Dextromethorphan: Works on the CNS to suppress cough centers in the brain in the medulla oblongata. When coughing is suppressed, the throat does not lose moisture.	**Mechanism of Action of Expectorants—Guaifenesin**: Thin the mucus and lubricate the irritated respiratory tract.
(2) Mechanism of Action of Codeine: Codeine is a centrally acting agent that elevates the threshold for cough in the medulla oblongata. As a result, dry, unproductive coughs become more productive and less frequent. It may be combined with an expectorant.	
Side effects: Drowsiness or tranquilization, constipation, over-drying of respiratory secretions, and upset stomach. At high doses, can cause nausea, itchy skin, visual and audial hallucinations, loss of motor control, and a feeling of being very "stoned and out of it."	**Side effects**—rare, but may include vomiting, diarrhea, stomach upset, headache, skin rash, and hives.

TABLE 13-7 Comparison of Cough Formula for Nonproductive versus Productive Coughs (*continued*)	
Indications—Nonproductive Cough	Indications—Productive Cough
Contraindications—Patients with hypertension, kidney problems, diabetes, or glaucoma must seek approval from their doctor; increases the effects of those conditions. Pregnancy; patients with persistent lingering cough, excessive phlegm, chronic cough due to bronchitis, smoking, asthma or emphysema.	**Contraindications**—Pregnancy; patients with persistent lingering cough, excessive phlegm, chronic cough due to bronchitis, smoking, asthma, or emphysema.

There is current research negating that premise and showing evidence that zinc has cold-fighting properties due to its effect on the immune system itself.

Note: Vitamin C as a preventative measure for the common cold: To date there is no conclusive data that has shown that large doses of vitamin C prevent colds. While the vitamin may reduce the severity or duration of symptoms (there is no definitive evidence), it may also cause severe diarrhea (dehydration is a danger for the elderly and children) and change blood and urine glucose test results. Combinations of oral anticoagulant drugs and vitamin C can produce abnormal results in blood-clotting tests and change the coagulation of blood.

Asthma

A number of different factors can trigger an asthmatic attack. These triggers include air pollutants, allergy antigens, infection, emotional states, exercise, and exposure to cold. Approximately 17 million people have asthma caused by allergies to airborne pollutants that trigger their asthma attacks, which are most common in children. These airborne pollutants include dust, mold, mites, pollen, and animal dander. Mast cells, found in the wall of the bronchi, are involved in the release of many naturally occurring chemical transmitters. Together with nerve impulses, these chemicals help the smooth muscle tissue of the wall of the bronchi to contract. The contractions constrict or narrow the air passageways of the respiratory tract, restricting the flow of air and producing difficulty in breathing. In addition to the narrowing of the bronchi, breathing becomes more difficult and the condition worsens because mucus production increases, and concurrently restricts airflow. When mucus increases, this is called bronchial congestion; when the smaller branches are involved, it is bronchiole congestion.

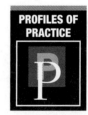

PROFILES OF PRACTICE

Asthma affects over 15 million people and is responsible for as many as 1.5 million ER visits and 500,000 hospitalizations each year.

BRONCHOCONSTRICTION

This is a term used for the action of the smooth muscles encircling the airways or tubes, tightening them and causing them to go into spasm. The actual interior wall will constrict because the tissue will become inflamed. This inflammation further constricts the airflow. The narrowing of the bronchi during an asthmatic attack may be fatal if the person cannot get the passageways opened quickly. Albuterol and other *bronchodilators* are often the drug of choice for quick relief and restoration of airflow.

Studies have shown that 71 percent of patients responded to allergy shots, which reduced symptoms, lung inflammation, and the need for medications and improved lung function. Allergy shots alter the underlying disease process by gradually reducing the sensitivity to allergy triggers.

Symptoms of an asthma attack include coughing excessively, shortness of breath (SOB), a feeling that one cannot catch one's breath, feeling like something may be stuck in the throat, a tightness or pain in the chest, wheezing (the name give to the sound made when a person with asthma coughs or breathes).

Diagnosis may include chest X-ray to rule out other diseases, blood tests, sputum studies, physical exam listening to the sounds and noting symptoms, and spirometry test. A spirometry breathing test measures the amount of air intake and rate at which air can pass through airways. Slower speed and lessened amount of air will pass through airways if they are narrowed because of inflammation. This results in changes in normal spirometry values.

ALLERGIC ASTHMA

If a child has allergies, he is more likely to develop asthma. More than 70 percent of people with asthma also suffer from allergies, according to the National Institutes of Health, and research suggests that allergic triggers play a large role in triggering airway inflammation and asthma symptoms.

Allergies and allergic asthma are both allergic diseases caused by exposure to an allergic substance, or allergen. Exposure to an allergen triggers an allergic cascade of events that results in a runny nose/itchy eyes (allergy) or bronchial constriction/wheezing (asthma). Asthma symptoms can include coughing, wheezing, shortness of breath (or rapid breathing), chest tightness, occasional fatigue, and slight chest pain. Earaches are very common in young children, and they can be caused by allergic disease. Otitis media is an infection associated with fluid in the middle ear. Allergic rhinitis or sinusitis sometimes precedes otitis media. Otitis media can cause temporary hearing loss. If the condition becomes chronic, and happens when the child is learning to speak, language development may be impaired.

TREATMENT

Treatments of asthma with oral and nasal inhalers are divided into those used for quick relief to immediately open up the airway passages; those used for prophylactic maintenance to decrease and prevent swelling, irritation, and inflammation on a daily basis; and those used to prevent the release of histamines and leukotrienes so that the asthma attack will not start. Those which open up the passageways are usually stimulant inhalers, while those for prevention of inflammation are usually anti-inflammatory corticosteroids. The aim of treatment is to reduce this inflammation and to prevent further injury to the airway. There are also oral medications that can prevent the inflammation. According to *Understanding Asthma* by Glaxco-SmithKline, there is mounting evidence that, if left untreated, asthma can cause a long-term decline of lung function.

There are many substances, called biochemical mediators, inside of the mast cell. These mediators can be released during allergenic exposure. A severe allergenic response is called asthma. Two of the most common mediators released from the mast cell that cause allergies are leukotrienes and histamine. Leukotrienes are potent mediators that are released from mast cells, eosinophils, and basophils. Leukotrienes work to contract airway smooth muscle, increase vascular permeability, increase mucus secretions, and attract and activate inflammatory cells in the air passageways of patients with asthma. Among the many other mediators that are released during respiratory inflammation are eosinophilic chemotactic factor of anaphylaxis (aka ECF-A), various prostaglandins, cytokines, such as TNF (tumor necrosis factor), and interleukins.

One of the most important prostaglandin mediators involved in asthma is the slow reacting substance of anaphylaxis known as SRS-A. Leukotrienes B,C,D, and E are also released. LTC, LTD, and LTE help to make SRS-A. The effects of SRS-A last longer than histamine, creating mucosal edema and leukocyte infiltration and causing major bronchoconstriction.

The autonomic nervous system plays an important role in COPD, especially in asthma. Stimulation of the sympathetic nervous system Beta-2 receptors by epinephrine creates bronchodilation, while stimulation of the parasympathetic nervous system, specifically the activation of the vagus nerve by irritants, causes bronchoconstriction.

Emphysema

Emphysema is a COPD (chronic obstructive pulmonary disease), which describes a condition resulting from something that is continually blocking the oxygen external exchange in the lungs. It affects people worldwide and is associated with a limitation of activity due to a lack of oxygen. Approximately 3 million Americans have emphysema, which ranks 15th among chronic conditions that contribute to limitations on physical activity. Almost half of individuals with emphysema report that their daily activities have been limited by the disease. Forty percent more men are affected by emphysema than women. There were 17,787 deaths attributed to emphysema in 1999.

Emphysema is defined as the destruction of air sacs (alveoli) in the lungs, where oxygen from the air is exchanged for carbon dioxide in the blood. The external exchange is interrupted when the thin, fragile air sacs become permanently and irreversibly damaged as a protein called elastin is destroyed. The alveoli become less able to transfer oxygen to the blood system. In addition, bronchioles are less able to dilate and often collapse due to a lack of elastin.

Together these two evils cause one of the symptoms of SOB, shortness of breath. As alveoli are destroyed, the lungs continue to lose the elasticity needed to keep the airways open. The alveoli stay full of air and carbon dioxide, but are unable to exhale the waste and inhale the much-needed air to extract the oxygen from. Another symptom is great difficulty exhaling, which leads to the characteristic fully expanded chest, known as a "barrel" chest.

Other symptoms include the inability to perform normal daily activities or exercise. Chronic breathing problems, such as bronchitis and or asthma, may also develop before emphysema is diagnosed. The causes of emphysema are long-term exposure to pollutants that irritate the alveoli such as tobacco smoke, asbestos, pollution, coal dust, and chemical fumes. About 80–90 percent of all COPD, including emphysema, is related to cigarette smoking. About 50,000 to 100,000 Americans living as of 2001 were born with a deficiency of a protein known as alpha 1-antitrypsin (AAT), which can lead to an inherited form of emphysema called alpha 1-antitrypsin (AAT) deficiency-related emphysema.

Treatment of emphysema, like asthma and other COPDs, may include oral inhaler bronchodilators and routinely used drugs designed to relax and open air passages in the lungs rather quickly. Sometimes, antibiotics are given for secondary bacterial infection, such as pneumococcal pneumonia. In this disease, coughing to expel air dries out the mucus lining of the respiratory tract and the viscous mucus immobilizes the cilia and bacteria (and other pollutants), which then become trapped and colonize. The progressive inflexibility of the alveoli contributes to worsen this infection at this stage. Breathing exercises to tone the diaphragm and other breathing muscles constitutes what is known as pulmonary rehabilitation.

Prevention is the main key to eliminating the environmentally caused emphysema. Preventive measures include the following:

- Do not ever smoke. If you are a smoker, quit smoking.
- Maintain good, health-conscious habits of sound nutrition, exercise, and adequate sleep to ensure a good immune system to fight respiratory infection.
- Exercise to build endurance levels and to improve the immune system's ability to fight infection.
- Get flu and pneumonia immunizations.
- Avoid areas of environmental pollution and dust.

The prognosis is difficult to predict, as patients with less damage to the lung have better chances than those with more damage; yet it is possible for patients with extensive lung damage to live for many years. Death may occur from pneumonia, respiratory failure, cardiac problems, or other complications.

Cystic Fibrosis

Cystic fibrosis (CF) is a genetic disease in which a defective gene causes the body to produce an abnormally thick, sticky mucus. This disease affects approximately 30,000 children and adults in the United States. The abnormally thick, sticky mucus clogs the lungs, obstructs the pancreas, and leads to life-threatening lung infections, breathing difficulty, and digestive problems. These thick secretions block the pancreas, preventing digestive enzymes from entering the intestines, and in turn prevent metabolism or the chemical breakdown and absorption of food nutrients. According to the CF Foundation's National Patient Registry, the median age of survival for a person with CF is 33.4 years, and 95 percent of men with CF are sterile.

Symptoms include: very salty-tasting skin; persistent coughing with or without phlegm; wheezing or shortness of breath; an excessive appetite with poor weight gain; and greasy, bulky stools. Symptoms may vary partly because more than 1,000 mutations of the CF gene exist.

Treatments include the following:

- chest physical therapy, a form of airway clearance performed with vigorous clapping on the back and chest to dislodge the thick mucus from the lungs on a routine daily basis
- antibiotics, such as tobramycin inhalant solution, to treat infections
- bronchodilator and corticosteroid inhalers
- nutritional supplements
- mucolytics to thin out the thick mucus

Mucolytics thin out the sticky, viscous (thick) mucus that causes the breathing and digestive problems associated with CF. The viscosity of the mucus is dependent upon the amount of mucoprotein. The more mucoprotein there is, the greater the number of disulfide bonds there will be, making the mucus thicker. N-acetylcysteine, the generic of Mucomyst and Airbron, breaks the disulfide bonds in mucin, which thins the mucin and makes it more easily dislodged from the lungs by the MCE or mucociliary elevator.

N-acetylcysteine is also used as an antidote in acetaminophen overdose to prevent or mitgate hepatic injury (damage to the liver). Toxic effects of this poisoning are inevitable if not treated in time and include hepatic necrosis, renal tubular necrosis, hypoglycemic coma, and thrombocytopenia. But the potential for severe, irreversible hepatic failure, damage, and necrosis is most often the main concern. Clinical and laboratory results of hepatic toxicity may not be measurable until 48 to 72 hours after the initial oral overdose administration. Signs and symptoms of acute APAP OD is dose related and may include nausea, vomiting, diaphoresis, and general malaise. Finding an empty or spilled bottle of Tylenol next to an unconscious person, especially a child, is a good indicator that he is overdosed.

TREATMENT OF APAP OD

The stomach should be emptied promptly by lavage or by induction of vomiting (emesis) with syrup of ipecac. If an acetaminophen overdose is suspected, a serum acetaminophen assay should be performed as quickly as possible to ascertain how much drug has been taken, but no sooner than four hours following ingestion for an accurate reading. Liver function studies should be obtained immediately and q 24 hours. The antidote should be administered as early as possible, within 16 hours for optimal results, and up to 24 hours after the overdose ingestion.

Adverse effects of acetylcysteine may include hemoptysis, stomatitis, nausea, vomiting, and severe rhinorrhea. Interestingly, bronchoconstriction has also been reported with acetylcysteine therapy. The recommended dose of acetylcysteine is 3 to 5 ml of the 20 percent solution diluted with an equal volume of water or saline, or 6 to 10 ml of the 10 percent solution administered three to four times daily.

Another agent, Pulmozyme®, Recombinant Human Deoxyribonuclease I (rhDNase, Dornase alpha), is an enzyme that cleaves DNA left behind by neutrophils in the lungs. When a neutrophil dies, its DNA leaks out, which then comes into contact with mucin, making it very thick. A patient with cystic fibrosis is affected greatly by this natural process. The mechanism of action is one of hydrolysis; when this recombinant human DNA enzyme is inhaled, it hydrolyzes or cuts the neutrophil DNA apart and subsequently thins out the mucin for an easier removal by the MCE (mucociliary elevator). This agent is an inhalation treatment.

Side effects may include chest pain or discomfort, hoarseness, and sore throat. *Less common* are difficulty breathing; fever; redness, itching, pain, swelling, or other irritation of eyes; runny or stuffy nose; upset stomach, rare hives, or welts; itching; redness of skin; and skin rash.

Allergies

The treatment of allergies with respiratory responses includes antihistamines and anti-tussives to alleviate the symptoms and mast cell stabilizers to prevent initial allergic reactions and reccurrence.

ANTIHISTAMINES

If a patient has taken the antihistamine *before* exposure to the allergen, such as pollen, the drug will get into the H-1 receptor site. When the person is exposed to the pollen, the mast cell will release histamine-1, which will try to find H-1 receptors. But the antihistamine is already bound to the H-1 receptor sites, blocking or inhibiting the histamine from getting in. Thus, no allergic reaction will occur.

If a patient has been exposed to the allergen or pollen first, the receptor sites are already occupied by histamine. If a person takes antihistamines *after* exposure to the allergen, the drug will wait until the histamine, a protein, degrades and exits the receptor site. Since there are both more histamine-1 and antihistamine waiting to get into open receptor sites, while the person is still exposed to the allergen, the antihistamine will race the histamine-1 to get into the receptor site first. Antihistamines always win the race! This race is the mechanism of action known as competitive inhibition. Once inside of or attached to the H-1 receptor site, the antihistamine does not fit perfectly, but fits well enough to bind, preventing or blocking the histamine from getting in. This blocking is known as the inhibition. Since the antihistamine cannot fit like a key in a lock, there is *no turn*, no chemical change, and no allergic reaction. Think of this as a jigsaw puzzle piece that looks like the right color, right size, and right shape to be placed in the puzzle, but just does not fit exactly, so it does not snap into place. Contraindications are that individuals with prostate problems or glaucoma should avoid antihistamines, unless they have authorization from their physician.

MAST CELL STABILIZERS USED TO PREVENT ALLERGIES

The use of antihistamines is one way to treat allergies, as it stops histamine-1 from entering or binding to the nose, eye, skin, or other body cell, causing an allergic reaction. Mast cell stabilizers prevent the allergen from attaching to the mast cell, thereby preventing the histamine-1 from being released from the mast cell (see Table 13-8). If histamine is not released from the mast cell, then it cannot be free to seek the new binding receptor site of a body cell. For example, if no histamine is available to bind to the nose receptor site, the nose will not become itchy, have congestion, or become runny. In other words, mast cell stabilizers act prophylactically and prevent allergic responses. They are considered anti-inflammatory agents.

Nedocomil may also have more anti-inflammatory properties than cromolyn sodium. Mast cell stabilizers are generally used most often in prevention of asthma attacks, but can be used to prevent allergic rhinitis. Mast cell stabilizers are available for use in the nose, lungs, and GI tract. Other names for mast cell stabilizers are mast cell inhibitors and mediator-release inhibitors.

TABLE 13-8 Mast Cell Stabilizers	
Mast Cell Stabilizers	For Respiratory Tract
Generic	Trade®
cromolyn sodium	Intal®, Rx Inhaler
	Nasal Crom®, OTC nasal spray
	Crolom®, Rx eye drops
	Opticrom®, Rx nasal spray
nedocromil	Tilade® oral inhalation
	For gastrointestinal tract
cromolyn sodium	Gastrocrom®

There are three drawbacks to using these products, as follows:

- They must be used about four times a day.
- They take one to four weeks to take initial effect or give relief.
- They mainly work on nasal and respiratory allergies for asthma.

However, the side effects are so few and the drug is so gentle that the DOC, Intal®=cromolyn sodium, has been used successfully on infants and children and is now an over the counter remedy known as Nasalcrom®. A new mast cell stabilizer, Tiladec®=nedocromil, has been shown to be more advantageous still, with possibly a longer duration. Renal and hepatic function may decrease; therefore, the dosage should be decreased in such renal or hepatic function impaired patients. Due to the propellants in the inhalant canisters, these canisters should be used with caution by patients with coronary artery disease or a history of cardiac arrhythmias. If a patient develops eosinophilic pneumonia (or pulmonary infiltrates with eosinophilia), this treatment should be discontinued.

The benefits of the mast cell stabilizers are as follows:

- They stop the allergic response before it begins, without causing drowsiness, irritability, or a decreased ability to think or focus, such as in a learning activity.
- They do not reverse allergy symptoms that are already present, but they do prevent new exposure to new allergens, thus preventing allergic symptoms.
- They can be used for weeks or months at a time without the fear of rebound effects or threat of addiction that decongestants may pose.

Sodium cromolyn and nedocomil inhibit mast cell degranulation and activation by creating a protective barrier around the allergy cells in the nose and respiratory tract, so that pollen, mold, dust, and animal dander cannot bind or attach to them. The exact MOA is not fully understood, but it is believed that cromolyn indirectly inhibits calcium ions from entering the mast cell and triggering release of cellular contents. The mast cell stabilizers inhibit both the early and late phases of bronchoconstriction induced by inhaled antigens.

In clinical trials, they have been shown to be effective in mitigating the response induced by cold air, environmental air pollutants, exercise, sulfur dioxide, and other sources. It is important to note the following:

- Mast cell stabilizers do not exert bronchodilation, anticholinergic, antihistaminic, or glucocorticoid effects.
- Mast cell stabilizers are *not* used in any acute phase of severe bronchoconstriction.

Treatment of COPD

Mast cell stabilizers have no role in the treatment of acute asthma attack or status asthmaticus. Late phase responses may occur without detectable immediate IgE mediated mast cell reactions in asthma. Cases of severe asthma should be treated with both corticosteroids and quick relief bronchodilators (see Table 13-9).

There are three types of bronchodilators and three types of anti-inflammatory drugs used for COPD. Based on their specific mechanism of action, they may be used for asthma, emphysema, or bronchitis. Therefore, there are three separate mechanisms by which drugs can cause bronchodilation. Bronchodilators act to either immediately open up the airway passages, prevent the allergen attachment to the mast cell, or stop the prostaglandin synthesis.

Oral administration of bronchodilators includes ephedrine, albuterol and terbutaline. Note that oral epinephrine is unavailable because it is rapidly broken down in the digestive system before it can reach the lungs.

BRONCHODILATORS

Beta adrenergic inhalers act within approximately 15 minutes. One exception are those that contain salmeterol because it is a long-acting bronchodilator and not designed to give an immediate effect. The mechanism of action of these drugs is to mimic or stimulate epinephrine stimulation of the Beta-2 receptors of the respiratory tract, directly relaxing smooth muscles and causing immediate bronchodilation (see Table 13-10).

XANTHINES

The exact mechanism of action of these respiratory smooth muscle relaxants is unknown. However, the following is a list of some of the ways that xanthines are believed to work:

- Increase levels of energy-producing camp (cyclic adenosine monophosphate).

TABLE 13-9	Routes of Administration and Classification of Drugs Used in COPD
Drug Classification	**Route of Administration**
A. Bronchodilators—relax smooth muscle in airways	
1. Beta-adrenergics	Inhaled, subcutaneous, oral
2. Xanthines (aka Xanthine derivatives)	Oral or IV (*not* inhaled)
3. Anti-cholinergics	Inhaled only (*not* PO)
B. Anti-inflammatory Agents—decrease cellular response of inflammation	
1. Corticosteroids	Oral, IM, IV
2. Mast cell stabilizers (aka mediator-release inhibitors)	Inhaled *only*
3. Anti-leukotriene drugs	Oral only

TABLE 13-10 List of Beta-Adrenergic Bronchodilator Inhalers

Trade® Beta-Adrenergic Bronchodilator Inhalers	Generic Beta—Adrenergic Bronchodilator Inhalers
Prinatene Mist® (also available Sub Q and PO)	epinephrine
Foradil®	formoterol
Isuprel®	isoproterenol
Bronkosol®	isoetharine
Alupent®, Metaprel®	metaproterenol
Bricanyl®, Brethine® (also available Sub Q and PO)	terbutaline
Tornalate®	bitolterol
Maxair®	pirbuterol
Serevent®	salmeterol
Advair Diskus®	salmeterol + fluticasone combination
Combivent®	albuterol + atrovent combination

- Competitively inhibit phosphodiesterase (PDE), an enzyme that chemically breaks down camp.
- Inhibition of PDE results in increased camp levels, smooth muscle relaxation, bronchodilation, and airflow via air passages.

The result of these actions is an increased CNS and cardiovascular stimulation, force of contraction, kidney secretion, and diuretic effect. Side effects include nausea, vomiting, anorexia, gastroesophageal reflux during sleep, sinus tachycardia, extrasystole, palpitations, ventricular dysrhythmias, and transient increased. Some xanthines, such as Theophylline, may cause increased nervousness when used with the herbs St. John's Wort, ma huang, or ephedra.

ANTICHOLINERGICS

Anticholinergics work by blocking the effects of ACH, acetylcholine, by competing for the ACH receptor site. Bronchoconstriction is prevented while airway passages dilate. The side effects include dry mouth or throat, gastrointestinal distress, headache, coughing, and anxiety (see Table 13-11).

ANTI-INFLAMMATORY AGENTS

Corticosteroids are not quick acting and are used prophylactically. The resultant action of corticosteroids is decreased inflammation of the airway passages, allowing the patient to breathe easier. The mechanism of action is one of inhibition: "Corticosteroids act, at least in part, by recruitment of histone deacetylases (HDACs) to the site of active inflammatory gene transcription. They thereby inhibit the acetylation of core histones that is necessary for inflammatory gene transcription." Glucocorticoids exert their effects by binding to the glucocorticoid receptor (GR), which then inhibits or increases gene transcription through processes known as transrepression and transactivation, respectively. In this manner they also work to reduce the immune response (see Table 13-12).

TABLE 13-11 Various Treatments for Asthma

Type of Drug and Trade Name	Generic or Other Name	Availability	UAD
Natural Xanthines	caffeine, tea, cocoa, choclolate	PO	100 mg = 1 cup coffee
Methyl Xanthines and Derivatives Theodur®, Bronkodyl®, Slo-Bid®	theophylline	PO, and PO extended release 100, 125, 200, 300 mg tabs/caps	13 mg/kg/day NTE 900 mg dose/day 1 TR cap q12hr
Choledyl®	oxtriphylline (64% theophylline)	PO, 100, 200 mg tablets, 400 & 800 SR tablets, elixir and pediatric syrup also available	4.7 mg/kg/8 hrs 1 SR tab q12hr
various manufacturers	aminophylline (79% theophylline)	given as intravenous administration ONLY for respiratory distress. Also avail PR/supp	Infusion of 0.4–0.6 mg/kg /hr
Anti-cholinergics Atrovent® Combivent®	ipratropium bromide albuterol + atrovent	Inhaler Inhaler	2 puffs qid NTE 12/d 2 puffs qid, NTE 12/d

Oral thrush, or thrush mouth, is the common term for a yeast infection called candida albicans that occurs in the back of the throat of patients who use corticosteroid inhalers. The main symptom is a white film located at the back of the throat, tongue, and tonsil area. Antifungal mouthwash may be used to treat this infection (all yeast are fungi, but not all fungi are yeast). This common side effect occurs because steroids alter the local bacteria and fungal population of the mouth, enhancing fungal growth. Using a space inhaler or rinsing the mouth very thoroughly after each corticosteroid use will help to prevent it.

MAST CELL INHIBITORS

Mast cell inhibitors are also known as Mast cell stabilizers, mediator-release inhibitors, or prophylactic drugs. As discussed previously in the Allergy section, Intal® (cromolyn sodium) and Tilade® (nedocromil) have benefits that include reduction in asthma symptoms, improved peak expiratory flow rates, and decreased need for short-acting beta-2 agonists.

TABLE 13-12 Corticosteroids

Trade	Generic	Availability	UAD
Inhalers			
Vanceril®, Beclovent®	beclomethasone	MDI, Intranasal form for rhinitis	1–2 puffs tid–qid, NTE 20/d
Pulmicort®	budesonide	DPI (dry powder inhaler)	1–2 puffs of QD (200 mcg/inhalation) NTE 4/day (800 mcg /d)
Aerobid®	flunisolide	MDI, Intranasal form for rhinitis	2–3 puffs bid to tid, NTE 12/d
Flovent®	fluticasone	MDI	2 puffs bid (44 mcg each), NTE 10/d (440 mcg/day)
Advair Diskus®	salmeterol + fluticasone combination	DPI, 100/50, 250/50, and 500 /50 mcg fluticasone/salmeterol per inhalation with 60 blisters each	1 puff bid, strength depends upon other concomitant therapy
Azmacort®	triamcinolone	MDI, PO, TOP, SC, ID, IM	2 puffs tid–qid, NTE 16/d
Oral corticosteroids			
Medrol®, Medrol DosePak®	methylprednisolone	PO, 2, 4, 6, 8, 16, 24, 32 mg tablets, also available IM, SC for neoplasia and adrenal insufficiency	**4–48 mg qd** Note that reduction in dose should be gradual to decrease the risk of adrenal insufficiency
Deltasone®, Meticorten®	prednisone	PO only	**5–10 mg/day** Note that reduction in dose should be gradual to decrease the risk of adrenal insufficiency
Dexone®	dexamethasone	PO 0.5, 0.75, 1.5 and 4 mg tablets, IM	0.75 to 9 mg/day
Injectable			
SoluCortef®	hydrocortisone	IV, IM, Infusion Sterile Powder 100, 250, 500, 1000 mg Act–O Vial	100–500 mg for 48–72 hrs, over 30 seconds to 10 minutes, q 2, 4, or 6 hrs, then decreased gradually to a maintenance dose

TABLE 13-12	Corticosteroids (*continued*)		
Trade	Generic	Availability	UAD
SoluMedrol®	methylprednisolone	IV, IM, and Infusion Sterile Powder 40 mg, 125 mg, 500 mg, 1 gram Act–O Vial	30 mg/kg over 30 minutes, MR q 4 to 6 hrs × 48 hrs at least 30 minutes. Dosage must be discontinued gradually
Decadron®	dexamethasone sodium phosphate	Injection, 4 mg of dexamethasone phosphate in 1-ml ampoule	For anaphylactic shock: 10–100 mg IV (1 mg/kg slow IV bolus)

ANTI-LEUKOTRIENE DRUGS

Anti-leukotriene drugs, aka leukotriene receptor antagonists (LTRAs) are of two types. This is the first new class of drugs to fight asthma in over 30 years. Leukotriene inhibitors may be used to reduce the low-dose regimens of corticosteroid inhalers. The long-term effects of leukotriene inhibitors therapy is yet to be determined. It is speculated that, in the future, IV formulations of these agents may be useful in emergency situations. Leukotrienes are substances released when a trigger, such as cat hair, mold, or dust, starts a series of chemical reactions in the body. Histamine-1 is also released. Leukotrienes attach to the allergen and then to the mast cell, causing inflammation, increased mucus production, and bronchoconstriction. The patient will experience coughing, wheezing, and shortness of breath.

The mechanism of action of the new class of anti-leukotriene agents is to block or inhibit the leukotrienes from attaching to the receptors on the cells in the lungs (mast) and in blood (basophils) circulation. The result is that a decrease in neutrophil and leukocyte infiltration to the lungs decreases inflammation in the lungs, where asthma symptoms are mitigated and prevented. The specific MOAs of these new drugs will be further explained (see Table 13-13).

Toxic effects of antileukotriene agents unfortunately exists. The LTRAs may cause liver dysfunction, and, therefore, the liver assessments must continue during therapy with this agent. Side effects for Accolate® and Zyflo® may include headache, dyspepsia, diarrhea, dizziness, and insomnia. The toxic effect is liver dysfunction. Montelukast has fewer side effects and no liver toxic effects.

Another drug, atropine, may also be used to fight allergic reactions and anaphylactic shock because it has anti-secretory properties. It decreases the amount of nasal and respiratory secretions in the body. A future drug to combat moderate or severe allergic asthma is undergoing Phase III trials. A recombinant humanized monoclonal antibody (rhuMAb-E25) forms complexes with free IgE and blocks its interaction with mast cells and basophil.

There are many medications in many different dosage forms and routes of administration for respiratory diseases. Medications taken orally almost always have a much higher systemic concentration (concentration in the entire body and blood system) than inhaled medications. Therefore, an inhaled route is better and the preferred route whenever possible. The idea behind an inhaler is that the full dose is delivered to the lungs, where it is immediately absorbed by the lung tissue, taking a local effect. Excess drug that may be absorbed by the bloodstream, then distributed to the rest of the body, is minimal. The lungs

TABLE 13-13   Mast Cell Stabilizers and Antileukotrienes

Trade	Generic	Mechanism of Action
Mast Cell Stabilizers		**Prevent attachment of**
Intal®, Nasal Crom (OTC)	cromolyn sodium	MDI, 2 × 1 mg puffs QID, takes 2–4 weeks before results are seen. NTE 8 mg/day
Tilade®	nedocromil	MDI, 2 × 2 mg puffs QID, NTE 16 mg/day
Leukotriene-receptor-blocking drugs (LTRAs)		
Accolate®	zafirlukast	MOA = selectively blocks receptors of leukotrienes D_4 and E_4. LTD_4 and LTE_4 are components of slow-reacting substance of anaphylaxis (SRS-A).[32]
Singulair®	montelukast	MOA = binds with high affinity and selectivity to the $CysLT_1$ receptor rather than prostanoid, cholinergic, or β-adrenergic receptors, and inhibits the actions of LTD_4 at the $CysLT_1$ receptor without any agonist activity.[32]
Anti-leukotrienes block the synthesis of leukotriene		
Zyflo®	zileuton	MOA: Block the synthesis of leukotriene by specifically inhibiting the enzyme that causes the formation of leukotrienes: LTB_4, LTC_4, LTD_4, and LTE_4, from arachidonic acid.

receive an immediate, high concentration of the drug, while the rest of the body receives very little drug. One advantage to oral medication is that some are available as time-release formulations so that a tablet may require only aq12hr dosing, but the inhaled medication may require q4–6hrs. Keeping track of the number of doses used on an inhaler compared with the number it can deliver is the surest way of telling whether or not the inhaler is empty. One way to do this is to mark the beginning date of the inhaler and the end date of the inhaler, if all doses were given.

Products that once relied on CFCs (chlorinated fluorocarbons), such as air conditioning units, refrigerators, and most aerosol products, have been either totally banned or modified to use alternative chemicals that do not damage the ozone layer. However, metered dose inhalers have been granted an "essential use" exemption to the worldwide ban. This allows the manufacturers a few more years to develop new alternative propellants and devices. The FDA has approved a new non-CFC inhaler, Proventil HFA (albuterol), which uses hydrofluoralkane instead of CFC propellant.

SUMMARY

The respiratory system is crucial to sustain life because it is responsible for providing all cells of the body with the oxygen necessary to perform their specific functions. It is the system involved in the intake of oxygen through inhalation, and the excretion of carbon monoxide through exhalation. The respiratory system is divided into two parts, the upper and lower respiratory tracts. The upper respiratory tract consists of the nasal cavity (nose), paranasal sinuses, pharynx (throat), and the larynx. The lower respiratory tract is made up of the trachea, two lungs, two main bronchi (one to each lung), secondary and tertiary bronchi, bronchioles, alveolar ducts, and alveoli.

The most common disease of the respiratory system is the common cold. Uncomplicated common colds are generally treated with over-the-counter medications including antihistamines, decongestants, cough suppressants, analgesics, antipyretics, and anti-inflammatories. The aim in treatment is to provide relief of symptoms. The pharmacy technician should also be familiar with common-sense treatment measures such as increased fluid intake, bed rest, gargling with warm salt water, etc., and be able to assist the pharmacist in advising patients suffering from the common cold.

Of course, there are many more serious diseases of the respiratory system, one of which is asthma. Asthma affects over 15 million people and is responsible for as many as 1.5 million ER visits and 500,000 hospitalizations every year. If left uncontrolled, asthma can cause a long-term decline in lung function.

Other respiratory diseases, ranging from allergies to life-threatening Chronic Obstructive Pulmonary Disease (COPD) and their treatments are thoroughly discussed in this chapter. Since many respiratory diseases are treated with some form of inhalation therapy, it is important for you as a pharmacy technician to be able to assist the pharmacist in educating clients in the proper, safe use of inhalation products.

CHAPTER REVIEW QUESTIONS

1. Name the 10 parts of the respiratory system.

2. Name the respiratory disease states that have been discussed in this chapter.

3. What other condition can Mucomyst® be used for, and why?

4. Match the following drugs with their correct classifications:
   1. hydroxyzine
   2. loratidine
   3. ventolin
   4. zafirlukast
   5. cromolyn sodium
   6. Robitussin DM®
   7. Robitussin®
   8. Mucomyst®

   a. _____Antihistamine for allergies
   b. _____Mast cell stabilizer for asthma
   c. _____Cough suppressant for dry cough
   d. _____Mucolytic for cystic fibrosis
   e. _____Expectorant for wet cough
   f. _____Bronchodilator for COPDs
   g. _____Antileukotriene for asthma
   h. _____Antianxiety for pre-op

5. Match the following drugs with their correct trade and generic names:
   1. Atarax®
   2. ClaritIn®
   3. Phenergan®
   4. Zytrec®
   5. Allegra®
   6. Robitussin DM®
   7. Robitussin®
   8. Mucomyst®

   a. _____promethazine
   b. _____acetylcysteine
   c. _____fexophenadine
   d. _____loratidine
   e. _____guaifenesin
   f. _____cetirazine
   g. _____guaifenesin + dextromethorphan
   h. _____hydroxyzine

6. Match the following classifications or drugs with the correct mechanism of action:
   1. pseudoephedrine
   2. Robitussin DM®
   3. Tilade®
   4. albuterol
   5. Singulair®
   6. loratidine

   a. _____relaxes smooth muscle and dilates the bronchi
   b. _____strengthens the mast cell wall and prevents the release of histamine
   c. _____blocks the binding of leukotrienes to lung cells
   d. _____blocks the binding of histamine-1 to nose cells
   e. _____suppresses the cough by working on the medulla in the brain
   f. _____stops postnasal drip by binding to the alpha receptors in the blood vessels

7. Which lasts longer, the effect of histamine or the effect of SRS-A?

8. Which are the most important receptors in bronchoconstriction?

9. A genetic disease in which a defective gene causes the body to produce an abnormally thick, sticky mucus is known as:
   a. Cystic fibrosis
   b. Pneumonia
   c. Bronchitis
   d. Emphysema

10. Name the three supportive functions of the lymphatic system.

11. What is the estimated composition of air by volume?
   a. Nitrogen 87%, oxygen 12%, carbon dioxide .30%
   b. Nitrogen 67%, oxygen 22%, carbon dioxide .3%
   c. Nitrogen 57%, oxygen 32%, carbon dioxide .03%
   d. Nitrogen 78%, oxygen 21%, carbon dioxide .03%

12. The tiny air sacs of the lungs as known as what?
   a. broccoli buds
   b. bronchial tubers
   c. aveoli
   d. capillaries

13. What is the primary function of the diaphragm?

14. Vitamin C can help cure the common cold.
   a. true
   b. false

15. What are the two most common mediators released from the mast cell that are known as allergies?

Resources and References

1. http://www.radiation-scott.org/deposition/respiratory.htm
2. Rocky Mountain Poison Center toll-free (1-800-525-6115)
3. Function of the Respiratory System http://www.ama-assn.org/ama/pub/category/7165.html
4. http://www.saburchill.com/chapters/chap0020.html
5. Circulatory system likened to a "Freeway System" (analogy) is a brainstorm of Jeanetta Mastron in 1996 while teaching pharmacology to pharmacy technician students, which she has been doing since 1995 in tutoring sessions and has been used by her in her lectures ever since. Original author's quote. She holds the copyright.
6. About ischemia. http://www.ischemia.com/about.html
7. About air. http://www.engineeringtoolbox.com/24_212.html

8. Pulmonary Gas Laws.
   http://www.mtsinai.org/pulmonary/books/scuba/sectiond.htm

9. Respiratory system parts resembling a "tree" has been documented in many science text books; however, likening it to an "upside down tree" or "broccoli" is a brain child of Jeanetta Mastron as of 1996 while teaching pharmacology to pharmacy students, which she has been doing since 1996 in a tutoring session and has been used by in her lectures ever since. Original author's quote. She holds the copyright.

10. About alveoli.
    http://www.mrothery.co.uk/exchange/exchange.htm

11. What is a yawn?
    http://www.msnbc.com/news/205574.asp?cp1=1

12. About the diaphragm.
    http://www.breathing.com/articles/diaphragm-development.htm

13. What is a hiccup?
    http://www.tipsofallsorts.com/hiccup.html#facts

14. About the lungs.
    http://www.nym.org/healthinfo/docs/072/doc72.html

15. Hyaline in bronchi and trachea.
    http://www.smd.qmul.ac.uk/biomed/kb/microanatomy/respiratory

16. About vitamin C and the common cold (some paraphrasing and some quotes).
    http://www.niaid.nih.gov/factsheets/cold.htm

17. Common Cold Center—Coughing.
    http://www.cf.ac.uk/biosi/associates/cold/medicat.html

18. Cure for the Common Cold?
    http://www.quantumhealth.com/news/articlecold.html

19. All about Allergies.
    http://allergies.about.com/

20. Health on the Net Foundation: Separating the Common Cold from an Allergy.
    http://www.hon.ch/News/HSN/508858.html

21. Statistics on asthma.
    http://www.acaai.org/powerpoint/online/slide1.html
    http://www.acaai.org/powerpoint/online/slide8.htm

22. Statistics on allergy shots.
    http://www.acaai.org/powerpoint/online/slide11.htm

23. Statistics on emphysema.
    http://www.wrongdiagnosis.com/e/emphysema/intro.htm

24. Antihistamines for the common cold.
    http://www.update-software.com/abstracts/AB001267.htm

25. Decongestants for the common cold.
    http://www.update-software.com/abstracts/AB001953.htm
26. PPA removal.
    http://www.ucdmc.ucdavis.edu/ucdhs/health/a-z/77Allergic/doc77decon.html
27. Safety checker on ephedra and pseudoephedrine.
    http://www.gnc.com/health_notes/Drug/Ephedrine.htm
28. London Toxicology Group on Dextromethorphan on the Streets.
    http://ramindy.sghms.ac.uk/~ltg/dxm.htm
29. About Reye's Syndrome.
    http://www.thearc.org/faqs/reyes.html
30. Relationship of Jigsaw Puzzle Piece to Lock and Key Theory has been
    documented in many pharmacology text books; however, likening it to
    a "jigsaw puzzle piece that 'snaps' in place" is the brain child of Jeanetta
    K. Mastron while teaching pharmacology to pharmacy technician
    students since 1996 in tutoring sessions and has been used by her in
    her lectures ever since. Original author's quote. She holds the copyright.
31. Drug Facts and Comparisons—"Nasal Decongestants." See 1997
    edition.
32. Tilade and Nasalcrom drug information.
    http://www.rxlist.com
33. PNAS excerpt, Mechanism of Action of Corticosteroids.
    http://www.pubmedcentral.nih.gov/articlerender.fcgi?artid=124399
34. Specific MOAs of LTRAs.
    www.rxlist.com
35. Asthma general information.
    http://www.radix.net/~mwg/inhalers.html
36. Treatment of allergic asthma with monoclonal anti-IgE antibody.
    rhuMAb-E25 Study Group.
37. American Academy of Allergy, Asthma, and Immunology.
    http://www.aaaai.org/
38. Holland, Norman and Michael Patrick Adams. *Core Concepts in
    Pharmacology*. Upper Saddle River, NJ: Pearson Education, 2003.
39. Adams, Michael Patrick, Dianne L. Josephson, and Leland Norman
    Holland, Jr. *Pharmacology for Nurses—A Pathophysiologic Approach*.
    Upper Saddle River, NJ: Pearson Education, 2005.

The Cardio, Circulatory, and Lymph Systems

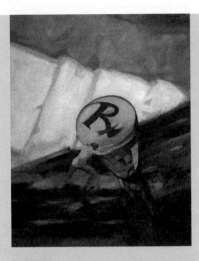

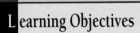
Learning Objectives

After completing this chapter, you should be able to:

- List, identify, and diagram the basic anatomical structure and parts of the heart.

- Explain the function or physiology of the heart and the circulation of the blood within the body.

- List and define common diseases affecting the heart and the causes, symptoms, and pharmaceutical treatment associated with each disease.

- Explain the mechanisms and comprehend how each class of drugs work in order to mitigate symptoms of the following heart diseases: CHF, arrhythmias, angina pectoris, MI, HTN, and CAD.

- Describe the indication for use, mechanism of action, and antidotes used for anticoagulants.

- Define and utilize key terms.

INTRODUCTION

The heart is both an organ and a muscle, with the main purpose of providing oxygenated blood throughout the body by a pumping mechanism. The heart is located just to the left of the sternum (breastbone) in the mediastinum between the two lungs and is about the size of a fist. This incredibly unique muscle pumps about 4,300 gallons of blood a day, even though the human body only contains about 5.6 liters of blood.

Diseases in which serious complications will result can interrupt this life sustaining function. The pericardium is a double layer of serous and fibrous tissue, a fluid filled sac that surrounds and protects the heart. It permits free movement during contraction, yet contains the heart in the chest cavity. The heart sits inside the pericardial cavity. The endocardium is the innermost layer of the three layered walls of the heart that covers the inside surface of the heart.

Anatomy of the Heart

The circulatory system is composed of organs and blood vessels that transport oxygenated blood to all parts of the body. This system is made up of the following organs and blood vessels: heart, lungs, veins, arteries, and capillaries. The septum divides the heart into two parts, the right and the left sides.

The heart is composed of four chambers. The top two chambers, or atria, that receive blood from the body or lungs are called the right atrium and left atrium. The bottom two chambers that pump blood to the lungs and the body are known as the ventricles. The right ventricle pumps deoxygenated blood to the lungs to pick up oxygen and drop off waste. The left ventricle, the strongest chamber, pumps oxygenated blood to the rest of the body and back to the heart. Therefore, damage to the left ventricle causes more severe problems for the heart and body when compared with problems that may arise from potential damage to any one of the other three chambers of the heart.

A nurse or physician can listen to the sounds of the opening and closing of the valves with a stethoscope to determine functionality of the heart. The sounds are referred to as "lup-dup, lup-dup. . . ." There are four valves in the heart that help to prevent the back-flow of blood and direct blood flow forward in one direction as follows: (See Figure 14-1.)

- Tricuspid valve, located between the right atrium and the right ventricle

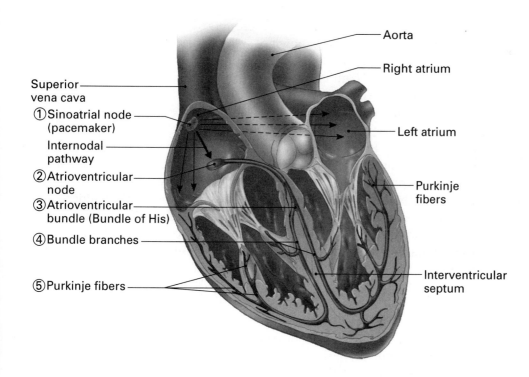

Figure 14-1 The heart

- Pulmonary valve, located between the right ventricle and the pulmonary artery
- Mitral valve, located between the left atrium and the left ventricle (aka the bicuspid valve)
- Aortic valve, located between the left ventricle and the aorta

The Function of the Heart

Every cell in the body needs oxygen in order to live and function. The purpose of the heart is to deliver the oxygen-rich blood to every cell in the body.

PUMPING OF BLOOD

The roads or tubes that oxygenated blood travels through are called *arteries*. The largest artery is the aorta, which branches off the heart, divides into many smaller arteries, and then divides into the smallest, called arterioles. The roads that carry the deoxygenated blood are called veins. *Veins* take deoxygenated blood back to the heart, then to the lungs to pick up more oxygen. Capillaries form a network of tiny streets or blood vessels connecting arterioles, carrying oxygenated blood and nutrients to venules, the smallest veins that carry deoxygenated blood and metabolic waste. In its passage through the capillaries of the body, the blood deposits the materials necessary for their growth and nourishment into the tissues, and at the same time receives from the tissues the waste products resulting from their metabolism.

The pumping action of the heart is provided by the heart muscle known as the myocardium. This muscle that surrounds the heart causes the contractions of the four chambers to push or force blood through the heart valves to the body, and this process is known as systemic circulation.

The heart itself needs its own supply of blood, which it receives from the two, right and left, coronary arteries. These arteries branch off into three other arteries known as the left anterior descending (LAD), circumflex (Cx), and right coronary artery (RCA). The right and left coronary arteries branch off from the aorta, the largest and main artery of the body, right after the blood leaves the left ventricle and semi-lunar aortic valve. The aortic arch leads to three larger arteries: the left subclavian artery, the left carotid artery, and the brachiocephalic artery. These carry oxygenated blood *up and away*, taking fresh blood back from the heart to the head, neck, and shoulder areas.

Contractility, or the ability and the degree of contraction, is determined by the alteration of the contractile force of the myocardium. This alteration results from the change in the availability of calcium or the sensitivity of the myofilaments to calcium. Any stimulus that alters contractility induces a change in steady-state Ca–Ca homeostasis and/or increased filament sensitivity to calcium. A change in calcium coming in is the net influx, while calcium going out is the efflux of calcium.

For example, an increase in contractility increases Ca influx (per unit time) and calcium loading of the sarcoplasmic reticulum (SR). At the new steady-state loading of the SR, more calcium is delivered to the myofilaments, and more force is developed. The contribution of Ca from outside versus SR varies as a function of the state of contractility.

Relaxation of the heart entails the removal of calcium to the extracellular space, where the Na^+Na^+–Ca^{++} exchanger and $Ca^{++}Ca^{++}$–ATPase fine-tunes the resting level. The sarcoplasmic reticulum $Ca^{++}Ca^{++}$–ATPase sets the resting level. Under steady-state conditions, Ca influx and efflux during the cardiac cycle are said to be equal or in homeostasis.

The atria fill with blood at the same time and then contract, pushing the blood through the valves into the ventricles. While being relaxed, they fill up with the blood, then contract simultaneously to push the blood out of the heart through the pulmonary valve and aortic valve into the lungs and the rest of the body, respectively. Therefore, the heart beats top to bottom, not right to left or diagonally, with two pumping actions from left to right within one pumping system.

BLOOD

Blood, a liquid tissue, is known as the fluid of life, growth, and health. The average adult has approximately 5.6 liters of blood coursing through blood vessels in the body, which constitutes about 7% of our body mass. Blood serves as a carrier of oxygen, nutrients, hormones, disease fighting cells, and other substances to all parts of the body and transports waste to the kidneys for filtration and to lungs during expiration. Blood contains live cells such as red and white blood cells, known as *erythrocytes* and *leukocytes*. A drop of blood contains millions of RBCs and only 7,000 to 25,000 WBCs. Red blood cells are red because they contain a protein chemical called hemoglobin that contains the element iron, which makes the blood bright red in color. As blood passes through the lungs, oxygen molecules attach to the hemoglobin. As the blood passes through the body's tissues and organs, the hemoglobin releases the oxygen to the cells. Immediately, the empty hemoglobin molecules bond with the tissue's carbon dioxide or other waste gases, transporting it away. (See more on the composition of blood in The Immune System, Chapter 15.)

BLOOD FLOW

It is important to know the pattern of blood flow to understand the normal circulation of blood within the body. When you understand the normal circulation of blood, you can then understand the abnormal flow that leads to various disease states of the heart or circulatory system. Only then can you understand and prepare drugs and procedures to prevent, reverse, or mitigate such diseases, or offer suggestions for treatment. (See Figure 14-2.)

There are two kinds of blood, venous and arterial. Venous blood contains waste, or CO_2, and is considered impure, dirty, spent, used, high carbon dioxide, deoxygenated, blue, or purple. Veins carry deoxygenated blood to the heart to be sent to the lungs, where the external exchange occurs. (See The Respiratory System, Chapter 13.)

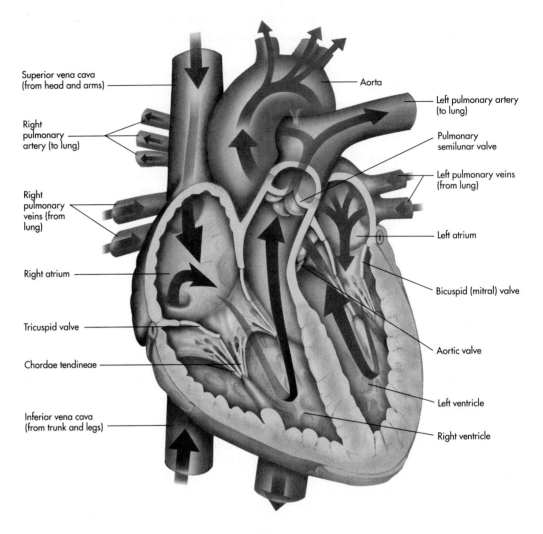

Superior vena cava (from head and arms)

Right pulmonary artery (to lung)

Right pulmonary veins (from lung)

Right atrium

Tricuspid valve

Chordae tendineae

Inferior vena cava (from trunk and legs)

Aorta

Left pulmonary artery (to lung)

Pulmonary semilunar valve

Left pulmonary veins (from lung)

Left atrium

Bicuspid (mitral) valve

Aortic valve

Left ventricle

Right ventricle

Figure 14-2   The flow of blood through the heart
(Mulvihill, Mary Lou; Zelman, Mark; Holdaway, Paul; Tompary, Elaine; Turchany, Jill, Human Diseases, A Systemic Approach, 5th Edition, © 2001. Reprinted by permission of Pearson Education, Inc., Upper Saddle River, NJ)

Arterial blood contains nutrients and O_2 and is considered pure, clean, fresh, new, oxygenated, and bright red. Arteries carry oxygenated blood to the body to feed and nourish it.

The one exception to the rule that veins carry high CO_2 blood to the heart and the arteries carry high O_2 blood to the body is that the pulmonary arteries take high CO_2 blood out of the heart to the lungs, and the pulmonary veins take high O_2 blood out of the lungs to the heart. The heart itself requires its own blood supply to get its own supply of oxygen and nutrients. The blood that goes through the chambers does not do this. The blood that leaves the left ventricle to the aorta does this via the coronary arteries. The famous right and left coronary arteries are the aorta's first branches. The openings of the coronary arteries lie behind the flaps of the aortic semi-lunar valves. The aortic arch leads O_2-rich blood to the brachiocephalic, the carotid, and the subclavian arteries up and away from the heart back to the head and shoulders.

Venous, deoxygenated blood leaving the lower part of the body enters the right atrium of the heart via the inferior vena cava, while the deoxygenated blood from the upper part of the body enters the RA via the superior vena cava. Then it goes from the RA through the tricuspid valve, preventing the back-flow of blood, continuing in one direction to the right ventricle, through the semi-lunar pulmonary valve into the pulmonary artery, which branches, taking deoxygenated blood to the right and left lungs. (See Figure 14-3.)

Blood is cleaned, or waste CO_2 is dropped off, while O_2 is picked up during respiration, and the external exchange occurs (as discussed in The Respiratory System, Chapter 13). The CO_2 is exhaled out of the body, while the clean, oxygenated blood travels out of the lungs via the pulmonary vein to the left atrium of the heart, which then goes through the bicuspid valve, also known as the mitral valve, to the left ventricle. Arterial oxygenated blood then leaves the heart via the semi-lunar aortic valve to the aorta, the largest and main artery of the body.

Some of the blood goes back to the heart via the three arteries that branch off of the aortic arch—the brachiocephalic, the carotid, and the subclavian arteries—and through the narrower coronary arteries to feed the heart its own blood supply and oxygen. The rest of the blood flows through a succession of narrowing arteries, from the aorta to arteries to arterioles, then enters the capillaries as oxygenated blood, dropping off the oxygen and picking up the diffused waste called carbon dioxide, or CO_2. This is known as the "internal exchange." The deoxygenated blood then leaves the capillaries, flowing through a succession of widening veins, as it enters the venules (the smallest of veins), then the veins, and finally the superior and inferior vena cavas back to the right atrium, starting the circulation process all over again.

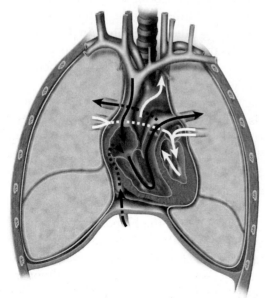

Figure 14-3   Pulmonary circulation

The Conduction System

The conduction system, or electrical system of the heart controls the speed of the heartbeat. The spontaneous contractions of the heart muscle cells are coordinated by the *sinoatrial (SA) node*. This specialized type of nodal tissue provides the energy in the form of electricity to the heart and is characteristic of both muscle and nervous tissue. The SA node sends the electrical impulses, which, in turn, causes the muscles to contract.

This conduction tissue has an unusual characteristic known as autorhythmicity that allows the heart to generate its own electrical stimulation. The electrical impulse, generated within the SA node, is known as the natural pacemaker, and it continues through the atrioventricular (AV) node, known as the electrical bridge, into the common Bundle of His (aka AV bundle), through the left and right bundle branches and Purkinje fiber.

This conduction of electrical impulse results in the contraction of the atria immediately followed by contraction of the ventricles. Therefore, coordination of the contractions of the heart chambers is dependent upon both the SA node and autorhythmicity. An electrocardiogram (ECG, EKG) that records the electrical activity of the conduction system yields a characteristic wave pattern form on a printout of graph paper. In general descriptive terms, the P-wave represents electrical activity in the atria and the beginning of their contractions(s); the large deflection (the QRS wave) represents electrical activity in both ventricles and the beginning of their contraction(s); while the T-wave represents electrical recovery in both ventricles. In the healthy human, as the electrical impulse moves through the heart, the heart contracts about 60 to 100 times a minute. This is known as the "heart rate." Each contraction represents one heartbeat. The atria contract about 1/10 of a second before the ventricles, so that their blood empties into the ventricles before the ventricles contract. This delay occurs when impulses reach the AV node. The impulses are then sent down the atrioventricular bundle, or Bundle of His, a bundle of fibers that branch off into two bundles. The impulses are then carried down the center of the heart to the left and right ventricles where the atrioventricular bundles divide further into the Purkinje fibers. When the impulses reach these fibers, they trigger the muscle fibers in the ventricles to contract.

The cardiac cycle is the pattern of events that occur when the heart beats. There are two phases of this cycle: (1) diastole, when the ventricles are relaxed; and (2) systole, when the ventricles contract.

During the diastole phase, both the atria and ventricles are relaxed, and the atrioventricular valves (tricuspid and mitral) are open to allow blood to pass into both ventricles. Deoxygenated blood from the superior and inferior vena cava flows into the right atrium and from the pulmonary vein into the left atrium. The SA node contracts, prompting the atria to contract. The right atrium empties all of its blood into the right ventricle, while simultaneously the left atrium empties its contents into the left ventricle. The tricuspid and bicuspid (mitral) valves prevent the blood from flowing back into the atria.

During the systole phase, the right ventricle receives electrical impulses from the Purkinje fibers and contracts simultaneously with the left atrium. The atrioventricular valves close, and the semi-lunar pulmonary and aortic valves open. The deoxygenated blood is pumped into the pulmonary artery, and the oxygenated blood is pumped into the aorta. The pulmonary valve prevents the blood from flowing back into the right ventricle, while the aortic valve prevents the back flow of blood from the aorta back to the left ventricle.[5, 6]

Nerve Supply to the Heart

The nerve supply from the two divisions of the autonomic nervous system (ANS)—the sympathetic (SNS) and parasympathetic (PSNS) nervous systems—functions to regulate the heart rate and the force of contraction of the heart. Even though the heart can commence and maintain its own heartbeat, the ANS regulates the speed and force of contraction. The SNS neurotransmitter, norepinephrine (NE), increases the heart rate and force of contraction, while acetylcholine (ACH), the PSNS neurotransmitter, decreases the heart rate and force of contraction. These actions are opposite to each other, depending upon the degree of body activity. The more activity correlates with more NE (↑ SNS), and less ACH, likewise less activity, correlates with more ACH (↑ PSNS) and less NE. This homeostasis is usually achieved when one division adjusts its activity so that a relatively stable condition is maintained.

Nerve fibers reach the heart from the cardiac autonomic plexus, which lies beneath the arch of the aorta. Fibers are distributed from the cardiac plexus to the sinu-atrial and atrio-ventricular nodes, the myocardium, and the coronary arteries. (See more on this in The Nervous System, Chapter 19.)

Diseases of the Heart

There are two main, common diseases affecting the heart. This section will explore the complications that can occur and the pharmaceutical treatment for each. The two diseases are congestive heart failure, also known as CHF, and coronary artery disease, also known as CAD.

CONGESTIVE HEART FAILURE (CHF)

In this disease, the heart pumps out less blood than it receives. It is caused by a decreased contractile ability of the myocardium (heart muscle). This is known as a lack of force of contraction. Another way of saying this is that the heart receives more blood than it can pump out. The myocardium is not strong enough to push out the blood from the atria through the valves into the ventricles. This causes a backup of blood in the atria and a weakened and enlarged heart. Think of the word congestion, the backup of blood, as traffic is the backup of cars. Blood accumulates inside the atria, which then enlarges the heart. This enlargement weakens the heart muscle as it tries to contract the heart more and more to push more and more blood, and as it gets stretched out with the enlargement due to more blood in the upper chambers.

The result of less blood leaving the atria to enter the ventricles is less blood available to leave the ventricles to go into the lungs and to the rest of the body. Therefore, there is less CO_2 leaving the lungs and less O_2 entering the blood for an external exchange, since there is less blood in the lungs. Blood accumulates inside the upper chambers, causing an enlargement of the

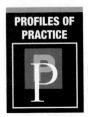
heart. Less blood to the body means less oxygen available to feed the organs and body parts, which means parts of the body may die or become "necrotic."

COMPLICATIONS OF CHF—ISCHEMIA, MYOCARDIAL INFARCTION, AND ARRHYTHMIAS

Some conditions that occur because of the incidence of CHF are ischemia, myocardial infarction, and arrhythmias. A prolonged cessation of blood flow or supply is called an ischemia.

Ischemia is a condition in which the oxygen-rich blood is stopped, blocked, or restricted to a specific part of the body. Cardiac ischemia refers to lack of blood flow and oxygen to the heart muscle, or myocardium. If ischemia is sustained (or lasts too long), it can cause a heart attack, also known as a myocardial infarction, and can lead to heart tissue damage or death. In most cases, a temporary blood shortage (oxygen deprivation) to the heart causes the pain called angina pectoris.

The resulting condition is damaged or dead tissue because it has not received oxygen. If this necrotic tissue is in the heart or cardiac muscle, then the necrosis is called an infarct. "Heart attack" is the layman's term for MI, or myocardial infarction. This death or damage to the heart can be fatal if the area of the infarct is large enough (a massive heart attack). Some people can survive two or three MI's, if the areas of the MI's are small and do not overlap to a large area of damage.

The area or tissue of a myocardial infarct will never return to functional cardiac muscle. Therefore, the functionality of the heart muscle is reduced with each successive MI. Since blood is accumulating, or pooling, in the atria or upper chambers of the heart, the blood will have nowhere else to go except to back up into the blood vessels that it came from in the first place. The right side of the heart will back blood up to the inferior vena cava. This right-sided failure will lead to fluid buildup in the abdomen, abdominal organs, and extremities (legs, ankles, feet, and arms). The backup of blood or congestion from the right side of the heart may also lead to two other complications: phlebitis and *thrombophlebitis*, a formation of blood clots in the veins and cardiac arrhythmias, or irregular heartbeat, which can lead to sudden death.

Cardiac arrhythmias, irregular patterns in the beating of the heart or cardiac cycle, can also occur as a result of the side effects of some medications, and not from cardiac diseases alone (see Table 14-1). The left side of the heart will back blood back to the lungs eventually. Symptoms will be shortness of breath, or SOB, pulmonary edema (fluid collects in the pulmonary vessels or lungs), and interference with the external gas exchange. A person would die of fluid (blood) in the lungs.

TYPES OF ARRHYTHMIAS

Atrial fibrillation, or AFib, is a rapid and irregular heartbeat in which the ventricles contract abnormally, caused by signals in the atria. Blood accumulates in the atria. A blood clot may form as a result of atrial fibrillation, leading to stroke or myocardial infarction.

Ventricular fibrillation occurs when irregular electrical signals in the ventricles cause rapid contractions of the heart. This is common after MI and

TABLE 14-1   Characteristics of Arrhythmias

Symptoms of Bradycardia—A Slow Heartbeat	Symptoms of Tachycardia—A Fast Heartbeat
Fatigue	Heart palpitations
Slow heart action	Rapid heart action
Dizziness	Dizziness
Lightheadedness	Lightheadedness
Fainting spells	Fainting spells

can occur from electrocution or drowning. It is a life-threatening condition that should be treated immediately with defibrillation electric shock to the heart followed by anti-arrhythmic drugs. It accounts for about 90 percent of all sudden cardiac deaths. (See Figure 14-4.)

Atrial flutter is less common than atrial fibrillation. The main difference is that more-organized and more-rhythmic electrical impulses cause atrial flutter, short circuits that exists in the right atrium.

Premature ventricular contraction occurs when an abnormal electrical signal from the ventricles causes the heart to beat prematurely (early). More common in children and teenagers, it may not require treatment. When the PVCs are caused by disease or injury, they could lead to ventricular tachycardia and also fibrillation.

Ventricular Fibrillation

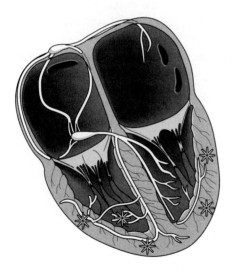

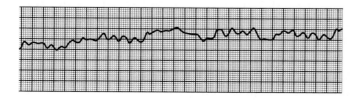

Figure 14-4   EKG of ventricular fibrillation (*Colbert, Bruce J., Mason, Barbara J.,* Integrated Cardiopulmonary Pharmacology, *1st Edition,* © 2002. Reprinted by permission of Pearson Education, Inc. Upper Saddle River, NJ)

Supraventricular tachycardia or *SVT*, is a broad term that includes many forms of arrhythmia originating above the ventricles. SVTs cause a burst of rapid heartbeats that begin and end suddenly and can last from seconds to days. These bursts of rapid beats often start when the electrical impulse from a premature heartbeat begins to circle repeatedly through an extra pathway. During SVTs, the heart will beat 140 to 200 times a minute, even though this is usually not life-threatening. (See Figure 14-5.)

Heart block occurs when the electrical communication between the atria and ventricles is interrupted. The ventricles subsequently contract less often than the atria, leading to episodes of dizziness, fainting spells, or stroke. Severe cases require an artificial pacemaker; less severe cases are treated with drugs such as isoproterenol.

In general, right-sided congestive heart failure occurs before left-sided. Left-sided is considered much more serious than the progression of right-sided CHF. The heart requires its own supply of oxygenated blood so that it does not die. Since the oxygenated blood flow to the aorta and body has been impeded in left-sided CHF, the blood flow to the heart via the coronary arteries, the heart's own supply of oxygenated blood, has also been impeded. Due to this ischemia, the heart could sustain a myocardial infarction, as discussed earlier.

Multifocal Atrial Tachycardia (supraventricular)

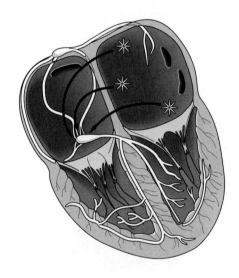

Figure 14-5 EKG of tachycardia *(Colbert, Bruce J., Mason, Barbara J.,* Integrated Cardiopulmonary Pharmacology, *1st Edition,* © 2002. Reprinted by permission of Pearson Education, Inc. Upper Saddle River, NJ)

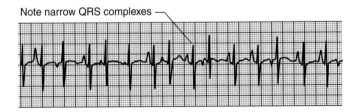

Note narrow QRS complexes

Symptoms of CHF include upright posture or leaning forward, anxiety and restlessness, cyanotic and clammy skin, persistent cough, rapid breathing, fast heart rate, and edema of the lower limbs.

CORONARY ARTERY DISEASE (CAD)

Coronary artery disease occurs when there is a lack of, or insufficient, blood flow to the heart via the right or left coronary artery. There are two types of *CAD*, atherosclerosis and arteriosclerosis.

Atherosclerosis is the buildup of fatty deposits, high in cholesterol, known as plaque, that hardens the walls of the arteries. Soon the lumen will become occluded due to this plaque. Blood clots also form, since the wall is no longer smooth, but an irregular surface that the platelets may stick to easily. This will impede blood flow and lead to ischemia, which may lead to angina, MI, stroke, or pulmonary embolism. Athersclerosis is often caused by a diet high in cholesterol and by stress, and aggravated by injury to the arterial wall and by smoking.

Arteriosclerosis is a term used to describe several diseases that involve the cardiovascular system and the many arteries and vessels which make it up. Arteriosclerosis is often referred to as "hardening of the arteries." Arteriosclerosis occurs over a period of many years, during which the arteries of the cardiovascular system develop areas that become hard and brittle. Vessels become thickened. There is a loss of elasticity. This occurs because of the deposition of calcium in their walls. Arteriosclerosis is the actual stiffening of the arteries themselves. The arteries will become inflexible and will not constrict or dilate as they should, when they should. During exercise the arteries should constrict, and during rest they should dilate. A *stenosis*, or narrowing of the lumen, may occur. A person can have one condition without the other, or both can coexist. Arteriosclerosis can lead to hypertension, MI, and stroke. All the organs that are fed by the sclerotic arteries (hardened) can suffer damage and fail to function properly. Arteriosclerosis is usually caused by normal aging; genetics and diet can also contribute.

Because there is less blood to get through the arteries and because blood hits the narrowed lumen strongly to try to get through, blood pressure goes up. Therefore, HTN is a complication of CAD. Fatal heart attacks, known as massive myocardial infarctions, may result from coronary blockage due to arterioscleross or atherosclerosis. Because clots and plaque can break off and travel, stroke or pulmonary embolism may also result.

Treatment for Diseases of the Heart

Pharmaceutical treatment of Congestive Heart Failure (CHF) involves the administration of drugs from various drug classifications. The following classification of drugs will be discussed: (1) Cardiac Glycosides, (2) Diuretics, (3) Vasodilators, (4) ACE Inhibitors, (5) Beta-Adrenergic Blockers, and (6) Phosphodiesterase Inhibitors.

CARDIAC GLYCOSIDES

Cardiac glycosides are used to increase the force of myocardial contraction, without causing an increase in the consumption of oxygen (see Table 14-2). The most common cardiac glycoside is the digitalis derivative known as digoxin = Lanoxin®. Cardiac glycosides have been used for hundreds of years and are derived from the digitalis purpurea or digitalis lanata plant. Cardiac glycosides are not to be confused with amino glycosides, which are potent antibiotics. Cardiac glycosides increase blood flow and kidney filtration, thereby reducing sodium and other electrolytes, which reduces fluid retention, a main culprit in CHF. The main mechanism of action is acceleration of calcium cations inside the myocardium by first blocking the enzyme ATP (adenosine triphosphate), which in turn shuts off the Na^+/K^+ pump. This pump would normally remove Na^+ ions from inside the heart muscle. Since the sodium ions will now be brought into the heart muscle, they will be exchanged with Ca^{++} ions.

Calcium ions will be brought into the myocardium, which will increase the synthesis of actinomycin and the force of contraction of the heart muscle. With a greater force of contraction, more blood can be pumped out of the heart. Deslanoside also acts on the AV node by slowing and delaying the electrical transmission through the heart, which helps restore normal rate and rhythm. A patient taking cardiac glycosides should never take grapefruit and grapefruit juice because it decreases absorption rates.

Low potassium levels in the serum increase the toxic effects of the glycosides to the heart. Hypokalemia may increase the potential for arrhythmias, ventricular fibrillation, or sudden death. Hyperkalemia, high potassium serum level, blocks the therapeutic effects of cardiac glycosides. Hypercalcemia, high calcium serum level, increases the therapeutic effects of cardiac glycosides, and this can increase the force of contraction and speed to create arrhythmias also. (Treatment of arrhythmias will be discussed later in this chapter.)

A patient is started on a rather high dose of digoxin and then maintained on about $\frac{1}{4}$ of the original dose. This is called digitalization, to produce a rapid high blood level, somewhat like a loading dose.

DIURETICS

Diuretics are used to eliminate excess sodium and water via the urinary tract. Since wherever sodium goes, water follows, retention of sodium means a retention of water. A retention of water increases the amount of blood volume

TABLE 14-2 Cardiac Glycosides: Increase Force of Contraction		
Trade	Generic	Dose
Lanoxin®	digoxin	0.125–0.5 mg PO/IV
Cedilanid-D®	deslanoside	Injection: 0.2 mg/1 ml IM, IV
Purodigin®, Crystodigin®	digitoxin	0.05–0.2 mg PO/IV

and causes an edema. Both lead to and aggravate the congestion and problems with blood circulation associated with CHF.

Less sodium means less water in the blood, which means less volume of blood to back up to the abdomen or the lungs, which means less pumping of the heart and less force of contraction required. Since diuretics reduce the volume of blood, they also would reduce the amount of blood that would hit the walls of the blood vessel, therefore reducing high blood pressure or hypertension.

By promoting water loss, diuretics are used to treat both HTN and CHF. The layman's term for a diuretic is a "water pill." Potassium serum levels must be monitored when a patient is taking diuretics. (See more on diuretics in Chapter 16, The Renal System.)

Examples of diuretics include the following:

- Thiazide diuretics produce mild to moderate diuretic effects and are the most common type of diuretic used for CHF (see Table 14-3).
- Organic Acid Diuretics are also called "Loop" diuretics because they work in the Loop of Henle, an area within the kidneys (Renal System, Chapter 16). These diuretics have a moderate to potent diuretic effect. Used often in acute CHF, they are given IV (parenteral administration) for rapid relief of edema and pulmonary congestion (see Table 14-4).

Potassium sparing diuretics allow water loss without loss of the important electrolyte, potassium (see Table 14-5). Low levels of potassium lead to a weak heart muscle with less ability to contract and to pump, exacerbating the CHF condition. Any diuretic that has some amount of a K^+ sparing diuretic added as a combination drug is considered a K^+ sparing drug in total.

TABLE 14-3 Thiazide Diuretics: Mildly Reduce Blood Volume		
Trade	Generic	Dose
Diuril®	chlorothiazide	PO 250 mg—1 gm, 1–2 doses, NTE 2 gm/day
Hydro-Diuril®	hydrochlorothiazide (HCTZ)	25–200 mg PO, qd, bid, or tid NTE 200 mg/day

TABLE 14-4 Organic Loop Diuretics—Potent, Reduce Blood Volume		
Trade	Generic	Dose
Lasix®	furosemide	PO 29–80 mg in 1 or more divided doses, NTE 600 mg/day. IV and IM available also
Demadex®	torsemide	PO 10–20 mg qd NTE 200 mg/day
Bumex®	bumetanide	PO 0.5–2 mg NTE 10 mg/day, IV available also

TABLE 14-5 Potassium Sparing Diuretics: Prevent Potassium Loss		
Trade	Generic	Dose
Dyrenium®	triamterene	100 mg bid PO, NTE 300 mg/day
Aldactone®	spironolactone	250–0100 mg PO, in divided doses, NTE 200 mg/day
Dyazide®	triamterene + HCTZ	1–2 tablets qd, NTE 4 tablets per day
Aldactazide	spironolactone + HCTZ	NTE 4 × 25–25 tabs/day or 2 × 50–50 tabs/day

VASODILATORS

Vasodilators are used to increase the amount of blood pumped by the heart, with less effort. These drugs widen the roads or dilate blood vessels that the blood travels through, so that more blood can exit the heart, preventing or mitigating congestion. This action increases cardiac output. Vasodilators have a stronger effect on arteries than they do on veins, but will work on both.

Vasodilators relax the arterioles, causing them to dilate so that more blood can pass from the ventricles to the lungs and from the aorta to the rest of the body. Vasodilators dilate blood arterioles, lowering blood pressure, which decreases the work and oxygen consumption of the heart. So the heart does not have to work as hard or pump as hard.

Vasodilators can be used alone or in combination with cardiac glycosides and diuretics to treat CHF. Vasodilators lower blood pressure and decrease O_2 consumption (decrease cardiac output). Nitrobid relaxes smooth muscle, which causes venous dilation and results in a decreased work load on the heart. It also dilates the arteries leading to the heart, which helps improve oxygen supply to the heart. Direct acting vasodilators work directly on the blood vessels in the arms and legs as a peripheral vasodilator for moderate to severe HTN (see Table 14-6).

These drugs are used in conjunction with diuretics and/or another antihypertensive drug of a different classification. Coronary vasodilators are used in the treatment of chest pain, called angina pectoris, caused by an obstruction of a coronary artery, which has decreased the blood supply to the myocardium (see Table 14-7). These drugs can be used in a sudden onset, called acute angina, to stop the pain and allow for immediate dilation of the coronary artery to give oxygen to the heart muscle. They can also be used prophylactically to manage the ongoing disease, known as chronic angina, and to prevent acute attacks of angina pectoris. Nitrates, beta blockers, and calcium channel blockers are coronary vasodilators that help in the prophylactic management of angina.

TABLE 14-6	Vasodilators: Direct Peripheral Acting	
Trade	**Generic**	**Dose**
Apresoline®	hydralazine	PO 10–50 mg qid, NTE 300 mg/d
Isordil®	isorsorbide dinitrate	PO 2.5–30 mg qid, ac & hs, NTE 160 mg/d

TABLE 14-7	Vasodilators: Dilate Coronary Arteries Treating Angina Pectoris	
Trade	**Generic**	**Dose**
Nitrostat®	nitroglycerin SL	NTE 3 Tablets in 15 minutes
Nitrobid® NTG PO tablets	PO 2.5 mg bid-tid. NTE	26 mg PO qid
Nitro-Dur®	NTG Trans Dermal Patch	NTE 0.8 mg/hr × 12/day
Nitrol®	NTG ointment	NTE $\frac{1}{2}$ inch (7.5 mg) tid
Nipride®	nitroprusside, IV infusion	NTE 500 μg/kg, not faster than 2 μg/kg/min
Capoten®	captopril (see other ACEIs)	PO 6.25–12.5 mg tid, NTE 450 mg/d
Minipress®	prazosin	PO 1–20 mg in divided doses, NTE 40 mg/d

ACE INHIBITORS

A specific class of antihypertensive drug known as angiotensin converting enzyme inhibitors, or ACEIs, are now thought to be one of the best treatments for CHF (see Table 14-8). ACEIs are considered the top DOC (drug of choice) for CHF. ACE inhibitors lower high blood pressure and are thought to reshape the heart, downsizing it, while increasing the vitals.[7]

Side effects include a very annoying dry cough. Many ACEIs have the suffix of "pril." Renin is made in the kidneys, which then helps to make Angiotensin I (AI) in the blood vessels. AI has no effect on blood pressure. With the help of an enzyme called ACE, Angiotensin I (AI) is changed (converted) to Angiotensin II . Angiotensin II (AII) is a natural vasoconstrictor, which commences the synthesis and release of aldosterone, cardiac stimulation, and renal reabsorption of sodium (see Table 14-9).

When AII binds to AT1 receptors in the blood vessels, vasoconstriction occurs, and these characteristics of AII lead to high blood pressure. Drugs in the class of angiotensin converting enzyme inhibitors block the conversion of AI to AII by combining with the enzyme known as ACE, the angiotensin converting enzyme. By attaching or binding to this enzyme, the enzyme is unable to convert AI to AII. Without AII, there is no AII to bind to the AT1 receptors in the blood vessels, the blood vessels will not constrict, and blood pressure will not go up.

TABLE 14-8 Angiotensin Converting Enzyme Inhibitor

Trade	Generic	Dose
Aceon®	perindopril	PO 2–8 mg qd-bid, NTE 16 mg/d
Accupril®	quinapril	PO10–020 mg qd, NTE 40 mg/d
Altace®	ramilpril	PO 2.5–5 mg bid, NTE 10 mg/d
Capoten®	captopril	PO 6.25–12.5 mg tid, NTE 450 mg/d
Capozide®	captopril + HCTZ	NTE 150 mg captopril and 50 mg HCTZ/day
Lotensin®	benazepril	PO 10–40 mg, qd–bid, NTE 80 mg/d
Lotrel®	benazepril + amlodipine	NTE 80 mg benazepril/d and 20 mg amlodipine/day
Mavik®	trandolapril	PO 1–4 mg/d NTE 8 mg/d
Tarka®	trandolapril + verapamil	NTE 8 mg/d trandolapril and 480 mg/d verapamil
Monopril®	fosinopril	PO 5–40 mg qd, NTE 40 m
Prinivil®, Zestril®	lisinopril	PO 10 mg qd, NTE 80 mg/d
Prinizide®, Zestoretic®	lisinopril + HCTZ	NTE 80 mg lisinopril/d and NTE 50 mg HCTZ/d
Univasc®	moexipri	PO 3.75–7.5 mg qd, NTE 15 mg/d
Uniretic®		NTE 15 mg/d moexipril and
	moexipril + HCTZ	50 mg HCTZ/d
Vasotec®	enalapril	PO 2.5 mg qd-bid, NTE 40 mg/d
Vaseretic®, Lexxel®	enalapril + felodipine	NE 40 mg/d enalapril and NTE 10 mg/d elodipine
Teczem®	enalapril + diltiazem	NTE 40 mg/d enalapril and NTE 360 mg/d diltiazem

TABLE 14-9 Angiotensin II Receptor Blockers (aka Angiotensin II Antagonists)

Trade	Generic	Dose
Atacand®	candesartan	PO 2–32 mg qd, NTE 32 mg/d
Avalide®		
Avapro®	irbesartan	PO 150 mg qd, NTE 300 mg/d
Benicar®	olmesartan	PO 20 mg qd, NTE 40 mg/d
Cozaar®	losartan	PO 25–100 mg qd, NTE 100 mg/d
Diovan®	valsartan	PO 80–320 mg qd, NTE 320 mg/d
Hyzaar®		
Micardis®	telmisartan	PO 40 mg qd, NTE 80 mg/d
Tevetan®	eprosartan	PO 400 qd–bid, NTE 800 mg/d

BETA-ADRENERGIC BLOCKERS

Beta-adrenergic blockers are used to block Beta-1 and Beta-2 receptors from receiving the sympathetic neurotransmitters norepinephrine (NE) or epinephrine (EPI). Beta-1 receptors are found in the heart and are stimulated by both NE and EPI. Beta-2 receptors are found in the lungs and are stimulated by EPI, but not by NE. When the heart Beta-1 receptor is stimulated by NE or EPI, the following occur with changes first in the heart and then in the lungs:

- Heart rate increases.
- Pulse rate increases.
- Vasoconstriction increases.
- Blood pressure increases.
- Force and rate of contraction of the heart increase.
- Breathing rate increases.
- Bronchodilation increases.
- Oxygen consumption increases.

Likewise, when Beta-2 receptors in the lungs are stimulated by EPI, the following occur with changes first in the lungs and then in the heart:

- Bronchodilation increases.
- Breathing rate increases.
- Heart rate increases.
- Pulse rate increases.
- Vasoconstriction increases.
- Blood pressure increases.
- Force and rate of contraction of the heart increase.
- Oxygen consumption increases.

By blocking the Beta-1 and/or Beta-2 receptors from the sympathetic neurotransmitters NE or EPI, the following will occur instead:

- Heart rate decreases.
- Pulse rate decreases.
- Vasoconstriction decreases.
- Blood pressure decreases.
- Force and rate of contraction of the heart decrease.
- Oxygen consumption decreases (prevents ischemia and angina).
- Breathing rate decreases.
- Bronchodilation decreases.

If a patient is diagnosed with hypertension, angina, or cardiac arrhythmias, Beta-1 blockers will mitigate these conditions (see Table 14-10). (See Chapter 15, The Nervous System, for more about the sympathetic activity and response.) Selective beta blockers that block only Beta-1 receptors in the heart are used primarily for HTN (see Table 14-11). Beta blockers may affect insulin and glucose levels. Inderal® is also used for migraine headaches, glaucoma, cardiac arrhythmias, and post MI.

In addition to beta blockers, an adrenergic neuronal blocker such as Aldomet® = methyldopa is a centrally acting antihypertensive agent. This drug interferes with the manufacturing of NE at nerve endings. Less NE is released, but methyldopa is stored as a false transmitter and is released like natural NE, as needed. Drowsiness may occur upon initial therapy. Other neuronal agents include the following:

- Serpasil® = reserpine
- Ismelin® = guanethidine
- Hylorel® = guanadrel

TABLE 14-10   Nonselective Beta-Adrenergic Blocking Agents

Trade	Generic	Dose
Blocadren®	timolol	20–40 mg/day in divided doses
Corgard®	nadolol	80–240 mg/day in a single dose
Inderal®	propanolol	120–480 mg/day in divided doses
Normodyne®	labetolol	100–400 mg/day in divided doses
Visken®	pinolol	15–60 mg/day in divided doses

TABLE 14-11   Selective Beta-Blocking Agents

Trade	Generic	Dose
Brevibloc®	esmolol	IV infusion for supraventricular tachycardia
Lopressor®	metoprolol	150–450 mg/day in divided doses
Sectral®	acebutolol	400–1200 mg/day in divided doses
Tenormin®	atenolol	50–100 mg/day in a single dose
Zebeta®	bisoprolol	2.5–20 mg/day in a single dose

TABLE 14-12   Phosphodiesterase Inhibitors

Trade	Generic	Dose
Ionocor®	inamrinone	IV 0.75 mg/Kg bolus, NTE 10 mg/Kg/day
Primacor®	milrinone	IV 50 mcg/Kg over 10 min, then 0.375–0.75 mcg/Kg/min

Phosphodiesterase inhibitors increase cardiac contractility by increasing intracellular levels of cyclic AMP, by blocking the enzyme phosphodiesterase in cardiac and smooth muscle. This creates positive inotropic response and vasodilation (see Table 14-12).

Hypertension

As discussed earlier, once AII is made by ACE, converting AI to AII, it binds to AT1 receptors in the blood vessels, causing vasoconstriction and high blood pressure. Angiotensin receptor antagonists block AII from getting into the AT1 receptors in the blood vessels. The mechanism of action that ARBs, angiotensin receptor blockers[4] do this by is "competitive inhibition" or by racing AII to get into the AT1 receptors first. If AII wins, Bp goes up; and if ARBs win, Bp goes down. ARBs usually win. These drugs are considered the new kids on the block. ARBs may increase blood levels of potassium. Rifampin reduces the blood levels of losartan, and DIFLUCAN® = fluconazole reduces the conversion of losartan to its active form; this decreases the effects of losartan.

Treatment of Coronary Artery Disease

CAD, especially atherosclerosis, creates a condition in which blood clots will form. The blood contains platelets that help the blood to clot when necessary. As more blood with more sticky platelets runs through the "tunnels" of the coronary arteries, the platelets aggregate (attract and stick to each other). Blood clots "snowball," getting larger and larger, until the lumen is eventually occluded, causing an ischemia and angina. To prevent blood clots from getting bigger or forming in the first place, anticoagulants are given that reduce the number of platelets, while antiplatelets are given to reduce the amount of stickiness that the platelets have. Think of a platelet as a piece of adhesive tape. The more tape there is, the more stickiness there will be. To reduce stickiness, you can use less tape pieces or reduce the amount of adhesive on each piece of tape. Doing both reduces even more stickiness (ability to clot).

ANTIPLATELET AGENTS

Also called platelet aggregation inhibitors, these drugs reduce and prevent platelet aggregation by interfering with the extrinsic and intrinsic pathways (see Table 14-13). Since they reduce the ability of the blood to *coagulate*, the chance of internal and external hemorrhage exists. Blood in the urine, hematuria, or feces; tarry stools; or heavy menstrual bleeding are indicators of this side effect.

The patient's blood clotting ability, urine, and stools should be monitored. GI upset and bleeding may also lead to GI ulcers; therefore, platelet inhibitors should be taken on a full stomach and at least two hours apart from antacids.

Of the second generation subclassification of thienopyrindines, Ticlid has been known to cause blood dyscrasias such as thrombotic thrombocytopenia, neutropenia/agranulocytosis, and thrombotic thrombocytopenic purpura.

Thrombotic thrombocytopenic purpura, TTP, a life threatening condition, differs from the autoimmune disorder ITP, immune thrombocytopenic purpura. TTP is a drug-induced condition characterized by thrombocytopenia, microangiopathic hemolytic anemia, neurological findings, renal dysfunction, and fever. Early symptoms of TTP are weakness, aphasia, convulsions, jaundice, hematuria or dark urine, pallor, and petechiae. Many oral IIb/IIIa inhibitors, called super-aspirins, that were under investigation have been withdrawn after reports surfaced of significantly high mortality rates, often from sudden death (not from actual heart attacks), and high rates of major bleeding. Studies are ongoing.

ANTICOAGULANTS

Anticoagulants are sometimes erroneously called "blood thinners." Anticoagulants *cannot* dissolve existing blood clots, but they can prevent them from getting bigger or forming in the first place (see Table 14-14).

TABLE 14-13   Comparison of Anti-Platelet Agents

Anti-Platelets Agents

First Generation Subclassification: Platelet Inhibitors	Second Generation Subclassification: Thienopyrindines	Third Generation Subclassification: Parenteral Glycoprotein II/IIIa Platelet Inhibitors Also known as: Glycoprotein II/IIIa Receptor Antagonists
aspirin = acetylsalicylic acid	Ticlid® = ticlopidine Note: not used as much as Plavix because it causes blood disorders such as thrombocytopenia	ReoPro® = abciximab
Persantine® = dipyridamole	Plavix® = clopidogrel	Centocor® = abciximab Aggrastat® = tirofiban Integrilin® = eptifibatide
Mechanism of Action The MOA of ASA is the inhibition of cyclo-oxygenase, which prevents prostaglandin G2 from forming, which, in turn, prevents thrombaxane A2, a potent platelet aggregator and vasoconstrictor[18]		Glycoprotein II/IIIa Receptor antagonists block certain receptors on the platelets responsible for the clumping and therefore block the platelet activity[19]
Side Effects Bleeding gums, poor healing of scratches or sores, bruises, hematuria or heavy menstrual bleeding, GI upset with external or internal bleeding	Bleeding gums, poor healing of scratches or sores, bruises, hematuria or heavy menstrual bleeding, GI upset with external or internal bleeding	Bleeding gums, poor healing of scratches or sores, bruises, hematuria or heavy menstrual bleeding, GI upset with external or internal bleeding
Toxic effects anemia	Rare but serious blood disorders or discrasias thrombocytopenic purpura, which results in anemia, neurological changes, acute onset of altered mental status, and renal failure	anemia
Special Considerations and Warnings Blood must be monitored to dose PIs properly and to avoid anemia or blood disorders (especially with Ticlid)[17]	Blood must be monitored to dose PIs properly and to avoid anemia or blood disorders (especially with Ticlid)[17]	Blood must be monitored to dose PIs properly and to avoid anemia or blood disorders (especially with Ticlid)[17]

Antigoagulants do not thin out the blood. Warfarin is the generic oral DOC, while heparin is the parenteral DOC.

Warfarin is an oral anticoagulant used in the long-term prevention or management of venous thromboembolic disorders, including deep vein thrombosis, pulmonary embolism, and clotting associated with atrial fibrillation and prosthetic heart valves. It is also used after MI to prevent reinfarction, venous thromboembolism, and death. The trade name of warfarin is Coumadin®, and it works by prevention of the synthesis of clotting factors II, VII, IX, and X. Warfarin dosages are monitored by INR and prothrombin time (PT) values. An INR of 3.0 should be reported immediately. Signs of bleeding are usual indications for treatment with vitamin K. Warfarin takes several days for onset, with a long duration of two to five days after it is discontinued.

Heparin is a parenterally administered anticoagulant used *prophylactically* to prevent DVT and pulmonary embolism; to treat acute DVT, thrombophlebitis, and pulmonary embolism; and to prevent clotting during cardiac and vascular surgery, extracorporeal circulation, hemodialysis, blood transfusions, and in blood samples for laboratory tests. Heparin is a mucopolysaccharide found in bovine (cattle) and porcine (pig) lung and intestinal tissue. Heparin combines with antithrombin III to inactivate clotting factors IX, X, XI, and XII. This inhibits the conversion of prothrombin to thrombin, preventing the formation of Fibrin, one of the main clotting ingredients, thereby inhibiting the formation of a clot. Heparin also interferes with platelet aggregation and inhibits thromboplastin so that more thrombin cannot be manufactured. Heparin must be administered *parenterally* by intravenous or subcutaneous injection or by IV infusion. It is destroyed by gastric juices and cannot be given orally. The onset of action of heparin is immediate when given IV, and within 20–30 minutes when given subcutaneously, but it has a short duration and must be given continuously while needed. It may be given intravenously or by subcutaneous injection.

Bioequivalence is still a main issue among different manufacturers of warfarin and unfractionated heparin (UFH). It is still considered sound judgment not to switch manufacturers of products during therapy of an individual patient once therapy has begun. Likewise, it is sound judgment not to switch from trade Coumadin® to generic warfarin. Low molecular weight heparins (LMWH) are also not interchangeable at this time of writing. Both UFH and LMWHs inactivate factor Xa by interacting with antithrombin. The UFH inactivates factors IIa and Xa, while LMWHs exert their anticoagulant effect by inhibiting factor Xa, but minimally affect thrombin (factor IIa)[20].

Some advantages of LMWH's over UFH are as follows:

- Longer half-life yields less frequent dosing, predictable anticoagulant response
- Reduces time in hospital stays and therefore is cost efficient
- UFH has less bioavailability because it binds to more blood components and has greater variability in patient response to each dose.
- Lower incidence of LMW heparin-induced thrombocytopenia than UFH
- The smaller molecule, from the removal of some endogenous porcine mucopolysaccharides, lends to subcutaneous absorption.

TABLE 14-14	Anticoagulants: Doses Vary with Blood Monitoring Results		
Trade	Generic	Usual Dosage Form	O.D. Antedote
Coumadin®	warfarin	PO	Vitamin K
No Trade	heparin sodium	IV, SC	Protamine Sulfate
Low Molecular Wt. Heparins			

Currently approved LMWH's include the following:

- Fragmin® = dalteparin
- Lovenox® = enoxaparin
- Innohep® = tinzaparin

The disadvantage of LMWHs is that there is *no* specific antidote for them, as there is for heparin sulfate. Protamine sulfate reverses only about 60 percent of the anti-factor Xa activity of low-molecular-weight heparin.

TISSUE PLASMINOGEN ACTIVATORS

Tissue Plasminogen Activators, t-PA, and other thrombolytic enzymes chemically break down blood clots by reversing the clotting order and interfering with the synthesis of various clotting factors (see Table 14-15). The main use of these agents is for the management of acute, severe thrombolytic disease such as MI, pulmonary embolism, and iliofemoral thrombosis.

Tissue plasminogen activators must be administered by parenteral infusion within the "safe window of opportunity" to avoid intracranial hemorrhage. This window of opportunity is usually less than three hours from the onset of symptoms, but some thrombolytics may be used within six hours of the onset of symptoms. A fatal error occurs if a thrombolytic is given for an MI caused by a *stenosis* instead of a clot. Therefore, due to their potency and possible adverse reactions, they are used in ER for acute myocardial infarctions, acute ischemic stroke, and pulmonary embolism caused by blood clots only. Quick, expensive blood testing and ECG must be performed *before* a thrombolytic can be administered. This takes precious time away from the "safe window of opportunity," but it is well worth it. Thrombolytics stimulate the synthesis of fibrinolysin, which breaks down the clot into soluble products. These drugs are extremely expensive—thousands of dollars just for the product alone, not including diagnosis, ER personnel ordering and administering the drug, and pharmacy preparing the drug. The expiration of the recently compounded thrombolytic is usually 8 to 24 hours. Because of the expense and short shelf life of the compounded drug, thrombolytics are usually made as needed just before use.

Contraindications include previous stroke, major surgery, head injury, or a history of stomach ulcers or abnormal bleeding problems. Patients who have previously had an injection of streptokinase should not receive a further dose of streptokinase for life, unless it is within four days of the first dose. Streptokinase has antibodies that will reduce the effectiveness of a second dose. A second heart attack will require administration of alternative thrombolytic drug.

Thrombolytics should not be given if no ST segment elevation is present in the ECG waver pattern. Possible side effects include N/V; bleeding at injection site, gums, or other areas; and large bruises.

TABLE 14-15	Thrombolytics and Tissue Plasminogen Activators		
Trade	Generic	Type	Dose
Abbokinase®	urokinase	thrombolytic	4400 IU/Kg @90 ml/hr over 10 min, then 4400 IU/Kg/hr @ 15 ml/hr for 12 hours
Eminase®	anistreplase	thrombolytic	30 U IV over 2–5 min
Strepase® Kasbikinase®	streptokinase	thrombolytic	1.5 MU IV over 60 min
Activase®	alteplase recombinant	t-PA, thrombolytic	15 mg IV bolus, then 50 mg over 30 min, then 35 mg over 60 min
Retivase®	retiplase recombinant	r-PA, thrombolytic	10 U IV bolus over 2 min, repeated 30 min later
Metalyse®	tenecteplase	TNKase	30–50 mg IV bolus over 5 sec (based on weight)

Stages of Clot Formation

There are three basic stages of clot formation, with an intricate domino effect of the many clotting factors. The fourth stage returns everything to normal to maintain homeostasis of the blood, by breaking down the clot to its soluble components.

STAGE I

Thromboplastin is made *intrinsically* and *extrinsically*. The intrinsic system involves the following:

- introduction of a foreign object into the blood vessel endothelium (needle into blood vessel)
- Protein factors necessary for coagulation are present in the circulating blood.
- intrinsic system activated Factors IV (calcium)

The extrinsic system involves the following:

- activated as a result of injury (cut in skin)
- Coagulation is activated by release of tissue thromboplastin.
- thromboplastin not normally found in circulating blood

STAGE II

Thromboplastin converts Prothrombin to Thrombin.

- Prothrombin is synthesized in the liver in the presence of vitamin K.
- Prothrombin converted to thrombin in presence of calcium and Factor V.

STAGE III

Thrombin converts Fibrinogen to Fibrin, which forms the clot.

- Thrombin acts as a catalyst to convert fibrinogen to fibrin.
- Fibrinogen is synthesized in the liver in the presence of calcium.
- The gel-like substance of fibrin traps more calcium and platelets to form the clot.

STAGE IV

Fibrolysin dissolves the clot to attain homeostasis.

- Dissolution of the clot occurs.
- It begins when plasminogen and fibrinokinases are present in the blood and then are converted to fibrinolysin.
- This process occurs spontaneously and can be accelerated by the thrombolytic agents TpA, alteplase, retiplase, streptokinase, and urokinase.

ANTIDOTES FOR OVERDOSE OF ANTIPLATELETS OR ANTICOAGULANTS

Warfarin overdose   Vitamin K is a natural precursor to the synthesis of some clotting factors. Vitamin K is found in cabbage, cauliflower, spinach, other green leafy vegetables, cereals, soybeans, and egg yolks. It is also made by the bacteria that line the gastrointestinal tract. Vitamin K may reduce the effectiveness of the oral anticoagulant warfarin. Because of this, Vitamin K may also be used as an antidote to stop hemorrhage or when too much warfarin has been given, causing excessive bleeding. Bleeding can be internal or external. Note the locations and clotting factors on the coagulation pathway where vitamin K is required, particulary factors VII and IX and Prothrombin.

> Note: Here is a quick note about factor VIII that has little to do with diseases of the heart, but pertains to the subject of clotting factors. Hemophilia A is the most common hereditary disorder affecting blood coagulation. It is caused by a lack of plasma protein factor VIII. Heme = blood philia = loving. Hemophilia is a hereditary bleeding disorder. Hemophilia A and B are among the several types of hemophilia.[16]

The disorder is caused by an inherited, sex-linked recessive trait. The defective gene is located on the X chromosome. Females have two copies of the X chromosome "XX," and, therefore, if the factor VIII gene is on one defective X chromosome, there is a good chance that there will not be a defective gene on the other X chromosome. Males, however, carry only one X chromosome, "XY." Therefore, if the factor VIII gene on that chromosome is defective, the offspring will be born with the disease.[16]

Females with one defective factor VIII gene are carriers of this trait. Fifty percent of the male offspring of female carriers have the disease, and fifty percent of their female offspring are carriers. All female children of a male hemophiliac are carriers of the trait. While some cases of hemophilia go unnoticed until later in life when trauma, surgery, or injury occurs, many cases show the classic symptoms of severe bleeding. Hemorrhage may be internal or external. Hemophilia A affects about 1 out of 5,000 men.

Heparin overdose   The current and only antidote is protamine sulfate. Heparin's clotting ability centers around clotting factor called factor IXa. Protamine sulfate is used for the emergency reversal of heparin-induced bleeding. Activated partial thromboplastin time (aPTT) of more than 100 seconds may require administration of protamine sulfate. Excessive bleeding may need immediate reversal.

Thrombolytic enzyme overdose   Aminocaproic acid and tranexamic acid can be used in the case of a thrombolytic enzyme overdose. The fibrinolysis–inhibitory effects of aminocaproic acid are exerted principally via inhibition of plasminogen activators and to a lesser degree through antiplasmin activity. Tranexamic acid competitively inhibits the activation of plasminogen to plasmin.

NEW DIRECT THROMBIN INHIBITORS

Current traditional anticoagulant therapy has been used to prevent the production of thrombin or its activity. However, new direct thrombin inhibitors inactivate bound thrombin by binding to the enzyme and blocking its interaction with its substrates of fibrin. There are two receptor sites on the thrombin IIa.

The active site directed thrombin inhibitor, argatroban, binds to the thrombin without displacing the fibrin, which inactivates the thrombin so that it cannot form a clot. Bivalent direct thrombin inhibitors, hirudin and bivalirudin, displace thrombin from fibrin during binding and the inactivation process.

These new agents may have a potential advantage over heparin because DTIs produce a more predictable anticoagulant response, as they do not bind to plasma proteins, as heparin does. Therefore, there is greater capability for maintained, accurate response.

ANTIHYPERLIPIDEMICS OR HYPOLIPIDEMICS

These are drugs that help prevent the progression of coronary artery disease by lowering plasma lipid levels. Some are also useful in treating diabetes insipidis and in prevention of stroke and MI. Cholesterol comes from dietary sources and is made in the body by the liver. The cholesterol in the liver is derived from three main sources. The liver can synthesize cholesterol, take up cholesterol from the lipoproteins that are in the circulating blood , or take up cholesterol absorbed by the small intestine. Intestinal cholesterol is derived primarily from cholesterol secreted in the bile and from dietary cholesterol. The body uses cholesterol for building cellular structures and for making steroid hormones such as biles salts.

ADRENOCORTICOSTEROIDS

These are mainly used to fight inflammation and aid fluid balance. Extra cholesterol sticks to the walls of blood vessels and clogs them, with fatal effects to the heart and brain, causing myocardial infarction and stroke, respectively.

Cholesterol

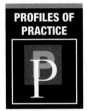

PROFILES OF PRACTICE

Risk for high blood cholesterol increases with age, until the age of 65.

The first line of defense in the fight against high cholesterol is diet and exercise. Screening for hyperlipidemia is a regular physical examination *must*, since there are no symptoms. When this fails to bring down the VDL and VLDL to the normal amounts, or if HDL decreases, a prescription medication must be employed. Normally good cholesterol known as HDL (high density lipids) carries away bad cholesterol known as LDL and VLDL from the artery wall (see Tables 14-16 through 14-18). *Hyperlipidemia* occurs when there is a higher than normal amount of LDL.

- LDL leaves the blood and is deposited between the smooth muscle cells of the artery.
- Macrophages, a specific type of white blood cells called phagocytes, eat up the LDL and then turn into "foam cells."
- Foam cells will ultimately rupture and form a lipid layer, known as "plaque," within the artery.
- The increase in lipids or fats made in the liver or from dietary sources can cause plaques to grow over time, leading to obstructions of the lumen of the blood vessel.
- If the obstructive clot or thrombus occurs in the coronary arteries it could result in a myocardial infarction.
- If the obstruction occurs in arteries of the brain it could lead to a stroke or transient ischemic attack.

There are various steps to the synthesis of cholesterol. Therefore, there are drugs with various mechanisms of action to lower or reverse cholesterol synthesis. The first-line treatment is a low-fat diet and exercise, but a statin may need to be added if the cholesterol remains too high. The most frequently prescribed drugs are called "statins," as they have been found to be highly effective in lowering LDL cholesterol. The statins are a group of drugs that suppress cholesterol synthesis by inhibiting the enzyme HMG CoA reductase.

Although various statins such as pravastatin, lovastatin, and simvastatin share their mechanism of action, there are some differences in their pharmacokinetics and their effects on plasma lipids. They are all metabolized in the liver via the cytochrome P450 enzyme system (which has implications for drug interactions).

For patients with existing coronary heart disease, those with high cholesterol concentrations are most likely to benefit from treatment with a statin. Statin treatment is generally long term. Commonly prescribed statins include lovastatin, simvastatin, pravastatin, fluvastatin, and atorvastatin. Currently, atorvastatin is regarded as the most effective in lowering LDL cholesterol, while fluvastatin is the least effective.

Niacin works indirectly to reduce total cholesterol by reducing the production of building blocks for low-density lipoprotein, "bad" cholesterol, and increasing production of high-density lipoprotein, "good" cholesterol. Bile acid sequestrants that work by fibric acid derivatives are also known as fibrates.

TRIGLYCERIDES

Triglycerides are a form of energy that is stored in adipose tissue and muscle, and gradually released and metabolized between meals as the body energy needs fluctuate. Triglycerides are often measured to depict fat ingestion and metabolism. The measurements can be used to rule out, or assess, coronary artery disease risk factors (see Table 14-19).

Fat is also called adipose tissue and lipids. Lipids are found in the adipose tissue, the liver, and the blood. Immediately after a meal, triglycerides can be found in the blood.

Chylomicrons are produced in the intestines and deliver dietary cholesterol and triglycerides. Usually, the fatty acids are removed from the triglycerides, which are found in the center of the chylomicrons, as they pass through various tissue, especially adipose and skeletal muscle. The remainder of chylomicron is then delivered to the liver, and they disappear from the blood within two or three hours. The remaining triglycerides, plus any triglycerides synthesized by the liver, are then secreted into the blood by the liver as VLDL (very low density lipids). High levels of triglycerides may indicate any of the following conditions:

Low protein in the diet with high carbohydrates—Unused, excessive intake of carbohydrates can cause an increase in the total caloric intake, causing obesity; while a lack of protein interferes with cell growth, renewal and development, structural and muscle building repair, composition or synthesis of hormones, blood, muscles, organs, and glands.

Cirrhosis is a chronic liver disease that has scarred liver tissue and results in liver dysfunction.

Uncontrolled diabetes—The pancreas is unable to make or secrete enough insulin to move glucose from the blood to adipose, fat, or muscle tissue in order for it to be used as fuel.

Hypothyroidism (aka Myxedema)—The thyroid gland in the neck is unable to make enough thyroid hormone, thyroxine (T4). This condition may also interfere with production of triiodothyronine (T3). Metabolism is interfered with in the adult, causing a variety of symptoms and complications such as cold intolerance, weight gain, fatigue, and thin, brittle hair and nails.

Nephrotic syndrome is characterized by large quanitities of protein in the urine, called "proteinuria," which leads to hypoproteinemia or hypoalbunemia. This is hyperlipidemia with elevated cholesterols, triglicerides and other lipids, and edema (see Table 14-20). The edema results not only from the loss of plasma proteins, but also from abnormal salt and water retention.

Pancreatitis is the inflammation or infection of the pancreas, leaving it unable to secrete the enzymes necessary to metabolize dietary fats and interfere with production of insulin, which may lead to or aggravate diabetes. It may be caused by a virus, specific pneumonia bacteria, excessive alcohol consumption, injury, gallstones, or gallbladder dysfunction.

Hypercholesterolemia is a familial (rare), genetically inherited disease with elevated LDL (low-density lipoprotein) cholesterol levels, which may result in myocardial infarctions at an early age.

Zetia® = ezetimibe is the newest breakthrough drug since the introduction of the statins to treat dyslipidemia, enabling a patient to reach lipid goals. It works in the digestive tract rather than in the liver. It does not affect fat absorption. Triglycerides are still excreted without any changes to the bowel. Dietary fat must be "packaged" into micelles prior to absorption. As a cholesterol absorption inhibitor, this drug blocks the transporter (micelles) of the dietary uptake. Ezetimibe selectively inhibits cholesterol absorption in the intestine by blocking the microvilli and villi from receiving cholesterol that is released from the micelles. The result is the prevention of cholesterol from entering the blood system or the liver, decrease in hepatic storage of cholesterol, and an increase in the clearance of cholesterol from the blood.

TABLE 14-16   Total Cholesterol Levels

Cholesterol Levels	Ranges for Most Adults
Optimal Cholesterol Level-**GOOD**	200 mg/dl or lower
Borderline High Cholesterol	200–329 mg/dl
High Cholesterol-**AT RISK**	240 mg/dl or higher

TABLE 14-17   "Good" Cholesterol Levels

HDL	Ranges for Most Adults
Low HDL-**AT RISK**	Less than 40 mg/dl
Borderline High HDL	40–59 mg/dl
High HDL-**GOOD**	60 mg/dl or higher

TABLE 14-18   "Bad" Cholesterol

LDL	Ranges for Most Adults
Optimal LDL-**GOOD**	Less than 100 mg/dl
Near or Above Optimal LDL	100–129 mg/dl
Borderline High LDL	130–159 mg/dl
HIGH LDL-**AT RISK**	160 mg/dl or higher

TABLE 14-19   Triglycerides

Triglycerides	Ranges for Most Adults
Normal Triglycerides-**GOOD**	less than 150 mg/dl
Borderline High Triglycerides	150–199 mg/dl
High Triglycerides	200–499 mg/dl
Very High Triglycerides-**AT RISK**	500 mg/dl or higher

TABLE 14-20	Antihyperlipidemics		
Trade	Generic	Type	Dose
Questran®	cholestyramine	Sequestrants	9 gm dose qd or bid, NTE
Questran Light®	cholestyramine	Sequestrants	4 doses/day
Colestid®	colestipol	Sequestrants	PO 2 gm qd, bid. NTE 16 gm/day
Welchol®	colesevelam	Sequestrants	PO 3 × 625 mg tab bid, NTE 7 × 625 mg tabs/day
Lopid®	gemfibrozil	Fibrate	PO 600 mg 30 minutes before the morning and evening meal
Tricor®	fenofibrate	Fibrate	PO 67 mg/day, NTE 3 × 67 mg or 1 × 200 mg cap/day
Abitrate®	clofibrate	Fibrate	PO1.5 to 2 gm a day.
Atromid-S®	clofibrate	Fibrate	divided into bid, tid qid

The cholesterol stays in the small intestine until the cholesterol is moved through to the large intestine, leaving essentially unchanged, without affecting bowel function, and without affecting the absorption of fat-soluble vitamins.

Ezetimibe does not inhibit cholesterol synthesis in the liver or increase bile acid excretion. Instead, ezetimibe localizes and appears to act at the brush-border of the small intestine, where ti inhibits the absorption of cholesterol, leading to a decrease in the delivery of intestinal cholesterol to the liver. This causes a reduction of hepatic cholesterol stores and an increase in clearance of cholesterol from the blood; this distinct mechanism is complementary to that of HMG-CoA reductase inhibitors.

As inhibitors of hepatic HMG-CoA reductase, the enzyme catalyzing the rate-limiting step in hepatic cholesterol synthesis, statins decrease synthesis of cholesterol by the liver, which results in two important effects: (1) the up-regulation of LDL receptors by hepatocytes and consequent increased removal of apolipoprotein (apo) E- and B-containing lipoproteins from the circulation, and (2) a reduction in the synthesis and secretion of lipoproteins from the liver. The net effect of statin therapy is to lower plasma concentrations of cholesterol-carrying lipoproteins, the most prominent of which is LDL.

Importantly, however, statins also increase the removal of and reduce the secretion of remnant particles, specifically, very low density lipoprotein (VLDL) and intermediate-density lipoprotein (IDL). This means that in patients who have an elevation of both LDL-C and triglycerides (indicating increased levels of triglyceride-rich VLDL and IDL remnants, as well as LDL), a statin is one of the therapies of choice because of its ability to effectively lower LDL-C and non-high-density lipoprotein cholesterol (non-HDL-C) levels.

Treatment of Arrhythmias

A change in the force or the speed of contraction can occur in one atrium or one ventricle, or in both atria or ventricles at one time at irregular intervals, due to cardiac diseases such as congestive heart failure, coronary artery disease, hypertension, or MI or as a result of the side effects of some medications.

The most serious arrhythmia is ventricular fibrillation, which presents a medical emergency because the ventricles cannot contract efficiently to maintain adequate blood circulation; MI or death may ensue. Anti-arrhythmic drugs restore normal rhythm patterns, but do not cure the cause of the irregular heartbeat.

These drugs are grouped into four classes by the effect that they have on the cardiac cycle (see tables 14-21 and 14-22).

CLASS I ANTI-ARRHYTHMIC AGENTS

These drugs cause local anesthetic effects, slow down the heart rate, slow conduction velocity, prolong the refractory period, and decrease automaticity of the heart by blocking the influx of sodium ions to excitatory membranes during depolarization and excitation.

CLASS II ANTI-ARRHYTHMIC AGENTS

Beta-adrenergic blockers slow down the heart rate, slow conduction velocity, prolong the refractory period, and decrease automaticity by blocking the release of sympathetic neurotransmitters and their activity. By antagonizing the effects of NE (norepinephrine) at Beta-1, (cardiac) receptors work particularly well on ventricular myocardium.

CLASS III ANTI-ARRHYTHMIC AGENTS

These block the efflux of Potassium (K^+) ions during repolarization phases 1–3, prolonging the refractory period and decreasing the frequency of *arrhythmias*.

CLASS IV ANTI-ARRHYTHMIC AGENTS

Calcium channel blockers or antagonists block the pathways for calcium entry to excitable membranes of the heart and blood vessels that develop action potentials. This action decreases the SA node activity, slowing down the heart rate and conduction velocity of the AV node. Supraventricular tachycardia often respond to class IV anti-arrhythmic agents.

The Lymphatic System

There is no separate body system known as the lymphatic system. What is called the lymphatic system is closely connected to the cardiovascular system.

STRUCTURAL COMPONENTS

These two closely related body systems work in tandem and are joined by a capillary system through which lymph and blood move. Blood circulates in the closed revolving circulatory system, while lymph moves in one direction to eliminate waste such as bacteria, old blood cells, debris, and cancer cells. (See Figure 14-6.)

TABLE 14-21   Other Cardiac Drugs

Class I Anti-arrhythmic Agents—Local Anesthetic Effects

Mexitil®	(mexiletine)	PO 150–250 mg q 8 to q 12 hrs, NTE 450 mg q 12 hrs used to treat life-threatening arrhythmias
Norpace®	(disopryamide)	PO 100–200 mg tid, qid, NTE 600 mg/day. May produce the anticholinergic effects of dry mouth, constipation and urinary retention, and blurred vision
Procanbid®	(procainamide)	PO 250–500 mg qid, available SR tablets and IV
Quinadex® Quinaglute®	(quinidine)	PO 200–400 mg bid, tid From cinchona bark, also for malaria, may cause cinchonism (OD causes tinnitus, H/A, dizziness, salivation, and hallucinations)
Rhythmol®	(propafenone)	PO 150–300 mg tid, NTE 900 mg/day
Tambocor®	(flecainide)	PO 50–150 mg q 12 hr, NTE 400 mg/day
Tonocard®	(tocainide)	PO 400 mg q 8 hr, NTE 2400 mg/day
Xylocaine®	(lidocaine)	No effect on AFib

Class I Anti-arrhythmic Agents—Beta-1 Blockers

Brevibloc®	(esmolol)	2500–50000 mg/IV @10 ml/hr Beta–1 cardioselective adrenergic receptor blocker
Inderal®	(propranolol)	PO 40 mg bid, NTE 640 mg/day

Class I Anti-arrhythmic Agents—Block K^+ Efflux

Betapace	(sotalol)	PO 80 mg bid
Bretylol	(bretyllium)	Varies, IM 5 to 10 mg/KG body wt q 6 hrs
Cordarone	(amiodarone)	Varies—NTE 1600 mg/day for first 3 wks, then NTE 800 mg/day thereafter. Also blocks Alpha, Beta, Ca^{++} ions. Used when all else fails, very potent, and some local anesthetic quality

Class I Anti-arrhythmic Agents—Calcium Channel Blockers

Calan® Isoptin®	verapamil
Cardene®	nicardipine
Cardizem® Tiazem® Tiamate®	diltiazem
DynaCirc®	isradipine
Lotrel®	amlodipine
Nimotop®	nimodipine
Norvasc®	amlodipine
Plendil®	felodipine
Procardia® Adalat®	nifedipine
Vascor®	bepridil

TABLE 14-22	Common Cardiac Drugs	
Type of Drug	**Function**	**Examples**
Anti-arrhythmics	temporarily correct slow or fast heartbeat	Cordarone® = amiodarone, Norpace®, disopyramide, Xylocaine® = lidocaine Procan® = procainamide, Rythmol® = propafenone, Inderal® = propranolol, Betapace® = sotalol
Beta blockers Calcium channel blockers	reduce the heart's workload increase blood flow through the heart and help prevent blood vessel constriction by blocking calcium ions	Calan®, Isoptin®, Verelan® = verapamil, Cardizem® = diltiazem, Adalat®, Procardia® = nifedipine
Anticoagulants or antiplatelets	work as blood thinners	aspirin, Coumadin® = warfarin Ticlid, Plavix, Aggrestat

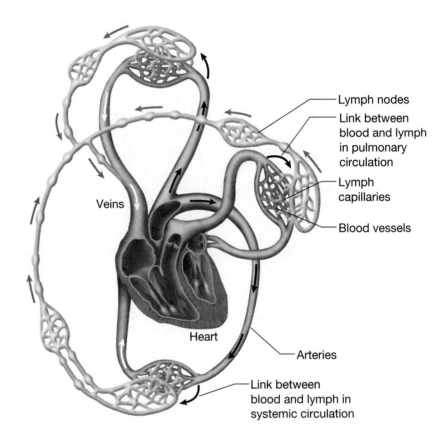

Figure 14-6 The lymphatic system and the circulatory system

Some medical experts consider this lymphatic system to be part of the blood circulatory system because lymph comes from blood and returns to blood, and because its ducts are very similar to the blood vessels (veins and capillaries) of the blood system. Others consider it the main component of the immune system. Throughout the body, wherever blood vessels are located there are lymph vessels, and the two systems work together.

Lymph fluid is not pumped as the heart pumps blood. The lymphatic system uses the contraction of skeletal muscles to move the fluid through the lymph vessels. Bone marrow produces certain cells called lymphocytes, monocytes, and leukocytes. Lymph nodes are areas where lymphocytes concentrate along the lymphatic veins. (See Chapter 15, The Immune System, for more details.)

The lymphatic system supports the immune system in the following ways:

- filters out organisms that cause disease
- produces specific white blood cells
- manufactures antibodies
- distributes fluids and nutrients in the body
- drains excess fluids and protein so that tissues do not swell or become inflamed

The Lymphatic Route

The lymphatic system includes lymph, lymph vessels, lymph nodes (sometimes incorrectly called lymph glands), lymphatic ducts, and specialized organs—the spleen, thymus, and tonsils. Lymph is a transparent, watery fluid that contains proteins, fats, and white blood cells called lymphocytes. Lymph leaks out of the blood vessels into spaces of body tissues and is stored in the "lymphatic" system before it flows back into the bloodstream.

Lymph is made when blood plasma filters out of capillaries into body tissue spaces, known as interstitial space, and is then called interstitial fluid. Most of this liquid will enter back into the capillaries and return to the blood circulatory system. The interstitial fluid that does not return to the blood supply enters the lymphatic capillaries and becomes lymph. The lymph then enters larger lymphatics, or lymph vessels, and then finally enters the blood via veins in the neck area. In this way, lymph carries products of cellular breakdown and bacterial invasion to be eliminated via this "system." The right lymphatic duct drains lymph fluid from the upper right quarter of the body above the diaphragm, while the thoracic duct, about 16 inches long and located in the mediastinum of the pleural cavity, drains the remaining lymph from the rest of the body. The right lymphatic and thoracic ducts come together and drain into the inferior vena cava entering the right atrium of the heart. There are more than 100 tiny oval structures called lymph nodes located mainly in the neck, groin, and armpits, which are clustered all along the lymph vessels. The roles of the lymph nodes are to act as barriers to infection by filtering out and destroying toxins and germs and to make white blood cells.

The spleen is the largest mass of lymphoid tissue in the body. It is located in the upper left corner of the abdominal cavity under the diaphragm. There is much uncertainty about its true function and purpose. The function of the spleen appears to be the synthesis of nongranular lymphocytes and monocytes. The splenic artery carries blood to the spleen from the heart. Blood leaves the spleen via the splenic vein, which drains into a larger "portal vein," which then carries the blood to the liver. Like the lymph nodes, the spleen contains antibody-producing lymphocytes. These antibodies weaken or kill bacteria, viruses, and other organisms that cause infection. White blood cells called macrophages in the spleen will destroy damaged blood cells and clear them from the bloodstream. (See Figure 14-7.)

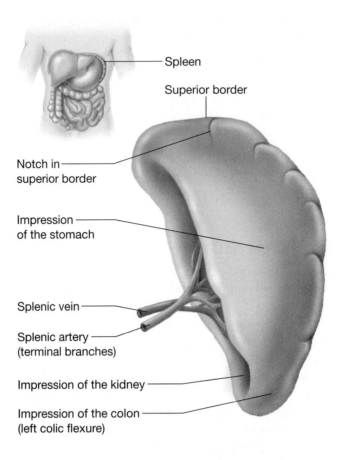

Spleen

Superior border

Notch in superior border

Impression of the stomach

Splenic vein

Splenic artery (terminal branches)

Impression of the kidney

Impression of the colon (left colic flexure)

Figure 14-7 The spleen

The spleen can act as the body's "blood bank" or reservoir. As much as 1 pint (500 ml) of the body's 5.6 liters (5,600 ml) can be stored at one time and released as quickly as needed. This may occur during strenuous exercise or after a hemorrhage.

The thymus, a body of lymphoid tissue, is a gland of the endocrine system that plays a role in the immune system. It is located in the upper part of the mediastinum behind the sternum and extends upwards into the base of the neck. It stops growing at puberty and begins to atrophy at that time. The thymus is stimulated by the hormone thymosin and helps the immune system of newborns by increasing T-cell maturation. An adult can live without the thymus gland, as other lymphoid tissue can compensate.

Diseases of the Spleen

The blood vessels of the spleen are lined with macrophages, which digest (eat up) debris in the blood such as worn out red blood cells and platelets. Mononucleosis is a disease caused by the Epstein-Barr virus, in which the macrophages in the spleen become overactive, trapping a higher than normal number of white blood cells. In the process, the spleen becomes swollen and may even rupture.

A patient with mononucleosis is directed not to be too active or be involved with contact sports for six months to one year, because injury to the swollen spleen could rupture it. A splenectomy would have to be performed. One can live without a spleen, but its absence decreases the body's ability to fight infection. "People who do not have a spleen are at particularly high risk of pneumococcal infections because of the spleen's role in fighting certain kinds of bacteria, such as pneumococcus." In addition, such patients without a spleen will need vaccinations against Haemophilus Influenza Type B, Meningococcus, and Pneumoncoccus.

A person can live without the spleen; the liver and the femur compensate by removing old damaged erythrocytes and manufacturing erythrocytes and leukocytes, respectively.

SUMMARY

The cardiovascular system, also called the circulatory system, is the system responsible for transporting blood to all parts of the body. The cardiovascular system consists of the heart, arteries and arterioles, veins and venules, and capillaries. The arteries are responsible for carrying oxygen-rich blood to the cells, and the veins carry the deoxygenated blood back to the heart and lungs. The lungs and respiratory system work in tandem with the cardiovascular system to sustain life.

In order to accomplish its primary purpose as a pumping mechanism to circulate blood to all parts of the body, the heart relies on a conduction, or electrical, system comprised of nodes and nodal tissues that regulate the various aspects of the heartbeat. In addition, the nervous system (which will be discussed in Chapter Nineteen) plays a vital role in regulating heart rate.

The two main common diseases affecting the cardiovascular system are congestive heart failure (CHF) and coronary artery disease (CAD). Congestive heart failure occurs when the heart pumps out less blood than it receives, resulting in a weakened and enlarged heart, and in less blood being pumped to feed the organs. Complications of CHF include ischemia (the blood supply to a specific organ is stopped, blocked, or restricted), myocardial infarction (the ischemia occurs within the heart itself), and cardiac arrhythmias (a disruption in the electrical conduction system of the heart). CHF is responsible for 40,000 deaths each year, as well as for 2.9 million doctor visits and 875,000 hospitalizations.

Coronary artery disease (CAD) refers to a lack of, or insufficient, blood flow to the heart. CAD is the result of atherosclerosis or arteriosclerosis. Many factors can contribute to CAD including, diet, stress, smoking, normal aging, and genetics. As a pharmacy technician, you need to be aware of these "life-style" factors that can lead to the development of CAD.

A thorough discussion, the treatment for diseases of the cardiovascular system is contained in this chapter. As you will note, although great strides have been made in the ability to treat CHF and CAD, cardiovascular disease remains the leading cause of death in the United States.

CHAPTER REVIEW QUESTIONS

1. Approximately how many gallons of blood are estimated to be pumped by the heart each day?
   a. 4,300
   b. 2,300
   c. 3,300
   d. 1,300
2. What is the purpose of the heart?
3. The average body contains how much blood?
   a. 7.6 liters
   b. 3.1 gallons
   c. 4.2 pints
   d. 5.6 liters
4. What is the name of the machine that records the electrical activity of the heart?
5. A type of arrhythmia in which a rapid and irregular heartbeat occurs when the ventricles contract abnormally due to signals in the atria is called:
   a. atrial flutter
   b. atrial fib
   c. atrial rhythm
   d. atrial wave
6. On which side, right or left, does congestive heart failure typically first take place?
7. What is arteriosclerosis?
8. What increases the toxic effects of the glycosides to the heart?
9. Can anticoagulants aid in the dissolving of clot formation, and if so how?
10. Explain how tissue plasminogen activators (t-PA) work.
11. Normally, how much lymph circulates through the body?
    a. one to two quarts
    b. one to two pints
    c. one to two gallons
    d. a or b, depending on the size of the person

Resources and References

1. Blood Statistics.
   http://ask.yahoo.com/ask/20000612.html
2. Blood Statistics.
   www.cardioliving.com/consumer/ Circulatory/Blood.shtm
3. Listen to the lup-dup sounds of the heart. See the cardiac cycle in action:
   http://www.jdaross.cwc.net/cardiac_cycle.htm
4. More on the sounds of lup-dup.
   http://www.backcsc.com/heart.html
5. Natural Pacemaker and the Electrical Bridge
   http://www.guidant.com/condition/heart/heart electrica.html
6. Read more about the cardiac cycle.
   http://www.medstudents.com.br/basic/cardfs/cardfs1.htm

7. Read more about the cardiac cycle.
   http://medlib.med.utah.edu/kw/pharm/hyper_heart1.html

8. Medical Treatments for Congestive Heart Simon Maybaum, MD; New York Presbyterian Hospital and Ainat Beniaminovitz, MD; Columbia

9. University College of Physicians and Surgeons Failure

10. Agenet on Nitrobid.
    http://agenet.agenet.com/?Url=link.asp?DOC/1339

11. Myofilaments, Sarcoplasmic Reticulum (SR)
    www.biology.eku.edu/RITCHISO/301notes3.htm

12. Nerve Supply of the Heart
    http://www.leeds.ac.uk/chb/HUMB2040/prac3thor.pdf

13. Endocardium and periocaridum
    http://www.medterms.com/script/main/art.asp?articlekey=3236

14. Phlebitis.
    http://www.zipmall.com/mpm-art-phlebitis.htm

15. Thrombophlebitis
    http://www.nlm.nih.gov/medlineplus/thrombophlebitis.html

16. Angina Pectoris
    http://www.leeds.ac.uk/chb/HUMB2040/prac3thor.pdf

17. Location of Lymph Nodes—a visual and interactive site
    http://www.innerbody.com/image/lympov.html

18. Survival with a Splenectomy
    http://www.merck.com/mrkshared/mmanual_home2/sec14/ch179/ch179a.jsp

19. Vaccinations for Patients with a Splenectomy
    http://www.mayoclinic.com/invoke.cfm?id=AN00615

20. Holland, Norman and Michael Patrick Adams. *Core Concepts in Pharmacology.* Upper Saddle River, NJ: Pearson Education, 2003.

21. Adams, Michael Patrick, Dianne L. Josephson, and Leland Norman Holland, Jr. *Pharmacology for Nurses—A Pathophysiologic Approach.* Upper Saddle River, NJ: Pearson Education, 2005.

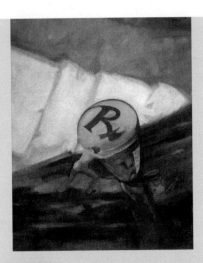

CHAPTER 15

The Immune System

After completing this chapter, you should be able to:

- List, identify, and diagram the three basic parts of a cell.

- Explain the function of the cell membrane wall and DNA in relation to common cell division and infection.

- List and define common diseases of infection and comprehend the causative pathogen or organism, symptoms, and pharmaceutical treatment associated with each disease.

- Describe the mechanisms of and comprehend how each class of drugs works in order to mitigate or destroy symptoms of the following immune system diseases or conditions: respiratory infection/pneumonia, HIV/AIDS, influenza, childhood diseases, cancer, malaria, diarrhea TB, and urinary tract infections.

- Describe the concept of autoimmune disease and relate it to the specifics of rheumatoid arthritis.

- Discuss the various uses of vaccines and how they work in the body.

- Explain why a vaccine for AIDS has not been developed as of 2004 and is difficult to develop.

INTRODUCTION

The immune system[1] functions to protect the body from foreign invaders that would otherwise destroy the body or parts of it via infection or cancer. There are numerous immune system responses to the attacks from these foreign invaders. The body's defense system is amazingly effective most of the time. To defend itself, the body has several defense barriers and defense mechanisms. These include the skin; moist germ-trapping linings of the breathing and digestive passageways (mucus and cilia); the mechanism by which blood clots (thrombi) seal wounds and leaks; white blood cells and other infection fighting substances; the thymus gland in the chest, which develops certain white blood cells; and small lymph nodes or glands spread all over the body that destroy invading substances.

Anatomy and Physiology
of the Immune System

The "first line of defense" is known as nonspecific defense mechanisms. These are the body's main fighting actions against disease.

THE BODY'S DEFENSE MECHANISMS

These mechanisms include physical barriers, natural deterrents (fluids or chemicals and immune cells that prevent or attack invaders), and the inflammatory process. The body's "second line of defense" is known as specific defense mechanisms. These are discussed next.

NONSPECIFIC DEFENSE MECHANISM

This mechanism effectively reduces the workload of the immune system by preventing entry and spread of microorganisms in the body.

- Physical or anatomical barriers include the following:
  - Mucus of the respiratory tract traps particles and microbes before they can infect the lungs (as discussed in Chapter 13, The Respiratory System).
  - Vertebral column, spinal cord fluid, and the meninges protect the central nervous system from injury or infection. (See The Nervous System, Chapter 19).
  - Skin protects the inside of the body from attack due to its hard, dry, dead skin cells along with salty and somewhat acidic pH. These work together to prevent MOs from reproducing and growing. (The effects of a lack of this protection are discussed in Chapter 9, The Skin.)
- Physiological deterrents to pathogens are found in natural body openings such as the following:
  - The vagina has acidic secretions so that it serves as a hostile environment that prevents the growth of many pathogens. In fact, if the vaginal fluid is too acidic it can kill sperm, rendering the female sterile.
  - The eyes have tears to continually flush irritants and MOs out of the eyes.
  - The eye, mouth, and nasal orafices are protected by various fluids (tears, saliva, or mucus) made of secretions that contain an enzyme which breaks down bacterial cell walls (lysozyme). (The necessity of the cell wall to any microorganism is discussed in Chapter 9, The Skin.)
  - Lysozyme is also present in blood, sweat, and some other tissue fluids, and also aids in prevention of MO growth.
  - Nonspecific immune system cells—phagocytes (or macrophages), special immune system cells, detect (or target), track, engulf, and

kill invading microorganisms, host cells, and debris. These phagocytic cells are part of the nonspecific immune system.

- Blood components or complement help in the following ways:
  - Clotting factors found in blood cause clotting at the site of injury site (scabbing), which can prevent pathogens from entry or invasion. This is a type of "perimeter" effect.
  - Proteins aid in inflammation and release of phagocytes. Proteins bind to the surface of the bateria/virus/host cells and destroy them (lyze or lyses). Recall that inflammation (previously discussed in Chapter 9, The Skin, Chapter 12, The Musculoskeletal System, and Chapter 13, The Respiratory System) can aid in prevention or recognition of invasion, but, unfortunately, uncontrolled inflammation may lead to more damage and possible death.

- The normal flora is a group of microorganisms naturally occurring in the body (mouth, skin, and GI tract). These do not cause disease, but serve to prevent infection from exogenous microorganisms by competing with them so that they cannot penetrate or invade the human host tissues.
  - Suppression of the natural endogenous or "good" microorganisms of the flora allows opportunistic exogenous or "bad" microorganisms to infect and cause disease.
  - An example of when the natural flora becomes suppressed is during antibiotic treatment, in some females, or in some cancer patients on chemotherapy.
  - It is said that the immune system or the patient is immunosuppressed when the person is susceptible to infection. Another term is immunocompromised.

SPECIFIC DEFENSE MECHANISMS

When the previously described nonspecific mechanisms of defense fail, the body initiates a second, or specific, line of defense: the immune system. The immune system has specialized protein molecules and cells that function to fight foreign invaders (see Table 15-1). Immune system molecules consist of two types of protein molecules called antibodies and complement. In simple terms, antibodies "finger" or mark the invading substance target, while the complement destroys it.

Antibodies, sometimes called *immunoglobulins*, have a concave area on the surface called a combining site. The epitopes of antigens fit perfectly into the combining sites of antibodies. When the two combine or bind to each other, the antigen is inactivated and unable to harm the body, by a process that makes a toxin non-poisonous or makes harmful substances stick together (agglutinate). Macrophages or phagocytes eat up or consume the disabled foreign invaders. The ability of the antibodies to disarm the foreign invaders is called the humoral immunity. Complement is a group of inactive enzymes, about 30 in the plasma, that is activated by the antibodies and antigen attachment. This attachment, or binding, changes the shape of the antigen. This then exposes two complement binding sites and in turn activates a complement enzyme to bind to one of the sites. Then another complement enzyme binds to the second complement binding site on the antibody. The whole time that the antibody is bound to the enzymes, it is also bound to the antigen. The function of the complement is to kill invading cells by "drilling" a hole in the cell membrane wall, which causes body fluid to fill the inside of the invading cell, bursting it open.

Immune system cells are "on the lookout for" invading cells that may have entered the body. Lymphocytes circulate within the body fluids, especially the blood and lymph, and may reside in the lymph nodes, lymphatic tissue, thymus gland, spleen, or liver. Lymphocytes are made in the bone marrow from primitive cells called hemopoietic (blood-forming) stem cells. There are two types of lymphocytes—the B-cells and the T-cells.

Lymphocytes

The B cells get their name from the first stage of development of B cells in the chicken bursa of fabricius. There is no such structure in the human, so it is called the bursa-equivalent structure, and therefore the B cell. The beginning of the B cell is when stem cells in the fetal liver become immature B cells. They continue to mature until the infant is about three to five months old. Then the immature cells insert one specific kind of antibody into their cytoplasmic membranes and leave the bursa-equivalent. They enter the bloodstream and are then carried to the lymph nodes, where they multiply, having the same specificity for the same antigen. If the B cell attaches to a specific antigen that fits into its receptor site, it will become an activated B cell. These activated B cells rapidly clone into either plasma cells or memory cells. Plasma cells rapidly and immediately make and secrete more antibodies in the blood. Memory cells secrete antibodies slowly. Memory cells continue to reside in the lymph nodes until an antigen that led to their production comes into the body again. It remembers this invader, which triggers it to become a plasma cell and secrete enormous amounts of antibodies into the blood. Stem cells in the liver first give rise to the T-cell just before and after birth. The T-cells are then carried to the thymus gland. T-cells undergo the first stage of development in the thymus gland; and thus the name T-cell. The T-cell undergoes a second change when it moves to the lymph nodes where it will reside. There it develops a specific protein shaped binding site that will attach to a specific kind of antigen. This binding sensitizes the T-cell and allows it to produce cell-mediated immunity, or resistance to disease organisms. (See Figure 15-1.)

Some T-cells release a toxin called lymphotoxin and kill the foreign invading cell. There are many lymphotoxins; however, two of them are chemotactic factor and macrophage activating factor. Chemotactic factor brings macrophages to invading substances, while macrophage activating factor tells the macrophages to destroy the cells by phagocytosis or by eating them.

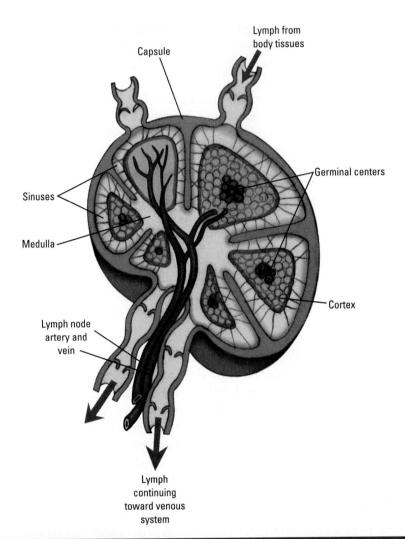

Figure 15-1 Lymph node

TABLE 15-1	Relationships Between Body Systems and the Lymphatic System	
System	The System's Role in and Effect on the Lymphatic System	The Lymphatic System's Effects on and Role in the System
Integumentary (Chapter 9)	(1) Provides a physical barrier to microorganisms. (2) Utilizes inflammation as a caution signal. (3) Aids in reduction and prevention of further inflammation.	Provides antibodies found in skin (IgA, IgG, etc.) to assist in immune function of protection
Digestive (Chapter 11)	(1) Provides important nutrients to the lymph tissues. (2) Digestive acid/enzyme cocktail that destroys microorganisms.	(1) The tonsils destroy infective bacteria and viruses of the mouth and throat (2) Lymph vessels carry absorbed lipid to bloodstream

TABLE 15-1	Relationships Between Body Systems and the Lymphatic System (*continued*)	
System	The System's Role in and Effect on the Lymphatic System	The Lymphatic System's Effects on and Role in the System
Musculoskeletal (Chapter 12)	(1) Muscles protect and cushion lymph nodes and vessels. (2) Muscles contract to help push lymph fluid through vessels, circulatory system, to elimination. (3) Lymphocytes and other immune cells are produced and stored in bone marrow.	(1) Assists in repair after injuries. (2) Assists in repair of bone (3) Macrophages. (phagocytes) fuse together to make bone cells.
Respiratory (Chapter 13)	(1) Lung cells present antigens to trigger the immune defense response. (2) Provides essential oxygen and eliminates carbon dioxide, both necessary for optimum immune cell function.	(1) Tonsils, lymphoid tissue, protect against infection at entry of the respiratory tract. (2) Lungs remove inhaled and deposited solid material and micro-organisms. (3) Provides a supportive role in maintaining and eliminating fluids.
Circulatory (Chapter 14)	(1) Distributes white blood cells and antibodies. (2) Clotting factors in blood make thrombi to assist as barriers to microorganisms.	(1) Fights circulatory and blood vessel infections. (2) Returns interstitial tissue fluid to circulation via veins.
Renal (Chapter 16)	(1) Eliminates waste produced by immune cell as a byproduct of reproduction, phagocytosis, and attack. (2) Acid pH of urine kills microorganisms.	Fights bladder and kidney infections.
Endocrine (Chapter 17)	(1) Adrenal gland corticosteroid hormones provide an anti-inflammatory effect. (2) Thymus hormone, thymosin, stimulates the development and maturation of lymphocytes.	Thymus gland secretes thymosin.
Reproductive (Chapter 18)	(1) Certain enzymes (lysozymes) and chemicals in vaginal and other body secretions kill bacterial microorganisms. (2) Reproductive hormones	(1) Presents antibodies to assist in immune system function. (2) The immune system, through cytokine and interleukin-mediated

System	The System's Role in and Effect on the Lymphatic System	The Lymphatic System's Effects on and Role in the System
	have been shown to regulate the immune system. (Estrogen has been shown to regulate the expression, distribution, and activity of immune chemicals called cytokines.) [3]	pathways, regulates the reproductive system by inducing the release of gonadotropins LH and FSH.[3]
Nervous (Chapter 19)	(1) Neurons have antigens that stimulate specific immune defense responses—the second line of defense.	(1) Produces cytokines, immune hormones that affect the function of the hypothalamus to produce other hormones.

Specific Mechanism of Defense

When the nonspecific mechanism of defense fails, the body initiates a second, or specific, line of defense. This specific immune response empowers the body to seek and then "target" *specific* pathogens and the body's own infected cells for destruction. It depends upon specialized white blood cells called lymphocytes, which include T-cells (produced from lymphocytes that matured in the thymus gland) and B-cells (produced from lymphocytes that matured in the bone marrow). There are two complementary parts of the specific immune response: the cell-mediated response and the antibody-mediated response.

- The cell-mediated response involves T-cells and is responsible for the following:
  - destroying body cells that are infected with a virus.
  - destroying cancerous cells (mutated cells growing rapidly).
  - T-cells activate other immune cells to be more efficient pathogen killers.

The antibody-mediated response involves both T-cells and B-cells and is necessary for the destruction of invading pathogens and for the elimination of toxins.

After a specific type of phagocytic cell, a macrophage, "engulfs" a pathogen, both the cell-mediated and antibody-mediated responses commence. Macrophages digest the pathogen. Then the macrophages "present" or exhibit antigens from the pathogen on their surface. Antigens are specific molecules that trigger an immune response. This exhibit of antigens is a "flagging" or a targeting that helps the macrophages stimulate specific helper T-cells to release signal molecules called lymphokines. The lymphokines, in turn, stimulate both the cell-mediated and antibody-mediated responses.

- In the cell-mediated response, the lymphokines released from the helper T-cells stimulate killer T-cells and phagocytic cells to help to destroy the pathogen infected cells.

- These natural killer T-cells attach themselves to the pathogen-infected cells and destroy them.
- Phagocytic cells produce toxin molecules that directly kill the pathogen.
- In the antibody-mediated response; the lymphokines activate specific B-cells to produce antibodies. Anitbodies are proteins that specifically seek and bind to antigens on the surface of the pathogens. This acts like a "flag" or signal to the phagocytic cells.
  - Other B-cells go on to become memory B-cells, which respond quickly by producing more antibodies upon future infection by the same pathogen. This reinfection can be years later. The memory of *healthy* B-cells lasts forever. The memory B-cell response is very quick, and the pathogen does not have time to reproduce enough pathogenic cells to cause disease before the host's body destroys it.
- Vaccination is explained by the mechanism of the memory response, which prevents even the first encounter of many diseases.

Cell Structure and Function

While this section is not meant to study each type of the human cell, it is presented to develop a better understanding of the cells of the pathogens that invade the body. With this general knowledge, it will be much easier to understand the mechanism of action of specific anti-infective agents. All cells at their essence have at least three things in common:

- cell membrane—a selectively permeable phospholipid membrane that allows some materials to pass into or out of the cell, while preventing others
- Cytoplasm—a fluid where cell respiration takes place; usually contains RNA
- DNA—the genetic code, floating freely in the cytoplasm of some cells or isolated inside the nucleus of other cells

Types of Infectious Organisms

There are many types of microorganisms that cause disease. These disease causing organisms are called pathogens. Pathogens are either animal or plant. Animal pathogens are parasites, bacteria, rickettsia, or viruses; while plant pathogens are fungi or yeast (a type of fungi).

ANIMAL MICROORGANISMS

The differences in pathogens can be observed under a microscope. They vary in shape, size, motility, and other characteristics.

Parasites can be bacterial, protozoal, or helminthes. Some parasites that can be treated topically (lice, scabies) have been discussed in Chapter 9, The Skin.

Human intestinal parasitic worms—The most common in the United States are pinworms, roundworms, and tape worms. Transmission usually occurs via ingestion of contaminated food or soil. Some types are large enough to be seen with the naked eye. Worm infections can cause perforating (make holes) of the intestines by burrowing. They can do this to the muscles, lungs, and the liver. They can damage or block certain organs by clumping together in balls, which can be mistaken for cancer tumors, and traveling into the brain, heart, or lungs. These worms rob the host of vital vitamins, mineral nutrients, and amino acids needed for human digestion, leaving some people anemic (anemia) or drowsy after meals. Worms can give off certain metabolic waste products that are poisonous to humans. This is called verminous intoxification. The toxins are not easily eliminated, usually being reabsorbed through the intestines. Having to work harder to remove the toxin, the immune system becomes suppressed, which leads to further fatigue and illness. Symptoms are diarrhea, loss of appetite, intense anal itching especially at night (worms lay eggs here), and abdominal cramping.

Protozoa are single celled eukaryotes that play a vital role in controlling the numbers of bacteria. Bacteria are necessary for maintaining soil, plants, and animal and human life. An example of a protozoa lives in the mosquito and is transmitted during a mosquito bite, causing malaria. There are four types, distinguished by their methods of obtaining food:

Ameboids are protozoa that most often consume algae, bacteria, or other protozoans.

Ciliates have a specialized opening in the outer edge to capture their prey.

Zooflagellates live through symbiotic relationships, meaning that their existence in another living creature is by mutual agreement. Each benefits from the co-existence.

Sporozoans are parasites that live inside a host and often cause disease to their host by robbing the host of its nutrients.

A common protozoal infection in women is *Trichomonas vaginalis*, or "trich," as it is commonly called. An overabundance of trichomonads grows out of control and develops into infections during times of stress, anxiety, and poor health. It usually is characterized by a yellow or yellowish-green discharge that is thin, foamy, and has a foul odor often described as "fishy." Because trichomonads travel through tiny lymph channels between the vagina and urethra, associated UTIs, such as cystitis, are common. It should be noted that this infection of the vagina should not be considered or treated as a fungal or yeast vaginal infection.

Bacteria—The three common shapes of bacteria are round (coccus/cocci), rod (bacillus/bascilli), or spiral. The organisms can love oxygen (aerobic) or not (anerobic). Bacteria are unicellular, prokaryotic microorganisms. Bacteria multiply by dividing or splitting into two parts, which is called binary fission. Bacteria is plural, and bacterium is singular.

- **Coccus** is spherical, oval, elongated, or flattened on one side. It measures about 0.5 micrometer (μm) in diameter and presents in one of the following arrangements after cell replication:
- Division in one plane produces the following:
  - **Coccus**—one bacterium

- **Diploccocus**—bacteria connected, two side by side
  - **Streptococcus**—aligned in a row or a chain, straight or curved
- Division in two planes produces a **tetrad** arrangement of four bacteria in a square.
- Division in three planes produces a **sarcina** arrangement, an "8-pack" cube.
- Division in random planes produces a **staphylococcus** arrangement, which appears like a bunch of grapes.

Staphylococcus aureus causes skin, respiratory, and wound infections. *Clostridium tetani* produces a toxin that can be lethal for humans.

- **Bacillus**, or rod shaped, measures **0.5-1.0 μm** and from **1-4 μm long** in three possible arrangements, as follows:
  - **Bacillus**, a single bacterium
  - **Streptobacillus**, a chain or a string of bacillus
  - **Coccobacillus**, an oval bacillus similar to oval cocci
- **Spiral** or wave-like shaped bacteria appear in one of the following arrangements:
  - **Vibrio** or comma shaped, or part of a wave
  - **Spirillium**, a thick rigid spiral wave
  - **Spirochete**, thin and flexible spiral wave

Rickettsia is a parasitic microogranism of the genus *Rickettsia/ Schizomycetes* bacteria, made up of small rod-shaped coccoids, that lives in the gut of arthropods (lice, fleas, ticks, and mites). They are transmitted to humans and other animals via a bite. The diseases that they cause have flu-like symptoms and include typhus, scrub typhus, Q-fever, and Rocky Mountain Spotted Fever in humans.

Virus is an ultramicroscopic infectious pathogen that can replicate itself only within cells of a living host, using the DNA and RNA of the host (some animal, some human hosts). Viruses consist of nucleic acid covered by protein; some animal viruses are surrounded by a membrane. Viruses are nonliving pathogens. Very tiny and surrounded by a capsid or protein coating, the basic virus contains only a few genes (DNA and RNA) to replicate. These intracellular parasites use the "machinery" inside the cell to replicate themselves. While most viruses are host-specific, some can cross, or "jump" species. It is thought that HIV jumped species. There are over 200 types of viruses that cause the common cold. These parasites last only about three to ten days in a healthy human. If the patient is immunosuppressed, the virus can stay longer, causing further damage to the immune system. Some viruses are damaging or fatal from the start. Viruses are difficult to cure because they are ever mutating and developing different strains that need different drugs to treat them. In addition, because the virus lives inside the host cells, attacking the virus usually means attacking the host's own cells. This leads to suppression of whatever system is affected. HIV, human immunodeficiency virus, is one such virus for which there is presently no cure.

HIV/AIDS

There are currently two types of HIV: HIV-1 and HIV-2. Unless specified otherwise, most references are to HIV-1, the most common worldwide. Both types are transmitted by sexual contact, through blood, semen, vaginal fluid, and from mother to child, and they appear to cause clinically indistinguishable AIDS. AIDS, or acquired immune deficiency syndrome, is the serious outcome of human immunodeficiency virus (HIV) infection, when the body's immune system is suppressed severely and cannot fight against opportunistic infections. People with AIDS often suffer with lung, brain, skin, eye, and other organ disease along with diarrhea, debilitating weight loss, candidiasis and other fungal infections, toxoplasmosis, dementia, and Kaposi's Sarcoma (a specific cancer). The presence of HIV antibody in the blood confirms that an individual has been infected with the AIDS virus. The FDA approved the first Oral Fluid Based Rapid HIV Test Kit (OraQuick®) on March 19, 2004, which provides rapid results in 20 minutes with over 99 percent accuracy. This test reduces the risk of health care workers who were once exposed to infected blood while taking blood from possible HIV-infected patients.

HIV-1 is subgrouped into two groups, M and O. M group has 10 subtypes, A-J. It is postulated that certain subtypes may be associated with specific modes of transmission. Consider the following examples:

- Subtype B is transmitted via homosexual contact and intravenous drug use (essentially via blood).
- Subtypes E and C are transmitted by heterosexual contact (via a mucosal route, as they are found to replicate in the cells of the pancreas—Langerhans) via vaginal mucosa, the cervix, and the foreskin of the penis, but *not* on the wall of the rectum.

Further subtypes are found more specifically around the world. For example, consider the following:

- Subtype B is mostly found in the Americas, Japan, Australia, the Caribbean, and Europe.
- Subtypes A and D predominate in sub-Saharan Africa. (In Africa, most subtypes are found, although subtype B is less prevalent.)
- Subtype C is found in South Africa and India.
- Subtype E is found in Central African Republic, Thailand, and other countries of Southeast Asia.
- Subtype F is found in Brazil and Romania.

Here are examples of very low prevalence in the following areas:

- Subtype G and H in Russia and Central Africa
- Subtype I in Cyprus
- Group O in Cameroon

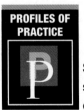

PROFILES OF PRACTICE

Some recent studies have concluded that subtype E spreads more easily than subtype B.

PROGRESSION OF HIV TO AIDS TO DEATH IN FIVE STAGES

- Stage 1—initial transmission and infection with HIV
- Stage 2—infected without presentation of signs or symptoms (10 or more years)
- Stage 3—signs and symptoms of HIV begin to show
- Stage 4—AIDS opportunistic infections to a CD4 cell count or a level below 200 per cubic millimeter of blood
- Stage 5—last and final stage of wasting to death

Retroviral Replication

HIV is a retrovirus. A retrovirus is a class of enveloped viruses that have their genetic material in the form of RNA and use reverse transcriptase to translate their RNA into DNA. The retrovirus family includes oncoviruses (such as HTLV-1) and lentiviruses (such as HIV-1 and HIV-2). In most animals and plants, DNA is usually made into RNA; hence, the word retro is used to indicate the opposite direction. Studying the replication process helps researchers to make drugs that interrupt the various stages of replication.

THE HIV REPLICATION PROCESS IN 11 STAGES

- Stage 1—HIV enters body via body fluids during lactation, sexual intercourse, or blood transmission. Vaccines would prevent this from happening.
- Stage 2—The gp 120 on the surface of the HIV attaches to the CD4.
- Stage 3—Attachment occurs with the help of one of two host cell co-receptors (either CCR5 or CXCR4). This attachment is called co-receptor bonding.
- Stage 4—Via endocytosis, the contents of HIV enters the CD4 (T-cell). This is known as fusion. Fuzeon® works here.
- Stage 5—HIV uses its own reverse transcriptase to change its single-strand viral RNA to double-strand viral DNA, making a copy of the viral RNA to do so. Drugs that work here are called reverse transcriptase inhibitors, both nonnucleoside and nucleoside RTIs.
- Stage 6—The double-strand viral DNA is then transported into the nucleus.
- Stage 7—The double-strand viral DNA is incorporated into, or mixed in with, the host cell's DNA by the viral enzyme integrase, making a *new* double-strand hybrid DNA. No integrase inhibitor drugs have been made to date, but there are a few in clinical trials. Keep your eye on Merck Sharpe Dome that announced in 2003 that it has an *integrase inhibitor drug* in the pipeline.
- Stage 8—The *new* double-strand hybrid DNA is transcribed (transcription) to a viral RNA. The RNA serves as a genome (the complete hereditary material) for new HIV viruses. Translation

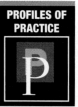

PROFILES OF PRACTICE

Why is there no vaccine for HIV yet? According to the AIDS 2004 XV International AIDS Conference July 11–16, designing an effective vaccine to protect people from HIV (human immunodeficiency virus) or from becoming ill if already infected by the virus is a high priority among worldwide efforts to control the epidemic. The search continues for an HIV vaccine that would be inexpensive, easy to store and administer, and would elicit strong, appropriate immune responses with long-lasting protection against HIV infection by exposure to infected blood and by sexual contact. In addition, such a vaccine would protect against exposure to the many different strains of HIV. One of the reasons a vaccine has not been found is that HIV continually evolves because of genetic mutation and recombination. Money to fund research has also been a problem. But the Global Fund has helped to address this issue and is making a big difference in recent years. According to the World Health Organization, more than 90 percent of all HIV transmission worldwide occurs sexually. To be effective, an HIV vaccine also may need to stimulate mucosal immunity. Unfortunately, relatively little is known about how the mucosal immune system protects against viral infection. Mucosal immune cells line the respiratory, digestive, and reproductive tracts, are found in lymph nodes, and are the first line of defense against infectious organisms.

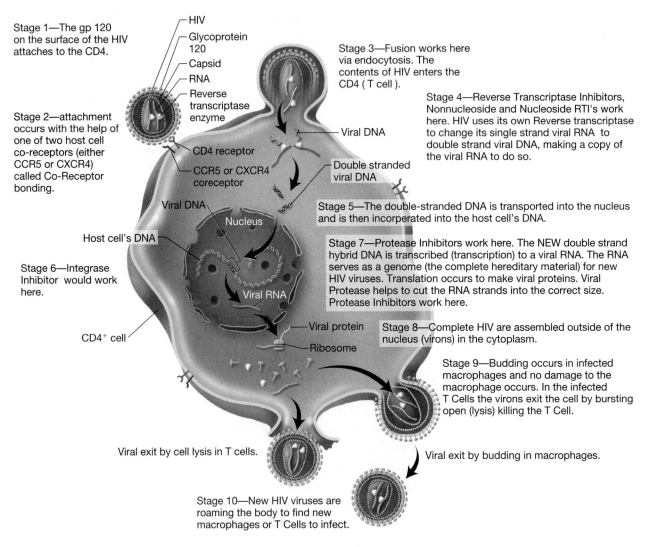

Stage 1—The gp 120 on the surface of the HIV attaches to the CD4.

HIV
Glycoprotein 120
Capsid
RNA
Reverse transcriptase enzyme

Stage 2—attachment occurs with the help of one of two host cell co-receptors (either CCR5 or CXCR4) called Co-Receptor bonding.

CD4 receptor
CCR5 or CXCR4 coreceptor

Viral DNA
Nucleus
Host cell's DNA

Viral DNA

Stage 6—Integrase Inhibitor would work here.

CD4$^+$ cell

Viral RNA

Viral protein
Ribosome

Viral exit by cell lysis in T cells.

Stage 10—New HIV viruses are roaming the body to find new macrophages or T Cells to infect.

Stage 3—Fusion works here via endocytosis. The contents of HIV enters the CD4 (T cell).

Stage 4—Reverse Transcriptase Inhibitors, Nonnucleoside and Nucleoside RTI's work here. HIV uses its own Reverse transcriptase to change its single strand viral RNA to double strand viral DNA, making a copy of the viral RNA to do so.

Viral DNA
Double stranded viral DNA

Stage 5—The double-stranded DNA is transported into the nucleus and is then incorporated into the host cell's DNA.

Stage 7—Protease Inhibitors work here. The NEW double strand hybrid DNA is transcribed (transcription) to a viral RNA. The RNA serves as a genome (the complete hereditary material) for new HIV viruses. Translation occurs to make viral proteins. Viral Protease helps to cut the RNA strands into the correct size. Protease Inhibitors work here.

Stage 8—Complete HIV are assembled outside of the nucleus (virons) in the cytoplasm.

Stage 9—Budding occurs in infected macrophages and no damage to the macrophage occurs. In the infected T Cells the virons exit the cell by bursting open (lysis) killing the T Cell.

Viral exit by budding in macrophages.

Figure 15-2   The HIV replication process

occurs to make viral proteins. Viral protease helps to cut the RNA strands into the correct size. Protease inhibitors work here.

- Stage 9—Complete HIV are assembled outside of the nucleus (virons) in the cytoplasm.
- Stage 10—Budding occurs in infected macrophages, and no damage to the macrophage occurs. In the infected T-cells, the virons exit the cell by bursting open (lysis), killing the T-cell.
- Stage 11—New HIV viruses are roaming the body to find new macrophages or T-cells to infect. (See Figure 15-2.)

HIV/AIDS Drugs

Reverse transcriptase and nonnucleoside and nucleoside reverse transcriptase inhibitors block the conversion of the HIV single-strand viral RNA to double-strand viral DNA, which then blocks the synthesis of copies of the viral RNA. There are two basic kinds of reverse transcriptase, nonnucleoside, as follows:

Nucleoside analogs are often called "nukes" and mimic the building blocks used by reverse transcriptase to make copies of the HIV genetic material. The fake building blocks interrupt or interfere with the copying.

Nonnucleoside reverse transcriptase inhibitors are called NNRTIs and prevent the reverse transcriptase enzyme from working.

Once the new double-strand hybrid DNA is transcribed (transcription) to a viral RNA, the RNA serves as a genome for new HIV viruses. Protease inhibitors block the protease enzyme, which blocks translation. This means that the HIV makes copies of itself that can't infect new cells. Studies have proven that PIs can reduce the amount of virus in the blood and increase CD4 cell counts.

The best known way to avoid drug resistance is to stop or reduce HIV production in the body. The less HIV there is in the body, the less chance there will be of creating anti-HIV drug resistant virus. It is recommended that protease inhibitors be taken in combination with at least two other anti-HIV drugs (see Table 15-2). This treatment protocol is known as highly active anti-retroviral therapy, or HAART. The implementation of HAART increases the anti-HIV effect, which prevents or overcomes resistance. Sometimes referred to as "protease boosting," drug resistance tests are ordered to determine which combination of drugs to use. The following is an example of one such combination, or "cocktail," given to HIV/AIDS patients:

Retrovir + Epivir + Crixovan Take for 4 weeks

Then: Retrovir 200 mg tid
          Epivir 150 mg bid
          Crixovan 800 mg tid

TABLE 15-2 Antiretroviral Drugs		
Anti-AIDS Drugs Classification	**Trade/Generic**	**Possible Side Effects**
Vaccine	In research	—
Attachment Inhibitors	In research	—
Fusion (fusion inhibitors)	Fuzeon® (enfuvirtide)	Itching, swelling, redness, pain, tenderness, hardened skin and bumps near the injection sites, Asthenia, insomnia, depression, myalgia, constipation, pancreas problems, numbness of feet and legs, dyspnea, fever, uremia, peripheral edema (feet)

TABLE 15-2   Antiretroviral Drugs (*continued*)

Anti-AIDS Drugs Classification	Trade/Generic	Possible Side Effects
Reverse Transcriptase Inhibitors		
Nucleoside Reverse Transcriptase	(1) Combivir® (zidovudine + lamivudine) AZT + 3TC (2) Emtriva® (emtricitabine) FTC (3) Epivir® (lamivudine) 3TC (4) Epzicom® (abacavir + lamivudine) ABC + 3TC (5) Hivid® (zalcitabine) ddC (6) Retrovir® (zidovudine) AZT or ZDV (7) Trizivir® (abacavir + zidovudine + lamivudine) ABC + AZT + 3TC (8) Truvada® (tenofovir DF + emtricitabine) TDF + FTC (9) Videx® (didanosine: buffered versions) ddl (10) Videx® EC (didanosine: delayed-release capsules) (11) Viread® (tenofovir disoproxil fumarate–DF) TDF or Bis(POC) PMPA (12) Zerit® (stavudine) d4T (13) Ziagen® (abacavir) ABC	(1) Headache (2) Nausea (3) Skin rash and skin discoloration on palms and soles (4) Lactic acidosis (5) Severe hepatomegaly with steatosis (6) Redistribution of body fat, peripheral wasting, facial wasting, breast enlargement, and cushingoid appearance have been observed in patients receiving antiretroviral therapy.
Nonnucleoside Reverse Transcriptase (NNRTI's)	(1) Viramune® (nevirapine) (2) Rescriptro® (delavirdine mesylate) (3) Sustiva® (efavirenz)	(1) Headache (2) Dizziness (3) Fatigue (4) Nausea, vomiting, diarrhea (5) Rash (may be severe) (6) Liver problems, which can be severe and life-threatening. Regular blood tests may be needed to monitor for liver problems. (7) Insomnia (8) Drowsiness (sedation)
Integrase Inhibitors	In the Pipeline	—
Protease Inhibitors	Agenerase® (amprenivir), Lexiva® (fos amprenivir), Crixivan® (ndinavir), Kaletra® (lopinavir/ritonavir), Norvir® (ritonavir), Invirase® and Fortovase® (saquinavir), Viracept® (nelfinavir), and Zrivada® (atazanavir)	↑ BP, Diabetes Lipodystrophy—inability to absorb fat Liver toxicity may worsen Hepatitis

To improve compliance and quality of life, and therefore decrease antiretroviral drug resistance, new drug delivery methods are being researched and developed. Replacing TID or QID oral tablets/capsules may involve new-time-release technology, allowing once a day or even once a week dosing or inhalants, while injections may be replaced by implants to be changed once a year or transdermal patches. Most HIV/AIDS drugs are made of molecules too large to pass easily through the skin or mucous membranes, but this is being addressed in current research.

Autoimmune Diseases

The Greek word auto means self. A person with an autoimmune disease has an immune system that mistakenly attacks itself. During the attack, it targets the cells, tissues, and organs of the person's own body. During the attack the immune system cells and molecules accumulate at a target site, and this gathering is broadly referred to as inflammation. In general, most autoimmune diseases affect women more often than men, especially women of working age and during their childbearing years.

Some autoimmune diseases hit specific populations. For example, lupus is more common in Hispanic and African-American women than in Caucasian women of European ancestry, while RA (rheumatoid arthritis) and scleroderma affect more residents of some Native American communities than the general population of the United States.

Autoimmune diseases are not contagious and are not related to AIDS or cancers (see Table 15-3). While many autoimmune diseases are inherited, it is also thought that some may be triggered by sunlight (lupus) or viruses that may have lain dormant for years, only to be reactivated and "protected" by the immune system, while the original antibody is attacked by the immune system (such as in the case of rheumatoid arthritis). Most autoimmune diseases are not curable, but are treatable to manage daily living with appropriate drug therapy.

Therapeutic agents that slow or suppress the immune system response in an attempt to stop the inflammation during an autoimmune attack are called immunosuppressive medications. These drugs include corticosteroids (prednisone), azathioprine, cyclosporin, cyclophosphamide, and methotrexate (MTX). Unfortunately, these medications also suppress the ability of the immune system to fight infection, and they have potentially serious adverse reactions.

The common pharmacotherapeutic goal in the care of patients with autoimmune diseases is to discover treatments that produce remissions, with few side effects. New research for agents that have therapeutic antibodies against specific T-cell molecules may produce fewer long-term side effects than the current chemotherapies that are now being used.

RHEUMATOID ARTHRITIS

Rheumatoid arthritis is thought to be genetic or autoimmune. Let us discuss the possibility of autoimmune disease under one theory. It is said that a virus such as influenza or chicken pox may have hidden dormant in the body for a long time. The virus is reactivated in later years, usually in the 40s or 50s. It attacks the synovial fluid of the joints first, hardening it, and thus changes its normal lubricating function.

Subsequently, the hardened synovial fluid and cartilage (soft bone) will hit against and erode each other during compression of joint activity. This will mimic arthritis joint pain and swelling. Eventually, the same virus will attack other tissue and organs, such as the pancreas or heart. The body had once made antibodies to this virus, which became reactivated when the virus was "awakened." However, the body's own immune system did not recognize the virus as a foreign substance; it recognized it as living in the body without incident for years. So, when the antibodies attacked it, the immune system made *new* and *different* antibodies, which now attack the old antibodies. Thus, the virus is free to survive, while the original antibody is demolished by the new antibodies.

TABLE 15-3   List of Common Autoimmune Diseases

Autoimmune Disease	Site of Action and Treatment	Notes
Multiple sclerosis	In the brain Rx: glatiramer acetate, interferon beta 1-a and interferon beta 1-b	**Nervous System** Patients with MS produce antibodies that attack the white matter in the brain and spinal cord, causing the myelin sheath, or coating of nerve fibers, to become inflamed in the brain and spinal cord, which results in signals that cannot be transported or passed along to the nerve.
Myasthenia gravis	In the muscles Tx: (1) Thymectomy or removal of thymus gland may improve immune system Fx. (2) Plasmapheresis—abnormal antibodies are removed from the blood (3) High-dose intravenous immune globulin, which temporarily provides the body with normal antibodies from donated blood	**Nervous System** Autoantibodies attack a part of the nerve that stimulates muscle movement.
Crohn's disease	In the gut or intestine Rx: (1) Remicade® (infliximab) a monoclonal antibody engineered as an inhibitor of tumor necrosis factor alpha, a protein that promotes inflammation in the body (2) Entocort EC® (budesonide) with high affinity of budesonide to glucocorticosteroid receptors, which mimics the potency of the anti-inflammatory effect of about 200-fold that of cortisol and 15-fold that of prednisolone	**Gastrointestinal System** Inflammation of the bowel both in the ileum (lower small intestine) and in the colon (large intestine), possibly caused by a reaction to a virus.

TABLE 15-3   List of Common Autoimmune Diseases (*continued*)

Autoimmune Disease	Site of Action and Treatment	Notes
Ulcerative colitis	In the large intestine (1) Anti-inflammatories, aka 5-ASA (mesalamine): Azulfidine® (sulfasalazine) Asacol® (sulfur free), Pentasa®, Colazal® (balsalazide), Rowasa® enema and Corticosteroids (2) Immunosuppressants: Imuran, 6-MP or cyclosporin. (3) Immune Modulators: Remicade® (infliximab)	**Gastrointestinal System** An irritable bowel disease: Inflammation due to ulcers of a part of the large intestine, or the entire colon and rectum, possibly due to a weakened immune response to bacteria.
Grave's disease	In the thyroid (1) PTU Propylthiouracil (2) Iodine (radioactive)	**Endocrine System** Immune cells "attack" both the eye muscles and the thyroid, leading to dysfunction of both. This may cause hyperthyroidism and increased thyrotoxicosis that lead to intolerance of heat, weight loss. May have exopthalmous wherein the eyes appear protruded or unusually "popped" out.
Autoimmune oophoritis and orchitis	In the gonads Tx: No known treatment or cure; however, hormone replacement therapy is used, but it cannot return fertility	**Endocrine System** Patients with oopheritis may have premature menopause before 40 years of age, or the ovaries are destroyed before the first menstruation (no Tx available). Patients with orchitis, an enlargement of the testis, in which infertility antisperm antibody can be detected.
Psoriasis	In the skin Tx: (1) Corticosteroids—Dovonex® (calcipotriene) (2) Coal tars, Anthra-Derm® (anthralin) (3) Topical receptor-selective retinoid—tazarotene (thought to normalize the proliferation of keratinocytes, as well as to decrease cutaneous inflammation). (4) Immunosuppressive dimeric fusion protein—Amevive® (alefacept), given FDA approval in 2003, primarily blocks the activation of an important type of immune system cell called T-cells, which normally help ward off foreign invaders and fight infection	**Integumentary System**—very small areas of skin or cover the entire body with a buildup of red and silvery scales called plaques; may be painful and unattractive. Epidermal cell kinetics with abnormal activation of immune mechanisms are thought to be the major contributors.

TABLE 15-3 List of Common Autoimmune Diseases (*continued*)

Autoimmune Disease	Site of Action and Treatment	Notes
Vitiligo	In the skin Tx: (1) Pallative with cosmetics and self-tanning products	**Integumentary System**—The body makes antibodies to its own pigment cells or melanocytes; creating patches of lighter skin. Cycles of pigment loss, followed by remission; when the pigment doesn't change, may continue indefinitely.
Pernicious anemia	In the blood (1) Restorative vitamin B12 shots, and Folic Acid	**Circulatory System** Pernicious anemia is caused by the inability of the body to absorb vitamin B12 from the digestive tract into the bloodstream, in which the ability to supply this vital nutrient to organs and bone marrow is compromised, and eventually attack of organs such as the liver, spleen, kidneys, heart, and the brain results.
Lupus or Systemic Lupus Erythematosus	Affects various tissues and organs, this also varies among individuals with the same disease. Lupus may be worsened or triggered by sunlight.	**Multiple Organs, including the Musculoskeletal System** Ultimate damage to specific tissues may be permanent. Example is destruction of insulin-producing cells of the pancreas, resulting in Type 1 diabetes mellitus. Immune cell complexes and inflammatory molecules can block blood flow and ultimately destroy organs such as the kidney.
Rheumatoid arthritis	In the joints and other tissues and organs Tx: (1) DMARDS = Disease—modifying antirheumatic drugs: MTX, leflunomide D-Penicillamine, sulfasalazine, gold therapy, minocycline azathioprine, hydroxychloroquine (and other antimalarials), cyclosporine, and biologic agents. DMARDS slow down the disease process by modifying the immune system in some way other than by inhibition of prostaglandin.	**Multiple Organs including the Musculoskeletal System** In rheumatoid arthritis, reactive oxygen intermediate molecules and other toxic molecules are made by overproductive macrophages and neutrophils invading the joints. The toxic molecules contribute to inflammation, which is observed as warmth and swelling, and participate in damage to the joint.
Scleroderma	In the skin and blood vessels Tx: Pallative only; no cure (1) Immunosupressants: cyclophosphamide (2) Nifedipine and calcium (3) Channel blockers (4) Antibiotics	Cytokines, proteins that may cause surrounding immune system cells to become activated, grow, or die, may also influence nonimmune system tissues. Some cytokines may contribute to the thickening of the skin and blood vessels resulting in scleroderma. Systemic sclerosis (scleroderma) is characterized by fibrosis of the skin, vasculature (blood vessels), and internal organs

Plant Microorganisms

Fungus is a plant-like filamentous or single-celled eukaryotic organism in the division of Thallophyta, characterized by a lack of chlorophyll, heterotrophic growth, and the production of extracellular enzymes. Fungi include yeasts, molds, mildews, and mushrooms. Fungi can be parasitic or saprobeic. Canker sores, ringworm, some kinds of molds, and mildews are fungal diseases. Common examples are *Candida* and *Aspergillus* fungi. Fungi feed themselves by secreting digestive enzymes that release organic molecules from the tree, soil, or organism (human) that it is living inside of. The fungus then absorbs those released organic molecules. Fungal infections love moisture, heat, and darkness. Tropical conditions grow fungus easily. Athletes' foot is an example of growth of fungus due to moist, hot, dark environment: the sneaker. Fungal infections of the blood are the hardest infections to cure. Many drugs used to fight fungal and yeast infection end in "azole." Examples are ketoconazole (which has many drug interactions), sulfamethoxazole, fluconazole, and itraconazole. Another antifungal is amphotericin B, which can have many side effects.

Yeast is a microscopic, dehydrated, hydrophilic single-cell organism of the fungus family, which produces alcohol and carbon dioxide as it grows and ferments, and eats sugar. *Candida albicans* or candidiasis is a yeast-like fungus that causes vaginal yeast infections. *Candida glabrata* is a more resistant yeast that also causes thrush and vaginal yeast infections. Antibiotics, taken to kill pathogenic bacteria, may also kill friendly bacteria, which are part of the "flora." These bacteria, such as lactobacilli, help to keep yeast in the vagina under control. Without lactobacilli, the balance of yeast in the vagina is disrupted and candida can take over.

Antibiotics have no effect on yeast itself; however, they can change the environment in the vagina just enough to cause a yeast infection (also known as vaginal thrush). If the body is left too weak after an illness such as a flu, or too busy fighting off another infection, the natural yeast in the body may not be "policed," and it may take the opportunity to multiply uncontrollably.

Diabetics have poor immune systems and are prone to many yeast infections. In addition, diabetes increases blood sugar levels, which may, in turn, increase the sugar in vaginal secretions. Diabetic women also tend to have high sugar levels in their urine. Vaginal yeast infections may exist because of the sugar in the urine that may be left outside the genital area, just outside of the vagina. Wearing tight or damp clothing, a change in the normally acidic vaginal environment (a pH of 4.0 to 5.0), and some foods may be contributing factors to growing vaginal yeast. Some practitioners suggest avoiding sugar, dairy products, coffee, tea, and wine that all contribute to thrush by increasing urinary sugar.

The following drugs are anti-fungals that work in similar ways to break down the cell wall of the candida organism until it disintegrates. They are available as vaginal suppositories (inserts) and topical cream applied with an applicator once at night for three or seven consecutive nights. It takes at least seven days before the yeast infection is cured, no matter which adminstration method is used. All of the applications in the specific package must be used.

- Femstat 3® (butoconazole nitrate)
- Gyne-Lotrimin® (clotrimazole)
- Monistat 7® (miconazole)
- Vagistat® (tioconazole)
- Oral Diflucan® (fluconazole), one 150 mg tablet taken by mouth, approved for yeast infections with just one dose

ANTIFUNGALS

The mechanism of action of an antifungal depends upon its subclass (see Tables 15-4 and 15-5). Imidazoles such as ketoconazole interfere with ergosterol synthesis, which alters the cell wall synthesis, increasing permeability. This allows outside material to enter the cell, and inside cell cytoplasm and nucleus to exit the fungal cell. This ultimately causes the collapse of the fungal cell and inhibits cell growth. Egrosterol is the vital, major component of the cell wall membranes of fungi and yeast.

Triazole antifungals such as ketoconazole fluconazole, itraconazole, and voriconazole are fungicidal agents that inhibit the fungal cell's ability to synthesize ergosterol. Voriconazole inhibits Cytochrome P 450 14-alpha lansosterol demethylation, while fluconazole inhibits CYP450 *and* is selective in blocking C-14 alpha-demethylation—both resulting in a blocking of the cell's biosynthesis of ergosterol. This allows increased permeability and leakage of the cell's inner contents. The fungal cell dies. Fluconazole inhibits fungal cytochrome P-450, the enzyme that is important in fungal ergosterol synthesis. This causes the cell walls to weaken and leak contents, and the fungal cell wall collapses upon itself.

Flucytosine competitively inhibits the cell for purine and pyrimadine. Biosynthesis of *purine* and *pyrimadine* nucleotides is an essential key process in all growing cells because these molecules are the direct precursors of DNA and RNA. Therefore, by blocking the cell's own production of purine and pyrimadine, production of DNA and RNA are also blocked. Flucytosine also metabloizes to 5-FU (5-flourouracil). 5-FU is then incorporated into the RNA of the fungal cell, where it blocks the synthesis of both DNA and RNA, leading to fungal cell death.

Amebicides/Antiprotozoal

Metronidazole is amebicidal, bactericidal, and trichomonicidal (see Table 15-6). Its selectivity for anaerobic bacteria is a result of the ability of these organisms to reduce metronidazole to its active form intracellularly, which then disrupts DNA's helical structure, thereby inhibiting bacterial nucleic acid synthesis. This eventually results in bacterial cell death. Metronidazole is equally effective against dividing and nondividing cells. The electron transport proteins necessary for this reaction are found only in

TABLE 15-4 Table of Antifungal Agents

Drug Name	Availability	UAD	Notes
flucytosine (Aancobon®)	250 and 500 mg capsules	50–150 mg/kg in four divided doses, Q 6 hrs	(1) Warning: Monitor with renally impaired patient. (2) Usually given with Amphotericin B to increase therapeutic action, but may also increase toxicity. (3) May cause bone marrow depression.
griseofulvin (Fulvicin®), griseofulvin ultramicrosize (Fulvicin PG® and Gris- Peg)	250 and 500 mg tabs 125, 165, 250, and 330 mg tablets	Depends upon wt and diagnosis. One tablet daily.	Photosensitivity and Lupus-like syndrome. PCN cross sensitivity may be possible.
amphotericin B, desoxycholate (Fungizone)®	Powder for injection: 50 mg vials	Depends upon wt and diagnosis. 0.25–1.5 mg/kg/day, 4 gram max daily dose, given 4–12 weeks	Only used for life threatening systemic fungal infections due to drug interactions and toxic effects. Monitor renal patients. May cause respiratory reactions and nephrotoxicity.
Amphotericin B, Lipid based (Amphotec®)	Powder for injection: 50 mg single dose vials	Depends upon wt and diagnosis 3–6 mg//kg/day	Reserved for life threatening systemic fungal infections. May cause: N/V/D, H/A, anxiety, asthma, convulsions, MI, anemia, leukemia, more.
ketoconazole (Nizoral)	200 mg tablets	200–400 mg QD	Side effects: H/A, dizziness. Toxic effects: May cause anaphylaxis on first dose, hepatoxicity. Gastric acidity. Contraindicated with triazolam (may cause CNS depression and psychomotor impairment, or suicidal tendencies). Contraindicated with antacids, which may reduce the effect of ketoconazole delay administration by 2hrs.
fluconazole (Difucan®)	50, 100, 150, and 200 mg tablets Powder for PO suspension: 10 mg/1 ml and 40 mg/1 ml when reconstituted Injectable: 2 mg/ml	200 mg day 1, then 100 mg QD For vaginal candidiasis one 150 mg tablet QD × 7 days	Double the daily dose on day 1 for a loading dose. Caution with renally or hepatically impaired patients. May cause hepatoxicity. Has 26% incidence of adverse reactions associated with 150 mg QD for vaginal candidiasis.

TABLE 15-4   Table of Antifungal Agents (*continued*)

Drug Name	Availability	UAD	Notes
Itraconazole (Sporanox)	100 mg tablet 10 mg/ml PO suspension Powder for injection: 10 mg/ml	100–200 mg QD Take capsules whole, with food to increase absorption.	Do not give to CHF patients, may increase CHF symptoms.
voriconazole (V-fend®)	50 and 200 mg tablets Powder for Injection: 200 mg SDV Take 1 hour before or 1 hour after meal/empty stomach	PO: 50–300 mg Q12 hr UAD 200 mg Q12 hr	Increase dosage of voriconazole if co-administered with phenytoin.
terbinafine (Lamsil®)	250 mg tablet	250 mg QD × 6 or 12 weeks	Do not give to patients with liver damage, transplants. May cause renal or hepatic function impairment and Stevens-Johnson Syndrome. Inhibits CYP450 enzyme. Caution in use with drugs that also interact with CYP450: MAOI's, TCA, SSRI's, beta blockers.

TABLE 15-5   Common Antifungal Agents

Drug	Uses	Basic Mechanism of Action
Amphotericin B	Systemic fungal infections	Alters permeabilization of cell membrane
Azoles such as clotrimazole, miconazole, fluconazole	Local candidiasis and dermatological infections. Systemic fungal infections	Inhibit sterol synthesis
Flucytosine	Serious fungal infections	Competes with uracil

anaerobic bacteria. Metronidazole's spectrum of activity includes protozoa and obligate anaerobes, including the following: *Bacteroides* group (including *B. fragilis*), *Fusobacterium*, *Veillonella*, the *Clostridium* group (including *C. difficile* and *C. perfringens*), *Eubacterium*, *Peptococcus*, and *Peptostreptococcus*. The protozoan coverage includes *Entamoeba histolytica*, *Giardia lamblia*, and *Trichomonas vaginalis*. It is not effective against the common aerobes, but it combats *Gardnerella* (*Haemophilus*) *vaginalis*.

Important Note: Patients receiving metronidazole and drinking alcoholic beverages may experience disulfiram-like side effects, which include nausea

TABLE 15-6　Common Antiprotozoal Agents

Drug	Uses	Mechanism of Action
imidazoles such as metronidazole, tinidazole	entamoeba, giardia, trichomonaiasis	Interferes with several metabolic pathways, disrupts DNA's helical structure
pyrimethamine	malaria, toxoplasmosis	Inhibits folic acid reduction
pentamidine	pneumocystis, trypanosoma rhodesiense/gambiense	Inhibits aerobic glycolysis
chloroquine, quinine	malaria	Inhibits nucleic acid synthesis

and vomiting, headache, flushing, and abdominal cramps. It is possible for these effects to last two to three weeks after the last dose of metronidazole has been taken. Disulfiram is the generic name for Antabuse® (and is used as an antialcoholic treatment. It also causes cramping with the slightest amount of alcohol, such as that in mouthwash.

Prions

In the last 20 years, researchers have noted that some degenerative disorders of the brain and spinal cord (CNS) are related to infectious particles that consist only of protein. These pathogenic proteinaceous particles are called prions (pree-ons). Prion induced diseases include Creutzfeldt-Jakob disease (in humans), bovine spongiform encephalopathy ("mad cow disease," in cattle), and scrapie (in sheep).

Prion diseases usually cause brain tissue to become perforated. While some prion diseases are genetic in origin, others are apparently due to transmission by ingesting infected tissue or unintended consequences of medical procedures or surgeries, such as organ or skin transplants.

There is no cure for this neurological disease. Since Creutzfeldt-Jakob disease affects the brain, the progressive symptoms include insomnia; depression; confusion; personality and behavioral changes; and problems with memory, coordination, and sight. The affected person rapidly develops dementia, involuntary and irregular jerking movements, and finally the loss of all mental and physical functions. The end result is coma and death. This usually takes about one year. The disease generally affects people between the ages of 50 and 75. Variant Creutzfeldt-Jakob affects younger people, from 18 to 53 years old. The symptoms present similarly to other brain disorders like Alzheimer's or Huntington's disease, making diagnosis difficult.

Gram Staining

The Gram stain is a method to identify and separate two main types of bacteria. This important staining technique is named after the Danish bacteriologist who originally devised it in 1844, Hans Christian Gram. It is almost always the first test performed for the identification of bacteria in cultured samples of the C&S

(Culture and Sensitivity) lab tests. The main stain of the Gram Stain method is crystal violet, but it is sometimes substituted with methylene blue. The microorganisms that retain the crystal violet–iodine complex appear purple/brown or blue under examination with a microscope. These microorganisms that stain blue or purple are commonly classified as Gram-positive (or Gram non-negative). Other bacteria not stained by crystal violet, that appear to stain red are referred to as Gram-negative. The theory of Gram staining is based on the ability of the bacteria cell wall to retain the violet dye during a solvent treatment. The cell walls of Gram-positive microorganisms have a higher peptidoglycan (a protein) and lower lipid found in the cell wall compared with the content of Gram-negative bacteria, and thus retain the dye.

The fairly simple procedure is outlined as follows:

1. Smear a sample of bacteria on a slide.

2. Soak the slide in a violet dye.

3. Treat it with iodine.

4. Rinse the slide with alcohol.

5. Counterstain with a pink dye called safranine.

Methods of Transmission

Pathogens can be transmitted by three main routes: ingestion, inhalation, and physical contact. Sexually transmitted diseases are transmitted via physical contact. The most common form of transmission of pathogens is via unwashed hands. Microorganisms can survive on inanimate objects such as desks, pencils, or door knobs for a very long time. However, the HIV virus is very unstable—living outside of the human host is not easy for this virus. Washing your hands is the number-one method of the prevention of transmission of pathogens. Aseptic technique is the number-one thing that you can do to prevent pathogens from entering the drug that you are working with, whether you are preparing an intravenous admixture or placing capsules into a prescription vial.

Anti-infectives

Anti-infectives is an umbrella name under which various types are then subclassified (see Table 15-7). Some anti-infectives treat bacteria only (antibacterials), while others treat viruses only (antivirals) or fungi only (antifungals). Other anti-infectives treat more than one type of pathogen. Another word for anti-infective is antimicrobial (against the growth of a microorganism or microbe).

Resistance

Resistance is the ability of a microorganism to live and grow despite the fact that an antiinfective or antimicrobial drug is present. Resistance is a result of genetic mutation during the replication or cell division process that causes

TABLE 15-7	Anti-infective/Antimicrobial
Antimicrobial, Anti-infective	General term to treat any pathogen or disease-causing microbe
Antibiotic or Antibacterial	Treat Bacteria penicillins, cephalosporins, macrolides, floroquinolones, lincosamides, oxalodinones, tetracyclines, aminoglycosides, vancomycin
Antifungal or Antimycotics	Treat Fungi sulfmethoxazole, imidazole, miconazole, clotrimazole, griseofulvin
Antiviral	Treat Viruses foscarnet, gancicovir, amantidine, ribavirin, rimantadine, zanamivir
Antiherpes, a specific antiviral	Treat Herpes acyclovir, famciclovir, valacyclovir
Antiprotozoal	Treat Protozoa pentamidine, atovaquone, eflornithine
Antimalarial, a specific antiprotozoal drug Anthelminitics, a specific antiprotozoal drug	Treat parasites that cause malaria Treat worm infestations pyrantel, praziquantel, and benzimidazoles
Amebicides	Treat amebic infections metronidazole, iodoquinol, and chloroquines
Antituberculosal drugs	Treat tuberculosis isoniazid, rifampin, rifabutin, ethambutol, pyrazinamide, streptomycin, rifapentine
Antiretroviral agents	Treat HIV (1) Protease Inhibitors: amprenavir, indinavir, nelfinavir, ritonavir, saquinavir (2) Nucleotide Analog Reverse Transcriptase Inhibitors: tenofovir (Viread®) (3) Nucleoside Reverse Transcriptase Inhibitors: didnaosine (ddi, Videx®), lamivudine (3TC, Epivir®), stavudine (d4T, Zerit®), zalcitabine (ddC, Hivid®), zidovudine (AZT, Retrovir®), abacavir (Ziagen®) (4) Nucleoside Analog Reverse Transcriptase Inhibitor Combinations: Combivir® = 3TC + AZT, Trizivir® = (abacavir + 3TC) (5) Nonnucleoside Reverse Transcriptase Inhibitors: nevirapine (Viramune®), delavirdine (Rescriptor®), efavirenz (Sustiva®)
Leprostatics	Treat Leprosy dapsone, clofazimine (Lamprene®)

the bacteria (or other pathogen) to evade or avoid the mechanism that a drug uses to destroy the pathogen. (A pathogen such as a bacteria, fungus, or virus becomes resistant to a drug; a person does not become resistant to a drug or a pathogen). The ability of the bacteria or pathogen to survive the mechanism of destruction of the antibiotic, or resistance, is promoted by certain factors, described as follows:

- Contributing to the problem is the fact that bacteria and other pathogens are remarkably resilient and can develop ways to evade drugs meant to kill or weaken them. The increasing use of antibiotics contributes to this action and is called *antibiotic resistance, antimicrobial resistance,* or *drug resistance.*

- Food-producing animals given antibiotic drugs for therapeutic, disease prevention, or production reasons can harbor microbes that become resistant to drugs used to treat human illness. This results in harder-to-treat human infections.

- According to the FDA[6], the following facts apply:

  - About 70 percent of nosocomal bacteria, which cause infections in hospitals, are resistant to at least one of the most commonly prescribed antibiotics.

  - Some organisms are resistant to all FDA approved antibiotics and can be treated only with experimental and potentially toxic drugs.

  - Research has shown that antibiotics are given to patients more often than recommended by federal guidelines.

    - Some patients ask their doctors for antibiotics for a cold, cough, or the flu, all of which are viral in etiology and do not respond to antibacterials.

    - Some patients who are prescribed antibiotics do not take the full dosing regimen, which contributes to resistance. Here nonresistant bacteria are killed first, as resistant bacteria multiply and become stronger. Soon the prescribed antibiotic will no longer work, and a stronger antibiotic will be needed. If the patient stops taking the prescribed drug this time, a stronger antibiotic may not be available next time.

    - Antibiotic resistance problems must be detected as soon as they emerge, and actions must be taken to contain them; otherwise, the world will be faced with previously treatable diseases that will once again become untreatable. It will be as it was in the days before antibiotics were first discovered and used. It is important to note that only four years after drug companies began mass-producing penicillin in 1943, pathogens began to appear that could resist it.

    - 1943—The first bug to battle penicillin was *Staphylococcus aureus,* causing pneumonia or toxic shock syndrome from wartime infected wounds.

- 1967—American military personnel in Southeast Asia were acquiring penicillin-resistant gonorrhea from prostitutes.
- 1967—*Streptococcus pneumoniae*, called pneumococcus, surfaced in a village in Papua New Guinea, causing PCN resistant pneumonia.
- 1979 to 1987—According to the CDC, only 0.02 percent of pneumococcus strains are penicillin-resistant.
- 1983—A hospital-acquired intestinal infection caused by the bacterium *Enterococcus faecium* appears.
- 1987—First Vancomycin resistant enterococci is reported in England and France.
- 1989—Vancomycin resistant enterococci is discovered in a New York hospital.
- 1994—A full 6.6 percent of pneumococcus strains are resistant.
- 2002—The CDC reports a Michigan patient with diabetes, vascular disease, and chronic kidney failure who developed the first *S. aureus* infection completely resistant to vancomycin.
- 2003—Epidemiologists report in the *New England Journal of Medicine* that 5 to 10 percent of hospital patients acquire an infection during their stay.
- 2003—Study in the *New England Journal of Medicine* found the incidence of sepsis (blood and tissue infections) almost tripled from 1979 to 2000.

Antibiotic resistance results when bacteria acquire genes conferring resistance in any of the following three ways:

- In spontaneous DNA mutation, bacterial DNA (genetic material) may mutate (change) spontaneously. Drug-resistant tuberculosis occurs this way.[6]
- In a type of microbial sex called transformation, one bacterium may take up DNA from another bacterium. Penicillin-resistant gonorrhea results from microbial sex, or transformation.[6]
- Most powerful is resistance acquired from a small circle of DNA (a plasmid) that can "hop" from one type of bacterium to another. A single plasmid can provide a great number of different resistances. In 1968, 12,500 people in Guatemala died in an epidemic of Shigella diarrhea because a pathogen harbored a plasmid carrying resistances to four antibiotics.[6]

Solutions to Resistance

1. Avoid using antibiotics unnecessarily. Use only when bacterial infections warrant use. Do not use for viral or fungal infections.

2. Complete antibacterial regimen; do not have leftover pills.

3. Use the most specific antibiotic possible, which is targeted or has a "narrow spectrum." This kills the offending bug without sparking resistance among other bacteria that live in the patient, as broader-spectrum drugs might do.

4. Use the common antibiotics first; if they work, do not go to second line defense drugs, if it is not necessary. Reserve them for the times when the first generation does not work.

5. Reduce hospital-transmitted infections by improving infection control in hospitals. This will kill the bugs before they get inside patients.

6. Invent new antibiotic drugs that have new mechanisms for killing microbes, and find new drugs that improve the action of existing antibiotics.

7. Invent vaccines against common microbial diseases to prevent initial infections.

8. Reduce the widespread use of antibiotics in animal feeds.

Pathogens exist in huge numbers. They have short generation times and the ability to swap genes, which makes them so flexible and dangerous. While there may be no ultimate cure for resistance, it can be slowed down.

Mechanisms of Action of Various Anti-infectives   Antibacterial agents will not work for colds, flu, or other infections caused by viruses (see Table 15-8). Attempting such treatment may lead to resistance. The mechanism of action of antibacterial agents varies, depending upon the specific agent being discussed. The first and second generation of PCNs work by interfering with the production of the cell membrane wall of the bacterial cell. They interfere with the protein synthesis, which gives integrity to the cell wall. Without the cell wall protein, the cell wall cannot grow; however, the bacteria cell contents (cytoplasm and nucleus) continues to grow. The contents inside of the bacterial cell have nowhere to go, so the cell wall bursts and the membrane collapses upon itself.

Penicillinase resistant penicillins contain beta-lactamase inhibitors, or are themselves able to destroy the beta-lactamase enzymes that certain bacteria produce to avoid destruction by antibacterials. Such bacteria are resistant to staph infections.

Side Effects of Most Anti-infectives   Pseudomembranous colitis has been reported as a result of antibacterial agents and may range in severity from mild to life-threatening. Therefore, it is important to consider this diagnosis in patients. Treatment with antibacterial agents alters the normal flora of the colon and may permit overgrowth of clostridia. Research studies show that a toxin produced by *Clostridium difficile* is one primary cause of "antibiotic-associated colitis."

Oral contraceptives (birth control pills) containing estrogen may not work properly with concomitant antibiotics, especially with tetracyclines. Unplanned pregnancies may occur. Women should use additional means of birth control while taking antibiotics.

TABLE 15-8   Comparison Overview of Various Anti-infectives

Anti-infective Classification	Common Side Effects	Toxic Effects	Drug, Food, and Herb Interactions	Special Notes Cross-Hypersensitivity
Antibacterials	(1) Rash (2) GI disturbances (4) N/V/D (5) Stomach pain (6) Vaginal itching or discharge	Anaphylactic Shock	(1) ↓ BCP's effect (2) Avoid taking with hot drinks, because the heat from the drink may stop the medicine from working, or make it work too fast. (3) Cross-hypersensitivity to a similar drug/classification.	(1) Patient must tell Doctor or Dentist before having surgery with a general anesthetic that he has been taking an AB. (2) ABs may cause incorrect results with some urine sugar tests used by pts with diabetes.
Penicillins (PCNs)	Most Common	Anaphylactic Shock	(1) Drugs that ↓ effect of PCNs: Chloramphenicol, EES, Sulfonamides and TCNs MTX. These drugs increase chance of side effects.	(1) Take PCNs with a full glass of water on an empty stomach (either 1 hour before or 2 hours after meals). (2) May be taken with food or milk to avoid GI upset. PCNs are high in sodium content.
Cephalosporins	(1) Most Common, plus: (2) Joint aches and pain	(1) Anaphylactic Shock for PCN Cross - Hypersensitive pts (2) Severe or bloody diarrhea and/or black, tarry stools (3) Chest pain (4) Chills, cough, fever (5) Painful or difficult urination (6) Shortness of breath (7) Sore throat, sores, ulcers, or white spots on lips or in mouth	(1) Drugs that ↑ chance of bleeding: Anticoagulants, dipyridamole sulfinpyrazone, ticarcillin, valproic acid, heparin, and thrombolytic agents Furosemide. These drugs may ↑ blood levels of cefuroxime. (2) Avoid acidic fruit juices/drinks (example, grapefruit juice or orange juice) within 1 hour of taking this medication.	(1) Hypersensitivity to PCN
Tetracyclines (TCNs)	(1) The common, plus: (2) May cause the teeth to become discolored and/or mottled.	(1) Photosensitivity, which may cause a skin rash, itching, redness, or other discoloration of the skin, or a severe	(1) Drugs that ↓ TCN effects: Antacids or calcium supplements Cholestyramine Iron and Magnesium containing medicine	(1) Patient must tell Doctor or Dentist before having surgery with a general anesthetic that he has been taking TCN.

TABLE 15-8   Comparison Overview of Various Anti-infectives (*continued*)

Anti-infective Classification	Common Side Effects	Toxic Effects	Drug, Food, and Herb Interactions	Special Notes Cross-Hypersensitivity
		sunburn and thinness of skin, which could lead to skin cancer. (2) Slows down the growth of bones, especially in children	(2) Antagonistic effect: PCNs decrease TCN effect.	(2) Do not give to children under 8 yrs old.
Macrolides	(1) The most common, plus: (2) Stomach upset or cramps (3) Sore mouth or tongue (4) Fever (5) Loss of appetite	(1) Rare: anaphylactic shock	(1) PCN may decrease the effect of EES. (2) May increase blood levels of theophyllin, warfarin, digoxin, dilantin, and tegretol.	(1) Abnormal liver tests or liver dysfunction can also occur with erythromycin.
Quinolones, aka fluoroquinolones	(1) Most common, plus: (2) Headache (3) Restlessness	(1) Rare: Status epilepticus and coma (2) Anaphylactic shock (3) Loss of consciousness (4) Photosensitivity	(1) Do not take with food or drink that has a lot of calcium, such as milk, yogurt, or cheese. (2) Caffeine or stimulant drugs will increase GABA inhibitory affect.	(1) Take with a full glass of water on an empty stomach (either 1 hour before or 2 hours after meals). (2) If food must be eaten, avoid calcium. (3) Avoid antacids— take 4 hrs before or after when taking Cipro, others 2 hrs before or after. (4) Also a GABA inhibitor: Do not give to pts with a pre-existing neurological problem or seizures.
Sulfur containing antibiotics, e.g. trimethoprim-sulfamethoxazole	(1) Most common, plus: (2) Tiredness (3) H/A (4) Dizziness	(1) Depression (2) Weakness (3) Eyes light sensitive (4) Yellow eyes/skin, dark urine (5) Abdominal pain (6) Ringing in the ears Rare: Gastrointestinal problems, damage to kidneys, and anemia	Some diuretics and anticoagulants	(1) Cross-hypersensitive to furosemide, BCPs, acetazolamide, thiazide diuretics, oral antidiabetics, antiglaucoma, phenazopyridine (e.g., Pyridium). Foods with preservatives or dyes. All above contain sulfur.

ANTIBACTERIALS

Penicillins   Penicillins are divided into four groups of varying spectrum of activity: Natural PCNs, penicillinase resistant PCNs, amino PCNs, and extended-spectrum PCNs (see Table 15-9). There are four generations of penicillins; each covers a broader spectrum of pathogens. To date, there is no penicillin that is taken orally, is penicilinase resistant, and has a broad spectrum. Therefore, in some cases combination therapy is required. There are more allergies to penicillins than to any other drug classification. The usual reaction is a rash or GI disturbance. The worst case is a severe allergy that is actually an anaphylactic shock; epinephrine must be administered within 5-20 minutes, or the person may die. The reaction to the PCN that is anaphylactic is a swelling in the airway passages such as the mouth, tongue, throat, nose/nasal tissue, or in the respiratory bronchi, bronchioles, or air sacs. When this happens, oxygen supply is cut off and death may result if the patient is not treated in time.

Cephalosporins are chemical cousins to penicillins (see Table 15-10). For this reason, any patient to have a known reaction to penicillin must be monitored if they are given a cephalosporin, as there is a 5 to 20 percent chance that they may also be allergic (cross sensitivity) to these anti-infectives. However, a better choice may be to give the PCN allergic patient macrolides such as erythromycin, tetracyclines, or quinalones. Much depends upon the culprit pathogen. C&S tests are employed for this purpose. Carbapenums are used for stronger bacteria, but only when PCN is not effective or safe due to the cross-sensitivity to penicillin and potential for the adverse reactions of pseudomembranous colitis, heart failure, arrhythmias, or kidney or hepatic failure.

Certain enzymes produced by some bacteria provide resistance to specific antibiotics. They are produced by both Gram-positive and Gram-negative bacteria and found on both chromosomes and plasmids. These enzymes inactivate the antibacterial activity of the drugs, which means the bacteria will survive while the drug is altered and rendered inactive; meanwhile, the patient's infection gets worse and the patient may die.

Scientists were challenged with making a drug that would be impervious to, or not affected by, these enzymes. The beta-lactamase enzymes are also called penicillinases. A drug or agent that destroys or interferes with the ability of the penicillinase or beta-lactamase is known as a beta-lactamase inhibitor.

Beta-lactamases work by hydrolysis of the beta-lactam ring of the basic penicillin structure, which adds a molecule of H_2O to the Carbon-Nitrogen bond, opening up the ring, thus making the penicillin drug ineffective. Most ESBLS (extended spectrum beta-lactamase enzymes) remain susceptible to beta-lactamase inhibitors.

MOA of Penicillin - PCN's   Penicillins work by binding to the proteins in the cell wall, inhibiting them from making the cell wall or to continue growth. The cytoplasm continues to grow and then bursts out of the cell along with the nucleus, destroying the bacteria cell.

Cephalosporins   Discovered in 1948, cephalosporins are grouped into "four generations" by their antimicrobial properties. Each newer generation of cephalosporins has significantly greater Gram-negative antimicrobial

TABLE 15-9   Four Groups of Penicillins

Groups of Penicillins	Examples	Spectrum	Specific Infections	Important Notes
Natural PCN's First Generation PCNs:	(1) pen G benzathine (Bicillin® IM (2) pen G Potassium IM, IV (3) pen G sodium IM, IV (4) pen V potassium (Pen V K®, V-Cillin K® Pen-Vee K®) PO	Gram + (1) Streptococci (2) Pneumococci	Ear, throat, gonorrhea, syphilis	While still used, it is the least effective.
Penicillinase-Resistant Penicillins	(1) cloxacillin (Tegopen®), PO (2) dicloxacillin (Dynapen®), PO (3) methocillin (Staphcillin®) IM, IV (4) nafcillin (UniPen® and Nafcil®), IM, IV (5) oxacillin (Prostaphlin®) PO, IM, IV	Staph (resistant) or *Staphylococcus aureus*	Endocarditis, abscesses, difficult to treat pneumonia	Are effective against PCNase producing organisms that are difficult to treat and do not respond to other 1st, 2nd, 3rd, and 4th generation PCNs.
Aminopenicillins: Second Generation PCNs	(1) ampicillin (Omnipen®), PO, IM, IV (2) amoxicillin (Amoxil®) PO (3) bacampicillin (Spectrobid®), PO	Gram + and Gram − organisms: (1) *E. coli*, (2) *Proteus Mirabilis* (3) *Haemophilus influenzae*	Ear, urinary, and respiratory tract infections	(1) Amoxicillin is well absorbed and causes less or no GI disturbance or diarrhea. (2) 2nd gen are not active against PCNase producing organisms.
Extended-Spectrum Penicillins Third Generation PCNs:	(1) carbenicillin (Geocillin®) (2) ticarcillin (Ticar®)	Broader than 2nd generation with Gram + and − coverage: (1) *Pseudomonas aeruginosa* (2) *Proteus vulgaris*	Difficult to Tx respiratory and urinary tract infections	(1) May require additional combination therapy with antibiotics such as aminoglycosides (2) Not resistant to PCNase.

TABLE 15-9 Four Groups of Penicillins (*continued*)

Groups of Penicillins	Examples	Spectrum	Specific Infections	Important Notes
Fourth Generation PCNs:	(1) mezlocillin (Mezlin®) IM, IV (2) piperacillin (Pipracil®) IM, IV	Broader than 3rd generation with Gram + and – coverage: (1) *Klebsiella pneumoniae* (2) *Bacterioides fragilis* (anaerobe) (3) *Pseudomonas aeruginosa* (4) *Proteus vulgaris*	Serious infections of skin, urinary and respiratory tract	(1) Made with Monosodium salts, reduce Na^+ intake. Great for CHF, HTN, or diabetic Patients. (2) To date require IV therapy (3) May require combination therapy

TABLE 15-10 Other Antibacterials Related to Penicillins

Classification	MOA	Examples	Spectrum and Specific Indications	Important Notes
Beta-Lactamase Inhibitors: clavulanic acid sulbactam tazobactam	Beta-lactamase inhibitors work by blocking the beta lactamase enzyme, inactivating it, thereby not allowing the molecule to hydrolyze the basic PCN beta–lactam ring.	(1) **calvulanic acid** + Amoxicillin (Augmentin®) (2) **calvulanic acid** + ticarcillin= (Timentin®) (3) **subactam** + ampicillin (Unasyn®) (4) **tazobactam** + piperacillin (Zosyn®)	Otitis media, and acute otitis media caused by PCNase or beta-lactamase producing bacteria: strains of *H. influenzae*, *Streptococcus pneumoniae*, *M. catarrhalis*, *Klebsiella pneumoniae*, *E. coli*, *Enterobacter* sp., *S. Aureus*, etc.	(1) Used for suspected resistance to PCNase (2) Mainly active against rapidly dividing bacteria
Carbapenums	Work similarly to PCNs: Interfere with the synthesis of cell wall by binding to penicillin protein binding targets.	(1) meropenem (Merrem®) IV (2) imipenem-cilastatin (Primaxin®) IM, IV (3) ertapenem (Invanz®) IM, IV	Complicated intra-abdominal infections due to clostridum, *E. coli*, *Peptostreptococcus*, *Bacterioides fragilis* (anaerobe), and bacterial meningitis due to *S. pneumonaiae*, *N. meningitides*, *H. Influenzae*	Structurally related to PCNs. Can be used against PCNase resistant PCN organisms.

TABLE 15-10   Other Antibacterials Related to Penicillins (*continued*)

Classification	MOA	Examples	Spectrum and Specific Indications	Important Notes
Monobactams	Work similarly to PCNs: Interfere with the synthesis of cell wall by binding specifically to protein 3 (PBP 3)	(1) aztreonam (Azactam®)	Skin, urinary, and respiratory tract, gynecological and intra-abdominal infections. Enterococcus and Gram (−) bacteria	(1) Structurally related to PCNs (2) Can be used against PCNase resistant PCN organisms. (3) Unlabeled use for PCNase resistant PCN gonorrhea as an alternative to spectinomycin.

properties than the preceding earlier generation. Likewise, older generations have a greater Gram-positive coverage than the newer generations. The first generation is the oldest. The frequency of dosing decreases with increasing generation(s), as does palatability.

MOA OF CEPHALOSPORINS

Cephalosporins are chemical cousins to penicillins, and, like them, bind to the proteins in the cell wall, inhibiting them from making the cell wall or growing (see Table 15-11). The cell wall collapses after the cell contents burst out. The body's natural defenses also continue to fight infection.

TABLE 15-11   The Cephalosporins

Drug	Route and adult dose
First Generation	
cefadroxil (Duricef®, Ultracef®)	PO; 500 mg–1 g qd-bid (max 2 g/day)
cefazolin sodium (Ancef®, Kefzol®)	IM; 250 mg–2 g tid (max 12 g/day)
cephalexin (Keflex®)	PO; 250-500 mg qid
Second Generation	
cefonicid sodium (Monocid®)	IM; 1 g qd (max 2 g/day)
cefaclor (Ceclor®)	PO; 250 g–500 mg tid
cefamanadole nafate	IM; 500 mg–1 g tid-qid (max 12 g/day)
cefprozil (Cefzil®)	PO; 250–500 mg qd-bid
cefuroxime sodium (Ceftin®, Kefurox®, Zinacef®)	PO; 250–500 mg bid
Third/Fourth Generations	
cefotaxime sodium (Claforan®)	IM; 1–2 g bid-tid (max 12 g/day)
cefdinir (Omnicef®)	PO; 300 mg bid
cefixime (Suprax®)	PO; 400 mg qd or 200 mg bid
cefepime (Maximpime®)	IM; 0.5–1 g bid (max 3 g/day)
ceftriaxone sodium (Rocephin®)	IM; 1–2 g qd-bid (max 4 g/day)

TABLE 15-12 The Tetracyclines

Drug	Route and adult dose
tetracycline hydrochloride (Achromycin®, Panmycin®, Sumycin®)	PO; 250–500 mg bid-qid (max 2 g/day)
demeclocycline hydrochloride (Declomycin®)	PO; 150–300 mg bid-qid (max 2.4 g/day)
doxycycline hyclate (Doryx®, Doxy®, Monodox®, Vibramycin®)	PO; 100 mg on day 1, then 100 mg qd (max 200 mg/day)
minocycline hydrochloride (Dynacin®, Minocin®, Vectrin®)	PO; 200 mg as one dose followed by 100 mg bid
oxytetracycline (Terramycin®)	PO; 250–500 mg bid-qid

Tetracyclines Tetracyclines are used as systemic agents for antiacne, antibacterial, antiprotozoals, and as an antirheumatic agent. In addition, some unusual uses are as a diuretic, for the syndrome of inappropriate antidiuretic hormone, and as an intrapleural sclerosing agent (see Table 15-12). Use of TCNs with diabetes, renal, or hepatic disease may make the condition worse. Use of this substance when it is outdated, warm, or changed in taste or appearance may cause *serious side effects*. TCN may be used to treat various systemic diseases such as Lyme disease, malaria, shigellosis, and pneumothorax.

MOA of TCNs Tetracyclines are bacteriostatic and therefore slow down the growth and reproduction of bacteria. TCNs enter the bacterial cell, utilizing energy, and bind to a subunit of the ribosome, which blocks the protein synthesis of the cell membrane wall. The growth of the cell slows down, and replication is hindered. The body's own immune system takes over to kill the bacteria.

Macrolides These antibacterial agents are active against aerobic and anaerobic Gram-positive cocci, with one exception of enterococci. They are also active against some Gram-negative anaerobes (see Table 15-13). Erythromycin has been used orally in combination with an oral aminoglycoside in order to prepare the bowel before GI tract surgery.

MOA of Macrolides Macrolides are mainly bacteriostatic. Erythromycin can be bacteriostatic at low doses and bacteriosical at high doses. They inhibit the protein synthesis that is dependent upon ribonucleic acid (RNA). To do this, they bind to the P site of the 50S ribosomal subunit of susceptible pathogens and may also inhibit the RNA dependent protein synthesis by dissociating the peptidyl t-RNA from ribosomes.

TABLE 15-13 The Macrolides

Drug	Route and adult dose
erythromycin (E-mycin®, Erythrocin®)	PO; 250–500 mg qid or 333 mg tid
azinthromycin (Zithromax®)	PO; 500 mg for one dose then 250 mg qd for 4 days
clarithromycin (Biaxin®)	PO; 250–500 mg bid
dirithromycin (Dynabac®)	PO; 500 mg qd

Aminoglycosides   Aminoglycosides are potent bactericidal antibiotics that act by creating fissures in the outer membrane of the bacterial cell. They are active against aerobic, gram-negative bacteria and act synergistically against certain gram-positive organisms. Because of the antibacterial activity, spectrum, and the toxic effects, they are usually reserved for the treatment of severe infections of the abdomen, urinary tract, endocarditis, and bacteremia. They are given IV only for systemic conditions and topically for ocular infections. Toxic effects include neprotoxicity and ototoxicity. Toxic effects result because the body does not metabolize aminoglycosides due to inhibition of metabolic enzymes, such as those in the cytochrome P450 system. Renal toxicity is most often documented and is usually reversible when treatment is stopped. Nephrotoxicity results from renal cortical cumulation causing tubular cell degeneration and sloughing. Ototoxicity is usually irreversible.

Recent studies in animals have shown that aminoglycoside accumulation in the ear is dose-dependent, but can reach a saturation point at low serum levels. Therefore, toxicity to the cochlear organ of Corti and inner ear is dose dependent.

Aminoglycosides are associated with post-antibiotic effect. It is believed that at higher doses leukocytes have enhanced phagocytosis and ability to kill after exposure to aminoglycosides for longer periods of time after the dose is given. The once standard dosing of gentamicin 80 mg q8–12hr no longer is recommended. Correct multiple daily dosing of aminoglycosides often requires pharmacokinetics expertise and close monitoring of drug serum levels and renal function and is both labor- and lab-intensive. It is now recommended that single daily dosing be used. This method of high concentrations of aminoglycosides and long dosing intervals of q 24–48 hours is called "pulse dosing."

MOA of Aminoglycosides   The agents act by binding to the 30S subunit of the ribosome of the pathogen, interrupting protein synthesis and causing the bacterium to die (bacteriocidal) (see Table 15-14).

Fluoroquinolones   Fluoroquinolones are used to treat severe infections such as infections of the bone and joint, skin, urinary tract, serious ear infections, bronchitis, pneumonia, tuberculosis, inflammation of the prostate,

TABLE 15-14 Various Aminoglycosides	
Drug	**Route**
gentamicin sulfate (Garamycin®, G-mycin®, Jenamicin®)	IM
amikacin sulfate (Amikin®)	IM
kanamycin (Kantrex®)	IM
neomycin sulfate (Mycifradin®)	IM
netilmicin sulfate (Netromycin®)	IM
paromomycin sulfate (Humatin®)	PO
streptomycin sulfate	IM
tobramycin sulfate (Nebcin®)	IM

TABLE 15-15   Select Fluoroquinolones

Drug	Route and adult dose
ciprofloxacin (Cipro®)	PO; 250–750 mg bid
levofloxacin (Levaquin®)	PO; 250–500 mg/qd
ofoxacin (Floxin®)	PO; 200–400 mg bid
sparfloxacin (Zagam®)	PO; 400 mg on day one, then 200 mg qd

some sexually transmitted diseases (STDs) or infections (STIs), and some infections that affect people with AIDS (see Table 15-15). Some fluoroquinolones may weaken the tendons in the shoulder, hand, or heel, making the tendons more likely to tear. Some people feel drowsy, dizzy, lightheaded, or less alert when taking quinolones. Special attention to patients with renal, hepatic, CNS disease and sclerotic cranial arteries, epilepsy, and other seizure disorders is called for.

MOA of Fluoroquinolones   Fluoroquinolones act by inhibiting gyrase, an important enzyme for replication of DNA, during bacterial replication. Since bacteria cannot reproduce, they die off (bacteriocidal).

Sulfonomides   Antibiotics containing sulfur are called sulfa drugs or sulfonomides (see Table 15-16). Sulfonamides are used to treat urinary tract infections, bronchitis, middle ear infection, and traveler's diarrhea. They are also used for the prevention and treatment of *Pneumocystis carinii* pneumonia (PCP).

MOA of Sulfonomides   Sulfonomides competitively inhibit both PABA, para aminobenzoic acid, and the enzymatic substrate dihydropteroate to block the essential synthesis of folic acid of the bacterial cell.

TABLE 15-16   The Sulfonomides

Drug	Route and adult dose	Remarks
Septra Bactrim®, Bactrim DS® Sulfamethoxazole + trimethoprim	400 mg/80 mg or 800/160 mg tablets, 1 tab q 12 hrs	Must have plenty of water to prevent crystallization in the kidneys. May require a loading dose.
Sulfadiazine (various mgs generics)	500 mg tablets, 2–4 gm in 3–6 divided doses	Must have plenty of water to prevent crystallization in the kidneys. May require a loading dose.
Gantanol® (sulfamethoxazole)	500 mg tablets, 4 tablets (2 g) initially, then 2 tablets (1 g) three times daily	Must have plenty of water to prevent crystallization in the kidneys. May require a loading dose.
Gantrisin® (sulfisoxazole)	500 mg tablets, 4–8 gm in 4–6 divided doses	Must have plenty of water to prevent crystallization in the kidneys. May require a loading dose.

Tuberculosis, or TB, is a disease caused by bacteria called *Mycobacterium tuberculosis* very common in Latin America, the Caribbean, Africa, Asia, Eastern Europe, and Russia. These bacteria attack any part of the body, but usually attack the lungs. Once a leading cause of death in the United States, it was eradicated for the most part when scientists in the 1940s first discovered the drugs to combat TB, which are still used today. However, due to complacency and a decrease of funding of TB programs, there has been a resurgence of the illness.

New programs and funding have helped to decrease its presence, but there were 16,000 cases of TB reported in 2000 in the United States. The bacteria are spread by breathing the air that infected people cough or sneeze into. Usually, it is spread among people in close proximity, who see each other on a day-to-day basis. It is found most commonly in homeless shelters, migrant farm camps, prisons, jails, and some nursing homes in the United States. TB can be active in a person whose immune system is weak and cannot fight it off, or it can be the latent type of TB that hibernates alive, but inactive, in the body (especially in a person with a strong immune system). Symptoms are different for the two states of TB.

In TB disease, TB bacteria are actively multiplying and attacking different parts of the body. Symptoms include weakness, weight loss, fever, no appetite, chills, and sweating at night. Other symptoms of TB disease depend on where in the body the bacteria are growing. If TB disease is in the lungs (pulmonary TB), the symptoms may include a bad cough, pain in the chest, and coughing up blood.

Those most at risk for developing the TB Disease are patients who have the following conditions:

- substance abuse
- diabetes mellitus
- silicosis
- cancer of the head or neck
- leukemia or Hodgkin's disease
- severe kidney disease
- low body weight
- certain medical treatments, such as corticosteroid treatment or organ transplants

TB infection is characterized by having dormant hibernating bacteria in the lungs or other parts of the body, sitting ready to attack when the immune system becomes weak. There are no symptoms. People don't feel sick, they can't spread TB to others, and they can develop TB disease later in life if they do not receive treatment for latent TB infection. Diagnosis is usually with a positive skin-test reaction.

Diagnosis of TB disease usually begins with a positive skin test. This will indicate presence of TB. Further diagnostic tests usually include a chest X-ray and sputum test (phlegm). Because the TB bacteria may be found somewhere besides the lungs, blood or urine may also be tested.

Treatment: The DOC is INH taken for at least six to nine months, and longer if the patient has a weakened immune system (see Table 15-17). A toxic effect is that hepatitis may result from the use of INH. The effect is age-related, with a higher incidence in 50–64-year-olds. The use of alcohol can be dangerous and can increase the chances of hepatitis. Precaution statements on the label placed by the pharmacy technician should include a warning that the patient is not to drink alcoholic beverages (wine, beer, and liquor) while taking INH.

Side effects should be reported immediately and include the following:

- no appetite
- nausea
- vomiting
- jaundice (yellowish skin or eyes)
- fever for three or more days
- abdominal pain
- tingling in the fingers and toes

INH is available as 100 mg or 300 mg tablets. Other anti-TB drugs can be given in conjunction. Some regimens are listed in Table 15-17.

TABLE 15-17   Antituberculosis Regimens

Regimen 1	Regimen 2	Regimen 3
Daily INH, rifampin, and pyazinamide for 8 weeks. Subsequent administration of INH and rifampin daily or 2-3 times weekly for 16 weeks. Ethambutol or streptomycin should be added to the initial regimen until sensitivity to INH and rifampin is demonstrated Additionally, a fourth drug is optional if the relative prevalence of isoniazid-resistant *Mycobacterium turberculosis* isolates are present.	Daily isoniazid, rifampin, pyrazinamide, and streptomycin or ethambutol for 2 weeks Subsequent administration of same drugs twice weekly for 6 weeks Subsequently twice weekly INH and rifampin for 16 more weeks.	Three times weekly with INH, rifampin, pyrazinamide, and ethambutol or streptomycin for 6 months.

Antituberculin Drugs	Usual Maximum Daily Dose	Max Twice Weekly Dose
Isonizaid, INH	300 mg	900 mg
rifampin	600 mg	600 mg
pyrazinamide	2 gram	50–70 mg/kg
streptomycin	1 gram (>60 yrs old 750 mg)	20–30 mg/kg
ethambutol	2.5 gram	50 mg/kg

Because resistance to TB can develop rapidly, both mycobacteriocidal or tubercularcidal and tubercularstatic drugs should be given—rifampin and isoniazid/ethambutol, respectively.

Antivirals

The common cold and influenza are discussed in Chapter 13, The Respiratory System. In this chapter, more time will be spent on antiretrovirals for HIV/AIDS (see previous text) and vaccinations for influenza. Some oral antivirals can be used to prevent the onset of influenza if used within 24 to 48 hours after the onset of signs and symptoms. Amantadine should be continued for 24 to 48 hours after the disappearance of signs and symptoms.

MOA OF ANTIVIRALS

Antivirals change or metabolize to acyclovir triphosphate, after which acyclovir inhibits the virus-specific DNA polymerase, an enzyme important for viral growth, multiplication, and replication. Replication is interrupted, and the viruses die (see Table 15-18).

TABLE 15-18 Common Antiviral Drugs		
Drug	**Uses**	**Mechanism of Action**
acyclovir, famciclovir, valaciclovir	Herpes viruses	Nucleoside analogue
ganciclovir	cytomegalovirus—group of herpetoviruses inhabit the salivary glands, causing immunocompromised individuals (AIDS and transplant pts) to have retinitis, pneumonia, colitis, and/or encephalitis.	Nucleoside analogue
ribavirin	RS virus respiratory syncytial, common cause of acute bronchitis in small children.	Nucleoside analogue
amantadine, rimantadine	Influenza A	Inhibit virus uncoating and assembly
Antiretrovirals - used specifically for HIV		
azidothymidine	HIV	Nucleoside analogue
nevirapin	HIV	Protease inhibitor

NOTE: Because viruses use the host cell's machinery, they are very difficult to target. The viruses can morph and elude the antiviral drug.

Vaccines

Vaccines were first used by the Chinese and were called "variolation." They were observed by Lady Mary Wortley Montagu, wife of the British Ambassador to Turkey, who brought them back to England in the early 1700s. In the late 1700s, Edward Jenner experienced variolation as a child, survived, and later became a doctor who was told by a milkmaid that she could not catch smallpox because she had had cowpox. In 1796, Jenner infected a boy with cowpox. After his recovery, Jenner injected the pus from a smallpox lesion directly under the boy's skin. The boy never contracted smallpox. Thus the first inoculation was born.

Today's immunizations are either "killed" (also known as inactivated) vaccines or "acellular" vaccines. The acellular are taken from the antigenic part of the disease-causing organism, such as the capsule or flagella. These types of vaccines cannot cause disease and therefore can be used in immunocompromised patients. These vaccines do require booster shots every few years.

Another type of vaccine, called "attenuated," is a live microorganism weakened by aging it or altering the viral growth conditions. These are the most successful vaccines, but they carry a high risk of mutation to virulent strains. Therefore, these types of vaccines should not be used in immunocompromised patients. However, they are lifelong and do not require booster shots. Some vaccines are made from toxins that are treated with aluminum salts to become a toxoid. Another type of vaccine that uses a part of the organism and stimulates a strong immune system response are called "subunit vaccines." Bacteria or yeast host cells have had the genome of the infectious agent inserted into them (see Table 15-19).

TABLE 15-19   Various Types of Vaccinations

Type of Vaccine	Examples	Notes
Inactivated or killed vaccines	Typhoid vaccine Salk poliomyelitis vaccine	Organism is killed using formalin
Acellular vaccines	*Haemophilus influenzae* B (HIB)	Requires booster shots
Attenuated vaccines	Measles, mumps, and rubella	Highest risk of mutation Lifelong immunization Does not require booster shots
Toxoid vaccines	Diphtheria Tetanus DPT immunization = diphtheria + tetanus + pertussis (whooping cough) vaccine	Administered with an "adjuvant"—an agent which increases the immune response
Biotechnology and genetic engineering techniques	Hepatitis B vaccine	Safe for immunocompromised patients
Use of an organism similar to a lethal organism	BCG vaccine against *Mycobacterium tuberculosis*	

The national goal to fully vaccinate 90 percent of two-year-old children depends on the support of private health care providers. The 12 diseases that the VFC program currently provides protection against are as follows:

- diphtheria
- *Haemophilus influenzae* type b
- hepatitis A
- hepatitis B
- measles
- mumps
- pertussis
- pneumococcal
- poliomyelitis
- rubella
- tetanus
- varicella

Various Infectious Disease States

In addition to varying in appearance, microorganisms vary in the specific disease(s) that they cause. Table 15-20 is a chart with some of the most common diseases and their origins:

Malaria is a disease transmitted by parasites found in the malaria infected mosquito. Four types of malaria are common in large areas of Central and South America, Haiti and the Dominican Republic, Africa, the Indian subcontinent, Southeast Asia, the Middle East, and Oceania. These areas of risk are said to have about one million deaths per year that are caused by malaria. The United States sees only a few cases each year. The four types are *Plasmodium falciparum* (plaz-MO-dee-um fal-SIP-a-rum), *P. vivax*, *P. ovale* (o-VOL-ley), and *P. malariae (ma-LER-ee-aa)*.

Malaria is diagnosed by a staining of the blood that allows the parasite to be seen in the blood. The following outlines the progression of malaria transmission:

1. When a noninfected mosquito bites an infected person, it ingests microscopic malaria parasites from the person's blood.

2. Human is bitten by the malaria-infected mosquito.

3. Malaria parasites must grow in the mosquito for a week or more before infection can be transmitted to another person.

4. After a week, the infected mosquito then bites another person. The parasites go from the mosquito's mouth into the person's blood.

5. The malaria parasites now travel to the person's liver, enter the liver's cells, grow, and multiply. During this time the person does not yet feel sick.

TABLE 15-20 Origin of Various Human Infectious Diseases

Bacterial in Origin	Viral in Origin	Fungal in Origin	Yeast in Origin	Parasitic in Origin
Anthrax	Childhood diseases: Mumps, Measles, German Measles, and Chicken Pox	Athlete's Foot (*Tinea pedis*)	Vaginal yeast infections (*Candida albicans*, Candidiasis, Moniliasis)	Malaria
Cholera	Common Cold	Cryptococcal meningitis	*Cryptococcus neoformans*—An opportunistic infection occurs as a complication of AIDS or immunosuppressant drugs	Pediculosis
Diphtheria	Hepatitis	Histoplasmosis (found in bird or bat droppings, when inhaled causes severe eye disease or blindness)		Scabies
Dysentery	HIV (progresses to AIDS)	Jock itch, thigh area (*Tinea cruris*, *Trichophyton rubrum*)	Jock itch inclusive of penis and scrotum (*Candida albicans*)	
Meningitis (bacterial, not all)	Influenza	Ringworm		
Pneumonia (bacterial, not all)	Meningitis (viral, not all)	Sporotrichosis caused by *Sporothrix schenckii* found in thorny plants such as roses, hay, sphagnum moss; causes boils and open lesions		
Rocky Mountain Spotted Fever (rickettsia/ rickettsii) Bacteria spread by ixodid (hard) tick	Polio	Thrush (caused by a yeast-like fungus)		
Scarlet Fever	Pneumonia (viral, not all)	Toxoplasmosis		

TABLE 15-20 Origin of Various Human Infectious Diseases (*continued*)				
Bacterial in Origin	Viral in Origin	Fungal in Origin	Yeast in Origin	Parasitic in Origin
Some STDs: Syphillis Gonorrhea Chlamydia	Rabies			
Tetanus Toxic Shock Syndrome	Shingles Small Pox			
Tuberculosis (TB)	Warts and genital warts			
Typhoid fever (*Salmonella typhi*) Whooping Cough	Yellow Fever (spread by mosquitos)			

6. Malaria parasites then leave the liver and enter red blood cells from as little as eight days up to several months. In the red blood cells, the parasites grow and multiply.

7. The many multiplied parasites over-crowd the red blood cell and burst the RBC open, freeing the parasites to attack other red blood cells. This destroys the RBCs.

8. In addition, toxins from the parasite are released into the blood, making the person feel sick. Symptoms of malaria begin eight days to four months after being bitten and include fever, flu-like illness, tiredness, shaking chills, muscle aches, H/A, and N/V/D. Due to the loss of red blood cells upon their bursting: anemia and jaundice (yellow coloring of the skin and eyes) may result. Infection with one type of malaria, *Plasmodium falciparum*, may cause kidney failure, seizures, mental confusion, coma, and death, if not promptly treated.

9. A noninfected mosquito bites this infected person while the malaria parasites are in his blood. It will ingest the tiny parasites and then transmit them to another human after a week or so, continuing the proliferation of this disease. The cycle continues.

Treatment: Malaria can be cured with prescription drugs (see Table 15-21). The type of drugs used and duration of the treatment depend upon which type of malaria is diagnosed, where the patient was infected, age of the patient, and the progression of the disease state at the start of treatment. Antimalarial drugs should be taken before, during, and after travel to high-risk malarial areas. One drug in particular is reserved for travelers who cannot take other drugs: Primaquine can cause an hemolysis, a bursting of the red blood cells. This occurs in G6PD deficient persons and can be fatal. Travelers *must* be tested for G6PD deficiency (glucose-6-phosphate dehydrogenase) and have a documented G6PD level in the normal range before primaquine is used.

The main focus is on prevention:

- Vaccinations are given four to six weeks before foreign travel, and a prescription for an antimalarial drug is prescribed. This antimalarial drug must be taken exactly on schedule without missing doses.

Note: Halofantrine (also called Halfan) is widely used overseas to treat malaria. The CDC does *not* recommend the use of Halfan because of serious heart-related side effects, including *deaths*.

- Prevent mosquito and other insect bites by using DEET insect repellent on exposed skin and flying insect spray in the room where you sleep.

- Protective clothing: Wear long pants and long-sleeved shirts, especially from dusk to dawn, the time when mosquitoes that spread malaria bite.

- Bed nets dipped in permethrin insecticide should be employed if screened or air-conditioned housing is not available.

TABLE 15-21 Antimalarial Drug Regimens			
Travel to Africa, South America, the Indian Subcontinent, Asia, and the South Pacific	Antimalaria Drug Regimen	Travel to Mexico, Haiti, Dominican Republic, and certain countries in Central America, the Middle East, and Eastern Europe as their antimalarial drug is available as an alternative	Antimalaria Drug Regimen
Antimalaria Drug Malarone™ a combination of Mepron® (atovaquone) 250 mg/proguanil 100 mg	(1) UAD = 1 adult tablet once a day, with food or milk, same time each day. (2) First dose of 1 to 2 days before travel to the malaria-risk area. (3) Last dose once a day for 7 days after leaving the malaria-risk area.	Antimalaria Drug chloroquine (Aralen™)	(1) UAD = 500 mg once a week same day of the week. Take on a full stomach to lessen the risk of nausea and stomach upset. (2) First dose of 1 week before arrival in the malaria-risk area. (3) Last dose 4 weeks after leaving the risk area.
doxycycline (a type of TCN, various trade names)	(1) UAD = 100 mg once a day, same time each day. (2) First dose 1 or 2 days before arrival in the malaria-risk area.	Hydroxychloroquine sulfate (Plaquenil™)	(1) UAD = 400 mg once a week on the same day of the week. Take on a full stomach to lessen nausea and stomach upset.

TABLE 15-21   Antimalarial Drug Regimens (*continued*)

Travel to Africa, South America, the Indian Subcontinent, Asia, and the South Pacific	Antimalaria Drug Regimen	Travel to Mexico, Haiti, Dominican Republic, and certain countries in Central America, the Middle East, and Eastern Europe as their antimalarial drug is available as an alternative	Antimalaria Drug Regimen
	(3) Last dose 4 weeks after leaving the risk area.		(2) First dose 1 week before arrival in the malaria-risk area. (3) Last dose 4 weeks after leaving the risk area.
Mefloquine (Lariam™)	(1) UAD = 250 mg tablet once a *week*, on a full stomach with a full glass of liquid. (2) First dose 1 week before arrival in the malaria-risk area. Once a week on same day of week thereafter (3) Last dose 4 weeks after leaving the risk area		
primaquine (in special circumstances)	(1) UAD = 2 tablets (30 mg base primaquine) once a day. (2) Take the first dose 1–2 days before travel and last dose 7 days after leaving high risk area.		

Cancer

According to the American Cancer Society (ACS), cancer is a group of diseases characterized by the uncontrolled growth and spread of abnormal cells. If the spread is not controlled, it can result in death. It is important to note that increased growth rate alone is not cancer. The cells must be mutated or abnormal to the extent that normal cell function is altered or impaired. As some cells stop functioning normally, they may no longer serve a useful or purposeful function, and then they become cancerous cells. Normal cells reproduce in a regulated and systematic manner. However, during injury, normal cells will speed up their cell division and reproduction until the injury is healed. In comparison, cancer cells divide in a haphazard process. The result is that they typically pile up into a nonstructured mass or tumor. When the cancer cells become invasive, they destroy the part of the body where they originated and then spread to other parts of the body. When the cancer spreads, or metastasizes, this can become life threatening. Benign growths, in contrast, stay localized and are not cancer, even though the cells may grow or divide fast.

The most common types of metastatic cancers are the following:

bladder	melanoma
breast	non-Hodgkin's lymphoma
colon and rectal	ovarian
endometrial	kidney (renal cell)
pancreatic	prostate
leukemia	lung
skin (nonmelanoma)	

Cancer is treated by many methods:

Surgery: is usually the first line of treatment for solid tumors. In early stage cancer, it may be sufficient to cure the patient by removing all cancerous cells. Benign growths may also be removed by surgery.

Radiation: may be used in conjunction with surgery and/or drug treatments. The goal of radiation is to kill the cancer cells by damaging them with direct high energy beams.

Chemotherapy: uses cytotoxic agents, a wide array of drugs, to kill cancer cells. Chemotherapy damages the dividing cancer cells and prevents their further reproduction.

Hormonal Treatments: prevent cancer cells from receiving signals necessary for continued growth and division.

Specific Inhibitors: this relatively new class of drugs works by targeting specific proteins and processes used by cancer cells. Inhibition of these proteins prevents cancer cell growth and division. Some of these are described as follows:

- **Antibodies** are used to target cancer cells, depriving the cancer cells of necessary signals or causing the direct death of the cells. They may also be called specific inhibitors.

- **Biological Response Modifiers** are naturally occurring, normal proteins that stimulate the body's own defenses against cancer.

- **Vaccines**—The purpose of cancer vaccines is to stimulate the body's defenses against cancer, increasing the response of the body against the cancer cells.

DRUGS USED TO TREAT CANCER

1. **Alkylating Antineoplastic Agents** cause the disruption of DNA function and cell death by three methods:
   - binds or latches alkyl groups to DNA bases, preventing DNA synthesis and RNS transcription from the affected DNA

- causes a formation of cross-bridges leading to two bases linked together, which prevents DNA from being separated for synthesis or transcription
- induction of mispairing of the nucleotides, leading to mutations of the cancer cell. Nucleotide "A" always pairs with "T," and "G" always pairs with "C." Alkylated G bases may erroneously pair with Ts. If this altered pairing is not corrected it may lead to a permanent mutation.

2. **Antimetabolites** inhibit ribonucleotide reductase and DNA polymerase to decrease DNA synthesis, which is primarily killing cells undergoing DNA synthesis (S-phase) and under certain conditions blocking the progression of cells from the G1 phase to the S-phase. Although the mechanism of action is not completely understood, it appears that antimetabolites act through the inhibition of DNA.

3. **Hormones** cause too much estrogen or testosterone to be made. Prostate cancer is caused by too much testosterone activating cell growth in the prostate. Breast cancer can be caused by too much estrogen activating cell growth in the breast. In some cancers, the opposite hormone, an androgen, is given to suppress the culprit hormone. For example, estrogen may be given to prostate cancer patients.

4. **Biological response modifiers (BRMs)** are substances found naturally in small amounts in the body that help to fight infections. BRMs produced in the laboratory in large amounts are then injected into the body to treat cancer. BRMs are sometimes combined with chemotherapy drugs to help to improve the effect of the cytotoxic agents. Unfortunately, BRMs are not effective against most cancers. The following are general types of BRMs: cytokines, monoclonal antibodies, tumor vaccines, and other immunotherapy.

   a. Cytokines: An example is Interferon, which travels into the cells that are affected by a virus or a cancer and stops the virus or cancer from multiplying. Interferon has been used to treat viral infections like hepatitis A, B, C, and D; CML; melanoma; and breast cancer.

      1. A special class of cytokines are called colony-stimulating factors (CSFs). These agents are used to stimulate the bone marrow to recover after chemotherapy.

   b. Monoclonal Antibodies are designed to cause the body to attack a cancerous tumor in the same way that it responds to a viral infection. The antibody can be attached to a medication used in chemotherapy and targeted against a specific cancer or tumor. When the antibody attacks the tumor, the chemotherapy medication is then delivered directly to the tumor.

   c. Tumor vaccines are mostly experimental medications made from bits of tumors. It is hoped and expected that, when the tumor vaccine is administered, the body will attack the tumor and keep it from growing.

   d. Other immunotherapy—A type of bacteria called bacillus Calmette-Guerin (BCG) is injected into the body to treat certain types of bladder and melanoma cancers by causing the body to mount a general immune response. This causes the body to attack the cancer.

The side effects of most BRMs are similar to flu symptoms. These symptoms include high fever, chills, fatigue, nausea, vomiting, and loss of appetite.

5. **Antibiotics**—Antitumor antibiotics work by binding with DNA in order to prevent RNA synthesis, thus preventing DNA replication, which also prevents cell growth. Antitumor antibiotics prevent the DNA from mending or reattaching itself together, thus causing cell death. Antibiotics treat a wide variety of cancers, including testicular cancer and leukemia. Usually administered IV, some examples of this category are Mitomycin-C and Doxorubicin.

6. **Plant (Vinca) Alkaloids** work by preventing cell division by binding to tubulin, which prevents the formation of mitotic spindles. During metaphase, mitotic spindles hold the two sets of DNA the cell needs to divide. Cancer cells cannot divide without mitotic spindles. These drugs are derived from plants and are used to treat cancers of the lung, breast, and testes. Plant alkaloids such as Vincristine and Vinblastine are administered intravenously (see Table 15-22).

TABLE 15-22 Anticancer Agents		
Trade/Generic Name	**Treats the Following Cancers or Disorders**	**Classification or Type of Anti-neoplastic Agents**
Hexalen® (altretamine)	Ovarian cancer	Antineoplastic agent, miscellaneous
Arimidex® (anastrozole)	Breast cancer in postmenopausal females	
Imuran® (azathioprine)	Prevent your body's rejection of solid organ transplants and autoimmune diseases	Immunosuppressant Agent
Casodex® (bicalutamide)	Prostate cancer	Androgen
Busulfex®; Myleran® (busulfan)	Primary brain cancers, leukemias, and bone marrow disorders	Alkylating Agent
Xeloda® (capecitabine)	Breast CA	Antimetabolite
Platinol®; Platinol®-AQ (cisplatin)	Variety of cancers	Alkylating Agent
Cytoxan®; Neosar® (cyclophosphamide)	Variety of cancers Prevent rejection after organ transplants Treats autoimmune diseases	Alkylating Agent
Cytosar-U® (cytarabine)	Variety of cancers	Antimetabolite
Adriamycin PFS®	Variety of cancers	Antibiotic
Adriamycin RDF®; Rubex® (doxorubicin)	In combination with other cytotoxic agents	

TABLE 15-22 Anticancer Agents (*continued*)

Trade/Generic Name	Treats the Following Cancers or Disorders	Classification or Type of Anti-neoplastic Agents
Ellence® (epirubicin)	Breast cancer	Anthracycline
Toposar®; VePesid® (etoposide)	Variety of cancers	Podophyllotoxin derivative
Propecia®; Proscar® (finasteride)	Symptoms of benign prostatic hypertrophy (BPH)	Antiandrogen
Adrucil®; Carac™ Efudex®; Fluoroplex® (Fluorouracil)	Variety of cancers	Antimetabolite
Mylotarg™ (gemtuzumab ozogamicin)	Acute myeloid leukemia (AML)	Natural source (plant) Derivative antineoplastic agent
Gleevec™ (imatinib)	Chronic myeloid leukemia (CML) Specific gastrointestinal cancer	Tyrosine kinase inhibitor
Femara® (letrozole)	Breast cancer in postmenopausal women	Aromatase inhibitor, antiestrogenic agent
Megace® (megestrol acetate)	Endometrial cancer Breast cancers that have spread Appetite stimulant	Progestin
Rheumatrex®; Trexall™ (methotrexate)	Variety of cancers Psoriasis Arthritis	Antimetabolite
Onxol™ Taxol® (paclitaxel)	Variety of cancers	Natural source (plant) Derivative antineoplastic agent
Rituxan® (rituximab)	Non-Hodgkin's lymphoma	Monoclonal antibody
Nolvadex® (tamoxifen)	Breast cancer in women and men Prevention of breast cancer in women at increased risk Induce ovulation	Miscellaneous antineoplastic agent
Trelstar™ Depot (triptorelin)	Prostate cancer	Luteinizing hormone-releasing hormone analog Antineoplastic agent
Oncovin®[DSC]; Vincasar PFS® (vincristine)	Variety of cancers	Natural source plant (vinca alkaloids) derivative Antineoplastic agent
Navelbine® (vinorelbine)	Variety of cancers	Natural source (plant) derivative Antineoplastic agent (vinca alkaloids)

SUMMARY

The immune system is the body's defense system and its function is to protect the body from foreign invaders that might otherwise destroy the body or parts of it. These foreign invaders, called pathogens, include parasites, bacteria, viruses, rickettsia, and fungi or yeast.

The body's defense mechanisms are broken down into either "nonspecific" or "specific." The nonspecific defense mechanisms include physical barriers, such as the skin, and the linings of the respiratory and digestive systems. They also include the lining of the spinal column, clotting factors in the blood, and normal flora (microorganisms) in the digestive tract that compete with invading pathogens so that they cannot penetrate host tissues. Pharmacotherapeutic treatment of pathogens includes antibacterials, anti-infectives, antifungals, etc., and is an important part of your knowledge base as a pharmacy technician.

Specific defense mechanisms are defined by specialized protein molecules and cells. These include antibodies and their complements, and lymphocytes (B-cells and T-cells). A detailed discussion of the body's defense mechanisms is covered in this chapter.

In addition to fighting foreign invaders, sometimes the immune system is called upon to help defend against the autoimmune process. A person with an autoimmune disease, such as Lupus Erythematosus of Rheumatoid Arthritis, has an immune system which mistakenly attacks itself. The end result of this defense is often inflammation. These autoimmune diseases are treated both pharmacologically and non-pharmacologically. The pharmacotherapeutics goal of treatment is to reduce inflammation, or to stop or suppress the inflammatory process.

CHAPTER REVIEW QUESTIONS

1. Immune system molecules are composed of two types of protein molecules called:
   a. antibodies and complement
   b. mucus and cilia
   c. thrombi and epitopes
   d. immunoglobins and enzymes

2. The Gram staining technique was developed in:
   a. 1850
   b. 1972
   c. 1844
   d. 1800

3. The main stain of the Gram stain method is crystal violet, but it is sometimes substituted with:
   a. candy apple red
   b. methylene blue
   c. the green method
   d. both b and c

4. What is the function of the complement?
   a. to help build up white blood cells
   b. to kill invading cells
   c. to build up red blood cells

d. to bind to protein

5. List three ways that pathogens can transmit.

6. _____ are bacteria connected, two side by side.
   a. coccus
   b. diplococcus
   c. streptococcus
   d. staphylococcus

7. List three types of animal pathogens.

8. In the progression of HIV to AIDS, at which stage do signs and symptoms begin to show?
   a. stage 1
   b. stage 2
   c. stage 3
   d. stage 4

9. Tetanus is an example of which type of vaccine?
   a. toxoid
   b. alleviated
   c. inactivated
   d. acellular

10. List five types of metastatic cancer.

Resources and References

1. Immune System Notes
   http://www.langara.bc.ca/biology/mario/Biol1215notes/biol1215chap43.html

2. The Lymphatic System by Sheryle Beaudry-RN,C
   http://www.biblerevelations.org/Health/lymphatic_system.htm

3. McLaughlin Centre, Institute of Population Health, University of Ottawa Health Systems Concerns: Immune System Fact Sheet
   http://www.emcom.ca/health/immune.shtml

4. Introduction to Microorganisms
   http://www.sparknotes.com/biology/microorganisms/intro/summary.html

5. Resistance U.S. Food and Drug Administration, "The Rise of Antibiotic-Resistant Infections" by Ricki Lewis, Ph.D. 1995
   http://www.fda.gov/fdac/features/795_antibio.html
   http://www.niaid.nih.gov/factsheets/antimicro.htm

6. About cells
   http://staff.jccc.net/pdecell/cells/basiccell.html#introduction

7. The Complement System
   http://users.rcn.com/jkimball.ma.ultranet/BiologyPages/C/Complement.html

8. Women's Health, What is Thrush?
   http://www.womenshealthlondon.org.uk/thrush/thrush.html

9. The Body: An AIDS and HIV Information Resource
   http://www.thebody.com/treat/protinh.html

10. AIDS Meds.com
    http://www.aidsmeds.com/NRTIs.htm

11. HIV and AIDS Treatments
    http://www.hivandhepatitis.com/hiv_and_aids/emtriva.html

12. About Fuzeon
    http://www.fuzeon.com/1000/1120.asp?nav=about&a=2

13. PharmPK Discussion—Pulse dosing of aminoglycosides
    http://www.boomer.org/pkin/PK96/PK1996093.html

14. Holland, Norman and Michael Patrick Adams. *Core Concepts in Pharmacology*. Upper Saddle River, NJ: Pearson Education, 2003.

15. Adams, Michael Patrick, Dianne L. Josephson, and Leland Norman Holland, Jr. *Pharmacology for Nurses—A Pathophysiologic Approach*. Upper Saddle River, NJ: Pearson Education, 2005.

Things to do

16. Watch video on Internet: HIVInfosource
    http://www.hivinfosource.org/animation.html

17. Watch Video on Internet on Fuzeon
    http://www.fuzeon.com/1000/1110.asp?nav=about&a=1

18. Look at various Fungi
    http://images.google.com/images?hl=en&lr=&ie=UTF-8&oe=UTF-8&q=Fungi&btnG=Google+Search

19. A Look at Various Protists (microoganisms)
    http://images.google.com/images?q=Protists&ie=UTF-8&oe=UTF-8&hl=en&btnG=Google+Search

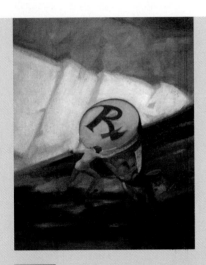

The Renal System

After completing this chapter, you should be able to:

- List, identify, and diagram the basic parts of the renal system, and the basic parts of the urinary system.

- Explain the function of the nephron, kidney, and bladder.

- List and define common diseases and conditions affecting the renal system, and the pharmaceutical treatment associated with each disease.

- Explain the mechanisms of each class of drugs in order to mitigate symptoms or destroy causes of the following renal system diseases or conditions: urinary incontinence, urinary tract infections, kidney stones, and edema.

- Describe and understand the concept of how homeostasis of water balance and electrolytes affects the body.

- List, define, and discuss the various diseases and conditions that are dependent upon and affected by a healthy renal system.

INTRODUCTION

The renal system is a fairly simple system with a few components; however, its condition has a grave impact on many parts of the body. Genitourinary tract infections, poor kidney filtration, and water imbalance can indicate or cause diabetes, high blood pressure, or dehydration. The proper functioning of the kidneys is essential to maintain life. The most commonly used drugs to treat diseases of the renal system are *antibacterial* and *diuretics*. The use of strong diuretics that help to remove excess water may lead to a loss of potassium, which may lead to muscle and heart problems. A delicate balance of electrolytes, kidney function, filtration, and waste removal must be maintained at all times during illnesses and while taking medications that affect or treat the urinary tract.

Anatomy and Physiology of the Renal System

The renal system, also called the urinary system, includes the two kidneys, two ureters, one bladder, and the urethra. The filtering system of the kidneys is composed of millions of microscopic kidney cells called *nephrons*. The waste that is created as food and drugs are continually metabolized is filtered through the nephrons of the kidneys and exits the kidneys as urine via the two tubes known as the ureters. The ureters lead the urine to the bladder where it is stored until it is released. The "kidney-bean" shaped kidneys, each about the size of one fist, are located in the backside (posterior) abdomen just above the waist. The right kidney is slightly lower than the left because of the location of the liver. The kidneys are protected by adipose tissue and the ribcage. (See Figure 16-1.)

The organs of the renal system are responsible for the following life-sustaining processes:

- filtering the "waste" known as urine from the blood
- removal of urine from the body
- maintenance of water balance

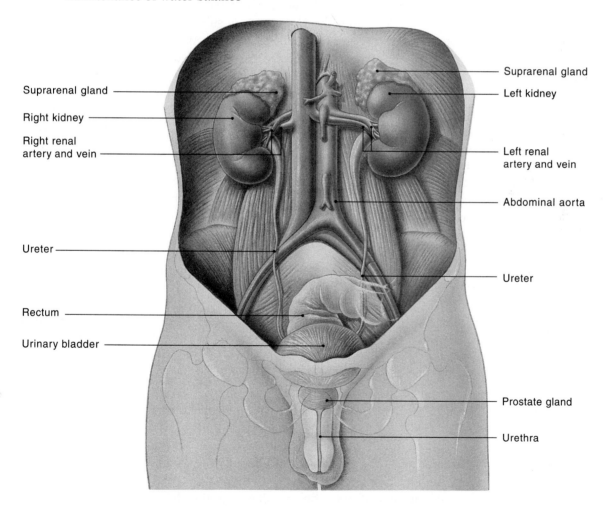

Figure 16-1 The renal system (*Holland, Norman; Adams, Michael Patrick,* Core Concepts in Pharmacology, *1st Edition, © 2003. Reprinted by permission of Pearson Education, Inc., Upper Saddle River, NJ*)

- maintenance of electrolyte balance
- maintenance of acid–base balance

The nephron is the main cell that filters the blood which enters the kidneys and is the smallest functional unit of the renal system (see Table 16-1). There are approximately one million nephrons in each kidney. Filtration, tubular reabsorption, and secretion are functions of the nephron that make urine. These functions enable blood to reabsorb the necessary substances, water, electrolytes, and nutrients. Approximately 25 percent of the blood in the body is being filtered by the kidneys at any one given moment, processing about 200 quarts of blood and clearing out about 2 quarts of waste. Waste includes excess fluid, minerals, toxic substances (urea), and substances that cannot be utilized by the body. When the nephrons, and therefore the kidneys, fail to filter, harmful toxic wastes build up in the body, which may flow back into the blood system, causing infection in the blood. The body may retain excess fluid, the blood pressure may rise, and the body may not make enough red blood cells.

The filter station of the kidney is inside of the nephron and is known as the glomerulus. It is housed and protected by Bowman's Capsule. The tubule that the filtrates flow into from the glomerulus is subdivided into three major parts: the proximal convoluted tubule, or PCT; the Loop of Henle, or LOH (also called the Loop of the Nephron); and the distal convoluted tubule, or DCT. The urine then flows into the collecting duct and finally out of the kidney via the ureters.

Tubular *reabsorption* is the act of transporting ions back into the blood. Facilitating the process of transportation and reabsorption is tubular secretion, in which ions, acids, and bases are secreted. Here again a *homeostasis* exists in the body, this time to ensure water balance, among other properties. Ions are reabsorbed when positively charged sodium, or Na^+, cations are exchanged for hydrogen cations; the Na^+ return to the blood, while the H^+ cations are secreted in the PCT and the DCT. The mineralcorticoid aldosterone, produced by the adrenal cortex, facilitates and regulates the secretion of K^+ cations in exchange for Na^+ cations in the DCT. When aldosterone gets into the aldosterone receptors of the distal tubule, it releases potassium ions into the tubule, and they are flushed out of the tubule along with urine into the collecting duct. Again, sodium ions are reabsorbed.

This process creates an *osmotic* gradient, in which more sodium ions are located in the blood, and less are in the urine or tubule. Remember that "wherever sodium goes, water follows." Therefore, water will follow the sodium ions in the blood, increasing the blood volume. This may exacerbate certain disease states such as CHF or HTN.

Tubular secretion serves to eliminate potassium ions, hydrogen ions, weak acids, and weak bases. The carbonic *anhydrase* system helps to accomplish this and to keep the blood at a proper pH. Carbonic anhydrase (CA) is an enzyme needed to convert carbon dioxide (CO_2) and water (H_2O) into carbonic acid, H_2CO_3, which then rapidly breaks down into hydrogen ions (H^+) and bicarbonate (HCO_3^-).

When the hydrogen ions are liberated, they become available to acidify urine. This allows the free bicarbonate (HCO_3^-) to be transported or reabsorbed back into the blood, reducing the acid by neutralizing the metabolic

TABLE 16-1 Actions of Selected Substances in the Nephron

Substance	Mechanism	Comments
Water	Reabsorbed by PCT and collecting ducts	Creates osmotic gradient
Sodium Ions (Na^+)	Reabsorbed by PCT and DCT	Cation exchange for H^+
Hydrogen ions (H^+)	Secreted by PCT and DCT	Na^+ and HCO_3^- go back into the blood. Acidifies urine to less than pH 7
Potassium ions (K^+)	Secreted by DCT	Cation exchange for Na^+, when aldosterone receptors are filled with aldosterone
Chloride ions (Cl^-)	Reabsorbed by Loop of Henle	Na ions follow Cl^- ions
Antidiuretic hormone	When released by pituitary, it opens the pores of the collecting ducts. Water immediately flows towards Na ions and is reabsorbed.	Causes urine to have a decreased amount of water

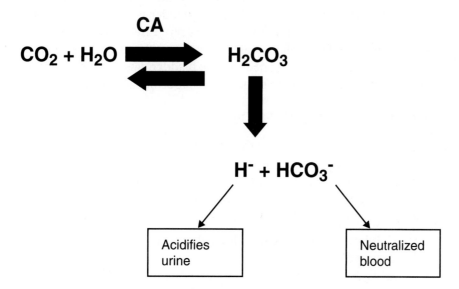

and toxic wastes, raising the blood pH to normal values. Metabolic acidosis can occur when CA is blocked.

The Bladder and Urine

The bladder capacity is about 350 to 550 cc of urine; about 150 cc brings a sensation of needing to void. Increased volume in the urinary bladder stretches its wall, which activates the micturition reflex. After voiding, it is normal to have about 50 cc left in the bladder.

Normal urine may vary in color from almost colorless to dark yellow. Some foods (beets and blackberries) and some drugs (anticoagulants) may color the urine red, while the urinary analgesic Pyridium turns the urine orange. Elavil, a tricyclic antidepressant, and vitamin B complex can turn the urine green or blue-green; and the anti-Parkinson drug, Levodopa, and iron compounds may turn the urine brown or black.

The urine specific gravity (similar to density) ranges between 1.006 and 1.03. (Higher numbers mean a higher concentration.) The value of specific gravity varies, depending on the time of day, amount of food and liquids consumed, and the amount of recent exercise.

The pH of urine is influenced by a number of factors. Generally, the normal pH range is from 4.6 to 8.0, with an average of 6.0. Usually, there is no detectable urine glucose, urine *ketones*, or urine protein. Glucose, ketones, and proteins can be detected in the urine in various disease states such as diabetes. There are usually no red blood cells, white blood cells, hemoglobin, or nitrites present in urine. While there may be a trace of urobilinogen in the urine, *bilirubin* is normally not detected in the urine.

Diseases of the Urinary System and Treatment

The urge to urinate varies upon how much liquid had been consumed and the capacity of the bladder. In most adults, the bladder can hold 10 to 20 ounces. The first signal occurs when the bladder is about one-half full. The average person should empty the bladder every three to six hours, to four to six times in a day. This will vary as a person ages. Usually, the first signal will subside if urination is postponed. As the bladder gets fuller and urination is further delayed, the signal or sensation will become stronger.

URINARY INCONTINENCE

Certain conditions may develop that may cause a person not to be able to hold one-half of the bladder's capacity or not hold the urine long enough before reaching a bathroom. This is known simply as incontinence, with three major types: stress, urge, and mixed. The majority of those who have incontinence are female. Causes are as follows:

- childbirth (supportive muscles and nerves of the urethra may be damaged)
- obesity
- hysterectomy (increases risk of incontinence by 30–40 percent)
- recurrent bladder infections
- medical illness (diabetes, lung disease, stroke)
- Certain drugs can relax the bladder too much and increase urinary flow (for example, first-generation, drowsy formula antihistamines (diphenhydramine and chlorpheniramine), some older antidepressants).

Treatment for incontinence will depend upon the cause. Pelvic muscle training exercises, called Kegel exercises, may prove to be beneficial in controlling the leakage of urine. Kegel exercises strengthen the muscles of the pelvic floor, thereby improving the urethral sphincter function. Various surgeries are available. Medications used to treat stress incontinence are aimed at increasing the contraction of the urethral sphincter muscle. Treatment with medications tends to be more successful in patients with mild to moderate stress incontinence. Alpha-adrenergic agonist drugs, such as pseudoephedrine, found in common over-the-counter decongestants, may be used to treat stress incontinence. They work by increasing the strength of the urethral sphincter, and improve symptoms in about 50 percent of patients. Additionally, the tricyclic antidepressant imipramine has similar properties, and so it may also be used to treat stress incontinence. Estrogen replacement therapy (ERT) can be used to decrease urinary frequency, urgency, and burning in postmenopausal women. ERT has also been shown to increase the tone and blood supply of the urethral sphincter muscles. However, the use of estrogen as a treatment for stress incontinence is controversial.

URINARY RETENTION

On the other hand, an inability to urinate is more common in men than in women. When about 1 cup (200–300 mL) of urine has collected in the bladder, a signal is sent via nerves in the spinal cord to the brain. The brain then returns a signal that starts contractions or spasms in the bladder wall. At this same moment, the internal sphincter muscle relaxes. These are the most likely causes of urinary retention:

- Blockage or obstruction of the urethra. The most common cause of blockage of the urethra in men is enlargement of the prostate, known as benign prostatic hypertrophy (often called BPH). The enlarged prostate gland presses against the urethra, blocking the outflow or passage of urine.
- Disruption or damage to the delicate and complex system of nerves that connects the urinary tract with the brain. Common causes include spinal cord injury, spinal cord tumor, herniated disk in the back, or an infection or blood clot that places pressure on the spinal cord.
- Inflammation and swelling caused by infections in the pelvic area, such as herpes, chlamydia, or PID, can interfere with nerves in the area, compressing the urethra. Infections of the spinal cord place pressure on the cord, leading to retention.
- Anesthetic effects during or post surgery is a relatively common and temporary cause.
- Other drugs that act to tighten the ureters, blocking the flow of urine, include ephedrine and pseudoephedrine found in nasal decongestants.

Treatment for urinary retention is the insertion of a Foley catheter and possibly antibiotics to avoid or treat urinary tract infection.

Other conditions that are associated with signs and symptoms of conditions of the renal system are as follows:

Anuria—a condition of no production of urine, and an excretion of less than 100 ml per day. If wastes are not eliminated from the body, the person may die from a toxemia or a septicemia.

Oliguria—a condition of scanty or decreased urine production, 100 to 400 ml/day

Dysuria—a condition that presents difficulty in urinating or painful urination

Hematuria—a condition of blood in the urine, possibly from an injured kidney or infection

Nephritis—an inflammation of the nephron, which causes the tissue of the whole kidney to become inflamed (as there are many nephrons). This inflammation is usually due to infection.

Pyuria—pus or bacteria in the urine

Uremia—a condition of urine in the blood. Nitrogenous waste is the byproduct of digestion of proteins and amino acids, and accumulates in the blood, when the filtration process is impaired. This may be due to glomerulonephritis.

URINARY TRACT INFECTIONS

Urinary tract infections are most common among women because the distance from the urethra to the anus is shorter. Keeping good hygiene, washing hands, wiping from the front to the back to avoid bringing *E. coli* to the front where the urethra is, wearing dry, cotton-crotch panties or cotton liners are some ways to avoid ascending urinary tract infections. Examples of some urinary tract infections are as follows:

Cystitis is an inflammation of the bladder that usually begins from the outer part of the body, since the cavity and urine are usually sterile. *E. coli* and *Staphylococcus* are the usual culprits. Following are some symptoms of cystitis: The urethra may begin to have a burning sensation along with burning upon urination; the bladder may feel full, and there may be the feeling of urgency and increased frequency to void.

Pyelonephritis is an inflammation of the kidney and upper urinary tract that is usually caused by a bacterial infection of the bladder or cystitis. The backflow of infected urine to the bladder goes up into the ureters and then into the kidney and nephrons. The following are causes of kidney infection: Pyelonephritis may result from urine that becomes stagnant due to an obstruction of urinary flow caused by a blockage, such as kidney stones, tumors, congenital deformities, or loss of bladder function from nerve disease. When no obstruction is present, the bacteria normally found in the feces, *Escherichia coli*, causes about 80 to 90 percent of acute bladder and kidney infections. Other bacteria that may cause both cystitis and pyelonephritis are *Klebsiella*, *Enterobacter*, *Proteus*, or *Pseudomonas*, *Mycoplasma*. Women who wear G-strings or thong underwear are more at risk of UTIs, as the thong can slip and bring *E. coli* from the rear to the front of the body. Sexual intercourse can bring bacteria present on the shaft of the man's penis in contact with the urethra of the female. Certain positions (non-missionary) can prevent this contact.

Symptoms of acute pyelonephritis include sudden onset of fever and chills, burning or frequent urination, aching pain on one or both sides of the lower back or abdomen, N/V/D, cloudy or bloody urine, tiredness, and fatigue. The flank pain may be extreme. The symptoms of chronic pyelonephritis include HTN, anemia, and protein and blood in the urine.

If left untreated, both cystitis and pyelonephritis can progress to a chronic condition that lasts for months or years and may lead to scarring and possible

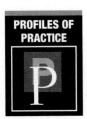

PROFILES OF PRACTICE

Incidence—approximately 30 percent of all women will experience a urinary tract infection in their lifetimes as compared with 3 percent of all males. The most common causes of UTI in the male are prostatic enlargement and diabetes. However, the incidence of UTI in men nears the incidence of UTI in women only in men over 60 years of age. There is evidence that circumcised male neonates have more UTIs than noncircumcised (intact) male neonates.

loss of kidney function. In a recent study, researchers found that a substance in cranberry juice keeps infection-causing bacteria from attaching to the walls of the urethra. Cranberry juice also makes the urine more acidic.[3]

The substances, "called condensed tannins, or proanthocyanidins, do this by stopping the bacteria from sticking to mucosal surfaces—the surfaces which line the bladder and bowel."[4] In addition to treatment to end the infection, treatment to manage the symptoms of burning and itching urethra can be performed with Pyridium (phenazopyridine). Treatment of a UTI with phenazopyridine should not exceed two days because there is a lack of evidence that the co-administration of phenazopyridine HCl and an antibacterial provides greater benefit than administration of the antibacterial alone after two days.

Treatment with an appropriate anti-infective is in order for UTIs. Table 16-2 outlines a few types of anti-infectives and the organisms that they treat.

TABLE 16-2 Anti-infectives for Urinary Tract Infections

Classification and approximate time discovered	Trade	Generic	Microorganism It Treats	Comments
Sulfonamides discovered by Gerhard Domagk in 1932	Bactrim®, Septra®	sulfamethoxazole/ trimethoprim SMX/TMP, SMZ/TMP	Bacteriocidal: *E.coli*, *Klebsiella*, *Staphylococcus*	(1) May cause resistance by over-use. (2) Causes crystallization in the kidneys. (3) Must ↑ fluid intake (4) Comparatively inexpensive
Penicillins discovered by Alexander Fleming in 1928, marketed by Howard Florey and Ernst Chain in 1941	(1) Veetids®, Pen Vee K®, (2) Omnipen® (3) Amoxil®	(1) Penicillin, penicillin V potassium (2) ampicillin (3) amoxicillin	Bacteriocidal: (1), (2), (3) *E. coli*, (2) *P. mirabilis*, *enterococci*, non-penicillinase producing *N. gonorrhoeae* (3) *E. coli, P. mirabilis*, or *E. faecalis*	Most commonly used
Aminoglycosides discovered in 1944 by Selman Waksman from a soil fungus, *Streptomyces griseus*	Nebcin® Garamycin®	tobramicin gentamycin	Complicated and recurrent UTIs caused by *P. aeruginosa*, Proteus spp (indole-positive and indole-negative), *E. coli*, *Klebsiella spp*, Enterobacter spp, Serratia spp, S. aureus, Providencia spp, and Citrobacter spp	(1) IV only, used in hospital setting for serious/life threatening upper UTI. (2) Sepsis (3) AR - Nephrotoxicity and ototoxicity (4) Must monitor blood level

TABLE 16-2 Anti-infectives for Urinary Tract Infections (*continued*)

Classification and approximate time discovered	Trade	Generic	Microorganism It Treats	Comments
Cephalosporins discovered in 1948 by E.P. Abraham, as a fungus in Sardinian sewage	Keflex®	cephalexin	UTIs and acute prostatitis, caused by *E. coli, P. mirabilis,* and *K. pneumoniae, Proteus mirabilis*	(1) Available in 1st, 2nd, 3rd, and 4th generations (2) Oral and injectable forms (3) Injectable forms are for serious UTIs (4) 5–15% of pts allergic to PCN have cross sensitivity
Tetracyclines Discovered in 1949[6] by Benjamin Duggar aureomycin	Sumycin®	tetracycline	Bacteriostatic: *Klebsiella, Staphylococcus*	(1) May cause teeth to become mottled yellow/gray/brown (2) Therefore, should not be given to children less than 8 yrs old or pregnant women (3) TCN causes bone deformities in children as it chelates with calcium (4) Causes photosensitivity (5) Take 1 hr before or 2 hrs after taking antacids, milk, or iron, which decrease absorption of TCN.
Combination PCN and Clavulanic acid	Augmentin®	amoxicillin/clavulanate (clavulanic acid)	*E. coli,* group D *streptococcus*	

TABLE 16-2	Anti-infectives for Urinary Tract Infections (*continued*)			
Classification and approximate time discovered	Trade	Generic	Microorganism It Treats	Comments
Quinolones

Discovered serendipitously at Sterling-Winthrop in the 1950s. Nalidixic introduced in 1962 | Cipro® | Ciprofloxacin | *E. coli*, *Pseudomonas*, *mycoplasma* | Newest class of ABs. Has extended spectrum, high cost. Do not take with milk or dairy products—blocks absorption |

A bit of history—an accidental toxic preparation of elixir sulfanilamide, containing ethylene glycol, a solvent, killed over 100 people, mostly children, and led to the passage of the 1938 Food, Drug, and Cosmetic Act.

KIDNEY STONES

Another word for kidney stones is urolithiais. This is a common and painful urinary tract disorder in which solid mineral deposits accumulate in the urinary tract, possibly obstructing urinary flow. It may also lead to UTIs. The pain of "passing" such a blockage or stone is considered excruciating. The mineral masses develop when waste is not dissolved completely in the urine. The microscopic, hard crystals that remain in the kidney are also called *calculi*, pleural for calculus. The most common waste substances that are found in the stones are calcium, oxalate, phosphate, and uric acid.

It is equally possible to have normal amounts of such solids in the urine, where the body does not produce enough water in the urine to dissolve them, as it is to have abnormally accumulated solids in the normal amount of urine, which is not enough to dissolve them. In addition, there may be a deficiency of certain chemicals that are normally present in the urine that help break down and dissolve the waste solids. These "helpers" are citrate, magnesium, and pyrophosphate. If calculi obstruct one of the ureters, they can cause the urinary tract to go into spasm, causing great pain. Large calculi can cause organ damage and even renal failure.

The male caucasian between 30 and 60 years old is the most prone to urolithiasis. Diet plays an important role, as does living in a warm climate near large bodies of water. Diets high in animal protein (meats) that increase uric acid levels in the body can lead to gout and kidney stones. The routine intake of rhubarb, spinach, pepper, cocoa, nuts, or tea can result in excess oxalate in people who have a high level of risk. Dehydration and diarrhea contribute to a deficiency of water available to dissolve the stones. The following chemical imbalances can contribute to the formation of kidney stones: (1) hypercalcemia: excess amounts of calcium; (2) hypernatremia: high levels of sodium; (3) hypocitraturia: low levels of waste-dissolving citrate.

People who also are diagnosed with hyperthyroidism or hyperparathyroidism are at a higher risk, because both conditions allow excess calcium to combine with phosphate or oxalate in the kidneys, resulting in the formation of calculi.

Treatment of urolithiasis is *pallative* with pain management, and preventative with diet, and consists of taking specific mineral and vitamin supplements and increasing fluid intake. Most calculi measure less than $1/4$ inch (4 mm) and spontaneously pass in the urine without need for any treatment. Stones that measure 5 to 7 millimeters can be passed without intervention about half of the time. When a stone exceeds 7 millimeters in diameter, however, some form of intervention is usually required.

Pain management depends upon the degree of pain. Oral analgesics for mild to moderate pain include diclofenac, acetaminophen with codeine, and propoxyphene HCL. Severe pain requires injections of narcotics such as morphine and Demerol. Since the narcotics can cause N/V/D, it is important not to let the patient get dehydrated if this side effect should occur.

Collecting and analyzing the stones can lead the physician to make specific diet and medication recommendations, such as staying away from high purine content foods (meats); taking the anti-gout drug allopurinol; increasing fluid intake, and using calcium citrate, magnesium, and cholestyramine to reduce oxalate levels. Taking potassium citrate supplement or citrus fruit such as lemons increases citrate levels to help dissolve waste. Taking a vitamin B6 supplement helps fight high levels of oxylate. Taking thiazide diuretics possibly reduces high urinary calcium levels. It should be noted that the patient should avoid decreasing calcium in the diet, as this may cause the formation of calcium calculi. Avoiding high fat diets is important. (See Chapter 8, The Musculoskeletal System, for a discussion of gout.)

EDEMA AND HYPERTENSION

Kidney damage can lead to hypertension, and HTN can lead to kidney failure. Consistently elevated blood pressure levels can lead to damage of the arteries in the body, the kidney arteries in particular. These arteries become thickened and narrowed with prolonged high blood pressure. When this happens, less blood gets to the kidneys, and that means a reduced oxygen supply to the kidneys. Kidney failure can lead to an excess of fluid in the body, called peripheral edema in the limbs, and ascites in the visceral or trunk of the body. This excess fluid leads to an excessive workload on the heart, which then raises blood pressure, and may lead to heart failure or myocardial infarction. Diuretics play an important role in reducing high blood pressure by reducing the volume of fluid in the body and in the blood. Certain disease states also require less blood volume, such as CHF (or congestive heart failure). (See Chapter 14, the Circulatory System.)

DIABETES MELLITUS AND THE KIDNEYS

Diabetes affects many organs of the body, including the eyes, kidneys, and blood vessels. Kidney damage, bladder problems, and UTIs are long-term complications affecting people with diabetes, and these complications can lead to renal failure. Diabetic kidney disease is also called diabetic nephropathy. End stage renal disease (ESRD), or nephropathy, requires the diabetic either to have dialysis, in which the blood is filtered through a machine several times a week to remove wastes such as urea, or to have a kidney transplant. Native Americans and African Americans are two racial groups who are at higher risk for developing ESRD than diabetics. Early warning signs of having protein in the urine can lead to early diagnosis and treatment. Familial ESRD, diet, high blood pressure, high blood glucose, and noncompliance are a few factors that lead to diabetic nephropathy.

Healthy Goals for the Diabetic:

- Blood sugar less than 126 mg/dl
- Hemoglobin A1C less than 7
- Blood pressure less than 130/80 mmHG
- Protein in urine (microalbumin)—have a professional check for this yearly, should be none

When the glucose in the blood becomes high, the body tries to get rid of the excess sugar by trying to eliminate it in urine. This leads to dehydration and is the reason why diabetics are usually excessively thirsty and urinate frequently. The effects of dehydration depend upon the degree of loss of water:

- Two percent body weight loss reduces performance significantly.
- Five percent body weight loss causes heat exhaustion.
- Seven to ten percent body weight loss results in heat stroke or death.

Diuretics

Diuretics increase urine output in various ways (see Table 16-3). Most diuretics inhibit or block sodium absorption to the blood system in the nephron, thus promoting the secretion of sodium. Recall that wherever sodium goes, water follows. Chloride also follows the sodium. The diuresis increases as sodium increases in the tubule. There are basically five main types of diuretics:

- osmotic diuretics
- loop diuretics
- thiazide and thiazide-like diuretics
- potassium sparing diuretics
- carbonic anhydrase inhibitors

If too much diuretic is taken, excessive water loss leads to dehydration and electrolyte loss, such as potassium loss. The K^+ ion is instrumental in muscular function. The heart is surrounded by a muscle called the myocardium. Without potassium, the heart fails to beat properly. Hypokalemia can lead to heart failure because it leads to dysrhythmias, or lethal arrhythmias, when the heart is beating out of normal sequence. Diuretics vary in the location of the action of the drug, or site of action.

Normally, about 98 percent of all that is filtered in the glomerulus is reabsorbed into the blood system. Osmotic diuretic compounds are filtered by

TABLE 16-3 Diuretics

Drug	Route and Adult Dose	Class
furosemide (Lasix®)	PO; 20–80 mg qd (max 600 mg/day)	Loop diuretic
bumetanide (Bumex®)	PO; 0.5–2 mg qd (max 10 mg/day)	Loop diuretic
ethacrynic acid (Edecrin®)	PO; 50–100 mg qd-bid (max 400 mg/day)	Loop diuretic
torsemide (Demadex®)	PO; 4–20 mg qd	Loop diuretic
hydrochlorothiazide (Hydrodiuril®, HCTZ®)	PO; 12.5–100 mg qd-tid	Thiazide/thiazide-like diuretic
bendroflumethiazide (Naturetin®)	PO; 2.5–20 mg qd-bid	Thiazide/thiazide-like diuretic
benzthiazide (Aquatag®, Exna®, Hydrex®)	PO; 25–200 mg qd or qod	Thiazide/thiazide-like diuretic
chlorothiazide (Diuril®)	PO; 250–500 mg qd	Thiazide/thiazide-like diuretic
hydroflumethiazide (Diucardin®, Saluron®)	PO; 25–100 mg qd-bid	Thiazide/thiazide-like diuretic
indapamide (Lozol®)	PO; 2.5–5 mg qd	Thiazide/thiazide-like diuretic
methylclothiazide (Aquatensin®, Enduron®)	PO; 2.5–10 mg qd	Thiazide/thiazide-like diuretic
metolazone (Zaroxolyn®, Mykrox®)	PO; 5–20 mg qd.	Thiazide/thiazide-like diuretic
polythiazide (Renese®)	PO; 1–4 mg qd	Thiazide/thiazide-like diuretic
quinethazone (Hydromox®)	PO; 50–100 mg qd	Thiazide/thiazide-like diuretic
trichlormethazide (Metahydrin®, Naqua®, Niazide®, Diurese®)	PO; 1–4 mg qd-bid	Thiazide/thiazide-like diuretic

glomerulus, but not reabsorbed into the blood system via the renal tubules. They work by creating an osmotic gradient. These diuretics are very potent and create no major change in sodium balance or acid–base balance. They must be given IV, and therefore in the hospital. They are usually used to treat glaucoma, edema, HTN, CHF, and uremia.

There is an abundance of sodium in the Loop of Henle (also called the Loop of the Nephron). Diuretics that work by blocking the sodium in the Loop of Henle are called loop diuretics. They are also known as organic acid or organic loop diuretics. These are very potent diuretics. Of the Loop Diuretics, Lasix (furosemide) is the most commonly prescribed.

The thiazide and thiazide-like diuretics are the most prescribed class. These act on the distal tubule to inhibit sodium reabsorption and increase water loss. Not as potent as the Loop Diuretics, thiazide diuretics are mainly used for mild to moderate HTN. Hydrodiuril®, known as hydrochlorothiazide or HCTZ, is a common thiazide diuretic.

Potassium sparing diuretics work by inhibiting K^+ secretion in the distal convoluted tubule (DCT) by inhibition of aldosterone in the aldosterone receptors of the DCT. No K^+ supplementation is required; in fact, taking K+ supplements may lead to toxic hyperkalemia. Very little diuretic effect is created. Since potassium is retained, these diuretics are usually used with thiazide or loop diuretics to prevent hypokalemia. Aldactone® (spironolactone) is a very common K+ sparing diuretic.

Carbonic anhydrase inhibitors work by inhibiting the enzyme carbonic anhydrase so that very little H^+ and HCO_3^- is produced. When this happens, there is no H^+ available for exchange with sodium ions. Consequently, Na^+ ions are excreted into the urine, and water follows. Because carbonic anhydrase is inhibited, no HCO_3^- is produced to buffer the blood, which can result in c. metabolic acidosis, a life-threatening condition. CA inhibitors are used to treat open angle glaucoma, acute mountain sickness. Currently there is only one CA Inhibitor, Diamox® (acetazolamide).

Because of the rapid and excessive water loss, potassium supplements are required with all diuretics except the osmotic and potassium sparing diuretics. Thiazide, thiazide-like, and loop diuretics and carbonic anhydrase inhibitors will cause hypokalemia.

SUMMARY

The renal system is a fairly simple system, yet its proper functioning is essential to maintaining life. The renal system, also called the urinary system, consists of two kidneys, two ureters, the bladder, and the urethra. The functions of the renal system are to filter waste (urine) from the blood and remove it from the body, to maintain water and electrolyte balance, and to maintain acid-base balance. Any dysfunction of the renal system can have grave impact on many parts of the body. Kidney damage can lead to hypertension, muscle problems, and serious cardiac disorders.

Common diseases of the renal system include urinary retention or urinary incontinence, kidney stones, and urinary tract infections. Approximately 30 percent of all women will experience a urinary tract infection in their lifetimes.

The two most commonly used drugs to treat diseases of the renal system are antibacterials and diuretics. This chapter contains a thorough discussion of the importance of the renal system in maintaining homeostasis, the incidence of diseases of the urinary tract, and the available drug therapies used to treat these conditions.

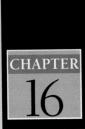

CHAPTER REVIEW QUESTIONS

1. Fill in the blanks to correctly label and identify
   the parts of the (a) kidney, (b) renal system,
   and (c) nephron:
   a. Kidney
   b. Renal system
   c. Nephron

a. Kidney

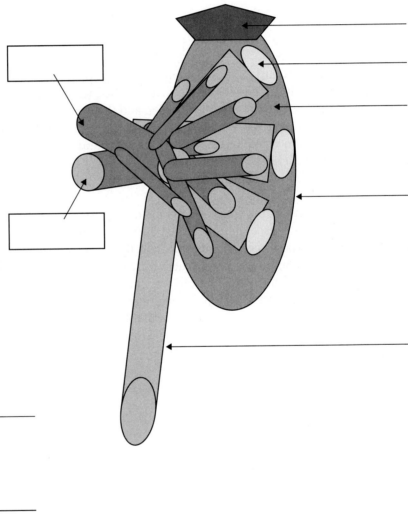

b. Renal system

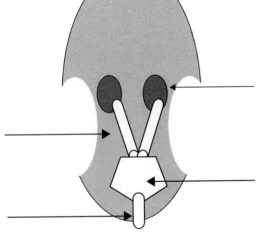

c. Nephron

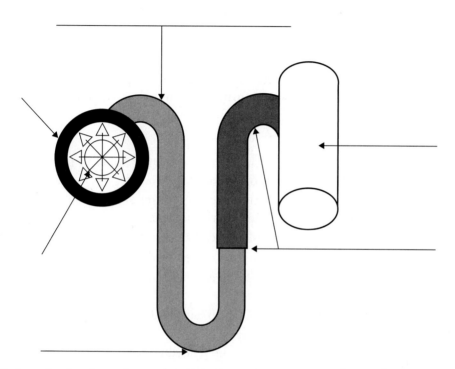

2. List the five basic functions of the kidneys.

3. Explain the function of the kidneys, nephrons, and bladder in detail.

4. Match the disease state with the causative factor and the correct pharmaceutical treatment.

   Diseases: (may be used more than once)
   urinary tract infection
   complicated and recurrent upper UTIs
   acute prostatitis

   Causative Factors: (may be used more than once)
   a. *E. faecalis*
   b. group D streptococcus
   c. *Klebsiella*
   d. *P. aeruginosa*
   e. *P. mirabilis*

   f. *Pseudomonas*
   g. *Staphylococcus*
   h. Rx Treatment
   i. Aminoglycosides: tobramicin, gentamycin
   j. Amoxicillin—a specific penicillin
   k. Augmentin®
   l. Cephalosporins: cefazolin
   m. Quinolones: ciprofloxacin
   n. Sulfonamides: sulfamethoxazole/trimethoprim
   o. Tetracyclines

5. Which of the following are symptoms of urinary tract infections?
   a. sudden onset of fever and chills, tiredness, and fatigue
   b. burning or frequent urination

c. aching pain on one or both sides of the lower back or abdomen

d. N/V/D

e. cloudy or bloody urine

f. all of the above

g. none of the above

6. Treatment of a UTI with phenazopyridine should not exceed two days because there is evidence that the co-administration of phenazopyridine HCl and an antibacterial counteract with each other.

a. true

b. false

7. Which applies to kidney stones?

a. Take thiazide diuretics to reduce high urinary calcium levels.

b. Take a vitamin B6 supplement to help fight high levels of potassium.

c. Increase fluid intake and use calcium citrate, magnesium, and cholestyramine to reduce oxalate levels.

d. All of the above

e. A and C only

f. A and B only

g. None of the above

8. Diabetics are dehydrated, have excessive thirst, and urinate frequently because the body is trying to eliminate high blood sugar levels via urination after blood is filtered in the kidneys.

a. true

b. false

9. High blood pressure is exacerbated by high sodium in the blood. Diuretics do which of the following?

a. inhibit or block sodium reabsorption

b. promote secretion of sodium

c. drag water with the sodium out of the tubule

d. flush toxins out of the tubule into urine

e. increase urine output, decrease blood volume and pressure

f. all of the above

g. none of the above

h. only a and d

10. Urinary incontinence is the inability to hold one's urine long enough to reach the bathroom.

a. true

b. false

11. Which of the following apply to urinary incontinence?

a. may be caused by relaxed supportive muscles and nerves near the urethra

b. may be caused by recurrent bladder infections

c. may be caused by diabetes, stroke

d. may be caused by diphenhydramine, treated with pseudoephedrine

e. may be treated with TCA or estrogen

f. may be caused by pseudoephedrine, treated with diphenhydramine

g. all of the above, except f

h. all of the above, except c

12. Urinary incontinence can be treated with pseudoephedrine to increase the strength of the urethral sphincter.

a. true

b. false

13. What happens when interruption of homeostasis of water balance and electrolytes occurs?

a. The body may retain water when Na^+ is reabsorbed, leading to high blood pressure, which may lead to hypertensive crisis or death.

b. The body may become dehydrated if too much Na^+ is secreted, which may shut down the ability of the body to remove toxins, and may cause death.

c. The heart muscle may not get enough K^+, rendering an irregular heart beat, possibly slowing the heart rate, which may lead to death.

d. The body may acidify the blood and urine, causing a life-threatening condition called metabolic acidosis.

e. The body may utilize N^+, Cl^-, and K^+ to inhibit urinary output, and death may result.

f. only a–d

g. only b–e

Resources and References

1. Control of the hydrogen ion activity (pH) in the body: http://www.usyd.edu.au/su/anaes/lectures/acidbase_mjb/control.html

2. Urinary Elimination, Newark College: http://www.newarkcolleges.com/professional/dmelick/pdf/Urination%20revised.pdf

3. Cranberry Juice: Helping to Keep Your Tracks Running Smoothly, University of Iowa Health Science Relations, first published November 2000: http://www.vh.org/adult/patient/urology/prose/cranberryjuice.html

4. Health Ask the Doctor BBC: http://www.bbc.co.uk/health/ask_doctor/cystitis_cranberry.shtml

5. RxList Pyridium HCl: http://www.rxlist.com/cgi/generic3/phenazopyridine_ids.htm

6. A Brief History of Infectious Diseases (Bayer): http://www.bayerpharma-na.com/healthcare/hc0112.asp

7. Circumcision and Urinary Tract Infection: http://www.cirp.org/library/disease/UTI

8. James C. Whorton. Nature Cures, the History of Alternative Medicine in America. Oxford University Press, 2002, R733.W495.

9. Read causes of cystitis that are related to sexual position and other issues. IVillage Sexual Health: http://magazines.ivillage.com/redbook/dh/health/articles/0,,284480_614819-3,00.html

10. National Institute of Diabetes and Digestive and Kidney Diseases (NIDDK), NIH: http://diabetes.niddk.nih.gov/

11. Holland, Norman and Michael Patrick Adams. *Core Concepts in Pharmacology*. Upper Saddle River, NJ: Pearson Education, 2003.

12. Adams, Michael Patrick, Dianne L. Josephson, and Leland Norman Holland, Jr. *Pharmacology for Nurses—A Pathophysiologic Approach*. Upper Saddle River, NJ: Pearson Education, 2005.

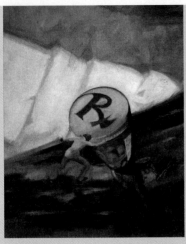

The Endocrine System

INTRODUCTION

The endocrine system is a collection of glands that produce hormones which help regulate the body's growth, metabolism, and sexual development and function. The hormones are released into the bloodstream and transported to tissues and organs throughout the body and, in fact, influence every cell in some way. Important to note is that the glands of the endocrine system are ductless. Because of this, their secreted hormones are released directly into the bloodstream and travel in the body to specific target organs, upon which they act.

The nervous system is considered the mass communicator of the human body, and hormones are the chemicals that do the communicating.

Endocrinology is the study of the chemical communication system that provides the means to control a large number of physiologic processes. It is also the study of hormones, their receptors, and the intracellular signaling pathways that they follow and call upon. As mentioned, cell types, organs, or processes are influenced, some more strongly than others, by hormone signaling. Growth from birth to adulthood involves the endocrine system, critical growth hormones, and other contributing hormones.

Many organs that are most known for their secretions of hormones will be discussed in this chapter, while others will be discussed in other chapters, such as The Gastrointestinal System, Chapter 11.

Anatomy of the Endocrine System

The endocrine "communication" system involves the hypothalamus, pituitary gland, other hormone producing cells or glands, hormones, and receptors. The major driving forces of the endocrine system are the hypothalamus and the pituitary gland. The glands that the pituitary gland controls are the thyroid, parathyroid, pancreas, adrenal glands, and gonads (testes and ovaries). During pregnancy, the placenta acts as an endocrine gland.

In the brain, part of the brain stem known as the hypothalamus controls the activity of the pituitary gland. The pituitary gland, the size of a large pea, is often referred to as the "master gland" because it controls many of the other glands. Hypophysis is another term for the pituitary gland. It is attached to the base of the hypothalamus in the brain. It is composed of two main sections, the anterior lobe and the posterior lobe. Each lobe contains a number of hormones, which may be released into the general blood circulation. The glands of the endocrine system are ductless. (See Figure 17-1.)

Some parts of the endocrine system secrete other substances besides hormones. The pancreas, for example, secretes digestive enzymes. The testes and ovaries secrete ova and sperm. Organs such as the stomach, heart, and intestines are involved in hormone production, but this is not their primary function.

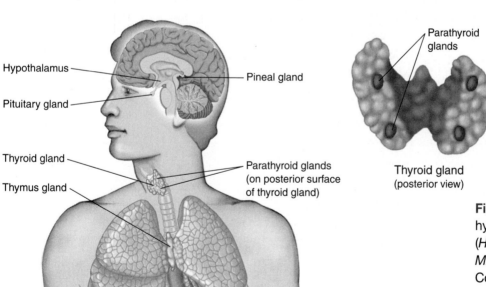

Figure 17-1 The hypothalamus (*Holland, Norman; Adams, Michael Patrick,* Core Concepts in Pharmacology, *1st Edition,* © 2003. Reprinted by permission of Pearson Education, Inc., Upper Saddle River, NJ)

Glands, Organs, and Secretions

Before we begin, the following is a list of the glands included in the endocrine system and the hormones each gland secretes. The majority of this list includes glands belonging to both males and females, with individual considerations toward the end. Looking at the list reveals how important this system is and how it is involved in every bodily function in some way. From top of the body to bottom, the glands are as follows:

- **hypothalamus**
  - thyrotropin-releasing hormone (TRH)
  - gonadotropin-releasing hormone (GnRH)
  - growth hormone-releasing hormone (GHRH)
  - corticotropin-releasing hormone (CRH)
  - somatostatin
  - dopamine
- **pituitary gland**
  - **anterior lobe (adenohypophysis)**
    - GH (human growth hormone)
    - PRL (prolactin)
    - ACTH (adrenocorticotropic hormone)
    - TSH (thyroid-stimulating hormone)
    - FSH (follicle-stimulating hormone)
    - LH (luteinizing hormone)
  - **posterior lobe (neurohypophysis)**
    - oxytocin
    - ADH (antidiuretic hormone)
- **pineal gland**
  - melatonin
- **thyroid gland**
  - thyroxine (T4)
  - triiodothyronine (T3)
  - calcitonin
- **parathyroid glands**
  - parathyroid hormone (PTH)
- **heart**
  - atrial-natriuretic peptide (ANP)
- **stomach and intestines**
  - gastrin
  - secretin
  - cholecystokinin (CCK)

- somatostatin
- neuropeptide Y
- **liver**
  - insulin-like growth factor
  - angiotensinogen
  - thrombopoietin
- **Islets of Langerhans in the pancreas**
  - insulin
  - glucagon
  - somatostatin
- **adrenal glands**
  - **adrenal cortex**
    - glucocorticoids—cortisol
    - mineralocorticoids—aldosterone
    - androgens (including testosterone)
  - **adrenal medulla**
    - adrenaline (epinephrine)
    - noradrenaline (norepinephrine)
- **kidney**
  - renin
  - erythropoietin (EPO)
  - calcitriol
- **skin**
  - calciferol (vitamin D_3)
- **adipose tissue**
  - leptin

males only:

- **testes**
  - androgens (testosterone)

females only:

- **ovarian follicle**
  - oestrogens
  - testosterone
- **corpus luteum**
  - progesterone
- **placenta** (when pregnant)
  - progesterone
  - human chorionic gonadotrophin (HCG)

Table 17-1 provides a brief description of the bodily function that a particular hormone helps control and where the hormone is produced.

Adrenal glands	Divided into 2 regions; secrete hormones that influence the body's metabolism, blood chemicals, and body characteristics, as well as influence the part of the nervous system that is involved in the response and defense against stress.
Hypothalamus	Activates and controls the part of the nervous system that controls involuntary body functions, the hormonal system, and many body functions, such as regulating sleep and stimulating appetite.
Ovaries and testicles	Secrete hormones that influence female and male characteristics, respectively.
Pancreas	Secretes a hormone (insulin) that controls the use of glucose by the body.
Parathyroid glands	Secrete a hormone that maintains the calcium level in the blood.
Pineal body	Involved with daily biological cycles.
Pituitary gland	Produces a number of different hormones that influence various other endocrine glands.
Thymus gland	Plays a role in the body's immune system.
Thyroid gland	Produces hormones that stimulate body heat production, bone growth, and the body's metabolism.

Source: AMA's *Current Procedural Terminology*, Revised 1998 Edition. CPT is a trademark of the American Medical Association.

Hormones

As previously mentioned, hormones are the chemicals that take the "messages" to the cells through the bloodstream.

Hormones transfer information and instructions from one set of cells to another. Each hormone affects only the cells that are genetically programmed to receive and respond to its message. There are many factors that can affect the level of hormones in the body at any time. Age, stress, infection, and changes in the balance of fluid and minerals in blood are only a few examples.

Hormones are divided into two groups according to their structure:

- steroids
  - slow acting
  - long lasting
  - usually end in "one"
  - examples—testosterone and progesterone
- peptides and amines
  - made of proteins
  - fast acting
  - short-lived
  - examples—insulin and ADH

Hormones control themselves by a means of feedback control, which means that when the hormone is in large supply, the gland stops making it. Feedback control is sort of a monitoring of supply and demand. When the level of hormone is low, the gland secretes the hormone until the level rises again (see Table 17-2).

TABLE 17-2 Hormones Secreted within the Endocrine System

Hormone(s) Secreted	Where the Hormone Is Produced	Hormone Function
Aldosterone	Adrenal glands	Regulates salt and water balance
Corticosteroid	Adrenal glands	Controls key functions in the body; acts as an anti-inflammatory; maintains blood sugar levels, blood pressure, and muscle strength; regulates salt and water balance
Antidiuretic hormone (vasopressin)	Pituitary gland	Affects water retention in kidneys; controls blood pressure
Corticotropin	Pituitary gland	Controls production and secretion of adrenal cortex hormones
Growth hormone	Pituitary gland	Affects growth and development; stimulates protein production
Luteinizing hormone (LH) and follicle-stimulating hormone (FSH)	Pituitary gland	Controls reproductive functioning and sexual characteristics
Oxytocin	Pituitary gland	Stimulates contraction of uterus and milk ducts in the breast
Prolactin	Pituitary gland	Initiates and maintains milk production in breasts
Thyroid-stimulating hormone (TSH)	Pituitary gland	Stimulates the production and secretion of thyroid hormones
Renin and Angiotensin	Kidneys	Controls blood pressure
Erythropoietin	Kidneys	Affects red blood cell (RBC) production
Glucagon	Pancreas	Raises blood sugar levels
Insulin	Pancreas	Lowers blood sugar levels; stimulates metabolism of glucose, protein, and fat
Estrogen	Ovaries	Affects development of female sexual characteristics and reproductive development
Progesterone	Ovaries	Stimulates the lining of the uterus for fertilization; prepares the breasts for milk production
Parathyroid hormone	Parathyroid glands	Affects bone formation and excretion of calcium and phosphorus
Thyroid hormone	Thyroid gland	Affects growth, maturation, and metabolism

The Glands

HYPOTHALAMUS

The hypothalamus is in charge of controlling many body functions, especially a number of hormones important to the female menstrual cycle, pregnancy, birth, and lactation (milk production). In the nervous system the hypothalamus mainly functions to keep the body in *homeostasis*, which means that it maintains the body's physical and chemical processes within the pre-set limits, or "status quo." Dynamic vital statistics such as blood pressure, body temperature, fluid and electrolyte balance, and body weight are held to a given, predetermined value called the set-point. Although this set-point can change over time, from day to day it is generally fixed.

To achieve homeostasis, one of the functions of the hypothalamus is to control the activity of the pituitary gland of the endocrine system. The hypothalamus produces hormones known as releasing factors. Releasing factors are sent to the anterior lobe via small blood vessels, which then connect the hypothalamus to the anterior lobe of the pituitary gland. The releasing factors stimulate the release of the hormones that are produced in the anterior lobe.

The hormones of the anterior lobe are known as tropic hormones. Tropic means "growth." The tropic hormones are released into the general blood circulation to control the activities of the other endocrine glands. Sometimes these hormones are called stimulating hormones because they stimulate other glands either to produce other hormones or to respond and perform an activity.

The hypothalamus also produces two hormones, which are stored in the posterior lobe of the pituitary gland. When needed, the hypothalamus will direct the master pituitary gland to release these two hormones, oxytocin and antidiuretic hormone (ADH). The posterior lobe sits behind the anterior lobe, also known as the neurohypophysis, and is a continuation of the hypothalamus.

The mechanism that controls the release of the tropic or stimulating hormones from the anterior pituitary gland is known as *negative feedback*. For example, the thyroid-releasing factor stimulates the release of thyroid-stimulating hormone (TSH), which in turn stimulates the thyroid gland to release the hormone thyroxine (also known as thyroid hormone). As a result, the concentration of thyroxine in the blood increases. When the thyroid hormone (T4) concentration rises above normal, this signals the hypothalamus to stop sending releasing factor. Since no releasing factor is sent to the pituitary gland, the gland does not send any more TSH (thyroid-stimulating hormone). Therefore, these mechanisms are inhibited.

Another example of the mechanism of negative feedback is when, after receiving a releasing factor from the hypothalamus, the anterior pituitary gland releases follicle stimulating hormone (FSH) in response. This FSH from the anterior pituitary gland stimulates the maturation of an egg in the ovary. When the egg has matured, the ovary releases negative feedback to the hypothalamus, which tells the brain that the "deed" is done. Hypothalamus responds by *not* sending any more releasing factor to the anterior pituitary gland. In turn, the inhibition of the Rheumatoid Factor causes the anterior pituitary gland to stop sending the FSH to the ovary.

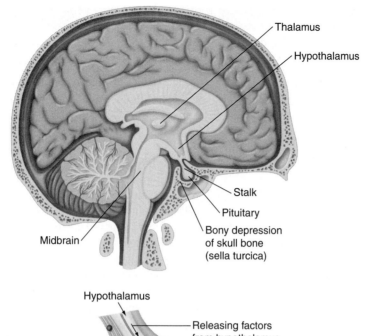

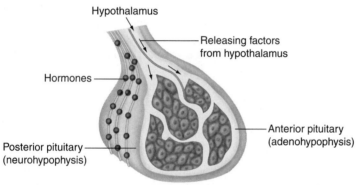

Figure 17-2   The pituitary gland (*Mulvihill, Mary Lou; Zelman, Mark; Holdaway, Paul; Tompary, Elaine; Turchany, Jill*, Human Diseases, A Systemic Approach, *5th Edition,* © 2001. Reprinted by permission of Pearson Education, Inc., Upper Saddle River, NJ)

THE PITUITARY GLAND

The main purpose of the hormones that are secreted by the anterior pituitary gland is to regulate the activities of the other endocrine glands (see Table 17-3). All of the hormones stimulate a specific endocrine gland, except the growth hormone. The growth hormone, known as somatotropin, regulates the growth and maintenance of all body tissues. An excess of growth hormone in a child results in gigantism, while a lack of GH in children results in pituitary dwarfism. A specific condition called acromegaly results when the lack of growth hormone is in the adult. If this happens, specific parts of the body grow to be unusually large, such as the head, hands, feet, jaw, arms, and legs. (See Figure 17-2.)

THYROID AND PARATHYROID

The thyroid gland is situated just below the "Adam's apple" or larynx. It is a small gland, weighing less than one ounce, located in the front of the neck. It is made up of two halves, called lobes, that lie along the windpipe and are joined together by a narrow band of thyroid tissue, known as the isthmus. The thyroid is directly regulated by the anterior pituitary and indirectly regulated by the hypothalamus.

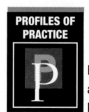

PROFILES OF PRACTICE

Every year, approximately 15,000 new cases of thyroid cancer are diagnosed.

TABLE 17-3 Anterior Pituitary Stimulating Tropic Hormones

Tropic or Stimulating Hormones	Target Gland or Body Part	Resultant Effect	Example
Growth stimulating hormone (GSH or GH)	All body tissues	GSH stimulates growth and repair	Child development, rebuild and repair muscle, bone, and other tissue.
Thyroid stimulating hormone (TSH)	Thyroid gland	TSH stimulates production and release of thyroxine (also known as the thyroid hormone, T4). An insufficient supply of this hormone can slow life-sustaining processes, damaging organs and tissues in every part of the body.	Aids in the rate of metabolism, cellular physical and chemical processes for body growth and maintenance: heart rate, digestion, physical growth, and mental development.
Adrenocorticotropic hormone (ACTH)	Adrenal cortex	ACTH stimulates production hormone and secretion of cortisol.	Aids in stress, injury, inflammation, anaphylactic shock.
Prolactin	Mammary glands	Milk production	Helps pregnant woman prepare milk in order to feed baby just after delivery, and continued lactation as required.
Follicle sstimulating hormone (FSH)	Male and female gonads (the testes and ovaries)	FSH stimulates the development of sperm and ovum	Matures sperm and egg for conception and healthy offspring.
Luteinizing hormone (LH)	Male and female (circulates in blood systems)	LH controls the production of sex hormones	Male androgens such as testosterone, the masculinizing hormone. Female estrogens, the feminizing hormone.

There are two types of cells that make up the thyroid tissue: follicular cells and parafollicular cells. The majority of the thyroid tissue consists of the follicular cells, which secrete iodine-containing hormones called thyroxine (T4) and triiodothyronine (T3). The parafollicular cells secrete the hormone calcitonin. The thyroid needs iodine to produce the hormones.

The thyroid is a very important gland that affects parts of the body functions that regulate growth, such as the following:

- **Thermogenesis**

  T4 and T3 produce heat by increasing the body's oxidative metabolism. This is accomplished by the synthesis of Na^+/K^+ ATPase.

- **Growth and Development**

  T4 and T3 are essential for growth in childhood. T4 and T3 stimulate growth by a direct effect on tissue and by having a permissive role on growth hormone action.

- **Nervous System**

  In childhood, T4 and T3 are essential for normal mylenation and development of the nervous system. Thyroid deficiency in childhood causes mental retardation. In adults, T4 and T3 deficiency causes lethargy and blunting of intellect. T4 and T3 excess causes restlessness and hypersensitivity.

- **Heart**

  Excess T4 and T3 can increase heart stroke volume and heart rate by increasing the heart's sensitivity to catecholamines. A deficiency of T4 and T3 has the opposite effect.

The thyroid gland takes iodine, found in many foods, and converts it into thyroid hormones: thyroxine (T4) and triiodothyronine (T3). Thyroid cells are the only cells in the body that can absorb iodine. The richest sources of iodine are seafoods and seaweeds (especially kelp). In the United States, the primary source of iodine is iodized salt.

Thyroid cells combine iodine and the amino acid tyrosine to make T3 and T4. T3 and T4 are then released into the bloodstream and are transported throughout the body, where they control metabolism. Every cell in the body depends upon thyroid hormones for regulating metabolism. The thyroid glands are responsible for the enhancement of growth and development and for nervous system maturation in children.

The normal thyroid gland produces about 80 percent T4 and about 20 percent T3; however, T3 possesses about four times the hormone "strength" as T4. When the level of thyroid hormones known as T3 and T4 drops too low, the pituitary gland produces thyroid stimulating hormone (TSH), which stimulates the thyroid gland to produce more hormones.

ADRENAL

Adrenal glands are located on the upper part of each kidney (Figure 17-3). The glands have an inner or center part known as adrenal medulla and an outer part known as adrenal cortex. The adrenal medulla, a part of the *sympathetic* nervous system, secretes EPI or epinephrine during sympathetic activation. Epinephrine is a catecholamine. Effects of epinephrine, and other catecholamines, will be further discussed in Chapter 19, The Nervous System.

The adrenal cortex secretes two types of hormones, which are divided into two main classes: the glucocorticoids and the mineralcorticoids. The hormones of the adrenal cortex, the adrenocorticosteroids, are generally referred to as corticosteroids, or steroids. As a pharmacological agent, the

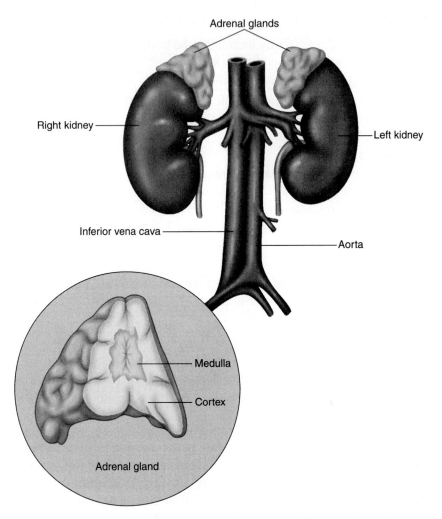

Figure 17-3 The adrenal glands
(*Mulvihill, Mary Lou; Zelman, Mark; Holdaway, Paul; Tompary, Elaine; Turchany, Jill,* Human Diseases, A Systemic Approach, *5th Edition,* © 2001. Reprinted by permission of Pearson Education, Inc., Upper Saddle River, NJ)

glucocorticoids, or glucocorticosteroids, are used frequently in the treatment of inflammatory or allergic conditions, such as arthritis or bee sting.

The following three factors induce the hypothalamus to secrete the releasing factor called adrenocorticotropin (ACTH): (ACTH is also called adrencocorticotropic hormone.)

Sleep Wake Cycle—Larger amounts of adrenocorticotropin from the anterior pituitary gland and cortisol, a glucocorticoid, from the adrenal gland are secreted while a person is awake. Smaller amounts of these hormones are present during sleep. During the wake period, cortisol requires body metabolism to meet the requirements of this active period. Coritsol is a natural anti-inflammatory substance.

Stress—Is the condition of the body when it is subjected to increased demands of physical or mental exertion. Stress may be induced by cold weather, exercise, infections, burns, surgery, and anxiety. Stress produces an increase in adrenocorticotropic hormone secretion (ACTH), which stimulates cortisol secretion from the adrenal gland. High amounts of cortisol give the body an increased ability to cope with the demands of stress.

Negative Feedback—The releasing factor and adrenocorticotropin stimulate the secretion and return of cortisol into the bloodstream. When the level of cortisol rises above normal, negative feedback begins, which stops the further release of releasing factors from the hypothalamus to the anterior pituitary gland, which in turn stops the further release of adrenocorticotropin (ACTH). This in turn stops the signal to the adrenal gland to release cortisol. Cortisol secretion is inhibited.

Glucocorticoids

The glucocorticoids regulate the metabolism of carbohydrates and proteins, especially during stress. Metabolism is a chemical breakdown. Carbohydrates are sugars and starches, which are metabolized into simple sugars, or monosaccharides. During periods of stress involving body injury, trauma, surgery, or wound healing, there is an increased requirement for glucose. Healing wounds and tissues in need of repair need to use more glucose than otherwise, and almost exclusively in repair stages. The brain normally uses only glucose.

Inflammation is considered the first step in the process of wound healing, as immune system mediators come to the rescue after an injury. However, sometimes the normal inflammatory response gets too overworked, as in an acute inflammatory reaction; or it becomes continual or is prolonged, as in a chronic inflammatory reaction. In this situation, inflammation becomes a disease in itself. Inflammation is also present in various types of allergic reactions, asthma, and anaphylactic shock. Therefore, the glucocorticoids are useful in treating these conditions. The glucocorticoids have potent anti-inflammatory effects. The synthetic glucocorticoids are frequently used to treat inflammatory and allergic conditions because they have a longer duration of action than naturally occurring adrenocorticosteroids.

ADMINISTRATION OF GLUCOCORTICOIDS

- PO—administered orally (Rx only).
- Top—topically—use in the treatment of inflammation and pruritic dermatoses.

While some topical steroids are available over the counter (OTC), the higher strengths are available by prescription only. The topical preparations are specifically labeled for temporary relief. They can be used for relief of minor skin irritations, itching, dermatitis, rashes, eczema, insect bites, poison ivy, cosmetics (perfumes), detergents, and itching in the anal and genital regions.

- IM—intramuscularly—used when frequent administration or IV is undesirable
- IV—intravenously—used in emergencies for immediate effect

Mineralcorticoids

The main function and purpose of mineralcorticoids is to regulate the electrolyte, or salt and fluid, balance of the body. Mineralcorticoids are essential for life. Therefore, a deficiency of mineralcorticoids requires replacement therapy so that the patient will not dehydrate, to maintain pH balance in the body, and to assist in the electrical needs of the body.

The most important mineralcorticoid is aldosterone. The site of action of aldosterone is in the distal tubules of the nephrons in the kidneys. Nephrons are the smallest working unit (cell) of the kidneys. The hormone aldosterone increases the reabsoprtion of sodium ions. Reabsorption means that the sodium leaves the tubule and returns to the blood supply. In this process, there is an exchange of potassium ions for sodium ions. The K^+ cations are led into the nephron tubule through the lumen (tunnel of the tubule) and transported into the urine. (See Figure 17-4.)

Water also is reabsorbed with the sodium. Consequently, normal sodium and water levels, which are isotonic, are maintained in the blood and other body tissues. *Isotonicity* is the characteristic of a solution in the body that has the same salt concentration as that of the blood. A therapeutic gonadal hormone used to treat Addison's disease and salt-losing adrenogenital syndrome is Florinef® (see Table 17-4).

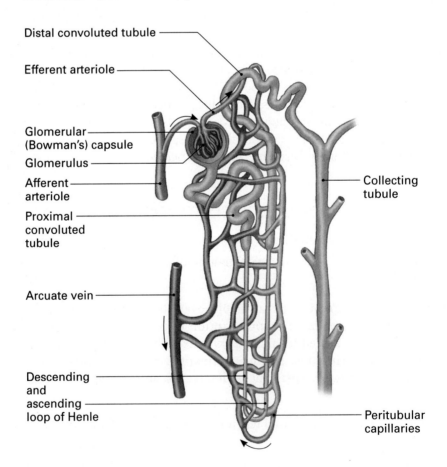

Distal convoluted tubule

Efferent arteriole

Glomerular (Bowman's) capsule

Glomerulus

Afferent arteriole

Proximal convoluted tubule

Arcuate vein

Descending and ascending loop of Henle

Collecting tubule

Peritubular capillaries

Figure 17-4 The nephron of the kidney

TABLE 17-4 Therapeutic Steroids

Examples of Corticosteroids

Trade®	Generic
Cortef®, Hydrocortone®, Corticaine®	Hydrocortisone used to treat Addison's disease
Destasone®, Orasone®	prednisone
Medrol®, Solu-Medrol® (inj)	methylprednisolone
Aristocort®, Kenalog®	triamcinolone
Celestrone®, Vanceril®	betamethasone
Decadron®, Hexadrol®	dexamethasone

Example of Therapeutic Mineralcorticoids

Florinef®	Fludrocortisone used to treat Addison's disease

The Gonads

The hormone released by the area of the brain known as the hypothalamus beginning at the onset of sexual maturity in both males and females is the gonadotropin releasing hormone, or GnRH. GnRH is needed for both sexual maturity and normal reproduction. It acts by stimulating the release of luteinizing hormone (LH) and follicle-stimulating hormone (FSH) from the anterior pituitary. LH and FSH act by stimulating the production of sex hormones in the gonads, known as the testes in males and ovaries in females.

Both LH and FSH are responsible for the development and secretion of sex hormones and the development of sex organs and secondary sex characteristics. Secondary sex characteristics are physical features that start to develop at puberty and serve to further distinguish males from females. The primary sex characteristics are the genitals.

Female Sex Hormones

The sex hormones of the female are estrogen and progesterone. Estrogen is responsible for the development of secondary sex characteristics as well as the formation of *osteoblasts*, inhibition of osteoclasts, and bone loss. Progesterone is another female hormone that prepares the lining of the uterus for the implantation of a fertilized egg and sperm. Two other pituitary hormones are involved in childbirth: Oxytocin, secreted by the posterior pituitary gland, but made by the hypothalamus, stimulates the uterus to start contracting at the beginning of labor. Prolactin signals the mammary glands in the female breast to start producing milk before the baby is born, in about the fourth to sixth month.

Dopamine serves as the major prolactin-inhibiting factor (stops prolactin secretion). Dopamine is secreted into portal blood by neurons and binds to receptors on lactotrophs, inhibiting both the synthesis and secretion of prolactin. Agents and drugs that interfere with dopamine secretion or receptor binding lead to enhanced secretion of prolactin. (This explains why some psychotropic drugs, such as tranquilizers and monoamine oxidase inhibitors (MAO inhibitors), as well as estrogen, cimetidine, and antihistamines cause gynecomastia and galactorrhea in the male. "In males, prolactin influences the production of testosterone and affects sperm production. In conditions where prolactin secretion is increased (hyperprolactinaemia), testosterone levels drop and sperm production is reduced or absent, resulting in male infertility." [11])

The female secondary sex characteristics are as follows:

- enlarged breasts
- higher pitched voice than males
- functional mammary glands
- smoother skin than males
- wider hips than shoulders, compared with males
- fat deposits mainly around the buttocks and thighs
- less or not as coarse body and facial hair, compared with males
- rounded shoulders

Male Sex Hormones

Male sex hormones or androgens are also known as the masculinizing hormones. The main sex hormone of the male, testosterone, is produced in the testes. The major functions of testosterone are to stimulate the development of male sex organs and to maintain the secondary sex characteristics.

At one time it was believed that men did not manufacture progesterone, also known as the pregnancy hormone. However, recently the important role of natural progesterone in promoting good health and well being for men was discovered. This hormone plays an integral part in maintaining a healthy prostate. In healthy men, progesterone is produced in the adrenal gland and the testes. [12]

The male sex organs are as follows:

- prostate
- seminal vesicles
- scrotum
- penis
- testes

The male characteristics are as follows:

- excessive facial and body hair
- vocal cord thickening, which lowers the voice
- developed Adam's apple
- distinct musculature
- squared shoulders
- fat deposits mainly around the abdomen
- coarser skin than females
- wider shoulders than hips, compared with females

Estrogen Replacement Therapy and Menopause

After menopause, estrone is the most active circulating estrogen and is then made in the adrenal glands only. Replacement therapy is the replacement of estrogen for post-menopausal women. It is prescribed for symptomatic treatment of the common symptoms associated with menopause, such as hot flashes and vaginal dryness, the prevention of bone fractures associated with *osteoporosis*, reduction of the risk of heart attacks and strokes, and excessive and painful uterine bleeding (see Table 17-5). Topical or vaginal cream is prescribed for vaginal or vulvar atrophy associated with menopause.

Estrogens reduce LDL cholesterol, the "bad" cholesterol, and increase HDL cholesterol, the "good" cholesterol, in the blood. When taken alone or in combination with a progestin synthetic progesterone, estrogens have been shown to reduce the risk of myocardial infarction and stroke by 40–50 percent. In addition, they have bone-promoting effects, which means that they reduce the risk for hip and knee fracture from osteoporosis by 20–30 percent.

Estrogens used in replacement therapy have been associated with an increased risk of liver disease through an unknown mechanism in patients receiving dantrolene. Women over 35 years of age and those with a history of liver disease are especially at risk. Estrogens increase the liver's ability to manufacture clotting factors, and those taking warfarin must have blood monitored for the reduced ability of the blood thinning effect. Blood clots are occasional, but serious, side effects of estrogen therapy and are dose-related; that is, they occur more frequently with higher doses. Cigarette smokers are at a higher risk than nonsmokers. Therefore, patients requiring estrogen therapy are strongly encouraged to quit smoking.

Estrogens can cause a buildup of the uterine lining (endometrial hyperplasia) and increase the risk of endometrial carcinoma. The addition of a progestin to estrogen therapy has been shown to prevent endometrial cancer from developing. There are conflicting data regarding an association between estrogen and breast cancer. It is not known at this time if the addition of a progestin to ERT reduces the risk of breast cancer, as it does for uterine cancer. There is no evidence that estrogens are effective for nervous symptoms or depression that might occur during menopause. Estrogens increase the incidence of gallbladder disease and abnormal blood clotting.

Some indications for estrogens are as follows:

- moderate to severe *vasomotor* symptoms associated with the menopause
- atrophic vaginitis
- kraurosis vulvae
- female hypogonadism
- female castration
- primary ovarian failure
- breast cancer, for palliative therapy only in appropriately selected women and men with metastatic disease
- prostatic carcinoma palliative therapy of advanced disease

TABLE 17-5   Estrogen Replacement Therapy Choices

From natural sources:	Trade Name	Dosage	Comments
Animal derived estrogen replacement has been considered more natural than plant derived estrogen.	Premarin® (conjugated animal estrogen)	(1) Available in 0.3, 0.625, 1.25 and 2.5 tabs 1 qd NTE 2.4 mg/d (2) Vaginal cream 1 app of $\frac{1}{2}$ gm to 1 gm/day (3) Injection 25 mg q 6 hrs prn hemorrhage	(1) Extracted from pregnant mares' urine and contains a mixture of different estrogens, not just one kind of estrogen. (2) Cream for short-term use for atrophic vaginitis, or kraurosis vulvae. (3) Injection for abnormal interuterine bleeding.
From Plant Sources Plant derived estrogens are chemically identical to animal estrogen made by the ovaries.	Estrace®		Estradiol is the most potent form of estrogen in premenopausal women.
	Estrasorb®	Apply two 1.74 mg packets to calf or thigh/day	Topical estradiol emulsion
	Estrogel®	Applied once daily on one arm from wrist to shoulder	Estradiol gel avoids first pass metabolism in the liver and minimizes application site skin irritation. The gel dries in as little as two to five minutes.
	ESTRING® (estradiol)	Soft, flexible vaginal ring with 2 mg estradiol delivery system, placed in the upper third of the vagina, by the physician or the patient and worn continuously for 90 days, then removed and replaced if continuation of therapy	(1) Discontinue during treatment for vaginal infection with vaginal antimicrobial therapy. (2) May not be suitable for women with narrow, short, or stenosed (constricted) vaginas, and prolapse (who are more prone to irritation of a tight fitting ring), or those with symptoms of vaginal irritation.[11]
	Alora® estradiol (transdermal system).	(1) Apply 0.025 mg/day twice a week to hips,	Continuous delivery for twice weekly dosing.

TABLE 17-5 **Estrogen Replacement Therapy Choices** (*continued*)

From natural sources:	Trade Name	Dosage	Comments
	Climara TDP	abdomen, or thigh NTE 1 mg/d, twice a week (2) Apply 1 TDP q week to abdomen, buttocks, inner thigh, upper arm, or hips as directed.	Applied to abdomen, hips, and thigh. 6.5, 12.5, 18.75, and 25.0 cm^2
Plant derived progesterones are chemically identical to animal progestins made by the ovaries.	Prometrium®		progesterone
Lab Modified Estrogens			
Laboratory modified, plant derived estrogens that have been chemically modified in a laboratory and are therefore not truly "natural"	Cenestin®	1. 0.625 NTE 1.25 mg QD	conjugated plant estrogens (1) & (2) Treatment of vasomotor symptoms due to menopause. Dosages for other conditions may vary.
	(1) Ogen® (2) Ortho-est®	1 × 0.625 (0.75 mg estropipate) tablet to 2 × 2.5 QD	Estrone estropipate
	(1) Estratab® (2) Menest®	Avail: 0.3–1.25 mg tabs, 1 tab qd (NTE 1.25/d)	Esterified estrogens (1) Dosage varies per patient and condition/indication (2) Given cyclically for short-term use only
Synthetic progesterones are known as progestins.	(1)Aygestin® (norethindrone acetate) (2) Provera®, Depo-Provera (MPA) (3) Cycrin® = medroxyprogesterone acetate (MPA)	(1) Avail 5 mg tab (2) & (3) avail 2.5, 5, & 10 mg tabs (2) Contraceptive injection 1 ml × 150 mg/90 days	Lab created progestins. (1), (2) amenorrhea, uterine cancer, and endometriosis (2) contraceptive injection All—dosing varies per indication.
Combination synthetic	(1) Prempro® (2) Premphase®	(1) 1 tab qd (2) 1 maroon tab qd	Combines norethindrone acetate or MPA with

TABLE 17-5   Estrogen Replacement Therapy Choices (*continued*)

From natural sources:	Trade Name	Dosage	Comments
progesterone and animal estrogens		days 1–14 & 1 blue tab/d days 15–28	Premarin®. Dosage varies with indications: postmenopausal vasomotor symptoms, prevention of osteoporosis
Combination synthetic progesterone and plant estrogens	Activella® (estradiol/norethindrone acetate)	1 tablet daily (1 mg/0.5 mg)	Prevention of osteoporosis, vasomotor menopausal symptoms

CONTRAINDICATIONS

Estrogens should not be used in women with any of the following conditions:

- undiagnosed abnormal genital bleeding
- known, suspected, or history of cancer of the breast, except in appropriately selected patients being treated for metastatic disease
- known or suspected estrogen-dependent neoplasia
- active or history of deep vein thrombosis or pulmonary embolism
- active or recent (within the past year) arterial thromboembolic disease such as stroke, or MI
- liver dysfunction or disease
- known hypersensitivity to ingredients of the particular estrogenic formula
- known or suspected pregnancy

Testosterone Hormonal Replacement

Testosterone also produces an anabolic effect that promotes the synthesis and retention of proteins, for muscle and bone, in the body. The more testosterone there is, the easier the body can build muscle and the more muscle can be built. In some diseases, the muscle will *atrophy* or become weak, in which case it needs to be rebuilt. Pharmaceutical anabolic steroids can help the patient with such a disease and, in addition, promote weight gain after surgery, trauma, or serious infection. Unfortunately, over-use of the steroids (as seen with the illegal use of them for athletic performance enhancement) can cause some irreversible effects.

The FDA has approved pharmaceutical steroids for the following uses:

- weight gain for chronic nutritional deficiencies or wasting syndromes such as those in cancer or AIDS patients
- relief of bone pain associated with osteoporosis

- corticosteroid-induced catabolism
- hereditary angioedema
- severe anemia
- metastatic breast cancer in women
- hypogonadism: hormonal replacement for hormonal deficiency states in males
- to stimulate the beginning of puberty in certain boys who are late starting puberty naturally
- cryptorchidism—failure of the testicle to descend

Angioedema is an autosomal dominant disorder characterized by returning episodes of swelling of the face, extremities, genitalia, bowel wall, and upper respiratory tract caused by deficient or nonfunctional C1 esterase inhibitor (C1 INH). Stanozolol cannot stop, but can prevent, slow the frequency of, and control the severity of attacks of angioedema and can increase blood serum levels of C1 INH and C4.

Anemia caused by the administration of myelotoxic drugs, or acquired aplastic anemia, congenital aplastic anemia, and myelofibrosis may respond to androgens. "Oxymetholone enhances the production and urinary excretion of erythropoietin in patients with anemias due to bone marrow failure and often stimulates erythropoiesis in anemias due to deficient red cell production."[3]

CONTRAINDICATIONS

The alcohol formulation suggests that patients also taking Antabuse® (disulfiram, avoidance therapy for alcoholism) or Agenerase® (amprenavir, protease inhibitor drug) should not use AndroGel®.[4] Oral testosterone or derivatives are contraindicated in male patients with carcinoma of the prostate or breast, and females with hypercalcemia or with carcinoma of the breast (see Table 17-6).

TABLE 17-6 Androgens	
Trade	Generic
Delatestryl®	Testosterone (parenteral) for testosterone replacement therapy
Oreton®	Methyltestosterone (oral capsules)
Halotestin®	fluoxymesterone (oral tablets)
Winstrol®	stanozolol (oral tablets) anabolic androgen for angio edema
Oxandrin	Oxandrolone for AIDS wasting syndrome (oral tablets), for bone pain, weight gain, post surgery/trauma, corticosteroid induced protein catabolism.
Testoderm®	Transdermal patches (scrotal)
Androderm®, Testoderm TTS®	Transdermal patches (abdomen, back, thigh, and arm)
Androgel®, Testim®	Topical gel applied to shoulders, upper arms, and/or abdomen.[4]

SIDE EFFECTS OF ANABOLIC STEROIDS

Too much testosterone or anabolic steroids signals the pituitary gland to stop producing the hormone gonadotropin. (This fact is the basis for research in a male contraceptive, as gonadotropin is necessary for spermatogenesis.) A domino effect occurs, causing testicular atrophy, a decreased size and function of the testicals and testes, lowered sperm count, sterility (reversible), painful, prolonged erection (priapism), prostate enlargement, and frequent or continuing erections. Upon cessation of steroid use, the natural ability to produce testosterone may remain completely shut down, possibly leading to a permanent imbalance of the hormone.

Side effects in both men and women include the following:

- edema and weight gain due to sodium and water retention
- Jaundice—increased concentration of bilirubin in the liver leads to jaundice. Bilirubin is a breakdown product of hemoglobin. Jaundice, a yellowing of the sclera or whites of the eyes and/or skin, occurs because red blood cells are being broken down too fast for the liver to process, because of disease in the liver, or because of bile duct blockage.
- hepatic carcinoma (cancerous tumor of the liver) after prolonged steroid use
- high cholesterol and associated diseases
- increased or decreased libido
- chills
- decreased glucose tolerance
- increased serum levels of low-density lipoproteins and decreased levels of high-density lipoproteins
- increased creatine and creatinine excretion
- In women, the following effects of masculinization are reversible if the drug is discontinued in time, except where those are noted with the word "permanent." (Long-term effects are irreversible.)
  - acne
  - hirsutism—growth of facial hair
  - permanent increases in body hair
  - permanent deepening of the voice
  - amenorrhea or other menstrual irregularities
  - permanent enlargement of the clitoris
  - uterine atrophy
  - shrinkage of breast size
  - masculinization of female fetuses in pregnant women[5]
- In men the following has been documented:
  - infertility in males
  - Impotence, after as little as 25 mg of testosterone a day for six weeks; spermatogenesis declines. Androgens will do the same even after drug withdrawal.

- increased frequency of erections
- pre-puberty penis enlargement
- testicular atrophy (shrinkage)
- decline in testicular function and decrease in spermatogenesis
- decrease in seminal volume
- chronic priapism (erections that last longer than four hours)
- epididymitis
- bladder irritability and decrease in seminal fluid volume
- gynecomastia, enlarged breast and nipple tenderness (on men)

PRECAUTIONS

It should be noted that, while the newer topical testosterone gels provide fewer side effects than oral or injectable testosterone, without protection these may cause severe side effects in other partners and family members by contamination. Therefore, the risk of testosterone transfer of a newly developed 2–5 percent testosterone gel preparation was evaluated.[6] Anabolic steroids may cause suppression of clotting factors II, V, VII, and X, and an increase in prothrombin time.

Note: See Chapter 18, The Reproductive System, for further specific details of the relationship of the endocrine system and the reproductive system.

Glandular Disease States

Some cancers, especially those involving the breast, uterus, and prostate gland, are dependent on the presence of sex hormones. The use of sex hormones opposite of those that are found in the tissue receptors most often appears to antagonize or inhibit tumor growth. Endocrine therapy is palliative (soothing) only.

EXAMPLES OF CANCERS THAT BENEFIT FROM ENDOCRINE THERAPY

Breast Cancer—Breast tissue has estrogen receptors. Breast cancer has more estrogen "feeding" the cancer cells. Therefore, adding more estrogen exogenously causes more breast cancer. Obese men have higher levels of estrogen in their bodies because fat cells produce estrogen from other hormones; they may also have fewer androgens. Taking an androgen as an anti-estrogenic therapy will lower the amount of endogenous estrogen; this is used in females. (See side effects of androgen steroidal therapy.) Androgen (and possibly progesterone) exerts a protective influence, is used to treat male breast cancer, and includes drugs tamoxifen (Nolvadex®) and megace (Megestrol®). Tamoxifen is an antiestrogen and works by blocking estrogen in the breast, which slows the growth and reproduction of breast cancer cells that depend on estrogen for survival.

Megace is an anti-androgen and blocks the effect of androgen (a male hormone) on breast cancer cells. It is uncertain to researchers why blocking androgen in the breast helps treat male breast cancer.

Polycystic ovary syndrome, PCOS, which involves enlarged ovaries containing many fluid-filled sacs, exhibits high levels of male hormones, or androgen, also known as testosterone. "Feeding" them more testosterone would only exacerbate the problem. Therefore, giving the female patient estrogen increases estrogen levels and helps lower the levels of male hormones. PCOS is not considered a cancer, per se.

Prostate Cancer—Researchers at the University of Connecticut Health Center have found that small amounts of estrogen help reduce the amount of bone loss caused by a common prostate cancer treatment. If the estrogen level in the body is high, the body doesn't make as much testosterone, so the cancer can't feed on it. Estrogens actually block prostate cancer growth, but only to a point.

Endometrial Cancer—Is a cancer dependent upon estrogen. Certain stages may be treated with estrogen antagonists such as aromatase inhibitors.

Endocrine System Disorders and Pituitary Abnormalities

Following are some of the abnormalities caused by defects related to the pituitary gland of the endocrine system:

PITUITARY GIGANTISM

This condition results from an excessive secretion of growth hormone (GH) in childhood, usually from a nonmalignant tumor of the pituitary gland. This causes the child to grow excessively and to be bigger in all areas of the body, height, weight, and size. The size is, however, proportionate. Treatment may be with surgical removal or radiation therapy of the pituitary tumor. Medications include somatostatin analogs, such as octreotide or long-acting lanreotide, which reduce growth hormone secretion. Also used, but less effective, are dopamine agonists, such as bromocriptine mesylate and cabergoline.

PITUITARY DWARFISM

This condition results from a lack of GH from birth or in childhood. The person may be somewhat short at birth, but usually the child's growth in height and weight is normal from birth up to the age when large amounts of growth hormone are needed, at six to twelve months old. That is when it may become apparent that the child is not growing normally.

The person may have hypoglycemia or low blood sugar because GH is not present to counter insulin, may have an exaggerated "puppet" or "baby-doll" face, and may be proportionately short with a chubby body build because the height as well as the growth of all other structures are decreased. Each case differs—either there is an unusually high deficiency of GH, or there may be no GH at all. It has been shown that patients with the form of isolated growth hormone deficiency develop anti-GH antibodies when growth hormone replacement is administered (exogenous GH). Thus, no treatment may be available when this happens.

There may or may not be a relevancy of the parent's stature to the child's dwarfism. Some syndromes are caused by genetic mutations at the moment of conception. Other syndromes are caused by the random combination of two recessive genes that may have been dormant for generations. (Examples of recessive genes are blue eyes or blond hair from parents with dark hair and eyes. The child must receive one recessive gene from each parent to show the trait.) The main course of therapy is growth hormone replacement therapy, with growth hormone, somatotropin, when there is lack of growth hormone in the body. A pediatric endocrinologist usually administers this type of therapy before a child's growth plates have "fused" or joined together. GH replacement therapy is rarely effective after the growth plates have been joined. This is usually before the age of 17. It is possible to see an increase in height of 4–6 inches (10–15 cm) in the first year of treatment[1]. Somatrem or Protopin® and somatropin or Humatrope®, among others, may be used.

ACROMEGALY

This is an excessive secretion of growth hormone during the adult years, characterized by enlarged bones of the cheek, hands, feet, and jaws, with a predominant forehead and a large nose. Ultimately, considerable disability with joint pain, cardiovascular disease, hypertension, insulin resistance, visual impairment, and severe headaches will result. The arms, legs, and hands are disproportionate to the rest of the body, being excessively large. But the person will have slender arms, sometimes exacerbated by atrophy of the muscles.

There is often a curvature of the spine associated with a deformity of the chest. The lower part of the sternum may project forward because the bones of the chest are increased in size. The cause is usually a tumor on the pituitary gland called a pituitary adenoma. Too much growth hormone after the age of 17 will lead to acromegaly, but seldom to gigantism, because the long bones of the limbs have fused and can't grow any more. Treatment includes surgical removal of the tumor. Medications that may decrease the secretion of GH and reduce the size of the tumor include the following:

- Somatostatin—a brain hormone that inhibits GH release
- Sandostatin® = octreotide—a synthetic form of somatostatin (analogue) used in the treatment of acromegaly
- Somatuline LA® = long-acting lanreotide LAR® = octreotide IM injection, a longer-acting, slow-release form of octreotide

Diabetes

It is estimated that approximately 6.6 percent of the population has diabetes, with about one-third of that number unaware of their serious medical condition. Diabetes is a disease in which the body does not produce or properly use insulin, a hormone that is needed to convert sugar, starches, and other food into energy necessary for daily life. The cause of diabetes is not certain, but both genetics and environmental factors such as obesity and lack of exercise appear to play roles.

There are 4 major types of diabetes, as follow:

- *Type 1 diabetes* results from the body's failure to produce insulin. It is estimated that 5–10 percent of Americans who are diagnosed with diabetes have type 1 diabetes.
- *Type 2 diabetes* results from insulin resistance (a condition in which the body fails to properly use insulin) combined with relative insulin deficiency. Most Americans who are diagnosed with diabetes have type 2 diabetes.
- *Gestational diabetes* affects about 4 percent of all pregnant women (135,000 cases) in the United States each year.
- *Pre-diabetes* is a condition that occurs when a person's blood glucose levels are higher than normal, but not high enough for a diagnosis of type 2 diabetes.

Many people remain undiagnosed because many of the diabetes symptoms seem harmless. Studies indicate that the early detection of diabetes symptoms and treatment can decrease the chance of developing the complications of diabetes.

Diabetes symptoms include the following:

- frequent urination
- excessive thirst
- extreme hunger
- unusual weight loss
- increased fatigue
- irritability
- blurry vision

Type 2 diabetes may be delayed, or even prevented from ever developing, through diet and exercise.

Most people with diabetes have high risk factors that impact other conditions, such as high blood pressure and cholesterol, which increase one's risk for heart disease and stroke. It is estimated that more than 65 percent of people with diabetes die from heart disease or stroke. With diabetes, heart attacks occur earlier in life and often result in death.

Diabetes is not something that should be taken lightly, and anyone can assess their risk through pre-diabetes screening. Diabetes is a major chronic disease that causes significant morbidity and mortality due to heart and circulatory conditions, renal failure, and blindness. By managing diabetes, high blood pressure, and cholesterol, people with diabetes can greatly reduce their risk. Treatment may include proper diet and exercise, oral hypoglycemics, insulin, or a combination of therapies.

Table 17-7 lists some oral agents used in the treatment of diabetes. Many medications are, and continue to be, developed that may be a combination of two of the following agents.

TABLE 17-7 Oral Hypoglycemics

Class	Example(s)	Primary Site of Action	Mechanism of Action
Biguanides	Glucophage© (metformin)	Liver	Reduce glucose release
Thiazolidinediones	Avandia© (rosiglitazone) Actos© (pioglitazone)	Muscle	Increase insulin sensitivity
Sulfonylureas	Glucotrol© (glipizide) Amaryl© (glimeprimide) Diabeta©, Micronase© (glyburide)	Pancreas	Increase insulin release
Alpha-glucosidase inhibitors	Precose© (acarbose) Glyset© (miglitol)	Intestine	Slow digestion of carbohydrates
Meglitinides	Prandin© (repaglinide) Starlix© (nateglinide)	Pancreas	Increase insulin release

Source: Today's Technician—Volume 5, Issue 1.

INSULIN

For some diabetic patients who are insulin dependent (type 1), there is an array of injectable insulins available. Which insulin is best for which patient is assessed by the health care provider.

Available insulins include the following:

- Rapid acting
  - Humalog (Lispro)
  - Novolog (Aspart)
- **Regular**
  - Novolin R
  - Velosulin BR
  - Humulin R
- **NPH**
  - Humulin N
  - Novolin N
- **Lente (L)**
  - Humulin L
  - Novolin L
- **Ultralente**
  - Humulin U
- **Pre-Mixed**
  - Humalog 75/25
  - Humulin 70/30
  - Novolin 70/30
  - Humulin 50/50
- **Peakless/Basal Action**
  - Lantus (glargine)

Compiled from Eli Lilly, Novo Nordisk, and Aventis product labeling information.

As with the oral medications, there are some combination insulins now available and still being developed. Research continues on insulin with the following considerations:

- rapid acting insulins
- short activity insulins
- intermediate acting insulins
- long acting insulins
- ultra long acting insulins
- Insulin Mixtures

Insulin delivery technology has developed the following innovations:

- insulin injection
- insulin pens
- insulin jet injectors
- external insulin pumps
- implantable insulin pumps
- transdermal insulin
- oral spray insulin
- inhaled insulin

DIABETES INSIPIDUS

Diabetes insipidus is a condition that results from a decrease or hyposecretion of ADH, the antidiuretic hormone. The symptoms for DI are the same as for diabetes mellitus, or DM (high amount of sugar in the blood). The symptoms include the following:

- polyuria—excessive urination
- polydipsia—excessive thirst
- polyphagia—excessive eating

The lack of antidiuretic hormone in patients with DI is caused by kidneys that don't concentrate urine very well, which means that their urine is more diluted. These patients will have to urinate very often, getting up as often as two or three times in the night. People with diabetes insipidus are thirsty all the time and may often want to drink liquids every hour (see Table 17-8).

Excessive urination may cause them to become dehydrated, making them feel lethargic and thirsty. When people feel tired or lethargic, they sometimes interpret that to mean that they need to eat. Two things can cause diabetes insipidus: (1) Hypothalamus doesn't make enough antidiuretic hormone, or ADH. (2) The kidneys don't work with ADH the way they should. Most people with diabetes insipidus acquire it after a head injury or after brain surgery; or they have a brain tumor. DI can also be congenital and run in families. DI can be drug induced, such as by lithium, which is used for bipolar disorder. About 25 percent of the time, however, the cause is unknown. Treatment for pituitary DI is with DDAVP nasal spray that contains a substance much like the body's natural ADH vasopressin. If a person taking DDAVP takes in too much liquid, the body will get overloaded with fluids, which will make the patient feel weak, dizzy, or bad all over.[3]

TABLE 17-8 Comparison of Diabetes Insipidus and Mellitus and Types

Factors	Diabetes Insipidus	Diabetes Mellitus Type I	Diabetes Mellitus Type II
Onset	Birth	Birth; may show up in childhood or adolescents; current trend being seen in older adults.	Adult onset, usually over 40 years old, but there is a trend in younger, overweight children
Mechanism of the Disease	Lack of ADH or vasopressin secreted by posterior pituitary gland	Beta cells of Islets of Langerhans do not manufacture insulin; creates the inability to transport sugar from the bloodstream into cells.	Beta cells of Islets of Langerhans do not manufacture enough insulin, or the muscles do not utilize insulin properly; creates the inability to transport sugar from the bloodstream into cells.
Other Names	Neurogenic, hypothalamic, pituitary, water diabetes	DM Type A Insulin-dependent IDDM Juvenile-onset diabetes Sugar	DM Type B Non-insulin-dependent NIDDM Adult-onset diabetes Sugar diabetes
Subtypes	Gestational Dipsogenic	N/A	N/A
Causes	Posterior pituitary is destroyed; tumors, infections, head injuries, infiltrations, and various inheritable defects.	Familial, congenital	Familial, acquired
Symptoms	Polydipsia, polyurea, polyphagia	Polydipsia, polyurea, polyphagia, weight loss, and tiredness	Polydipsia, polyurea, polyphagia, weight gain, sometimes asymptomatic
Notes	Rare	Accounts for 10% of DMs	Most common, 90% of all DMs
Danger	Dehydration, rapid heart rate, fatigue, headache, muscle pain, dry mucus membranes.	Too much glucose in the bloodstream and not enough glucose within the cells themselves. Result: cells attempt to derive energy from fat breakdown. Excessive breakdown causes production of harmful byproducts called	Too much glucose in the bloodstream and not enough glucose within the cells themselves. Result: cells attempt to derive energy from fat breakdown. Excessive breakdown causes production of harmful byproducts called

Factors	Diabetes Insipidus	Diabetes Mellitus Type I	Diabetes Mellitus Type II
		ketones. The accumulation of ketones causes the body's pH to become acidic (ketoacidosis), which makes the cellular environment inhospitable for normal metabolic functions. This condition can ultimately become life-threatening and requires aggressive medical therapy.	ketones. The accumulation of ketones causes the body's pH to become acidic (ketoacidosis), which makes the cellular environment inhospitable for normal metabolic functions. This condition can ultimately become life-threatening and requires aggressive medical therapy.
Treatment	DDVAP((desmopressin) Pitressin® (vasopressin) Diapid® (lypressin)	Insulin injections	Diet, exercise, oral hypoglycemics, and lastly with insulin injections
Complications	Dehydration, electolyte imbalance, rapid heart rate, high blood pressure, weight loss, dry skin, muscle pain	Diabetic retinopathy, glaucoma, HTN, renal impairment, neuropathy, heart disease	Diabetic retinopathy, glaucoma, HTN, renal impairment, neuropathy, heart disease

Abnormalities of the Adrenal Gland

Following is a discussion of some of the abnormalities that can occur in conjunction with the adrenal gland. See Table 17-9 (page 369) for an overview of endocrine system disorders.

CUSHING'S SYNDROME

Also known as hypercortisolism or hyperadrenocortism, this syndrome occurs when the body is exposed to high levels of the hormone cortisol for long periods of time. This may occur during long-term or high-stress situations; long-term therapy of glucocorticoid hormones, such as prednisone, for asthma, rheumatoid arthritis, lupus, and other inflammatory diseases; or from immunosuppression after transplantation and overproduction of natural cortisol. Cortisol performs vital tasks in the body by maintaining blood pressure and cardiovascular function, reducing the immune system's inflammatory response, balancing the effects of insulin in breaking down sugar for energy, and regulating the metabolism of proteins, carbohydrates, and fats. One of cortisol's most important jobs is to help the body respond to stress of all kinds. Considered rare, Cushing's Syndrome most commonly affects adults aged 20 to 50, but only affects 10 to 15 people per every million people each year. People at risk are those suffering from depression, alcoholism, malnutrition, and panic disorders who have increased cortisol levels. Symptoms vary and may include the following: upper body obesity, rounded face, increased fat around the neck, and thinning arms and legs. Children tend to be obese, with slowed growth rates. Purplish pink stretch marks may appear on the abdomen, thighs, buttocks, arms, and breasts. There may be weakened bones that fracture easily, fatigue, weak muscles, high blood pressure, and high blood sugar. Irritability, anxiety, and depression are common. Women can have excess hair growth on their face and body, with irregular menstrual cycles that may stop. Men have decreased fertility with diminished or absent libido.

The normal cycle would be as follows:

1. The hypothalamus sends corticotropin releasing hormone, or CRH, to the pituitary gland.

2. This releasing factor asks the pituitary to cause cortisol to be secreted by the adrenal gland.

3. CRH causes the pituitary gland to respond by secreting ACTH, or adrenocorticotropin, a hormone that stimulates the adrenal glands.

4. The adrenals, located just above the kidneys, receive the ACTH and respond by releasing cortisol into the bloodstream.

5. When the amount of cortisol in the blood is sufficient to meet the body's daily needs, the hypothalamus and pituitary release less CRH and ACTH. This is homeostasis.

Other causes of high cortisol relate to overproduction of, and therefore increased signaling to release, ACTH:

Pituitary Adenomas are benign, or noncancerous, tumors of the pituitary gland, which cause the pituitary gland to secrete increased amounts of ACTH. This form of Cushing's Syndrome is known as Cushing's disease, and it affects women more frequently than men, by a ratio of 5:1.

Ectopic ACTH Syndrome arises from benign or malignant (cancerous) tumors that are located outside of the pituitary gland and produce and secrete ACTH. Lung tumors are most common, but tumors of the thymus, pancreatic islet cell, and carcinomas of the thyroid are also known culprits.

Adrenal Tumors—Abnormalities or adrenal adenomas can also cause Cushing's Syndrome. Usual adult onset is 40 years old; most are noncancerous tumors of adrenal tissue, which release excess cortisol into the blood. Adrenocortical carcinomas are the least common cause of Cushing's Syndrome.

Treatment of Cushing's Syndrome varies, depending upon the cause, and ranges from surgery to use of synthetic cortisol to maintain and balance the amount needed in the body. Cortisol inhibitors, such as mitotane, aminoglutethimide, metyrapone, trilostane, and ketoconazole are also used.

ADDISON'S DISEASE

Also called hypocortisolism, this illness occurs in 1 out of 100,000 people when the adrenal glands do not produce enough of the hormone cortisol and, in some cases, the hormone aldosterone. For this reason, the disease is sometimes called chronic adrenal insufficiency. The disease is characterized by weight loss, muscle weakness, fatigue, low blood pressure, and sometimes darkening of the skin. Causes of cortisol deficiency are a lack of ACTH from gradual destruction of the adrenal cortex, the outer layer of the adrenal glands, by the body's own immune system, as seen with an autoimmune disease. This in turn may cause polyendocrine deficiency syndrome, in which many glands are affected. A secondary cause may be the long-term or over-use of glucocorticoids, such as prednisone, for asthma, ulcerative colitis, and rheumatoid arthritis.

The addition of exogenous cortisol sends a negative feedback to the hypothalamus to stop making releasing factor CRH, and, therefore, ACTH is not sent to the adrenal glands. This can be caused when someone suddenly stops taking the glucocorticoids or abruptly interrupts long-term therapy. Another cause is removal of a tumor of, or injury to, the pituitary gland. Symptoms range from darkening of the skin; penetrating pain in the lower back, abdomen, or legs; severe vomiting and diarrhea, followed by dehydration; low blood pressure; to loss of consciousness. Left untreated, an Addison's Disease crisis can be fatal. Treatment is by synthetic cortisol replacement with oral hydrocortisone tablets, taken once or twice a day. If aldosterone is also deficient, it is replaced with oral doses of a mineralocorticoid called fludrocortisone acetate (Florinef), which is taken once a day.

CRETINISM

An underactive thyroid gland, or congenital hypothyroidism, is caused by a lack of fetal or childhood thyroid hormone secretion. Cretinism may also be due to lack of iodine in the diet of the expectant mother, and therefore of the fetus. The result is babies who are born with, or children who later develop, mental retardation and a type of dwarfism. Other symptoms include coarse, dry skin and a slightly swollen tongue. Immediate treatment with synthetic thyroid hormone is imperative.

MYXEDEMA (SECONDARY HYPOTHYROIDISM)

This may also be caused by a deficiency of TH due to a lack of secretion of TSH from the pituitary gland, or lack of TRH from the hypothalamus in an adult. It is common among women. Usual symptoms are a coarse thickening of the skin and roughness that may be open with sores. Treatment includes synthetic thyroid hormone.

GRAVE'S DISEASE

This is also known as thyroid eye disease or thyroid orbitopathy (Figure 17-5). Made known by cartoon character "Popeye," it is characterized by the proptosis or protruding eye and swollen and congested eye muscles, which makes an affected eye appear larger than the other eye. The cause is *not* an overactive thyroid gland, as is commonly believed. Rather, those with Grave's disease often have an overactive thyroid gland, but not always. Grave's disease is an autoimmune disease, in which immune cells attack both the eye muscles and the thyroid, leading to dysfunction of both. Treatment of Grave's disease depends upon the severity of signs and symptoms. Dry eye due to exposure requires nonpreserved, lubricating eye drops. Acute episodes of inflammation result in double vision and optic nerve compression, and therefore corticosteroids such as prednisone are used.

Radiation therapy is also used for optic nerve compression to preserve vision, but, unfortunately, it may result in radiation retinopathy. Only when the disease is under control should surgical orbital decompression be employed to decrease proptosis and strabismus surgery be used to realign the eyes. Of course, the complication of hyperactive thyroid should be addressed with PTU (or propylthiouracil) or Propacil®.

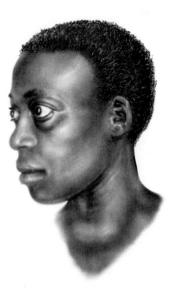

Figure 17-5 Eyes— signature characteristic of Grave's disease

ERECTILE DYSFUNCTION

Male sexual impotence is defined as the inability to sustain an erection for penetration, and it has many causes. A specific sequence of events such as nerve impulses in the brain, spinal column, and area around the penis, and response in muscles, fibrous tissues, veins, and arteries in and near the corpora cavernosa must take place in the proper order, in order for an erection to occur. It is much like a domino effect. Diseases—such as diabetes, kidney disease, chronic alcoholism, multiple sclerosis, atherosclerosis, vascular disease, and neurologic disease—account for about 70 percent of ED cases. Damage from these conditions to nerves, arteries, smooth muscles, and fibrous tissues is the most common cause of ED.

Researchers believe that psychological factors such as stress, anxiety, guilt, depression, low self-esteem, and fear of sexual failure cause 10 to 20 percent of ED cases. Those with an organic physical cause will also experience psychological factors. Smoking, which restricts blood flow in veins and arteries and reduces hormonal (testosterone) secretions, can contribute to ED. Sildenafil helps maintain an erection by blocking the action of an enzyme called phosphodiesterase type 5 in penile tissue. Researchers believe that Viagra (sildenafil) lacks specificity for certain forms of the enzyme phosphodiesterase, specifically type 1 and type 6, and that nonselective blockade of these enzymes may trigger some of the drug's adverse side effects, especially facial flushing and visual disturbances (seeing blue).

Levitra® (vardenafil) hydrochloride was approved in August 2003. Cialis (tadalafil) has been recently approved as of November 2003. Clinical trials proved an 88 percent response in men within 30 minutes and indicated that it lasted in the blood system for up to 24 hours. It has been dubbed the "weekend pill." Early tests show that Cialis® does not affect blood pressure as much as Viagra®. Following sexual stimulation, Cialis works by helping the blood vessels in the penis to relax, allowing the flow of blood into the penis. According to the package insert, Cialis® will not help sexual performance improve if the male does not have erectile dysfunction. Levitra works within 16 minutes, with physical stimulation, while Viagra takes longer, up to one hour. Levitra is to be taken from 30 minutes to 4.5 hours before desired intercourse. Levitra can be taken with food, while Viagra cannot. Levitra and Cialis have no vision or heart side effects.

HYPOTHALAMUS

The hypothalamus sends out releasing factors, or releasing hormones, "RH," to the pituitary gland, which responds by sending tropic, or stimulating, hormones.

1. TRH stimulates TSH.

2. CRH stimulates ACTH.

3. GHRH stimulates GH.

4. Somatostatin inhibits GH.

5. GnRH stimulates both LH and FSH (Gn = Gonadotropin).

PITUITARY GLAND

The pituitary gland, or master gland, sends a signal to the respective gland or body part to initiate its glandular function.

1. TSH stimulates the thyroid gland (thyroid hormone production).

2. FSH/LH stimulate the gonads—the ovaries and testes (gametogenesis and steroid production).

3. Growth hormone is sent to all body parts for linear growth and intermediate metabolism.

4. ACTH is sent to the adrenal gland to cause growth of the adrenal cortex and synthesis and secretion of cortisol.

5. Prolactin causes milk production in mammary glands during the fourth to sixth months of pregnancy and as long as suckling continues. Secretion from mammary glands, or milk lactation, first occurs after childbirth with the signal from oxytocin from the posterior pituitary gland. When dopamine, a prolactin-inhibitory factor, inhibits prolactin, milk is no longer produced or secreted.

Classes of pituitary hormones and their other, more technical names are listed as follows:

1. Somatomammotrophs
   a. Somatotrophs—GH, aka somatotropin
   b. Mammotrophs—aka lactotrophs—PRL

2. Glycoproteins
   a. Thyrotrophs—TSH, aka thyrotropin
   b. Gonadotrophs—LH and FSH
   c. Corticotrophs—ACTH, aka corticotropin
   d. POMC—ACTH, LPH, endorphins (not described in this book)

Disorder	Hormonal Change	Characteristics	Treatment
Gigantism	↑ GH in child	large stature, proportional	(1) Somatostatin analogs such as Sandostatin® = octreotide Somatuline LA® = Long-acting lanreotide Auto-gel SC, which reduces growth hormone secretion. (2) Also less effective dopamine agonists, such as bromocriptine mesylate and cabergoline.
Pituitary Dwarfism	↓ GH in child	small stature, proportional	Growth hormone such as Protopin® = somatrem or Humatrope® = somatropin
Acromegaly	↑ GH in adults	Enlargement of extremities and certain parts of the body, such as hands, feet, legs, arms, chin, head	Somatostatin analogs such as (1) Somatuline LA® = Long-acting lanreotide Auto-gel SC. (2) Octreotide®—synthetic somatostatin (3) Sandostatin® LAR® (octreotide) IM injection, a longer-acting, slow-release form of octreotide
Diabetes Insipidus	↓ ADH	HTN—blood glucose, polydipsia, polyphagia, polyuria	DDVAP® = desmopressin Pitressin® = vasopressin Diapid® = lypressin
Peripheral Edema	↑ ADH	Water and sodium retention, bloating	Exercise, elevate legs and ankles, mild K⁺ sparing diuretics such as spironolactone
Hypothyroidism, AKA Cretinism. Treat with synthetic thyroid hormone or iodine replacement.	↓ TH in child also caused by ↓ iodine in the fetus	Small stature, not proportional, short limbs, may be overweight, dry skin, thick tongue, and large nose.	Post-birth: Immediate treatment with synthetic thyroid hormone is imperative.
Myxedema	↓ TH in adult	Weight gain, cold	Treat with synthetic thyroid hormones: (1) Synthroid®, Levoxyl® = T₄ = L-thyroxine, levothroid, levothyroxine, (2) Cytomel® = triiodothyronine = liothyronine, (3) Armour Thyroid = synthetic desiccated animal thyroid hormones

TABLE 17-9   Endocrine System Disorders

TABLE 17-9   Endocrine System Disorders (*continued*)

Disorder	Hormonal Change	Characteristics	Treatment
Grave's Disease	↑ TH in adult	Weight loss, feels heat or warm	Propacil® = PTU or propylthiouracil
Cushing's Disease	↑ ACTH	May have a moon face, buffalo hump, obese torso	Surgical removal of the pituitary tumor, and possibly cortisol inhibitors such as mitotane, aminoglutethimide, metyrapone, trilostane, and ketoconazole
Cushing's Syndrome	↑ ACTH	May have a moon face, buffalo hump, obese torso	Tx varies due to cause: (1) Synthetic cortisol (2) Cortisol inhibitors such as mitotane, aminoglutethimide, metyrapone, trilostane, and ketoconazole.
Diabetes Mellitus	↓ Insulin	May have HTN, high blood glucose, polydipsia, polyuria, and polyphagia	Type 1—Insulin injections Type 2, diet modification, weight control, regular exercise, and oral hypoglycemic agents. (1) Sulfonylureas stimulate the beta cells to secrete more insulin Orinase = tolbutamide, Diabinese® = chlorpropamide. (2) Meglitinides Prandin® = Repaglinide (3) Biguanides decrease hepatic glucose output, reducing insulin resistance and lowering blood glucose. Glucophage® = metformin (4) Thiazolidinediones reduce insulin resistance and improve insulin sensitivity. (5) Alpha-glucosidase inhibitors block the breakdown of complex carbohydrates and delay the absorption of monosaccharides from the GI tract. Precose® = acarbose Glyset® = miglitol

TABLE 17-9 Endocrine System Disorders (*continued*)

Disorder	Hormonal Change	Characteristics	Treatment
Goiter	↓ Iodine	Enlargement of the thyroid gland in neck	Add iodine to diet
Addison's Disease	↓ Cortisol OR ↓ Aldosterone	Weight loss, muscle weakness, fatigue, low blood pressure	(1) Synthetic cortisol replacement: oral hydrocortisone tablets, Qd or BID. (2) Aldosterone replacement with an oral mineralocorticoid QD: Florinef® = fludrocortisone
Hirsutism	↑ Androgens OR ↑ Testosterone	Facial hair on females, unrelated to menopause	VaniqaTM® = eflornithine cream applied 5 minutes after hair removal.
Erectile Dysfunction	↓ Testosterone	Inability to obtain/maintain erection	Viagra® = sildenafil Levitra® = vardenafil Cialis® = tadalafil

SUMMARY

The endocrine system is a collection of glands that secrete hormones directly into the bloodstream to specific target cells. This system is a very complex one that interacts with many other body systems via the release of hormones that act as "messengers" from one set of cells to another. Some of the main functions of the endocrine system are the regulation of the body's growth, metabolism, and sexual development and function.

The "driving forces" of the endocrine system are the hypothalamus, located in the brain stem, and the pituitary gland, which is attached to the base of the hypothalamus. The hypothalamus directs the pituitary gland which, in turn, controls the thyroid, parathyroid, pancreas, adrenal glands, and the gonads (testes and ovaries). A complete review of these glands and their secretions, and their effects on body systems illustrates how important the endocrine system is to the proper functioning of the body. For example, every cell in the body depends upon thyroid hormone for regulating metabolism.

For the most part, the release of hormones is a "self-regulating" feedback mechanism that acts in a similar way to a "supply and demand" concept. There are many outside factors, however, that can influence the amount of hormones in the body at any given time. Such factors include age, stress, infection, and changes in fluid or mineral balance in the blood, to name a few.

Many of the diseases of the endocrine system discussed in this chapter will be very familiar to you already, i.e., menopause and diabetes (approximately 6.6 percent of the U.S. population suffers from diabetes). Less common disorders such as Grave's disease, Cushing's Syndrome, and Addison's Disease are also described, along with the various treatment modalities used to treat disorders of the endocrine system.

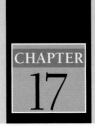

CHAPTER REVIEW QUESTIONS

1. What are the two major structures of the endocrine system that secrete hormones to control other endocrine glands?

2. What is homeostasis? Give one example.

3. Referring to the term Tropic hormones, what does "tropic" mean?
   a. warm
   b. homeostatis
   c. growth
   d. necessary

4. Which growth hormone is known for regulating growth and maintenance of all body tissues?

5. The adrenal cortex secretes two hormones divided into two classes known as:
   a. glucocorticoids and flucocorticosteroids
   b. mineralcorticoids and glucocorticoids
   c. ACTH and FSH
   d. estrogen and progesterone

6. Give three reasons it is necessary to keep appropriate levels of the mineralcorticoids.

7. During sleep, are there more or less of the adrenocorticotropin and cortisol hormones?

8. What effect does estrogen have on cholesterol?
   a. increases HDL and lowers LDL
   b. increases LDL and lowers HDL
   c. increases bad cholesterol and lowers good cholesterol
   d. no effect

9. Dopamine serves as the major prolactin-inhibitiing factor.
   a. true
   b. false

10. What are the two major functions of testosterone.

11. After menopause, estrone is made only in what gland?
    a. pituitary
    b. sebaceous
    c. hypothalamus
    d. adrenal

12. Grave's Disease is often misdiagnosed as what?
    a. overactive thyroid
    b. Cretinism
    c. menopause
    d. acromegaly

Resources and References

1. Carbohydrates: Fuel for Your Brain and Body:
   http://www.iemily.com/Article.cfm?ArtID=274

2. Pfizer package insert for Estring:
   http://www.pfizer.com/download/ppi_estring.pdf

3. Unimed package insert online:
   http://www.unimed.com/pdfs/Anadrol.pdf

4. FDA approves Androgel®:
   http://www.hivandhepatitis.com/recent/hormone/051700.html

5. Anabolic Steroids, by Nick Zaccardi, University of Massachusetts, Amherst, MA:
   http://www.wellnessmd.com/anabolics.html

6. "Interpersonal testosterone transfer after topical application of a newly developed testosterone gel preparation." Clinical Endocrinology (2002) 56, 637–641, 2002 Blackwell Science Ltd, 637:
   http://www.fsdinfo.org/pdf/Interpersonal_testosterone_transfer.pdf

7. Male Breast Cancer, Carol E.H. Scott-Conner, MD, PhD:
   http://aboutplastic.surgery.uiowa.edu/surgery/oncology/malebreastcancer.html

8. UConn Health Center Study Shows Prostate Cancer Patients Benefit from Estrogen Therapy:
   http://www.uchc.edu/ocomm/newsreleases02/jan02/prostatecancer.html

9. Obesity a Factor for More Aggressive Prostate Cancer, Disease Recurrence:
   http://www.mcg.edu/news/2004NewsRel/mterris.html

10. Endometrial Cancer Hormonal Therapy, Publish Date: January 3, 2003: Prolactin.
    http://sharedjourney.com/define/prolactin.html

11. 21st Century Nutrition Prosta-Health for Men:
    http://secure.21stcenturynutrition.net/Stanver/products/prosta.htm

12. Pituitary Dwarfism:
    http://www.ecureme.com/emyhealth/Pediatrics/Pituitary_Dwarfism.asp

13. Acromegaly and Gigantism: A Historical Portrait of a Disease:
    http://www.cladonia.co.uk/acromegaly/ampc.html

14. Medline Pulse: Diabetes Insipidus:
    http://www.nlm.nih.gov/medlineplus/ency/article/000377.htm

15. Medical Supervision of Individuals Using Anabolic-Androgenic Steroid (AAS) for Muscle Growth:
    http://www.mesomorphosis.com/articles/haycock/medically-supervised-steroid-use-02.htm

16. www.mmhs.com/clinical/ adult/english/endocrin/thygland.htm

17. Hitner Nagle *Pharmacology—An Introduction*, 5th Edition. McGraw Hill 2005.

18. Holland, Norman and Michael Patrick Adams. *Core Concepts in Pharmacology*. Upper Saddle River, NJ: Pearson Education, 2003.

19. Adams, M. P., Dianne L. Josephson, and Leland Norman Holland, Jr. *Pharmacology for Nurses—A Pathophysiologic Approach*. Upper Saddle River, NJ: Pearson Education, 2005.

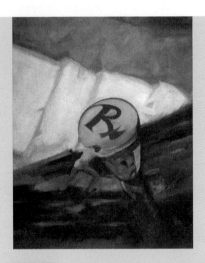

CHAPTER

18

The Reproductive System

Learning Objectives

After completing this chapter, you should be able to:

- List, identify, and diagram the basic anatomical structures and parts of the male and female reproductive systems.

- Describe the functions and physiology of the male and female reproductive systems and the hormones that rule them.

- List and define common diseases affecting the male and female reproductive systems and comprehend the causes, symptoms, and pharmaceutical treatment associated with each disease or condition.

- Explain the mechanisms and comprehend how each class of drugs works for the following reproductive system diseases: BPH, infertility, and vaginal infections.

- Describe and understand the indications for use and mechanisms of action of various contraceptives.

- Define and utilize key terms.

INTRODUCTION

The hormone released by the area of the brain known as the hypothalamus beginning at the onset of sexual maturity in both males and females is the gonadotropin releasing hormone, or GnRH. This hormone, GnRH, is needed for both sexual maturity and normal reproduction. It acts by stimulating the release of luteinizing stimulating hormone, LSH, and follicle-stimulating hormone, FSH, from the anterior pituitary. LSH and FSH act by stimulating the production of sex hormones in the gonads (the testes and ovaries).

The Female Reproductive System

The female reproductive system consists of two ovaries, two fallopian tubes, the uterus, and the vagina.(See Figure 18-1.)

ANATOMY AND PHYSIOLOGY

Reproductive Cycle   The menstrual cycle is made up of two states of being: ovulation and menstruation. An ovary normally matures and releases an egg (ovulation) about 11 to 17 days before the woman's next menstrual period, or approximately once every 28 to 30 days. The egg is released from the ovary into a fallopian tube and swept by tiny hairlike cells (cilia) and smooth muscle action into the uterus. Females are born with about 2 million oocytes, or eggs. By the time of puberty, only about 400,000 eggs remain. About once a month at the beginning of each monthly cycle, FSH causes one of the many underdeveloped ovarian follicles (eggs) to fully develop and mature. As the follicle gets larger, cells that are dedicated to producing the estrogenic hormones estriol, estrone, and estradiol become active.

Estradiol is the most abundant and most active of the estrogens. The main function of estradiol is to stimulate the development of the uterine lining and the mammary glands, readying the body for pregnancy. The estrogens are known as the "feminizing hormones" because they are responsible for the higher voice; breast development; softer, less square-looking shape, or curves; and less muscle, contributing to the appearance that is characteristic of women. Estradiol is the most potent form of estrogen in premenopausal women. Estrone, which accounts for most estrogen in postmenopausal women, is made in very small quantities by the ovaries, but the majority is converted from another

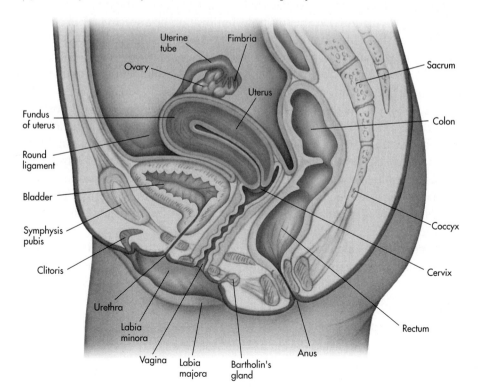

Figure 18-1   The female reproductive system (*Mulvihill, Mary Lou; Zelman, Mark; Holdaway, Paul; Tompary, Elaine; Turchany, Jill,* Human Diseases, A Systemic Approach, *5th Edition,* © 2001. Reprinted with permission of Pearson Education, Inc., Upper Saddle River, NJ)

hormone, androstenedione, in fat and other body tissues. Estriol—a weaker estrogen—is formed when estradiol and estrone are metabolized.

Progesterone, the second major type of female sex hormone made in the ovaries, develops the uterine lining, or endometrium, and the mammary ducts for lactation. In addition, progesterone is important for maintaining the uterine lining if implantation (pregnancy) should occur. Progesterone literally means "hormone for life."

If the female reproductive cycle is considered as a 28-day cycle (the average), during the first 12 days, estrogen has little effect. After that, estrogen is said to have a positive effect on the production of gonadotropins, causing a large increase in LH and a small increase in FSH. The sudden increase of LH causes the mature follicle to release the egg. Next, the ruptured ovarian follicle develops into the corpus luteum. The corpus luteum secretes estrogen and progesterone, which help to make the lining of the uterus strong where the conjoined sperm and egg would implant. If implantation has occurred, there will be continued high levels of estrogen and progesterone, which produces a negative feedback on the secretion of gonadotropins by the anterior pituitary gland, and pregnancy continues. If implantation does not occur, there is no need for progesterone; therefore, production will stop. The lining will shed, and the cycle will begin again. The unfertilized egg dissolves.

Midway through the cycle, after approximately 14 days of development, the follicle ruptures, releasing the egg, or ovum. This is known as ovulation and generally occurs 12–14 days before a woman's next period. If a woman has a 28-day cycle, ovulation occurs around day 14. If a woman has a cycle that is shorter or longer than that, ovulation occurs on a different day (day 7 or day 20), but will generally occur 12–14 days before she has a period. The egg passes into the fallopian tube. It takes about five days before the egg reaches the uterus. This "trip" is known as ovulation. During this time, fertilization by a sperm may occur in the first third of the fallopian tube. If implantation occurs when the egg is still in the fallopian tube, a fallopian (or tubal or ectopic) pregnancy will result. This ectopic pregnancy will require the immediate removal of the fallopian tube and/or ovary, leaving the female with reduced ability to conceive and to make the female hormones. A "slow trip" due to a scarred or clogged fallopian tube is the most common cause of an ectopic or tubal pregnancy. After ovulation, the follicle, which remained in the ovary, undergoes a change. LH (the luteinizing hormone) transforms the follicle into a corpus luteum, which continues to produce estrogen and begins to produce progesterone, the second major type of female sex hormone. A woman is most fertile around the time that she is ovulating. Some women can tell when they are ovulating by watching for changes in vaginal discharge or body temperature. Some women feel pain when the egg is released.

A condition called "PMS," or premenstrual syndrome, occurs during the phase before the periods, which most most women describe as uncomfortable. Other women find that the period itself is the worst part. Some women have both PMS and uncomfortable periods. Symptoms of PMS are as follows:

a. pain or cramping before and during periods
b. weight gain before and during periods, due to water retention or "bloating"
c. moody or irritable feeling before or during periods

d. breakout of acne or pimples before period is due

e. diarrhea, constipation, or upset stomach during periods

Contraceptives

There are several types of chemical contraceptives: estrogen and progesterone combinations and progesterone only (see Table 18-1). There are two main mechanisms of action of these contraceptives, prefertilization and post-fertilization mechanisms, described as follows:

- Major prefertilization mechanisms
  - prevent ovulation
  - thicken cervical mucus to provide a barrier to sperm, reducing likelihood of implantation
- major post-fertilization mechanisms
  - change the lining of the uterus to block implantation of the embryo

While most people define conception as the conjoining of an egg and sperm, it has been said that the blocking of implantation after the conjoining of the egg and sperm is an interference of conception. The low-dose progestins or progestin-only (POPs) contraceptives used to prevent pregnancy are also called minipills. Progestins can prevent fertilization by preventing the egg from fully developing and by thickening the cervical mucus that slows down the flagellation of the sperm (tail movement), preventing the sperm from entering the uterus. BCPs (birth control pills) also lower the midcycle LH and FSH peaks. The "sperm cannot 'swim' through the thick mucus and get into the uterus or fallopian tubes to fertilize the egg."[2] The progestin-only pills are about 93 percent effective; that is, 7 out of 100 women taking a POP will become pregnant each year.

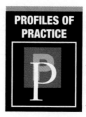

PROFILES OF PRACTICE

The federal law requires that all drugs that contain estrogen *must* be dispensed with the package insert. Therefore, a pharmacy technician must know which drugs contain estrogen. These drugs are usually Birth Control and Hormonal Replacement Therapy agents. Examples are Lo/Ovral®, Orto Evra Patch®, NuvaRing®, Prem-Pro®, and Premarin®.

TABLE 18-1	List of Birth Control Dosage Forms for Women	
Progestin Only Birth Control Pills	**Trade Name**	**Special Notes**
Oral Tablets—POP		
norethindrone tablets	Ortho-Micronor®	Can be given during lactation
norgestrel tablets	Ovrette®	Used normally as BCP. As an emergency contraceptive, 20 tablets are given within 72 hours and repeated within 12 hours.
Subdermal Implants—POP		
levonorgestrel—Implants	Norplant®	
Parenteral—POP		
medroxyprogesterone—injection	Depo-Provera® (1 ml of 150 mg)	Given every 13 weeks (3 months)
Transdermal Patch—POP		
estradiol cypionate/ medroxyprogesterone acetate	Lunelle®	Given monthly, injected into the arm, thigh, or rear.
Emergency Pregnancy Prevention		
levonorgestrel tablets	Plan B®	Used following unprotected intercourse or a suspected contraceptive failure. The first tablet should be taken as soon as possiblewithin 72 hours of intercourse. The second tablet must be taken 12 hours later.

TABLE 18-1 List of Birth Control Dosage Forms for Women (*continued*)

Progestin Only Birth Control Pills	Trade Name	Special Notes
Combination Progestin and Estrogen BCPs Both estrogen and progestin tablets	Alesse®, Levlen®, Lo/Ovral®, Nordette®, OrthoCyclen®, Ortho-Novum 7/7/7®, OrthoTri-Cyclen Lo®, Triphasil-28®, Trivora®, Yasmin®, and Seasonale®	Seasonale®, a new type of BCP, changes the menstrual cycle to have only 4 periods/yr. The active pills are taken 84 days in a row, followed by 7 days of non-hormonal pills. A woman has her period while taking the non-hormonal pills
Transdermal Patch—Combination norelgestromin (progestin) 150 mcg and ethinyl estradiol (estrogen) 20 mcg	Ortho Evra Patch®	Each small adhesive patch lasts 7 days
Vaginal Rings etonogestrel (progestin) 120 mcg and ethinyl estradiol (estrogen) 15 mcg	NuvaRing®	Inserted at home, a small (about 2 inches in diameter), flexible, colorless ring. Releases a continuous low dose of hormones to prevent pregnancy for that month. The ring is used for 3 weeks per month for continuous contraception. The fourth week, the ring is removed, to have a menstrual period. The exact position of the ring in the vagina is not critical for it to work.

Drug–Drug and Drug–Herb Interactions with Birth Control Pills   Antibiotics, antifungal, antiepileptic, and anticonvulsant drugs may interfere with the active ingredients of birth control agents. The drugs and herbs in Table 18-2 prevent the birth control drugs from working well, and the patient may become pregnant.

TABLE 18-2 Drugs and Herbs that Interact with Oral Birth Control

Classification	Examples (only)
Antibiotics	PCNs TCNs Rifampin Sulfa drugs nitrofuantoin (Macrodantin®)
Antifungals	fluconazole (Diflucan®)
Anticonvulsants	Phenobarbital carbamazepine (Tegretol®) primidone (Mysoline)® ethosuximide (Zarontin®) phenytoin (Dilantin®) and others
Herbs	St. John's Wort (herb): Some recent studies suggest that St. John's Wort may reduce the effectiveness of birth control

Note: If these drugs or herbs are taken for only a short period of time, another method of birth control should be used along with the birth control pills. Condoms with spermicide are a good alternative. If they are to be used long-term, the physician should be consulted.

Adverse reactions include the following:

- Side effects: weight gain, mild headaches, breast tenderness, N/V, HTN, decrease of libido
- Topical effects: vaginitis, skin irritation of the vagina, and vaginal discharge
- Toxic effects: SOB, chest pain, stomach or intestinal pain, severe lingering H/A, changes in vision (blurred, flashing lights or diminished vision), post discontinuation infertility for 3–12 months, blood clots (lung, brain/stroke), liver tumors, and gallbladder disease.

Contraindications apply to the following:

- women over age 35 who smoke
- women who are pregnant or suspect pregnancy or who are breastfeeding
- women with unexplained vaginal bleeding
- women with migraines
- women with active liver disease (hepatitis) or a history of liver tumors
- women with breast cancer or a history of breast cancer or of cancer of any reproductive organs
- women with a history of heart disease, stroke, or high blood pressure or blood clotting problems or diabetes
- women with moral objections to birth control that prevents an already conjoined egg and sperm from implantation

Important Note: The latest research shows that the risks of HRT outweigh the benefits, according to the 2002 HERS Study by cardiologist Mark A. Hlatky of Stanford University.

- **Risks:** Estrogen increases the risk of blood clots, gall bladder disease, uterine cancers and breast cancer.

- **Benefits:** Relief from frequent hot flashes is achieved with estrogen hormonal treatment. Hot flashes are sudden episodes of increased uncomfortable warmth, skin flushing, and sweating, which occur in about 70 percent of women during menopause. These hot flashes are sometimes severe enough to cause insomnia, fatigue, and irritability.

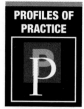

PROFILES OF PRACTICE

A 2000 study found that N–9 spermicides irritate the vaginal and rectal lining, which actually increases the recipient's exposure risk to an STI or HIV. (This study was reported as "Vaginal Microbicides, an Update" at the XIII World Conference on HIV/AIDS, Durban, South Africa, July 12, 2000.) Anyone using a product with N–9 who notices any genital irritation should discontinue use.

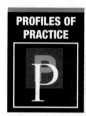

PROFILES OF PRACTICE

Microbicide products are being developed for use either vaginally or rectally to reduce the transmission of HIV and/or STIs. They may become available in many forms, including gels, creams, suppositories, films, a sponge, or a vaginal ring. Some microbicides will also offer contraceptive benefits. Microbicides are not available in 2004, but the public can expect to find microbicides on the market within the next five years.

TOPICAL CONTRACEPTIVES

Spermicides have the active ingredient of nonoxynol–9, which recently (August 2000) has been reported to cause the lining of the vaginal wall to thin or erode faster and may actually help bacteria and viruses to enter the flesh faster, when used often.[3] Spermicides are found in various forms, including creams, foams, gels, suppositories, and vaginal film. Apply and reapply spermicides before coitus (sexual intercourse) no earlier than the time stated on the directions, which varies from 20 minutes to 1 hour. It is important for the female to prevent the spermicide from dripping out of the vagina after intercourse so that it can be effective. While the use of a panty liner may help, lying down for 4–8 hours will better enhance the effectiveness of this product. Also, she should not douche for at least 8 hours after intercourse, because douching may interfere with the effectiveness of the spermicide. Spermicidal foam, the most effective spermicide, helps prevent pregnancy in two ways: The foam forms a physical barrier to the entry of sperm into the cervix, and the spermicide immobilizes and kills the sperm. Simple skin irritations and allergies to the ingredients other than the active ingredient can deter use, along with anticipation of coitus. Gels must be reapplied if not used within 20 minutes before intercourse. Vaginal filmstrips are good for one hour after insertion.

CONTRACEPTIVE DEVICES

Barrier Devices: Condoms—lamb intestine condoms do not provide protection from STDs or STIs. Latex condoms are the best for effective protection from transmission of bacterial and viral infections. The main drawback of these is allergic reactions by either the female or the male. Polyurethane condoms should be used if either partner is allergic to latex. Some condoms also contain a spermicide.

Condoms should never be used with greasy or oily substances such as vaseline, because these substances will cause the condom to weaken and burst. Personal water-based lubricants such as K-Y jelly are made for this purpose.

Female condoms—A polyurethane tube or sheath approximately 6.5 inches long, with an inner ring at the closed end that loosely lines the vagina, provides protection from unintended pregnancy and the transmission of STIs, including HIV/AIDS. This material does not cause allergies and does not have to be removed immediately after ejaculation. But it should be taken out before the woman stands up to avoid the semen spilling out. Upon removal, the outer ring should be twisted to seal the condom, so that no semen leaks out. Current standard directions indicate that it should only be used one time; however, clinical trials are underway to investigate multiple usage or re-use. It can be used with either oil- or water-based lubricants. The simultaneous use of both condoms is contraindicated because the condoms may cause friction, resulting in either or both condoms slipping or tearing, and/or the outer ring of FC being pushed inside the vagina (see Table 18-3).

TABLE 18-3 Male and Female Condom Comparison Chart

Male Condom	Female Condom
Brands: Trojan®, Lifestyles®, Durex®, Magnum®	Brands: Female Condom®, Reality® Femidom®, Dominique®, Femy®, Myfemy®
Nickname: Rubber	Nickname: FC
Rolled on the man's penis, fits snugly on the penis	Inserted into the woman's vagina, loosely lines the vagina
Lubricant: • Can include spermicide • Can be water-based only; cannot be oil-based • Located on the outside of condom	Lubricant: • Can include spermicide • Can be water-based or oil-based • Located on the inside and outside of condom
Requires erect penis	Does not require erect penis, can be inserted prior to sexual intercourse, not dependent on erect penis
Must be removed immediately after ejaculation	Does not need to be removed immediately after ejaculation, must be removed before the female stands.
Covers most of the penis and protects the woman's internal genitalia	Provides broader protection by covering both the woman's internal and external genitalia and the base of the man's penis.
Latex condoms can decay if not stored properly.	Polyurethane is not susceptible to deterioration from temperature or humidity.
Can be used *only* one-time, then discarded	Recommended as a one-time use product. Re-use research is currently underway. A WHO update in July 2002 is available at www.who.int/reproductive-health/rtis/reuse.en.html.
Disadvantage: must interrupt foreplay to use.	Can be inserted before foreplay, and intercourse occurs without interrupting foreplay.
Easy placement.	Disadvantage: Takes a while for the female to learn how to use it confidently. Takes practice. Makes a noise that can be silenced with use of more lubricant.

DIAPHRAGMS AND CERVICAL CAPS

Only a trained health-care provider must fit a woman for these devices. The size of the diaphragm is determined by a measurement of the vagina taken by the provider to securely fit. It matches the distance from the pubic bone to the posterior fornix of the vagina, or the largest size that is comfortable for the client. Cervical caps come in four sizes. A cap that is too small can injure the cervix, and one that is too large can slip off during intercourse. These devices may need refitting if a woman undergoes any of the following changes:

- gains or loses weight
- has a baby
- has 2nd or 3rd trimester abortion

These devices can also be used with spermicides. Diaphragms must be worn for at least six hours after intercourse. Since rubber deteriorates, the devices need to be periodically checked for small holes and replaced accordingly.

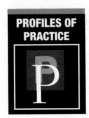

INTRAUTERINE DEVICES

Intrauterine devices (IUDs) are small, flexible devices composed of metal and/or plastic. These devices are inserted into a woman's uterus through her vagina during a doctor's visit. Approximately 15 percent of women of reproductive age currently use IUDs. These devices work to prevent pregnancy by a combination of mechanisms. They inhibit sperm migration in the upper female genital tract, which in turn inhibits ovum transport, and stimulates endometrial changes that will not support implantation. Most are unmedicated, but some are progestin-releasing IUDs (levonorgestrel or progesterone). These are safe for 5–10 years. IUDs have one drawback: They tend to cause heavy menstrual bleeding. These devices are 97 to 99.6 percent effective.

STDs—Sexually Transmitted Diseases

A sexually transmitted disease (STD) is a disease caused by a pathogen (for example, virus, bacterium, parasite, or fungus) that is spread from person to person primarily through sexual contact. STDs may also be referred to as sexually transmitted infections (STIs). They can be painful, irritating, debilitating, and sometimes life threatening. To date, there have been more than 20 sexually transmitted diseases identified.

STDs occur most commonly in sexually active teenagers and young adults. The risk of contracting an STD increases in those who engage in sex with multiple partners. It is estimated that approximately 200 to 400 million people worldwide are infected. STDs do not discriminate and are found among men and women of all economic classes.

STDs that have been identified include the following:

- bacterial vaginosis (change in the normal bacteria of the vagina)
- chlamydia trachomatis (bacterium that can cause an STI)
- genital warts (wart-like bumps)
- gonorrhea (bacterium that can cause an STI)
- hepatitis B (liver disease)
- hepatitis C (liver disease)
- herpes (virus)
- HIV/AIDS (Acquired Immune Deficiency Syndrome)
- lice and crabs (parasites)
- molluscum (viral infection)
- PID (Pelvic Inflammatory Disease)
- syphilis (bacterial infection)
- trichomonas (parasite)
- vaginal yeast (fungal infection)

Many STDs do not cause much harm or severe symptoms. However, some produce persistent asymptomatic or minimally symptomatic disease. The disease may be carried by some people for days, weeks, or even longer. During this time, an infected individual, or carrier, can spread disease.

Complications of STD infection include the following conditions:

- pelvic inflammatory disease (PID)
- inflammation of the cervix (cervicitis) in women
- inflammation of the urethra (urethritis)
- inflammation of the prostate (prostatitis) in men
- fertility and reproductive system problems in both sexes
- possible consequences to an infant infected while in the womb or during birth, including stillbirth, blindness, and permanent neurological damage

A person infected with an STD is more likely to become infected with HIV, and a person infected with HIV and another STD is more likely to transmit HIV.

Treatment and Prevention of STDs

The only sure way to avoid becoming infected with an STD is to practice monogamy with an uninfected partner. Viral STDs, such as genital herpes (HSV) and human immunodeficiency virus (HIV), can have symptoms managed with medication, but cannot be cured. Bacterial STDs, such as gonorrhea and chlamydia, can be cured with antibiotics. Fungal (such as vaginal yeast infection) and parasitic (such as trichomoniasis) diseases can be cured with antifungal and antihelminthic agents, respectively. Early diagnosis and treatment increase the chances for cure.

Mammary Glands and Childbirth

During the fourth or fifth month of gestation, prolactin is secreted by the pituitary gland. Prolactin causes the mammary, or "milk," glands to produce milk in the breast before the baby is born. Once the baby is born, the continued action of sucking on the nipple stimulates the pituitary gland to continue to secrete more prolactin, thus making more milk.

Oxytocin, secreted by the posterior pituitary gland, causes labor contractions. Immediately after the baby leaves the birth canal, oxytocin allows the milk that has been made by the signal of prolactin to be secreted. Once the baby is born, further sucking also causes oxytocin to be secreted by the posterior pituitary gland and causes the milk ducts to contract and relax, pushing the milk towards the nipple. Therefore, prolactin causes milk production, while oxytocin allows the milk secretion.

Current research shows that oxytocin may be responsible for the "bonding" attraction between mother and child, as well as between life partners. An example of oxytocin is Pitocin (used to induce labor).

At the end of the ovarian cycle (day 28), the corpus luteum will disintegrate if fertilization of the egg has not occurred, and the production of the female hormones estrogen and progesterone stops. Absence of the two hormones will cause the uterine lining to shed. This shedding begins what is known as menstruation. Simultaneously, a new follicle in the ovary begins to develop, and the cycle repeats again. Somewhere roughly between the ages of 40 and 55, the ovaries stop producing estrogen and progesterone, and monthly menstruation ceases. One year from the last period, or menstrual cycle, is known as menopause.

If, instead, pregnancy does occur, the corpus luteum continues to produce estrogen and progesterone until the placenta is developed, around day 12. The placenta, acting as an endocrine gland, then assumes the role of producing the hormones. The transitionary critical time usually occurs and is completed between the second and third month of pregnancy. If the corpus luteum disintegrates before the placenta can maintain the correct hormone level, the uterine lining, along with a fetus, will rupture and shed. This rupture causes hemorrhage, and the end result is known as a miscarriage.

During pregnancy, the levels of estrogen and progesterone are high. Constant high levels of estrogen and progesterone will continue to inhibit the release of FSH and LH. Therefore, during pregnancy no other follicle can develop; or, in other words, another egg will not mature and become released. The mechanism of action of oral contraceptives, transdermal contraceptive patch, and injectable hormonal contraceptive is to maintain a high level of hormone in the blood. The hormonal contraceptive will prevent the release of FSH by imitating what happens during pregnancy, preventing the development of another follicle or follicles. There is no egg available for fertilization.

LACTATION

Many other hormones, such as follicle stimulating hormone (FSH), luteinizing hormone (LH), prolactin, oxytocin, and human placental lactogen (HPL), also play vital roles in milk production.

Infertility

Infertility is the failure of a specific couple to conceive after one year of regular, unprotected intercourse. Infertility may occur as a result of a problem in either partner or because of a combination of problems in both partners.

DISEASE STATE, CAUSES, SYMPTOMS, OUTCOME IF LEFT UNTREATED

About 35 percent of all cases of infertility stem from problems in the man's system; another 35 percent arise from abnormalities in the woman's system; and about 20 percent of the time, both the man and the woman have fertility problems. In about 10 percent of the cases, no cause can be found. It is known that age often increases the risk of infertility. (See Figure 18-2.)

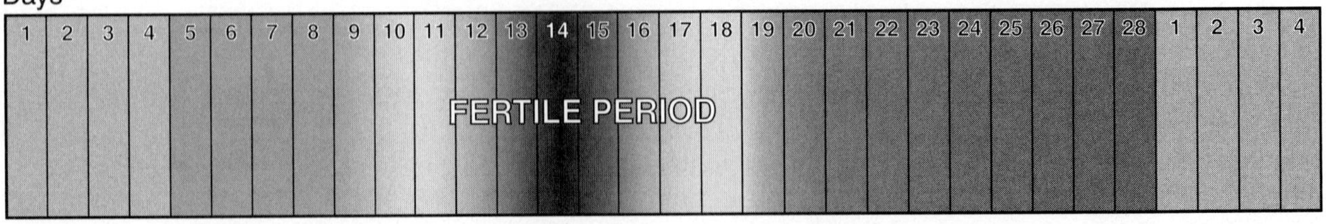

Days

FERTILE PERIOD

1 2 3 4 5 6 7 8 9 10 11 12 13 14 15 16 17 18 19 20 21 22 23 24 25 26 27 28 1 2 3 4

Figure 18-2   Fertility and the menstrual cycle

CAUSES OF INFERTILITY IN WOMEN

Pelvic Inflammatory Disease (PID) is the major cause of infertility worldwide, causing scarring, abscess formation, and tubal damage that result in infertility. PID is the most common cause of infertility worldwide. PID is an infection of the pelvis or one or more of the reproductive organs, including the *ovaries*, the *fallopian tubes*, the cervix, or the uterus. It may spread to the appendix or to the entire pelvic area. PID usually is caused by the same bacteria that cause sexually transmitted diseases or infections, such as gonorrhea or chlamydia. Chlamydia causes 75 percent of fallopian tube infections. PID may also develop from bacteria that thrive during abortion, hysterectomy, childbirth, sexual intercourse, use of an intrauterine (IUD) contraceptive device, or a ruptured appendix.

Spontaneous abortion has been associated with use of an electric blanket during the month of conception. Exposure to high levels of chemicals, toxic substances, high temperatures, and radiation, and persistent stress can lead to infertility. Along with smoking cigarettes and marijuana and taking caffeine and other drugs, many factors can lead to infertility.

Age—A woman's age (more accurately, the age of the eggs) can contribute to infertility. At age 25, the chance of getting pregnant within the first six months of trying to conceive is 75 percent; but it lowers to only 22 percent at age 40. This decrease in fertility appears to be caused by a higher rate of chromosomal abnormalities that occurs in the eggs as the woman ages.

Weight—30 percent of estrogen is made in fat cells; however, overweight patients have an overload of estrogen that throws off the reproductive cycle. Likewise, strict vegetarians, athletes, and dancers also have difficulties if they lack vitamin B12, zinc, iron, and folic acid. These deficiencies can lead to irregular periods and possibly complete shutting down of the reproductive process.

Endometriosis—A condition in which fragments of the lining of the uterus are found in other parts of the pelvic cavity. These pieces of endometrium respond to the menstrual hormonal cycle slowly increasing in number and size. Because the blood cannot escape, it builds up and leads to the development of small or large painful cysts, causing scarring and inflammation.

Hormonal changes in the female—About one-third of infertility cases can be traced to ovulation and hormonal problems.

Progesterone deficiency—Progesterone keeps the lining ready to accept implantation. Without it, or with decreased levels, implantation cannot occur, or an implanted embryo may abort.

Polycystic ovarian syndrome (PCO)—Occurs in six percent of women and is the major cause of infertility in American women. PCO increases androgen production, producing high LH levels and low FSH levels. This prevents the maturing of an egg, which does not get released. Inflammation and edema occur in the fallopian tube, creating a cyst, which creates more cysts.

Elevated prolactin levels—In women who are not lactating inhibit ovulation, and it may also indicate a pituitary tumor. Parlodel® is the drug of choice.

Medications—Certain medications can cause temporary infertility, such as prescription antibiotics, antidepressants, hormones, and narcotic analgesics, and OTC medications such as ASA and ibuprofen (when taken midcycle). Taking acetaminophen regularly may reduce estrogen and luteinizing hormone levels. In most cases, once the drugs are discontinued, fertility is often restored.

Antibodies to sperm—Some women have antibodies to sperm that attack them as if they were foreign bodies or substances.

PHARMACEUTICAL TREATMENT OF INFERTILITY IN WOMEN

If infertility persists untreated, it may affect the couple, breaking down communication as one or both partners feels guilty and depression sets in. Having to have intercourse at specific times of the menstrual cycle and times in which the female has a specific basal temperature can add more stress.

An example of an antiestrogenic drug is the fertility drug: Clomiphene = CLOMID® Serophene® = antiestrogenic non-steroidal antiestrogen.

Clomiphene tricks the brain and pituitary gland into "thinking" that there is less estrogen around. This stimulates pituitary production of FSH and LH, boosting follicle growth and the release of the egg.

Side effects include hot flashes, breast tenderness, mood swings, visual problems, thick cervical mucus, and luteal phase deficiency. The time from ovulation to onset of the next period is known as the "luteal phase," during which the "corpus luteum" (yellow body), the area where the egg was released, makes progesterone. Progesterone prepares the uterine lining for embryo implantation. A luteal phase deficiency or a short luteal phase occurs with a lack of progesterone production by the corpus luteum, or poor response of the endometrium to normal progesterone levels. This lack of progesterone or response to it may cause infertility.

Toxic effects: Long-term safety: Use for more than a year may increase the risk of ovarian cancer. The risk of multiple births and low birth weight increases with the use of fertility drugs.

The Male Reproductive System

ANATOMY

The prostate is situated at the base of the bladder and encircles the urethra. The organ is roughly the size and shape of a large walnut, with an average normal weight of 20–30 g. Secretions produced in the prostatic glands empty into the urethra during ejaculation via the prostatic ducts to make up a sizable volume of the ejaculate. While it is not fully understood what the function of this fluid is, it is speculated that the most likely functions include neutralization of the acidic environment in the vagina, and possibly providing a nutritional role for the spermatids (young sperm cells). While not absolutely necessary for fertilization, prostate solutions increase the chances of fertilization. A pair of organs which are located in the scrotum, thin mesothelial membrane, are responsible for the production of sperm, as well as the production of androgens. The testes are made up of thousands of tiny tubules supported by fibrous septae, and the entire gland is surrounded by a

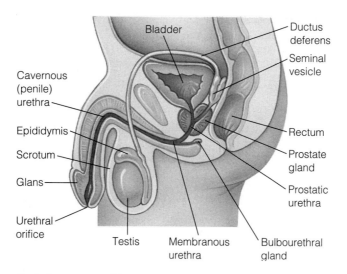

Figure 18-3 The male reproductive system (*Mulvihill, Mary Lou; Zelman, Mark; Holdaway, Paul; Tompary, Elaine; Turchany, Jill, Human Diseases, A Systemic Approach, 5th Edition, © 2001. Reprinted with permission of Pearson Education, Inc., Upper Saddle River, NJ)*

Labels on figure: Bladder, Ductus deferens, Seminal vesicle, Cavernous (penile) urethra, Epididymis, Rectum, Scrotum, Prostate gland, Glans, Prostatic urethra, Urethral orifice, Testis, Membranous urethra, Bulbourethral gland

thick fibrous capsule called the tunica albuginea. Mature sperm are stored in the epididymis. During ejaculation, the sperm are propelled along the vas deferens into the urethra.

DISEASES OF THE MALE REPRODUCTIVE TRACT

Infertility in Men Fertility in the male begins with the production of *gonadotropin-releasing hormone (GnRH)* in the hypothalamus, which instructs the pituitary gland to manufacture *follicle-stimulating hormone (FSH)* and *luteinizing hormone (LH)*. FSH causes sperm production, and LH stimulates the production of the male hormone *testosterone*. Both sperm and testosterone production occur in the *testicles*, or testes. The testicles are contained in the scrotal sac, also known as the *scrotum* where sperm are manufactured in the several hundred microscopic *seminiferous tubules*. The *Leydig cells* surround these tubules and manufacture testosterone. The life cycle of sperm is about 70–75 days. The ability of a sperm to move forward rapidly and straight, attained by its tail, known as flagella, is probably the most important factor that determines male fertility. During sexual excitement, nerves stimulate the muscles in the epididymis to contract, forcing the sperm into the vas deferens, and then through the penis. The seminal vesicles, clusters of tissue, contribute seminal fluid to the sperm. The vas deferens also collects fluid from the nearby *prostate gland*. The mixture of the fluids from the seminal vesicles, prostate gland, and the sperm is called *semen*. The two vas deferens join together to form the *ejaculatory duct*, containing the semen, which now passes down through the *urethra*. The urethra is the same pathway in the penis through which urine passes. During orgasm in a healthy male, the prostate closes off the bladder so urine cannot enter the urethra. The semen is forced through the urethra during *ejaculation*, the final stage of orgasm. Of the 100 to 300 million sperm that are in the ejaculate, about 400 survive the acid environment of the vagina, and only about 40 reach the egg.

Specific causes of infertility in men are listed as follows (see Table 18-4):

1. Smoking impairs sperm motility, reducing sperm lifespan.

2. Poor nutrition, with a deficiency of vitamin C, selenium, zinc, and folate, in particular, can contribute.

TABLE 18-4	Causes of Male Infertility	
Category	Medical Name	Description/Comment
Low sperm count—most common cause	oligospermia	Sperm count is less than 10 million sperm/mL of semen. Causes of temporary and permanent low sperm count vary and are numerous.
No sperm	azoospermia	Complete absence of sperm. This is relatively rare, affecting less than 1% of all men and 10% to 15% of infertile men. Causes: Obstruction or production failure of sperm in the testes, which can be caused by mumps, genetic disorders, radiation, or exposure to chemicals.
Low-quality sperm	dysspermia	Quality is determined by sperm motility (ability to move), due to its flagella or its morphology (shape and structure). The quality of the sperm is usually more significant than the count.
No semen production	aspermia	Ejaculation does not secrete any semen.

3. Bicycling causes pressure from the bike seat, which may damage blood vessels and nerves that are responsible for erections. Biking can expose the perineum to extreme shock and vibrations, increasing the risk for injuries to the scrotum.

4. Oxygen-Free Radicals (Oxidants). Unstable particles are released as a byproduct of many natural chemical processes in the body, such as infection. These oxidants negatively affect DNA in the sperm.

5. Chemicals—Exposure to pesticides, phylates (DEHP) used to soften plastics, hydrocarbons (benzene, ethylbenzene toluene, and xylene) can be a factor. Quality may be affected by exposure to heavy metals such as lead, cadmium, or arsenic.

6. Hypogonadism—Severe deficiency in gonadotropin-releasing hormone (GnRH), the hormone that signals the release of testosterone and other important reproductive hormones may play a role. Low levels of testosterone may result in defective sperm production. Tumors of the pituitary gland may also affect GnRH, FSH, or LSH levels.

7. Autoantibodies caused by infections or injury—the body thinks that the sperm are invading foreign bodies and creates antibodies to destroy them.

8. Retrograde ejaculation occurs when the muscles of the urethra do not propel the semen properly during orgasm. The sperm are forced

backward into the bladder instead of forward out of the urethra. Retrograde ejaculation is the consequence of several conditions, including diabetes, HTN, MS, spinal cord injury, tranquilizers, and HTN medication.

9. Cryptorchidism, associated with mild to severely impaired sperm production, is a failure of the testes to descend from the abdomen into the scrotum during fetal development. The testes are exposed to the higher degree of internal body heat.

Medications that Contribute to Male Infertility   Anabolic steroids, often abused by weight lifters and other athletes, severely impair sperm production. Other drugs that affect male fertility are the following:

- cimetidine (Tagamet®)
- sulfasalazine (Azulfidine®)
- methadone (Dolophine®)
- methotrexate (Folex®)
- phenytoin (Dilantin®)
- spironolactone (Aldactone®)
- thioridazine (Mellaril®)
- calcium channel blockers
- colchicine
- corticosteroids

Drugs that can treat male infertility caused by hormornal changes include the following:

Antibiotics—Infections interfering with infertility may be treated with antibiotics.

Antihistamines—Studies report that non-drowsy antihistamines that block mast cells may be beneficial for some cases of low sperm count. Mast cells release inflammatory immune factors that may reduce sperm quality. Overseas studies reported improved pregnancy rates with two agents, ebastine and tranilast. Similar antihistamines in the United States are cetirizine (Zyrtec®), fexofenadine (Allegra®), and loratidine (Claritin®).

Anti-erectile dysfunction agents (sildenafil (Viagra®), vardenafil (Levitra®), and tadalafil (Cilalis®)) may enhance fertility by increasing sperm motion and capacitation (the explosion of energy in the sperm that aids the act of fertilization).

Bromocriptine (Parlode®) is used to reduce excess prolactin manufactured by the pituitary in some infertile men.

Gonadotropin-releasing hormone (GnRH) is beneficial for men with gonadotropin deficiency and hypogonadism, and it is good for restoring sperm production post-chemotherapy.

Benign Prostatic Hypertrophy   Because of the relationship of the proximal urethra to the prostate, the urethra is susceptible to pressure from hyperplastic enlargement of the prostate. The prostate may be divided into anatomical zones: The centrally located zones are prone to hyperplasia in older men, while the peripheral zone is much more frequently affected by carcinoma.

As men get older, the prostate gland enlarges. Such an enlargement is called benign prostatic hyperplasia, or BPH. This is a benign, noncancerous growth. BPH is the most common benign tumor in men over the age of 50. The enlargement causes the following problems:

1. difficult urination called prostatismurinary problems

2. urinary blockage, urinary retention, or the inability to urinate

3. urinary frequency, a feeling of incomplete voiding, the sensation of incomplete bladder emptying

Other symptoms include hesitancy or slow initiation of urination (slow start), decreased force of the urinary stream (weak stream), and intermittence (stopping and starting) of the urinary stream. A variety of other symptoms may include frequent urination, nocturia (nighttime urination), and urgency to urinate.

Changes caused by prostate enlargement are gradual and may often be ignored by the patient. It is thought that from 20 to 30 percent of men will need medical or surgical treatment of BPH before they reach the age of 80.

Pharmaceutical Treatment of BPH   *5-Alpha reductase inhibitors*, such as finasteride (Proscar®) and dutasteride (Avodart™), prevent the conversion of testosterone to the hormone dihydrotestosterone (DHT). A treatment period of six months may be necessary to see if the therapy is going to work. Finasteride is available in tablet form, and dutasteride is available as soft gelatin capsules. These are taken orally once a day. Patients should see their physician regularly to monitor side effects and adjust the dosage, if necessary.

Side effects—Include reduced libido, impotence, breast tenderness and enlargement, and reduced sperm count. Long-term risks and benefits have not been studied.

Teratogenic effects—Women who may be pregnant must avoid handling dutasteride capsules and broken or crushed finasteride tablets. Exposure to the drugs may cause serious side effects to the male fetus. Intact tablets are coated to prevent absorption through the skin during normal handling. To prevent pregnant women from being exposed to the drug and teratogenic effects through blood transfusion, patients should wait at least six months after treatment with an 5-Alpha reductase inhibitor, to donate blood.

Alpha blockers relax smooth muscle tissue in the bladder neck and prostate, which increases urinary flow. They typically are taken orally, once or twice a day.

Commonly prescribed alpha blockers include the following:

- alfuzosin (UroXatral™), extended-release tablet taken once daily
- doxazosin (Cardura®), tablet taken once daily
- prazosin (Minipress®), capsules, one BID or TID

- tamsulosin hydrochloride (Flowmax®), capsules one QD
- terazosin (Hytrin®), capsules, one QD

Side effects include headache, dizziness, low blood pressure, fatigue, weakness, and difficulty breathing.

Non-pharmaceutical Treatment of BPH   *Prostatic stents* can be used to push back the surrounding tissue and widen the urethra. It can take less than 15 minutes to insert a stent, and it is done with regional or local anesthesia. The patient is usually discharged the same day or the next morning. It is necessary to remove one-third of all urethral stents because they may cause pain upon urination, or incontinence.

SUMMARY

The reproductive system is made up of internal reproductive organs, associated ducts, and external genitalia. Its primary function is the reproductive process. Sex hormones are produced in the gonads (in males, the testes, and in females, the ovaries).

While there are many diseases that can affect the reproductive system, as a pharmacy technician, you will most frequently encounter those conditions involving infertility, sexually transmitted diseases (STDs), and vaginal infections. The causes and treatments of these diseases are discussed in detail in this chapter.

You will also learn about the indications of use and the mechanism of action of various contraceptives. Of particular importance to you will be the drug interactions associated with the use of birth control pills.

CHAPTER REVIEW QUESTIONS

1. The most fertile time during the reproductive cycle is:
   a. day 1–day 14
   b. day 20
   c. mid-cycle, usually day 12–14
   d. end of the cycle

2. The main function of estradiol is:
   a. to stimulate the development of the uterine lining and the mammary glands
   b. to get the female's body ready for pregnancy
   c. to start menstruation, or the "period"
   d. A and B only

3. While estradiol stimulates the readying for pregnancy, progesterone is:
   a. the hormone for life
   b. the feminizing hormone
   c. maintaining the uterine lining if implantation should occur
   d. A and C only

4. Which hormone causes sperm and the ovum to develop and mature?
   a. FSH
   b. FCH
   c. LSH
   d. LH

5. Progestin or progesterone-only birth control pills, known as POPs, prevent:
   a. major pre-fertilization mechanisms such as ovulation and thickening of the cervical mucus to provide a barrier to sperm, reducing likelihood of implantation
   b. major post-fertilization mechanisms such as changes in the lining of the uterus to block implantation of the embryo

   c. major post-fertilization mechanisms such as ovulation and changes in the lining of the uterus to block implantation of the embryo
   d. major pre-fertilization mechanisms such as ovulation and changes in the lining of the uterus to block implantation of the embryo

6. Prolactin is secreted by the pituitary gland and makes the milk during the 4th and 5th months of pregnancy, while oxytocin is released during labor and allows the milk to flow through the mammary ducts post partum.
   a. true
   b. false

7. Spermatids develop into mature sperm in the:
   a. prostate gland
   b. penis
   c. epididymis
   d. chromosomes

8. Fertility in the male begins with the production of
   a. gonadotropin-releasing hormone (GnRH) in the hypothalamus
   b. follicle-stimulating hormone (FSH) from the pituitary gland
   c. luteinizing hormone (LH) from the pituitary gland
   d. both FSH and LH from the pituitary gland

9. What is the main factor that causes BPH?
   a. race
   b. age
   c. HTN
   d. diabetes

10. What occurs in BPH?
    a. The prostate gland enlarges.
    b. The neck of the bladder narrows.

c. frequent urination, nocturia, and urination hesitancy

d. all of the above

11. BPH can be treated with:

a. cardiac stents

b. 4–alpha reductase inhibitors

c. Alpha blockers

d. Beta blockers

12. Side effects of Alpha blockers are:

a. H/A, dizziness, and HTN

b. H/A, dizziness, and hypotension

c. H/A, fatigue, and hypertension

d. SOB, fatigue, and HTN

13. 5-Reductase Inhibitors such as Proscar® and Avodart®:

a. cause the conversion of testosterone to the hormone dihydrotestosterone (DHT)

b. prevent the conversion of testosterone to the hormone dihydrotestosterone (DHT)

c. convert DHT to testosterone

d. prevent the conversion of DHT to FSH

14. Which of the following may be used to treat BPH?

a. finasteride (Proscar®) and dutasteride (Avodart™)

b. finasteride (Avodart™) and dutasteride (Proscar®)

c. finesteride (Proscar®) and dutasteride (Avodart™)

d. finasteride (Proscar®) and dutesteride (Avodart™)

15. List the parts of the male and female reproductive systems, and give a brief explanation of each system.

Resources and References

1. When Do Humans Begin?
http://www.abortiontv.com/WhenDoHumanBeings.htm#I.%20Introduction
HYPERLINK "http://www.muschealth.com/breast/normal.htm"

2. http://www.uwo.ca/pathol/Path240/malegenital-03.ca.pdf

3. http://www.muschealth.com/breast/normal.htm

4. http://www.oxytocin.org/oxytoc/

5. http://www.muschealth.com/breast/normal.htm

6. Progestin-Only Birth Control Pills
http://scc.uchicago.edu/progestinbcpills.htm
http://patienteducation.upmc.com/Pdf/BirthControlPoc.pdf

7. CDC Statement on Study Results of Product Containing Nonoxynol-9, released at the XIII International AIDS Conference held in Durban, South Africa, July 9–14, 2000.
http://www.cdc.gov/mmwr/preview/mmwrhtml/mm4931a4.htm

8. Find Law on Estrogen and Package Inserts
   http://caselaw.lp.findlaw.com/scripts/getcase.pl?court=ny&vol=i99&in
   vol=0168

9. Shands at the University of Florida
   http://www.shands.org/professional/drugs/bulletins/0601.pdf

10. FDA Dockets of non-contraceptive, estrogen-containing drugs
    http://www.fda.gov/OHRMS/DOCKETS/98fr/092799d.txt
    http://a257.g.akamaitech.net/7/257/2422/14mar20010800/edocket.acc
    ess.gpo.gov/cfr_2002/aprqtr/pdf/21cfr310.517.pdf

11. Holland, Norman and Michael Patrick Adams. *Core Concepts in
    Pharmacology*. Upper Saddle River, NJ: Pearson Education, 2003.

12. Adams, Michael Patrick, Dianne L. Josephson, and Leland Norman
    Holland, Jr. *Pharmacology for Nurses—A Pathophysiologic Approach*.
    Upper Saddle River, NJ: Pearson Education, 2005.

Things to Do

13. Watch video on women's reproductive cycle and how the pill works.
    http://www.cnn.com/2000/HEALTH/women/12/14/contraceptives.ap/

The Nervous System

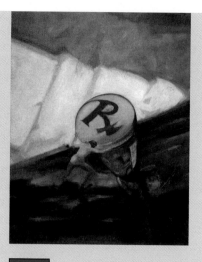

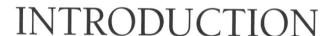

Learning Objectives

After completing this chapter, you should be able to:

- List, identify, and diagram the basic anatomical structure and parts of the basic unit of the nervous system and create a flow chart of the divisions of the peripheral and central nervous systems.

- Describe the function or physiology of neurons and nerve transmission and the various neurotransmitters.

- List and define common diseases affecting the nervous system and comprehend the causes, symptoms, and pharmaceutical treatment associated with each disease.

- Explain the mechanisms or conditions and comprehend how each class of drugs work in order to mitigate symptoms of the following nervous system diseases: mood disorders, Parkinson's, dementia and Alzheimer's disease, anxiety, insomnia, epilepsy, ADHD, schizophrenia, cancer, and severe pain.

- Describe and understand the paradigm effect of the use of stimulants for attention deficit disorder in children.

- Discuss the various uses of benzodiazepines and how they work in the body.

- Define and utilize key terms.

INTRODUCTION

There are two systems that control the body functions by communication with the billions of cells in the human body in order to keep it alive: the nervous system and the endocrine system (see Chapter 17). The endocrine system communicates in a slow manner via chemicals called hormones that are secreted by ductless glands into the circulatory system and carried by the blood to muscles, glands, and various other parts of the body. By contrast, the nervous system communicates messages very quickly through nerve impulses conducted from one part of the body to another by the transmission of chemicals called neurotransmitters from one nerve cell to another. The nervous system is complex and one of the least understood parts of the body.

Anatomy of the Nervous System

At its core, the brain has billions of individual connecting pieces and makes trillions of connections. It works on electrochemical energy, which allows a person to read this book, smile at a friend, remember a computer password or social security number, and decide between eating fish or chicken. The brain also controls emotions, sex drive, heart rate, breathing and respiration, appetite, and sleep. The specific function of these pieces known as nerve cells or neurons is to allow the brain to learn, reason, and remember.

The brain requires energy in the form of glucose, a sugar. Essential substances, such as vitamins and minerals, as well as sources of dietary carbohydrate energy, help the brain to function properly. The brain cannot turn off like a computer or radio. When you are asleep, your brain is still active, as if on an automatic pilot. This is the time when you digest and metabolize most of your food; and you are still breathing, but at a much slower rate.

The nervous system is tied into every other system in the body. It interacts with every system to ensure homeostasis. The chart in Table 19-1 will explain the function of the nervous system with each system.

Functions of the Nervous System

The nervous system is made up of the brain, spinal cord, numerous nerves of the body, and sensory organs (skin, eyes, and ears). The nervous system is divided into two parts called the *central nervous system* (CNS) and the *peripheral nervous system* (PNS). Like the CPU (central processing unit) of a computer that controls other devices, the CNS is the main area that controls all other nervous system functions, some directly and others indirectly via the peripheral nervous system. (See Figure 19-1.)

The CNS is made up of the brain and spinal cord. Remember that, if a particular nerve is not located in one of those two areas, then it must be in the peripheral nervous system; this will help you to understand and differentiate the two systems. The PNS is divided into two parts, the somatic and the autonomic nervous system.

The autonomic nervous system, or ANS, is further divided into two more parts called the sympathetic and the parasympathetic nervous systems. Many drugs will directly affect these two systems beneficially or cause adverse reactions. Therefore, comparing and contrasting these two subdivisions will become paramount to understanding how drugs for the nervous system work.

The nervous system has the following three basic functions:
The *sensory* or *afferent function* senses or recognizes the external changes in the environment such as cold or heat or internal changes in the body such as a decrease in potassium or calcium.

The *integrative* (or *CNS*) *function* processes the perceived information about the changes and interprets or explains the changes in the external and internal environments.

The *motor* or *efferent function* responds to the aforementioned interpretation and integration of the external and internal environments by making muscles move, groups of muscles interact, and glands secrete hormones or other chemicals into the bloodstream.

TABLE 19-1 Effect of the Nervous System on Each System of the Body to Ensure Homeostasis	
Interactive System	Nervous System
Respiratory	The brain monitors respiratory volume and blood gas levels. The brain responds by regulating the respiratory rate.
Heart–Cardiovascular	(1) Endothelial cells maintain the blood–brain barrier, protecting the brain from harmful substances. (2) Baroreceptors send information to the brain about blood pressure. The brain responds by regulating vasodilation, therefore regulating heart rate and blood pressure. (3) Cerebrospinal fluid drains into the venous blood supply, removing harmful waste from the brain.
Skeletal System	Bones provide essential calcium for the proper functioning of the NS. The skull and vertebrae protect the brain and spinal cord from injury. Sensory receptors in bone joints send signals about body position to the brain. The brain regulates the position of bones by controlling muscles.
Muscles	Muscle receptors send the brain information about body position and movement. The brain controls the contraction of skeletal muscle. The nervous system regulates heart rate (myocardium contractions) and the speed at which food moves through the digestive tract (peristalsis).
Digestive System	Digestion of food provides the building blocks of the hormones and neurotransmitters. The autonomic nervous system (ANS) controls the tone of the digestive tract via peristalsis. The nervous system (NS) responds to thirst and hunger and controls drinking and feeding. The NS controls the smooth muscles for peristalsis in order for the body to eat and eliminate food.
Endocrine System	The hypothalamus controls all other endocrine glands by controlling the pituitary gland. Reproductive hormones affect the development of the NS. Hormonal feedback to the brain affects the processing of neuronal information integration.
Lymphatic/Immune System	The brain stimulates the mechanisms of defense against infection.
Renal or Urinary System	The bladder sends sensory information to the brain, which controls urination and, therefore, hydration and thirst.
Integumentary System	Receptors in the skin send sensory information to the brain, which then regulates peripheral blood flow and sweat glands. Nerves control muscles that connect to hair follicles (erector pili).

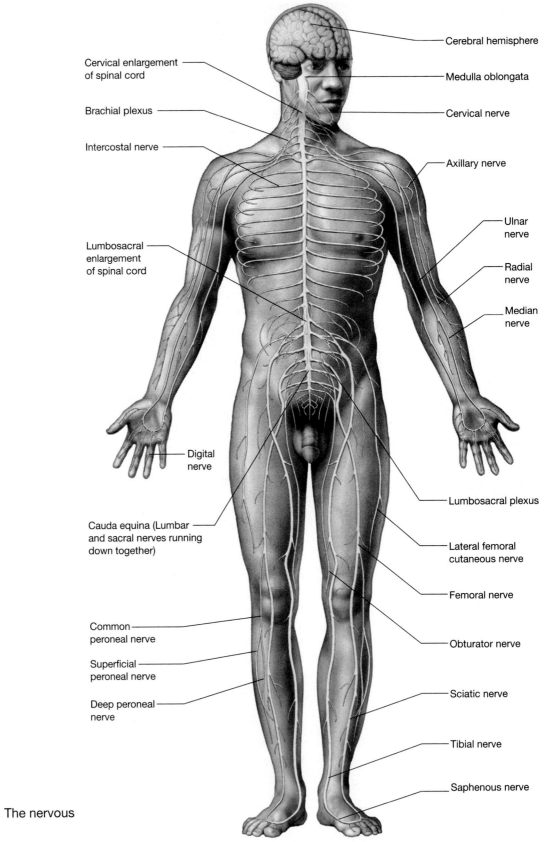

Cerebral hemisphere

Medulla oblongata

Cervical nerve

Axillary nerve

Ulnar nerve

Radial nerve

Median nerve

Lumbosacral plexus

Lateral femoral cutaneous nerve

Femoral nerve

Obturator nerve

Sciatic nerve

Tibial nerve

Saphenous nerve

Cervical enlargement of spinal cord

Brachial plexus

Intercostal nerve

Lumbosacral enlargement of spinal cord

Digital nerve

Cauda equina (Lumbar and sacral nerves running down together)

Common peroneal nerve

Superficial peroneal nerve

Deep peroneal nerve

Figure 19-1 The nervous system

THE NEURON

The smallest unit of the nervous system is a nerve cell called the **neuron**, which is about 10 microns wide. The brain is made up of approximately 100 billion neurons. Neurons are similar to other cells in the body, as they are surrounded by a membrane wall, have a nucleus that contains genes, and contain cytoplasm, mitochondria, and other organelles (Figure 19-2). However,

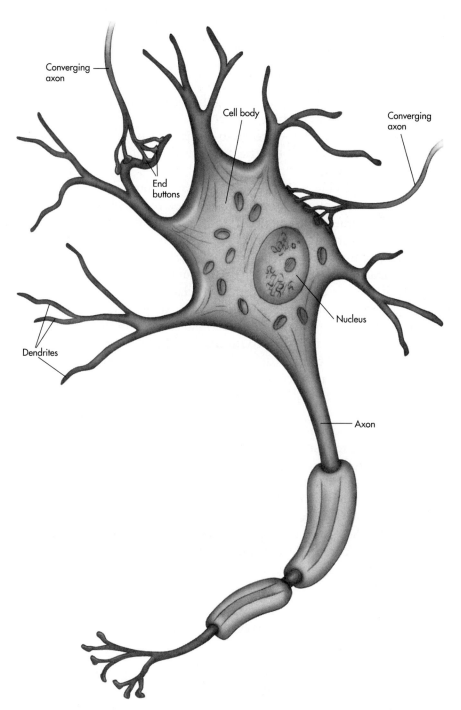

Figure 19-2   Neurons

neurons differ from other cells in that they have projections called dendrites and axons. These projections have the following specialized functions:

- Dendrites bring information to the cell body from the CNS.
- Axons take information away from the cell body to the CNS.

Nervous system cells communicate with each other through an electrochemical process. Computers send electrical signals through wires and fiber optics to control devices. The brain also sends electrical signals, but it sends them through the nerve cell or neurons. The neurons produce electrochemical hormones called neurotransmitters. These chemicals are stored in the ends of the nerve cells. The neurotransmitters are released at the end of the neuron and cross the space, called a synapse, between two different neurons. This crossing of the synapse is also part of the nerve transmission. Signals in neurons transfer information to other neurons by crossing the synapses to control glands, organs, or muscles. The neurotransmitters travel across the synapse to reach a receiving neuron where they attach themselves to special structures called receptors.

This results in a small electrical response within the receiving neuron. This response may be the "end" or terminal message, or it may be continued with second messengers. However, this small response does not mean that the message will continue to result in an action by the gland, organ, or muscle. Only when the total signal from all of the synapses involved in this message exceeds a certain level will a large signal, called an action potential, be generated and the message be continued.

Neuronal studies can encompass the function of groups of neurons or nerve cells, the role of neurotransmitters, what happens at ion channels on a neuronal and cell membrane, reproduction, or genetic basis of neuronal function. The nervous system uses neuronal circuits throughout the brain to store memory and undergoes continual modification so that a person can learn new things. The brain can actually "rewire" itself when necessary. After some kinds of brain injuries, undamaged brain tissue can take over functions previously performed by the injured area.

The changes in the environment that set off the nerve impulse to communicate with another neuron are called stimuli. The action of the impulse that triggers the release of a neurotransmitter to another neuron is called the "firing of neurons" and is both electrical and chemical in nature. There are about 50 neurotransmitters in the brain. These are made of amino acids by the body with the help of other proteins called enzymes and are stored in the neuron vesicles. Adding a substance that mimics the neurotransmitters to the body may help, or it may cause certain conditions or disease states. Most addictive drugs change the effect of neurotransmitters on neurons.

Neurotransmission and Receptors

A name for the constant exchange, or firing, of chemical messages between neurons is neurotransmission. Neurotransmission is achieved by three basic steps, as follows:

Step 1: Neurons release neurotransmitters. In the beginning, the resting neuron, or neuron 1, has a negative charge, with more negative ions inside the axon than outside the axon. The fluid outside the axon has a positive charge. Due to this difference in charges, the axon is said to be polarized.

When a neuron is excited, it fires a neurotransmitter, or chemical. During this time, several things happen to create an electrical impulse called an action potential:

- Positively charged sodium ions enter the axon, shifting the charge within the axon from negative to positive. This event is called depolarization of the axon. The axon is depolarized.

- In response to this action potential, or electrical impulse, the vesicles that store the neurotransmitters move to the edge of the axon and release neurotransmitters into the synapse.

- Subsequently, positively charged potassium ions flow out of the axon, causing the inside of the axon to return to a negative charge. The neuron is again polarized and at rest, waiting to fire another impulse.

Step 2: Neurotransmitters bind to receptors. The released neurotransmitters "swim" across the synapse until they "land," or meet the dendrites of the next neuron, neuron 2. This is called uptake. The neurotransmitters recognize molecules that are waiting to receive them, called receptors. Neurotransmitters "dock," or attach to these specific receptors in a chemical reaction, a process called binding. The neurotransmitter of the sending neuron (neuron 1) must fit like a key in a lock into the receiving neuron's receptor in order to generate a response. The neurotransmitters are then released by the receptors. Several things can happen next:

- Some neurotransmitters are broken down or destroyed by enzymes.

- Carrying proteins transport the neurotransmitters back to the axon from which they originally came, a process called *reuptake*.

- Neurotransmitters may be used again in a type of recycling of the chemical messenger.

Step 3: Binding passes on or continues (transduces) the neurotransmitter's message. The binding itself causes a set of chemical reactions within neuron 2, the receiving neuron. The same kind of impulse that was fired by the sending neuron continues in the nerve pathway from neuron to neuron until it reaches its terminal destination of a muscle, gland, or organ. The result of this can be a change in the way we respond, behave, think, feel, or react physically.

The Central Nervous System

The central nervous system is composed of the brain and spinal cord. The brain weighs approximately 1.3 to 1.4 kilograms or 2.8 to 3 pounds. To put that in perspective, consider that the brain of an elephant is about 6 kilograms, and the brain of a rhesus monkey is about 1 kilogram. The spinal cord is the main pathway for information connecting the brain to the peripheral nervous system and has 31 paired nerves: 8 cervical, 12 thoracic, 5 lumbar, 5 sacral, and 1 coccygeal. The main regions of these nerves are called the skull, the cervical vertebrae, the thoracic vertebrae, the lumbar vertebrae, and the sacral vertebrae (sacrum). The spinal cord is protected from injury by the cerebrospinal fluid (CSF), which is contained within a system of fluid-filled cavities called ventricles. Receptors in the skin send information to the spinal cord through the spinal nerves.

CSF provides the following services:

- **Protection**—the CSF protects the brain from damage by acting like a cushion to lessen the impact in the event of a blow to the head.
- **Excretion of waste products**—due to the one-way direction of the flow of CSF to the blood, it takes harmful metabolites of drugs and other toxic substances away from the brain.
- **Endocrine communication**—CSF serves as the vehicle to transport hormones to other areas of the brain. Hormones released into the CSF can be carried to remote sites of the brain.

The Brain

The head or cephalic region of the body has a bony structure, the skull, to protect the brain from injury. Futher protection is provided by the three layers of meninges: dura matter, arachnoid, and pia matter. The outermost, hardest layer is the dura matter. The arachnoid has spaces in it that resemble a cobweb and are filled with CSF for further protection.

The brain can be divided down the middle, lengthwise, into two halves called the cerebral hemispheres. (See Figure 19-3.) Each hemisphere of the cerebral cortex is divided into the following four lobes:

- The *frontal lobe* is concerned with higher intellect or reasoning, problem solving, parts of speech, movement or motor cortex, and emotion.
- The *parietal lobe* is related to the stimuli and perception of touch, pressure, temperature, and pain.
- The *temporal lobe* is related to perception and recognition of auditory stimuli for hearing and memory (involving the hippocampus).
- The *occipital lobe* is related to stimuli pertaining to vision.

The brain can be divided into three main parts for the purposes of this chapter: the cerebellum, the cerebrum, and the brain stem.

CEREBELLUM

This is located behind the brain stem and below the cerebrum. The main purposes of the cerebellum are to coordinate the movement of the body and maintain equilibrium and balance. Some drugs such as alcohol can depress the cerebellum, which then decreases body coordination and reaction or response time.

CEREBRUM

This is divided into two main parts:

- *Cerebral cortex* contains grey matter made up of the nerve cells known as neurons that control voluntary actions of the body. An electroencephalogram (EEG) is a recording of the electrical activity of the cortex and can be useful in diagnosing some brain disorders. The cerebral cortex is tied in with the somatic part of the peripheral nervous system.

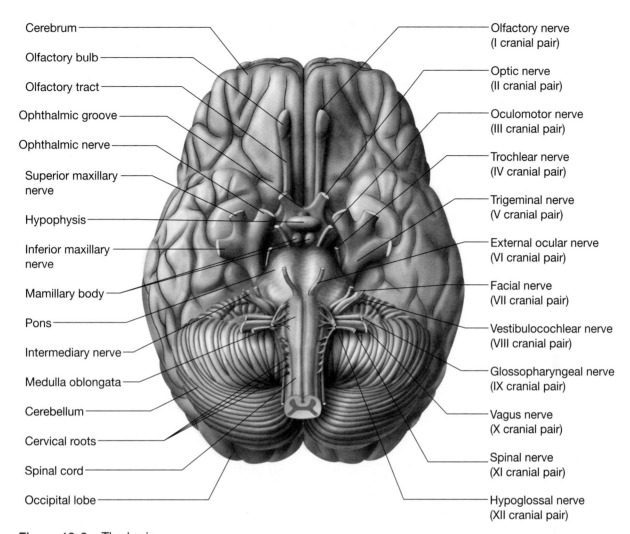

Cerebrum

Olfactory bulb

Olfactory tract

Ophthalmic groove

Ophthalmic nerve

Superior maxillary nerve

Hypophysis

Inferior maxillary nerve

Mamillary body

Pons

Intermediary nerve

Medulla oblongata

Cerebellum

Cervical roots

Spinal cord

Occipital lobe

Olfactory nerve
(I cranial pair)

Optic nerve
(II cranial pair)

Oculomotor nerve
(III cranial pair)

Trochlear nerve
(IV cranial pair)

Trigeminal nerve
(V cranial pair)

External ocular nerve
(VI cranial pair)

Facial nerve
(VII cranial pair)

Vestibulocochlear nerve
(VIII cranial pair)

Glossopharyngeal nerve
(IX cranial pair)

Vagus nerve
(X cranial pair)

Spinal nerve
(XI cranial pair)

Hypoglossal nerve
(XII cranial pair)

Figure 19-3 The brain

- *Cerebral medulla* contains white matter made up of myelinated axons of the neurons, which serve to conduct nerve impulses to and from different areas of the nervous system. Within the cerebral medulla is more grey matter known as the basal ganglia. The basal ganglia regulates motor activity or movement. Damage to the basal ganglia may result in disorders like Parkinson's disease.

The **brain stem**, an extension of the spinal cord, is divided into four main parts, as follows:

a. **Thalamus** sits at the top of the brain stem and regulates and evaluates the sensory impulses of pain, hot, cold, and touch. It directs the sensory information to the correct part of the cerebral cortex or regulates the response.

b. **Hypothalamus**, located just below the thalamus, controls body functions such as water balance, body temperature, sleep, hunger and appetite, sex drive, the autonomic nervous system, and some emotional and behavioral responses.

c. **Pons,** located below the hypothalamus, regulates respiration and is considered the "relay" station for nerve fibers that travel to other parts of the brain.

d. **Medulla oblongata**, the final part of the brain stem, is located at the base of the brain stem and the top of the spine. It contains the three vital centers that keep the body alive and functioning: cardiac (heart), respiratory (breathing), and vasomotor (blood vessels). Injury to this area of the brain usually results in death. The reflexes for gagging, swallowing, coughing, and vomiting are regulated by the medulla oblongata.

Reticular Formation

Located throughout the brain stem and cerebrum, a network of nerve fibers known as the reticular formation affects the degree of alertness. It is made up of two types of fibers, described as follows:

Excitatory fibers—when stimulated by external stimuli such as noises (traffic), bright lights, or danger, the degree of alertness is increased. Certain stimulant drugs such as Ritalin and caffeine can increase the reticular formation, or degree of alertness.

Inhibitory Fibers—an absence of external stimuli causes the inhibitory fibers to become more active, which decreases the activity of the excitatory fibers and, therefore, the degree of alertness. Inhibitory fibers are usually more activated during sleep or rest. Certain drugs such as alcohol and hypnotics or barbiturates can decrease the reticular formation.

The Limbic System

One of the least understood areas of the brain is the *limbic system*, a collection of nerve cells in various areas of the brain, especially the hypothalamus, that form a specific neural pathway. The limbic system is associated with such emotional and behavioral responses as sexual behavior, anger, rage, fear, anxiety, reward, and punishment.

Blood Brain Barrier (BBB)

The BBB is a semi-permeable membrane that allows some substances to cross, but prevents others from crossing. The following are the general properties of the BBB:

1. Water soluble or low lipid/low fat soluble molecules do not penetrate into the brain. Highly lipid/fat soluble molecules such as barbiturates rapidly cross through the BBB into the brain.

2. Large molecules do not easily pass through the BBB.

3. Highly electrically charged molecules are slowed down.

However, the BBB can be broken down. The following disease states can compromise the barrier:

- Hypertension (high blood pressure) can open up the BBB.
- Infectionious agents can open up the BBB.

- Hyperosmolitity—a high concentration of a substance in the blood can cause the BBB to open up.

The following physical changes can also break down the BBB:

- When the developmental stage is interrupted, the BBB is not fully formed at birth, leaving the BBB open.
- Exposure to microwaves can open up the BBB.
- Exposure to radiation can open up the BBB.
- Injury to the brain can open up the BBB. Examples are trauma, ischemia, inflammation, pressure.

The functions of the BBB are as follows:

- Protect the brain from "foreign invaders," or substances in the blood, that could injure the brain.
- Protect the brain from hormones and neurotransmitters in the rest of the body.
- Maintain a constant environment, or homeostasis, for the brain.

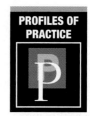

Diseases Affecting the Central Nervous System

Mental illness can affect anyone. Considered disorders, they may range from mild and temporary to serious and long-lasting. Pharmacotherapeutics has empowered many people with mental disorders to enhance their lives and reach their fullest potential. The first antipsychotic drug, chlorpromazine, was introduced in the 1950s. Psychotherapy and counseling can be more effective with the use of psychotherapeutic agents. People who were once too depressed to open up and talk to a psychiatrist begin to respond after a few weeks of treatment with psychotherapeutic drugs.

The following mental disorders may be treated psychotherapeutically: psychosis, depression, anxiety, obsessive-compulsive disorder, and panic disorder. While there is no cure for mental illness, these drugs will help the patient to have a better experience in daily living and to function more effectively.

The National Institute of Mental Health classifies the following four types of psychotherapeutic agents: antianxiety, antidepressant, antimanic, and antipsychotic medications.

Anxiety

Anxiety is associated with the following risk factors: genetics, brain chemistry, life events, and personality. Fewer than one-third of all those suffering from anxiety seek medical treatment; yet, it is a most treatable condition. There are many forms of anxiety, categorized as follows: generalized anxiety disorder (GAD), obsessive-compulsive disorder (OCD), panic disorder or panic attack, post-traumatic stress disorder (PTSD), social anxiety disorder (SAD), and specific phobias. Anxiety can hit anyone at any time, but is usually slowly progressive. Some anxiety occurs as a result of a traumatic or childhood event. Specific symptoms or behaviors interfere with work, social situations, or everyday tasks (see Table 19-2).

TABLE 19-2 Types of Anxiety

Type of Anxiety and Cause	Description	Symptoms
GAD—The person has unrealistic focus on or chronic worry about everyday living issues such as health, money, or work/career.	Uncontrollable worry about things that occur in daily living usually is considered GAD if it persists 6 months or longer; focus may shift from issue to issue.	trembling, muscular aches, insomnia, abdominal upsets, dizziness, irritability, easily tired, and have trouble sleeping.
OCD—The person has continuous and recurring thoughts (obsessions) that reflect exaggerated anxiety or fears. Obsessions can lead to performing a ritual or routine (compulsions).	Typical obsessions/compulsions are fear of germs (washes hands). Fear of improper performance or behavior (repeats phrases that are "magical"). Persistent doubts that everything is okay (checks things over and over again (is the iron shut off?)).	Symptoms are the compulsions that are manifested to relieve the anxiety: constant cleaning; checking if all is okay (doors locked); repeating phrases/words; spending time organizing; hoarding unnecessary items such as junk mail, old bills; unable to part with old, useless items (rooms get filled).
Panic Attacks—An abrupt or sudden onset of fear or discomfort.	Usually accompanied by fear of having a panic attack in the future after experiencing one. Usually has at least four of the symptoms. Most predominant feeling is a fear of impending doom.	Physical: palpitations, sweating, trembling, nausea or GI disturbances, chest pain or discomfort, tingling sensations, chills or hot flushes, dizziness, and lightheadedness. Emotional: a feeling of imminent danger or doom; a feeling of choking, creating a need to escape; sense of things being unreal, surreal, or depersonalization; fear of "losing it" or going crazy; fear of one's own death
PTSD—Experience of or witnessing a traumatic event such as criminal assault, a serious accident, a natural disaster, or a death.	The after-effects of exposure to a traumatic experience impede with normal function of everyday living. Is accompanied by intense fear, helplessness, and/or horror.	Relives the trauma, recurrent dreams or nightmares, possible loss of interest in previously enjoyed things/people, excessive response to being startled, irritability, anger
SAD—Extreme fear about being judged or ridiculed by others.	Extreme fear of social or performance situations and embarrassment that may occur. Fear that others will think poorly of them. Usually have anxiety in anticipation of a feared event.	Heart palpitations, faintness, blushing and profuse sweating, diarrhea, or panic attack. Leads to avoidance behavior.
Specific Phobias—Usually caused by an event in early childhood.	Suffer from an extreme fear of, or express an intense reaction to, a specific object or situation such as spiders, heights, being outdoors, being among the public/people.	The fear produces panic attacks, which lead to avoidance of everyday situations such as work, intimacy.

A lack of a specific neurotransmitter, Gamma-aminobutyric acid (GABA), is associated with anxiety. The more GABA there is, the less anxiety there will be; conversely, the less GABA there is, the more anxiety there will be. The specific drug used to treat anxiety depends upon the type of anxiety and the symptoms. It should be noted that counseling in the form of cognitive and behavioral therapy should be utilized in the treatment of anxiety, along with psychotherapeutics, for the greatest effect.

Barbiturates are not used as often for anxiety as they once were because they are highly addictive (CII) and there are better alternatives. Anxiety is normally pharmaceutically treated with benzodiazepines, but may also be treated with antidepressant drugs such as selective serotonin reuptake inhibitors (SSRIs), tricyclic antidepressants, monoamine oxidase inhibitors (MAOIs), beta blockers, or any combination of them.

Another antidepressant, Effexor XR, is a potent inhibitor of the reuptake of both serotonin and norepinephrine. An inability to fall asleep or stay asleep is a common symptom because the person has obsessive thoughts of anticipated or previously experienced events. The β-Adrenergic blockers, such as propranolol, reduce the autonomic symptoms of anxiety (including changes in breathing rate, heart palpitations, tremors, sweating, and shaking). Non-benzodiazepine hypnotic Ambien® (zolpidem) and Sonata (zaleplon) selectively bind only to omega-1 or BZ-1 receptors affecting the GABA-A receptor, and therefore do not produce as much anticonvulsant or muscle relaxant effect. However, an off-label use of these drugs is for anxiety, as they help the person who worries at bedtime and cannot fall asleep. Non-benzodiazepine anxilytic, Buspar® (buspirone), works at the 5-HT1A receptor subtype. Serotonin receptors (5-HT and subtypes) have long been associated with sleep. There are no muscle relaxant or anticonvulsant properties for either non-benzodiazeine.

BENZODIAZEPINES

Because benzodiazepines bind to all three BZ receptors, they can relax the muscle, which can lead to a feeling of total relaxation and sleepiness. They are used as hypnotics and sedatives in higher doses, and in lower doses when used as anxioytics. Proper dosing is important so that anti-anxiety drugs can be given during the day to prevent anxiety episodes and avoid sleepiness. These drugs are also used as anticonvulsants and anti-epilectics (see Table 19-3).

Benzodiazepines are used to treat many disorders other than anxiety, due to the sedation and hypnotic effects. Some of these agents and the conditions they treat are listed as follows:

- hypnotics for insomnia
- anticonvulsant for epilepsy
- muscle relaxant for muscle spasticity
- induction of sleep or anesthesia as pre-anesthetic or pre-surgery medication
- adjunct in alcohol withdrawal
- for various psychiatric diagnoses

Side effects are related to dosing and co-administration with drugs or alcohol. High doses taken with alcohol produce lethal effects. Benzodiazepines may cause dependence over long-term use, and are therefore classified as Class IV. Because of this, prescriptions for these drugs are now recommended only for short-term use. Research is currently underway to make more selective anxiolytic compounds such as partial agonists at the benzodiazepine receptor.

Mechanism of Action of Benzodiazepines The MOA of benzodiazepines is centered around GABA and GABA-A receptors. These drugs bind to the GABA-A receptors and potentiate (increase) the actions of GABA. When there is a lack of GABA, they act like GABA; and when GABA cannot cross the synapse, they increase the crossing and the binding of GABA into the GABA-A receptors.

Management of Benzodiazepine Overdose The primary use of Romazicon® (flumazenil) is as a benzodiazepine antagonist in the event of overdosage. Romazicon® competitively antagonizes the binding and allosteric effects of benzodiazepines at the BZ GABA-A receptors. Additional use is in the reduction of benzodiazepine effects in general anesthesia or diagnostic procedures. Fumazenil is available only for intravenous administration because it has a high first-pass effect (hepatic/liver). It should be noted that the physician must be certain of the cause of overdose because of the following adverse effects:

- In comatose patients, intoxicated with alcohol, flumazenil may increase risk of seizures.
- In patients comatose due to tricyclic antidepressant agents, flumazenil increases seizure risk.

MECHANISM OF ACTION OF BUSPIRONE

Buspirone has an anti-anxiety effect without marked sedation or euphoria. As an antagonist, it binds to the serotonin 5-HT1A receptor at post-synaptic sites. As an agonist, it binds at 5-HT1A presynaptic receptors. It has no direct effect on the GABA system.

Mood Disorders

DEPRESSION

Neurotransmitters are generally monoamines, which can be destroyed in the synaptic cleft by enzymes called monoamine oxidases. Another cause of depression is the excessive reuptake of neurotransmitters or reabsorption into the proximal nerve. Either event leads to a lack of the neurotransmitters serotonin, norepinephrin, and dopamine, and the result is depression. Thus it is postulated that clinical depression is related to decreases in concentration of the neurotransmitters. For this reason, pharmaceutical research and current drug therapy are centered around drugs that can either block the reuptake of neurotransmitters (for example, cyclic antidepressants and newer selective serotonin

TABLE 19-3 Table of Anti-anxiety Drugs

Trade/Generic Name	Availability	Usual Adult Dose
Benzodiazepines		
Xanax® (alprazolam) (CIV) used for GAD and Panic Disorder (PD)	0.25, .05, 1, and 2 mg PO tablets 1 mg/1 ml Intensol oral solution	**GAD Initial dose**: 0.25 to 0.5 mg given 3 times daily NTE 4 mg/day **PD**: NTE 10 mg/day (Average dose is 5–6 mg/day)
Ativan® (lorazepam) (CIV) used for GAD, pre-op medication	0.25, .05, 1, and 2 mg PO tablets 2 and 4 mg prefilled syringes 2 mg/1 ml concentrated oral solution	**GAD Initial dose**: 2 to 3 mg/day given BID or TID Usual range: 2 to 6 mg/day Largest dose at bedtime.
Librium® (chlordiazepoxide) (CIV) used for GAD	5, 10, and 25 mg PO tablets 100 mg powder for injection	**Mild anxiety** 5–10 mg TID or QID Severe anxiety 20–25 mg TID or QID
Valium® (diazepam) (CIV) used for GAD, pre-op medication	2, 5, and 10 mg PO tablets 5 mg/1 ml Injection (IV or IM) 5 mg/5 ml and 5 mg/1 ml oral solutions	2–10 mg PO BID, TID or QID 2–20 mg IV or IM Injection
Serax® (oxazepam) (CIV) used for GAD and alcohol withdrawl	10, 15 and 20 mg capsules	**Mild–Mod** 10 to 15 mg, TID or QID **Mod–Severe** 15 to 30 mg
Tranxene® (clorazepate) (CIV) used for GAD and alcohol withdrawal	3.75, 7.5, and 15 mg Tranxene–T Tablets 22.5 mg Tranxene–SD Tablets 11.25 mg Tranxene–SD Half Strength Tablets	**Tranxene T** – PO Tablets: 15 to 60 mg daily in divided doses Average daily dose 30 mg **Tranxene–SD and SD Half Strength** are given single dose QD
Non-benzodiazepines		
Buspar® (buspirone)	5, 10, 15, and 30 mg PO Tablets	Initial dose: 5 mg TID (15 mg/day) Average dose 20–30 mg/day in TID dosing, range 15–60 mg/day NTE 60 mg/day
Ambien® zolpidem (CIV)	5 and 10 mg PO Tablets	10 mg HS
Sonata® (**zaleplon**) (**CIV**)	5 and 10 mg PO Capsules	10 mg HS Range 5–20 mg HS
Antidepressants—TCA's		
Tofranil® (imipramine) in panic disorder	10, 25, and 50 mg PO Tablets	Panic disorder—**150–300 mg** (Note: Dose is higher than for depression, which is 50–150 mg/day)
Anafril® (clomipramine) used for OCD	25, 50, and 75 mg PO Capsules	Initial PO dose: 25 mg/day NTE 250 mg/day
Antidepressants—SSRIs		
Prozac® (fluoxetine) used for ODC	10, 20, 40 mg PO Pulvules 10 mg PO Tablet 20 mg/5 ml oral solution	20 mg QAM >20 mg/day in QD or BID dosing (morning and noon) recommended 20–60 mg/day NTE 80 mg/day

TABLE 19-3 Table of Anti-anxiety Drugs (*continued*)

Trade/Generic Name	Availability	Usual Adult Dose
Paxil® (paroxetine) Used for OCD, SAD, and Panic Disorder	10, 20, 30 and 40 mg PO Tablets 12.5, 25 and 37.5 mg Controlled-Release Capsules 10 mh/5 ml Oral Suspension	OCD and SAD 20 mg/day initial dose Average range for OCD and SAD: 20–60 mg dose. NTE 60 mg/day Recommended for OCD is 40 mg/day Panic Disorder: initial dose 10 mg, target dose 40 mg/day Controlled-Release for Panic Disorder 12.5–75 mg/day NTE 75 mg/day
Luvox® (flufoxamine) used for OCD	25, 50, and 100 mg PO Tablets	50 mg initial dose, range 50–300 mg/day Doses greater than 100 mg/day to be given in divided doses NTE 300 mg/day
Celexa® (citalopram) Unlabeled use for SAD Zoloft® (sertraline) used for OCD, PTSD, and Panic Disorder	10, 20, and 40 mg tablets 10 mg/5 ml Oral Solution 25, 50, and 100 mg PO Tablets 20/1 ml Oral Concentrate	Initial dose: 20 mg/day NTE 60 mg/day (**G**) OCD 25–200 mg QD PTSD and Panic Disorder 25–50 mg QD NTE 200 mg/day
Antidepressants—Other Effexor® (venlafaxine) Effexor XR used for GAD (Note: Only XR caps are used after initial dosing.) Serzone® (nefazodone) Unlabeled use for GAD May cause hepatic failure	25, 37.5, 50, 75, and 100 mg PO Tablets 37.5, 75, and 100 mg Extended Release Capsule (XR) 50, 100, 150, 200, and 250 mg PO Tablets	Initial dose: 37.5 mg–75 mg (XR Caps) Usual range 75–300 mg (XR caps) 225 mg/day (XR caps) Initial dose: 50 Usual range: 300–550 mg
β-Adrenergic blocker of cardiac arrythmias associated panic attacks and performance anxiety Tenormin® (atenolol) Unlabeled use for Panic Disorder	25, 50, and 100 mg PO Tablets	Initial dose: 25/50 mg/day Range: 25–100 mg/day (**F**)
Inderal® (propranolol) Unlabeled use for Panic Disorder	10, 20, 30, 40, 60, 80, and 90 mg tablets 60, 80, 120, and 160 mg Sustained-Release Capsules 4 mg/1 ml and Oral Solution 80 mg/1 ml Oral Concentrate 1 mg/1 ml Injectable	10–20 mg Initial dose 10–160 mg/day, in divided doses (TID and QID) **F**

reuptake inhibitors) or interfere with the breakdown of the monoamines within the synaptic cleft (monoamine oxidase inhibitors, or MAOIs).

There are many types of depression, including seasonal major depression (seasonal affective disorder), postpartum depression, bipolar disorder, and dysthymia (mild depression on most days of the year). Depression is very treatable.

People with depression have sympton that include a feeling of a "black curtain" of despair coming down over their lives, lack of energy and inability to concentrate, and feeling irritable for no apparent reason. If the symptoms occur for more than two weeks to six months and are interfering with daily life, the person may be clinically depressed.

Patients will show such changes in behavior as the following:

- constant feelings of sadness, worthlessness, hopelessness, or guilt
- irritability or tension
- decreased interest or pleasure in usual activities or hobbies
- changes in appetite, increase or decrease, with significant weight loss or weight gain
- a change in sleeping patterns, increase or decrease, such as difficulty sleeping, early morning awakening, or sleeping too much
- restlessness, fidgeting, or feeling slowed down
- decreased ability to make decisions or concentrate
- thoughts of suicide or death

There is no one specific known cause of depression, but rather it results from a combination of things. Risk factors for becoming depressed are listed as follows:

- Genetics play an important part in depression.
- Trauma and stress—negative issues like financial problems, the breakup of a relationship, or the death of a loved one can bring on depression. But it can also be caused by positive situations or after such changes in one's life as starting a new job, getting married, or graduating from school.
- Pessimistic personality, low self-esteem or a negative outlook can contribute. (Dysthymia can actually have the same characteristics.)
- Physical conditions—serious medical conditions or diseases such as cancer, HIV, heart disease, and unwanted sterility can contribute to depression, partly because of the physical weakness and stress they bring on. Depression can worsen medical conditions because it weakens the immune system and can make pain more intense. Depression can be induced as a side effect by medications used to treat medical conditions.
- Other psychological disorders such as anxiety disorders; schizophrenia; anorexia, bulimia, or compulsive eating disorders; and substance abuse often mask as or appear with depression.

Depression can make a person feel afraid and alone, without hope, as if things will never get better. It can change how the patient thinks and feels. Depression affects social behavior as it depletes a sense of physical well-being. Depression can affect anyone, of any age, at any time.

Once the illness is identified, most people diagnosed with depression are successfully treated. Pharmaceutical treatment can reverse much of that doomed feeling. Psychotherapy and medication are the two primary treatment approaches. Antidepressant medications can enhance psychotherapy for some people; but they cannot cure. The "blues" are considered transient and short-term, while depression is a prolonged condition lasting longer than two weeks and interfering with or interrupting a person's life and ability to carry out daily tasks and to enjoy activities that previously brought pleasure to them.

Antidepressants are not stimulants like coffee or amphetamines. But they do remove or reduce the symptoms of depression, helping the depressed person feel the way he did before the affliction. Antidepressants are also used for anxiety disorders, mainly blocking the symptoms of panic—rapid heartbeat, nausea, terror, dizziness, chest pains, and breathing problems. They can also be used to treat some phobias, which are also a type of anxiety (see Table 19-4).

Bipolar disorder (BD), which will be discussed in more detail in a separate section, is characterized by bouts of oscillating high and low moods. Therefore, the depression state of BD may require the use of an antidepressant. There are many types of antidepressants: selective serotonin reuptake inhibitors (SSRIs), TCAs, or tricyclic antidepressants, once the most commonly used, have many drug interactions. Monoamine oxidase inhibitors (MAOIs) were often used for atypical depressions that have symptoms of oversleeping, anxiety, panic attacks, and phobias. However, they have some major side effects and drug/food interactions. Both TCAs and MAOIs take two to four weeks to begin working. SSRIs have successfully replaced the use of MAOIs, except in some cases.

A major depressive episode is categorized. The category of a DSM-IV episode signifies a well observable and relatively persistent depressed or dysphoric mood that is present almost every day for at least two weeks, that usually interferes with daily living or functioning, and will include at least five of the following nine symptoms: depressed mood, insomnia or hypersomnia, loss of interest in usual activities, significant change in weight and/or appetite, psychomotor agitation or retardation, increased fatigue, feelings of guilt or worthlessness, slowed thinking or impaired concentration, and a suicide attempt or suicidal ideation.

Bipolar Disorder

Manic–depressive disorder, now called *bipolar disorder (BD)*, is characterized by peaks and valleys of severe highs (mania) and lows (depression). Episodes are referred to as mood swings. The spread between episodes may be hours, days, months, or years. In the manic state, the patient is overactive and over-talkative, displays a great deal of energy, and sleeps less. The manic patient cannot speak fast enough to catch up with his thoughts. He will have unrealistic thoughts; he may present an angry or irritable state, with false ideas about his importance to others or in the world at large. In a manic high, the patient uses poor judgment in business dealings and may plan and carry out careless romantic get-aways or "flings." If left untreated, mania may worsen, developing into a psychotic disorder. As discussed earlier, in the depressive cycle the patient presents a difficulty in concentration, lack of energy, lethargy, slow thinking and moving, more sleeping and eating. The patient has feelings of hopelessness, helplessness, despair, sadness, worthlessness, and guilt. This may be accompanied by thoughts of suicide.

TABLE 19-4	Antidepressant Comparative Chart			
Type/Trade/ Generic Name	Indication	Mechanism of Action	Side Effects and Toxic Effects	Usual Adult Daily Dose
SSRIs	Mild to Major Depression, Some anxiety disorders	Selectively block the reuptake of serotonin, weak effects on NE and dopamine reuptake	**Side Effects, Mild:** H/A, N/V, insomnia, tremor, and dry mouth. SSRIs have also been studied in the treatment of attention-deficit/ hyperactivity disorder (ADHD). **Toxic Effects:** Anemia, hives, skin rash, or seizures. Wait at least 14 days when switching to an MAOI. Contraindication: At this time of writing SSRIs have come under scrutiny.	Varies, see specific drug.
Celexa™ (citalopram HBr)	Mild to Major Depression	Same as SSRIs. Its chemical structure is unrelated to other SSRIs	**Above common side effects plus toxic effects:** Amenorrhea, polyuria, aggravated depression, suicide attempt, and confusion. Contraindication: Azole antifungals may increase plasma level of citalopram.	Start 20 mg QD, increase to 40 mg/day
Prozac® (fluoxetine)	Depression, OCD	Same as SSRIs.	**Above common side effects plus toxic effects:** Abnormal sweating, anxiety, change in appetite, H/A, N/V, seizure, nervousness, stomach, rash, cramps, or trouble sleeping.	20–40 mg/day
Luvox® (fluvoxamine)	Depression, OCD	Same as SSRIs	**Above common side effects plus toxic effects:** Breathing difficulties, coma, convulsions, arrhythmia, and N/V. Monitor liver and kidney functions.	100–200 mg/day

TABLE 19-4   Antidepressant Comparative Chart (*continued*)

Type/Trade/ Generic Name	Indication	Mechanism of Action	Side Effects and Toxic Effects	Usual Adult Daily Dose
Paxil® (paroxetine) Paxil CR	Depression, Panic Disorder	Same as SSRIs.	**Above common side effect plus toxic effects:** Blurred vision, dizziness, hypomania, H/A, palpitations, weakness, rash, sweating, taste disorders, tingling in hands. Monitor liver and kidney functions	20–40 mg/day 10–40 mg/day for renal and hepatic pts
Zoloft® (sertraline)	Depression, Panic Disorder, social phobia, obesity, or OCD.	Ditto	**Above common side effects plus toxic effects:** Hx of seizures, heart attack, kidney or hepatic disease, Parkinson's disease.	100–150 mg/day 50 mg TID
Miscellaneous Atypical Antidepressants				
Effexor® (venlafaxine)	Major Depression	inhibits serotonin and norepinephrine reuptake and weakly inhibits dopamine reuptake.	**Above common side effects plus toxic effects:** Suicidal attempts	Start 75 mg/day, in two or three divided doses. Increase to 150 or 225 mg/day. Taken with food.
Serzone® (nefazodone)	Depression, GAD	Occupies central 5-HT_2 receptors inhibiting the reuptake of serotonin and norepinephrine.	**Side effects:** Sedation and hypotension	Initial 100 mg BID Target dose: 300 to 600 mg/day in BID dosing
Desyrel® (trazedone)	Depression	Selectively blocks the reuptake of serotonin and potentiates the behavioral changes induced by the serotonin precursor 5-hydroxytryptophan.	**Side effects:** Sedation and hypotension	Initial dose: 150 mg/day individed doses NTE 600 mg/day
Wellbutrin® (bupropion) Wellbutrin SR® (bupropion) Wellbutrin XL (bupropion) used for GAD	Depression, GAD	Blocks more norepinephrine and dopamine than serotonin	Good news: No weight gain or sexual dysfunction Bad news: cannot be used by persons with risk of seizures, bulimia, or anorexia nervosa.	Immediate release Tabs: 300 mg/day, given TID dosing Sustained Release Tablets: 150 mg BID

TABLE 19-4 Antidepressant Comparative Chart (*continued*)

Type/Trade/ Generic Name	Indication	Mechanism of Action	Side Effects and Toxic Effects	Usual Adult Daily Dose
Zyban® (bupropion) 150 mg sustained release tablets	Non-nicotine aid to smoking cessation to treat depression associated with smoking withdrawals	Weakly blocks the neuronal uptake of serotonin and norepinephrine. Also, it inhibits the neuronal reuptake of dopamine to some extent.	**Above common side effects**	Sustained Release Tablets 150 mg BID
TCAs	Severe depression, depression that occurs with anxiety. Some TCAs have have broad anti-obsessional and anti-panic effects.	Strongly block the reuptake of serotonin and norepinephrine, while weakly blocking effects of dopamine	**Side effects:** Anticholinergic effects of dry mouth, blurred vision, constipation, and difficulty in urination; postural hypotension; tachycardia, loss of sex drive; erectile failure; photosensitivity; weight gain; sedation; increased sweating. Uncommon: jitteriness, irritation, unusual energy, and insomnia. Delayed onset of action from 2–12 weeks. May need to administer an amphetamine for first few weeks. Pt may experience more general anxiety the first few days up to three weeks.	Usually given in a single daily dose. Begin at lower doses to avoid jitteriness and insomnia. Tiyrate up to max dose. After improvement, may taper off gradually.
Elavil® (amitriptyline)	Panic attacks and depression	Same as TCAs	**Above common side effects, except** Less potential for insomnia. May be used for pts who are having trouble sleeping, because of its sedating effects. The sedating side effects can limit productivity and concentration during the day.	Start: 25–75 mg QHS and increase over two weeks to average of 200 and maximum of 300 mg. Taper off gradually.
Anafranil® (clomipramine)	Helps control obsessive-compulsive disorder by reducing the duration and	Same as TCAs	**Above common side effects plus contraindications:** Avoid administering to patients with certain abnormal electrocardiograms,	Start: 25 mg QD, UAD 150–300 mg QD. Taper off slowly over 3–4 week period.

TABLE 19-4   **Antidepressant Comparative Chart (*continued*)**

Type/Trade/ Generic Name	Indication	Mechanism of Action	Side Effects and Toxic Effects	Usual Adult Daily Dose
	intensity of symptoms and anxiety. May help as much as imipramine for panic attacks. Relieves depression		narrow-angle glaucoma, or with an enlarged prostate.	
Tofranil® (imipramine)	Panic Attacks	Same as TCAs	**Above common side effects**	Start: 10 mg QD Tirtate up to 250 mg QD
Norpramin®, (desipramine)	Depression, Panic Attacks	Same as TCAs	**Above common side effects, except** causes little or no drowsiness.	25–300 mg QD. Taper off gradually.
Pamelor® or Aventyl® (nortriptyline)	Depression, Panic Attacks	Same as TCAs	**Above common side effects**	Start: 10–25 mg QD, UAD 50–75 mg QD, as high as 150 mg QD, based on blood level. Taper off slowly.
Tetracyclic Agents	Major Depression	Two different actions for these two drugs in same classification.	See specific drug.	Start low, titrate up slowly, and taper off slowly.
Remeron® (mirtazapine)	Major Depression	Mirtazapine is a potent antagonist of 5-HT2 and 5-HT3 receptors and a moderate peripheral a_1 adrenergic antagonist.	Sleepiness, dizziness, weight gain, flu-like symptoms, inability to focus, GI upset, tachycardia in some pts. Contraindication: hypersensitivity to mirtazapine. Do not give with Ludomil or alcohol.	Start: Tablets 15 mg/day, increase up to 15–45 mg/day
Ludiomil® (maprotiline)	Major Depression and Manic-Depressive Disorders	Blocks NE at nerve endings.	**Side effects:** Anticholinergic effects. **Contrindications:** Do not give to pts with acute phase MI or recent MI; may cause seizures. Do not give within 2 weeks of MAOIs. May cause leukocytopenia or neutopenia.	Start: 25–75 mg QD, UAD 150 mg QD

TABLE 19-4   Antidepressant Comparative Chart (*continued*)

Type/Trade/ Generic Name	Indication	Mechanism of Action	Side Effects and Toxic Effects	Usual Adult Daily Dose
MAOIs	Major Depression	Blocks the enzyme, monoamine oxidase, from destroying the monoamines serotonin, norepinephrine, and dopamine.	Dietary restrictions: Interacts with tyramine containing foods, leading to HTN crisis or stroke. Avoid: beer, wine, herring, certain aged cheeses. Adverse effects: hypotension, ED, blurred vision, urinary retention, constipation, and dry mouth.	See specific drug.
Marplan® (isocarboxazid)	Major Depression	Isocarboxazid is a nonselective hydrazine monoamine oxidase (MAO) inhibitor.	**Above common side effects plus** orthostatic hypotension	Start: 10 mg increase to 40 mg/day
Nardil® (phenelzine)	Depression, "atypical," "non-endogenous" or "neurotic" depression	Potent MAO Inhibitor Leukopenia.	**Above common side effects, plus** Ataxia, shock-like coma,	15 mg TID
Parnate® (trancypomine)	Major Depressive Episode without Melancholia	Nonhydrazine MAO Inhibitor	**Above common side effects, plus** Anemia, leukopenia, agranulocytosis, and thrombocytopenia	Start 30 mg/day, increase to 60 mg/day
Eldpryl® (selegiline)	Specifically for depression associated with Parkinson's Disease (levorotatory acetylenic derivative of phenethylamine)	**MOA #1**—Inhibition of monoamine oxidase, type B. **MOA #2**—may increase dopaminergic activity	**Above common side effects, plus** Orthostatic hypotension	5 mg BID

The biological causes of mania are an excess of neurotransmitter norepinephrin, NE (and perhaps other neurotransmitters), while the depression is deficiency of monoamines (neurotransmitters) such as serotonin (S), NE, or dopamine (D). In addition, sodium, Na^+, is a conductor of nerve impulses. Lithium (Li^+) interferes with such conductions and impulses.

In mania there is an excessive amount of Li$^+$ ions, which helps to reuptake NE and D. Li$^+$ also appears to reduce the release of NE and D from the neurons. Someone who does not have enough lithium, or has too much sodium, will exhibit hyperexcitability of the nerves and signs of mania. Therefore, lithium, a mood-stabilizing drug, is given to reduce hyperexcitability of the nerves and hyperactivity of the patient. This allows the patient to have slower and more realistic thoughts. Sometimes, antidepressant drugs in addition are given to the patient to manage the lows.

Side effects of lithium include drowsiness, weakness, nausea, fatigue, hand tremor, and increased thirst and urination. Too much lithium contributes to complications of the thyroid, kidney, heart, or brain. Lithium increases the risk of congenital malformations in babies. Too much lithium may be toxic, and too little may not be effective. The difference in the two amounts is very small and is called a narrow therapeutic window or index. Therefore, blood levels must be monitored. Decreased salt (Na$^+$) intake or increased output may cause a lithium buildup that could lead to toxicity. Dehydration, fever, vomiting, and diuretics (coffee or tea) can contribute to this decrease of sodium and resultant lithium toxicity. Signs of lithium toxicity include drowsiness, mental dullness, slurred speech, blurred vision, confusion, muscle twitching, irregular heartbeat, and seizures. A lithium overdose can be life-threatening (see Table 19-5).

Benzodiazepines, lorazepam or clonazepam, can be given 2 to 4 mg tid IM or PO in acute management, these agents can boost the antipsychotic's effects so that high doses can be reduced, diminishing the possibility of toxicity.

Because of the toxicity associated with lithium, doctors are prescribing an alternative—anticonvulsant drugs. Anticonvulsants are also prescribed when lithium does not prove effective. Equally effective for nonrapid cycling bipolar disorder, and superior to lithium in *rapid-cycling bipolar disorder*, is valproic acid (Depakote®, divalproex sodium), a great alternative. Adverse side effects include gastrointestinal symptoms, headache, dizziness, double vision, anxiety, and confusion. Valproic acid has caused liver dysfunction in some cases; therefore, liver function tests should be performed before therapy and at frequent intervals. Research shows that anticonvulsant therapy is more effective for acute mania than for long-term management of bipolar disorder. Other anticonvulsants that are used that lack formal FDA approval for bipolar disorder include those outlined in Table 19-6.

TABLE 19-5 Lithium Carbonate for Bipolar Disorder			
Generic Name	Brand Name	Usual Dosage	Half life (hours)
Lithium Carbonate	Lithobid® Eskalith®, Lithotabs®	Acute episode 900–2400 mg/day Maintenance 300 mg PO bid or tid (blood level of 0.8 to 1.2 mEq/L)	8–35

TABLE 19-6   Anticonvulsants Used in Bipolar Therapy

Trade/Generic Name	Usual Daily Adult Dose	Usual Daily Adult Dose	Adverse Actions and Special Notes	Half life (hours)
Tegretol®, (carbamazepine)	100 mg tablet and chew tablet, 200 and 400 mg Extended Release tablets, 300 mg ER Capsule, 100 mg/5 ml Suspension	400–1200 mg (blood level: 6 to 12 mg/L) (B) Off-label use for BD (use for acute mania)	May cause aplastic anemia agranulocytois, requires blood monitoring	25–65 hrs
Neurontin®, (gabapentin)	100, 300 and 400 mg capsules 600 and 800 mg tablets 250 mg/5 ml solution	100–1200 mg/day usually in TID dosing NTE 3600 mg/day Off label use for BD, migraines, MS, and tremors	Side effect—dizziness, somnolence, and peripheral edema	5–7 hrs
Depakote®, (divalproex sodium) (aka valproic acid)	125, 250, and 500 mg Delayed Release tablets, 500 ER tablets, and 125 mg Sprinkle Capsules	750 mg initial dose, increased to effective dose (blood level: 40–40 mg/L) (B) NTE is 60 mg/kg/day. FDA approved for mania associated with BD per Facts and Comparisons 2000	Toxic effect: Hepatic failure; Liver Function must be monitored Teratogenic Effect: Spina Bifida	6–16 hrs
Lamictal® (lamotrigine)	25, 100, 150, and 200 mg tablets 2, 5, and 25 mg Chewable Dispersible Tablet Also in Special Starter Kits for those NOT taking enzyme inducing drugs or Valproic Acid for BD Patients ONLY	NTE 200 mg/day PO as monotherapy. (used for depressive phase of BD called BD-1) NTE 100 mg/day in combination valproic acid or 400 mg/day with carbamazepine	Side effects: H/A (25%), rash (11%), dizziness (10%), diarrhea (8%), and pruritus (6%). Toxic effects: Serious rashes or Stevens-Johnson Syndrome (0.8%) and Epidermal Necrolysis	Depends upon dosing
Topamax® (topiramate)	Availability: 25, 50, 100, 200 mg tablets, 15 and 25 mg Sprinkle capsules	Begin with low doses target 600 mg/day (E) NTE 1600 mg/d Note: Off-label use for rapid cycling and mixed bipolar states	Side effects: fatigue, somnolence, dizziness, nausea, abdominal pain	21 hrs
Klonopin®, (clonazepine) Class IV benzodiazepine	0.5, 1, and 2 mg K shaped perforated tablets	0.75 – 16 mg/day NTE 20 mg/day Off-label use for acute mania associated with BD per Facts and Comparisons 2000	Side effects: drowsiness and ataxia	18–50 hrs

MECHANISM OF ACTION OF LITHIUM

Many theories of the MOA of lithium exist. The most common is the Li^+/Na^+ exchange theory already discussed. According to a study by Hokin et al., 1998 cited in the University of Wisconsin News, ". . . the exact mechanism of action was not discovered until earlier this year. Researchers from the University of Wisconsin, Madison, indicated that lithium acts upon the stimulatory neurotransmitter of glutamate, providing a bi-directional force that ultimately results in a relative stasis in mood." This means that lithium has the ability to lower and increase amounts of glutamate simultaneously, creating a chemical balance for the patient. Furthermore, "In addition to inhibiting reuptake during depressive cycles it is believed that during the manic phase, when levels of glutamate are extremely high, lithium aids in increasing the reuptake process, thus doing double duty on the same neurotransmitter" (Hokin).

The exact mechanism of action of anticonvulsants for BD is unknown, but may involve the GABA (ergic) mechanisms and, ultimately, G-protein signaling systems. Goodwin and Ghaeni (1998) propose that carbamazapine functions by blocking the reuptake of norepinepherine, which prevents the sodium channel impulses from repeatedly firing and inhibits the enzymes that break down gamma aminobutyric acid (GABA). Thus, more of the neurotransmitters are made available during the manic and depressive episodes. It has been theorized that GABA has an antimanic mechanism that limits manic episodes by blocking the reuptake of GABA; it is by this same method that carbamazapine makes more norepinepherine available to reduce depressive episodes (Walsh, 1998). Goodwin and Ghaeni found that individuals diagnosed with bipolar disorders and prescribed carbamazapine in conjunction with lithium therapy were six times less likely to engage in suicidal behaviors when compared with individuals involved in other treatment options.

ALCOHOL WITHDRAWAL

Addiction to alcohol, known as alcoholism and alcohol dependence, is a disease that includes the following four symptoms:

- *Craving*—urge to drink, described by some as a need.
- *Loss of control*—unable to stop drinking once drinking has begun.
- *Physical dependence*—experiencing symptoms of withdrawal, such as nausea, shakiness, sweating, and anxiety after drinking stops.
- *Tolerance*—the requirement to drink greater amounts of alcohol to get the same "buzz" or "high."

Several withdrawal syndromes are observed over the first 48 hours of cessation from alcohol, or alcohol withdrawal, as follows: seizures, blood pressure changes, delerium tremens (hallucinations, tremors, and shaking caused by alcohol withdrawal; may be fatal), dehydration, malnutrition, ataxia, nystagmus (eye problem), cognitive chantes associated with Wernicke's Encephalopathy, and liver damage.

TABLE 19-7 Alcohol Withdrawal Treatment

Benzodiazepines	Indications	Usual Adult Dose
Serax® (oxazepam)	Alcohol Withdrawal, Short Acting	15 to 30 mg, 3 or 4 times daily
Valium® (diazepam)	Alcohol and Cocaine Withdrawal Long Acting	10–20 mg every 1–3 hours for first three doses
Librium® (chlordiazepoxide)	Alcohol Withdrawal, DTs, Long Acting	25–100 mg every 1–2 hours as needed
Arivan® (lorazepam)	Alcohol Withdrawal and DTs, (Delerium Tremens), Short Acting	2–4 mg IV Q1 hour prn until calm
Antipsychotics		
Haldol® (haloperidol)	Extreme agitation during withdrawal	2–4 mg IV Q 1 hour pm, until calm
Miscellaneous **Antialcoholic Agents** (Detoxification Helpers)		
ReVia® (naltrexone)	Alcohol antidote for the management of abstinence of alcohol, Narcotic Antagonist	Initial dose: 25 mg PO QD (1/2 50 mg tab) Maintenance dose: 50 mg tablet PO QD
Antabuse® (disulfiram)	Management of abstinence of alcohol in aversion therapy	Initial dose—500 mg PO QD Maintenance dose—250 mg PO QD Range 125–500 mg PO QD, NTE 500 mg/day

TREATMENT

A 12-step group support program, in conjunction with individual therapy and counseling, are essential in alcohol withdrawal. While thiamine and folate are routinely used to reverse common nutritional deficiencies, a few benzodiaepines that are used for anti-anxiety are also used for alcohol withdrawal (see Table 19-7). Benzodiazepines are sometimes used during the first few days after a person stops drinking to help him safely withdraw from alcohol. Extreme agitation during withdrawal may require other drugs such as barbiturates, antipsychotics, anticonvulsants, and antihypertensives. The smallest dosage necessary to manage symptoms should be given. The liver may undergo severe benzodiazepine toxicity if given a long-acting benzodiazepine for alcohol withdrawal. Note: 1 mg Lorazepam = 5 mg Diazepam = 25 mg Chlordiazepoxide. Antipsychotic Haldol (haloperidol) IV and benzodiazepine Ativan (lorzepam) can be given together to help control DTs (delirium tremens); however, haloperidol must be used with caution because of the risk of Torsade De Pointes (an uncommon type of ventricular tachycardia (VT), in which QT interval is increased markedly, causing sudden death).

Some drugs, such as ReVia® (naltrexone), help people remain sober. The combination of counseling and naltrexone can reduce the craving for alcohol and help prevent the return to alcohol abuse and relapsing into heavy drinking, but only *after* the patient stops drinking. This drug works by blocking the same receptors and areas that narcotics and alcohol block in the brain: the Mu receptors, limbic system, and reticular formation. This lessens the feeling of needing to drink alcohol so that the patient can stop drinking more easily. Side effects of naltrexone include nausea, headache, constipation, dizziness, nervousness, insomnia, drowsiness, and anxiety. Recommended dose is 50 mg daily. This drug was approved for this purpose in 1994; since then, research has shown mixed results.

Another drug, Antabuse® (disulfiram), discourages drinking by provoking the person to feel nauseated and flushed and develop sudden stomach cramps, headache, and vomiting when or if he drinks alcohol. This type of management of abstinence of alcohol is called aversion therapy. Alcohol treatment will work only when the patient wants to stop drinking. Along with medical treatment, sometimes counseling helps, sometimes time helps, and unfortunately sometimes nothing at all helps.

Smoking Withdrawal and Cessation

In 2000, the American Psychiatric Association updated the data on smoking as a mental disorder, not a habit. Diagnostic and Statistical Manual of Mental Disorders, 4th rev. ed. (DSM-IV-TR), pages 264–269, "Nicotine-Related Disorders . . . Nicotine Use Disorder 305.1 Nicotine Dependence . . . Nicotine-Induced Disorder 292.0 Nicotine Withdrawal. . . ."

Statistics from the last five years show that almost 25 percent of all adults continue to smoke, despite all the recognition and acceptance that smoking is detrimental to health. Smoking among 18–24 year olds increased to 33 percent between 1991 and 1997. While many people find that support groups or therapy help them quit smoking, others quit cold turkey. Still others have used some of the pharmaceutical agents on the market to help them curb the urge to smoke.

Nicotine inhaler—A nicotine oral inhalation system called Nicotrol Inhaler® is available by prescription, but requires the use of four inhalers a day, totaling 2000 puffs per day, to achieve adequate nicotine levels. This poses compliance problems. Side effects include mouth and throat irritation due to the oral delivery.

Nicotine nasal spray—Nicotrol NS®, available by prescription, requires four sprays per hour, or a maximum of 80 sprays per day. Common side effects are nasal and throat irritation and rhinorrhea.

Nicotine gum—Nicorette (nicotine polacrilex) is available OTC in 2-mg and 4-mg strengths. The most effective dose is the use of 10 to 15 pieces of 4-mg gum per day initially; after two weeks, most patients can benefit with the 2-mg strength. Nicotine gum should be chewed once or twice every few minutes and then placed between the cheek and the gum (buccal placement) until the next "chew." GI upset, caused by chewing the gum too quickly and swallowing nicotine with saliva, is a common side effect.

Nicotine Patch—Once prescription only, Habitrol, Nicoderm CQ, and Nicotrol are now available OTC. The Fagerstrom test score determines which strength of patch the patient should begin using. A score of 5 to 6 indicates the use of the 21-mg nicotine patch; a score of 3 to 4 means that the 14-mg nicotine patch is appropriate for initial therapy; and a score of zero to

2 indicates initial use of the 7-mg nicotine patch. Side effects are mild skin irritation just under the patch and possible sleep disruption. Alleviation of these results from rotating the patch site and removing the patch at bedtime. People who use the patch should know that concomitant smoking and nicotine patch use may cause sudden cardiac death.

ANTIDEPRESSANTS IN SMOKING CESSATION

The immediate release form of the antidepressant bupropion inhibits the uptake of monoamine neurotransmitters norepinephrine and serotonin and weakly blocks the reuptake of dopamine. The sustained release form weakly inhibits the neuronal uptake of norepinephrine, serotonin, and dopamine. It is believed that this MOA allows for the reduction in the urge to smoke. The most common side effects of bupropion include dry mouth and sleep interruptions. If depression is also present, the patient will benefit from the antidepressant effects of this drug. Note: Bupropion is sold as antidepressant Wellbutin XL for Anxiety/GAD, Wellbutin for depression, and Zyban for smoking cessation. The combined use of antidepressant, bupropion, and nicotine replacement agents appears to be the most effective treatment for nicotine dependence (nicotine withdrawal/smoking cessation). Zyban® (bupropion) should be dosed as follows: 150 mg per day for 3 days, 150 mg twice daily, 8 to 12 weeks.

ANTI-ANXIETY AGENTS IN SMOKING CESSATION

Anti-anxiety agents are also used to reduce the symptoms of anxiety associated with nicotine withdrawal and smoking cessation. Benzodiazepines enhance the effects of the brain chemical called gamma aminobutyric acid (GABA). This slows down nerve cell activity and decreases nerve excitement, thus causing relaxation and quieting the anxiety symptoms that accompany smoking withdrawal. Maintenance drug therapy can employ Xanax® (alprazolam) and other benzodiazepines. Xanax alprazolarm may be dosed as follows: 0.25 to 0.5 mg PO bid to tid. Maximum Daily Dose: 4 mg.

Psychosis

A person who is out of touch with reality is considered psychotic. Symptoms of a particular psychosis, schizophrenia, include the following: illogical thoughts or paranoia, such as the certain knowledge of being followed by someone all the time; hearing someone else's thoughts; hearing voices; seeing people, events, and things that aren't there (hallucinations); believing that they are someone else, usually of extreme importance or celebrity (such as the King of England or Britney Spears). They may have poor hygiene, spend much time alone, and pass the time at night awake, but sleep during the day. The patient may exhibit delusions of grandeur, but with a lack of insight and poor judgment.

Early antipsychotic drugs caused muscle stiffness, tremor, and abnormal movements. An irreversible adverse reaction called tardive dyskinesia (TD), characterized by involuntary movements, can affect about five percent of the patients using the older antipsychotics long term.

Newer drugs developed in the 1990s, called atypical antipsychotics, have lessened the side effects and improved compliance. The most common side effects are drowsiness, rapid heartbeat, dizziness upon moving from one position to another (sitting to standing, for example), weight gain, and decreased sexual function (ED) or libido (interest).

When these drugs take effect, the degree of effectiveness, and the side effects vary from patient to patient. In most cases, the drugs take effect within two to six weeks, and improvement can be noticed after a few days, up to several months.

Drug interactions are wide and include antihypertensive agents, antiepileptics, anticonvulsants, and anti-Parkinson drugs. One of the most commonly accepted theories on the causes of schizophrenia is a biological increase in the amount of the neurotransmitter dopamine in the brain. The causes of the increase in dopamine may be predisposed (genetic), drug-induced, condition- or disease-induced, or food- or food-allergy induced. Environmental stressors in early childhood and brain development are in current research. According to the U.S. Surgeon General in 2002, "The onset and course of schizophrenia are most likely the result of an interaction between genetic and environmental influences." Carl C. Pfeiffer, Ph.D., M.D., pioneered the treatment of mental illnesses with nutrition and found 29 possible causes of schizophrenia. His research showed *that an increase in copper, which decreases blood histamine (histapenia) and the low levels for histamine were found in over 50 percent of psychotic patients.* "It's been observed that geographical regions with low selenium levels in the soil and less sunshine have higher rates of 'schizophrenia.' Since some prostaglandins require selenium for their synthesis, it's believed prostaglandin deficiency may be a source of 'schizophrenia.'"

MECHANISM OF ACTION OF ANTIPSYCHOTIC DRUGS

One of the causes of pychosis has been well documented to be an increase in dopamine. Antipsychotic drugs attach to the dopamine D2 receptor, blocking its action, thereby decreasing dopamine activity. Unfortunately, conventional or traditional (that is, typical) antipsychotics do this, but also induce involuntary movements and elevate serum prolactin. When given within the accepted clinical effective ranges, atypical antipsychotics do not cause these adverse reactions. To understand how these drugs work, it is important to examine the atypical antipsychotic's mechanism of action and how it differs from that of the more typical drugs. The key difference in the mechanism is a physical one: The atypical antipsychotics (see Table 19.8) bind more loosely than dopamine to the dopamine D2 receptor; they also have dissociation constants higher than that for dopamine, while the conventional antipsychotics "bind more tightly than dopamine itself to the dopamine D2 receptor, with dissociation constants that are lower than that for dopamine."

It is also postulated that atypical drugs block 5-HT2A receptors (serotonin, another neurotransmitter) at the same time that they block dopamine receptors and that, somehow, this serotonin–dopamine balance keeps prolactin levels normal, spares cognition, and does not promote involuntary movement. Clozaril, introduced in 1990, was the first atypical antipsychotic. It has helped 25–50 percent of patients who had not responded to conventional antipsychotics. Unfortunately, Clozaril is associated with two percent agranulocytosis, which is a deficiency of a specific white blood cell. Agranulocytosis is potentially fatal, but reversible if diagnosed early. When affected by agranulocytosis, the immune system is decreased, rendering the patient susceptible to infection. Patients using Clorazil must have their blood checked regularly. Doctors now recommend that Clozaril be used only after at least two other, safer antipsychotics have been tried without success.

Conventional antipsychotics are becoming obsolete due to the side effects of involuntary movement. Experts usually recommend using a newer, atypical antipsychotic rather than a conventional one unless the patient is already doing well on the older treatment. If the person is noncompliant with multiple daily dosing, the once a day dosing of Haldol® or Prolixin® may be more suitable.

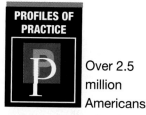

PROFILES OF PRACTICE

Over 2.5 million Americans suffer from psychosis.

CONVENTIONAL, TRADITIONAL, OR TYPICAL ANTIPSYCHOTIC DRUGS

- Haldol® (haloperidol)
- Stelazine® (trifluoperazine)
- Mellaril® (thioridazine)
- Thorazine® (chlorpromazine)
- Navane® (thiothixene)
- Trilafon® (perphenazine)
- Prolixin®, Permitil® (fluphenazine)

Newer, atypical antipsychotic drugs are being prescribed more often to reduce side effects, thus improving the quality of life for patients with psychosis.

Insomnia

Different individuals' requirements for sleep vary as do their feelings of satisfaction from sleep. Insomnia is described as an individual's complaint of inadequate or poor-quality sleep. Insomnia is characterized by one or more of the following complaints:

- difficulty falling asleep
- difficulty returning to sleep if awoken during the night
- waking up frequently during the night
- waking up too early in the morning

TABLE 19-8	Atypical Antipsychotic Drugs	
Trade/Generic Name	Availability	Dosage
Abilify® (aripiprazole)	10, 15, 20, and 30 mg tablets	1 tab QD (nrtm*)
Clozaril®, (clozapine) (given only when two other atypical antipsychotic drugs have not shown improvement or effectiveness)	25, 100 mg tablets	12.5 ($\frac{1}{2}$ 25 mg tab) QD or BID initial dose, 350 to 400 mg/day with TID dosing as target dose NTE 900 mg/day
Geodon®, Zeldox® (ziprasidone)	20, 40, 60, and 80 mg capsules	20 mg BID w/food initial dose NTE 80 mg BID
Risperdal® (risperidone)	0.5, 1, 2, 3, and 4 mg tablets M-Tab (disintegrating) R0.5, R1, and R2 1 mg/mL PO solution in 30 ml bottles	1 mg QD or BID initially, NTE 16 mg/day
Seroquel® (quetiapine)	25, 100 and 20 mg tablets	25 mg BID initial dose, with 300–400 mg daily dose in TID dosing as a target of Day 4. NTE 800 mg/day in TID dosing
Zyprexa® (olanzapine)	5, 10, 15, and 20 mg tablets	5–10 mg QD initial dose, NTE 20 mg QD

*nrtm means no regard to meals, may be taken with or without food

- poor energy or not feeling refreshed in the morning, as if there had been no sleep at all

Insomnia may cause problematic symptoms such as a lack of energy, tiredness, daytime sleepiness, difficulty in focus or concentration, impaired performance and irritability, and a tendency to feel anger. Those most likely to experience insomnia are as follows:

- Elderly people are most likely to have sleep problems, which occur more in people over 60 years of age. It has been incorrectly stated that the need for sleep decreases with age; in fact, it is the *ability* to sleep that decreases with age.

- Females, especially after menopause, are more likely to have insomnia than males.

- Those with a history of depression are also likely candidates.

Certain risk factors contribute to the increased likelihood of insomnia. They are anxiety, stress, specific diseases or conditions, the use of certain medications, intake of specific foods and drinks, sleep–wake scheduling problems, interruptions such as jet lag or a change in work shift schedules, nighttime activity, change in physical surroundings such as sleeping in a hotel room or even just a different bed, and a change in the environment such as noise, light, climate, or temperature alterations.

Chronic insomnia is multifaceted and results from a combination of factors. Common causes are physical or mental disorders, especially depression, arthritis, kidney disease, diabetes, hyperthyroidism, CHF, asthma, restless legs syndrome, sleep apnea, and narcolepsy.

To overcome insomnia, the individual could try making changes to his environment, schedules, medications that contribute, and diet (such as eliminating caffeine). Also, playing some soft music, reading a boring book to tire the eyes, doing homework, taking a warm bath, and drinking warm milk are good evening habits. Light exercise, yoga, hypnosis, relaxation techniques, and sleep restriction therapy may all work. Then, an over-the-counter sleep aid such as Nytol® (diphenhydramine 25 mg), Sominex® (diphenhydramine 50 mg), and Unisom® (doxylamine 25 mg), which are antihistamines, can help. Recall from Chapter 13, The Respiratory System, that the side effects of some OTC antihistamines are drowsiness and sleepiness. The antihistamine ingredient most commonly used is diphenhydramine. Some combination products have analgesics as well. When all else fails, prescription sedatives and hypnotics are available.

PRESCRIPTION HYPNOTICS, SEDATIVES, AND BARBITURATE MEDICATION

In layman's terms, hypnotics are sleeping pills, and sedatives are tranquilizers (see Table 19-9). A medical definition of a hypnotic is a drug that causes drowsiness, induces sleep onset, and/or maintains sleep. A medical definition of a sedative is a drug that calms and relaxes a person. Pharmacologically speaking, a hypnotic and a sedative are the same drug (same ingredients), which vary in amounts only to vary the degree of response. For example, a higher dose of a hypnotic would put someone to sleep very quickly, whereas a smaller dose of the same drug would merely calm him down, reducing nervous tension. Both hypnotics and sedatives decrease mental activity and nervous system function. Another way of saying this is that the nervous system is *depressed*. By this action, these agents can reduce anxiety, stress, irritability, and excitement. Since relaxation is essential to falling asleep—that is, the muscles and mind must relax—sedatives may lead a person to fall asleep by merely relaxing or calming the mind or loosening the muscles. Because of this, when a person takes a sedative close to his bedtime to calm his nerves, he will more than likely fall asleep rather than stay calmly awake.

Barbiturates are very addictive sleeping pills, but are chemically different from the many benzodiazepines that are considered hypnotics and sedatives. Barbiturates, hypnotics, and sedatives are depressants (see Table 19-10). The pupils become constricted, the vision is blurred, and breathing is shallow. Large doses of barbiturates can cause respiratory depression, coma, and death.

Barbiturates, hypnotics, and sedatives are used when the cause of insomnia is any emotional disturbance other than depression. Tolerance and addiction can result from long-term use; therefore, all patients should be counseled to use hypnotics only short term (two to four weeks) or episodically (no more than a few times a week). Because the depressed patient may be prone to suicide, he should be prescribed small quantities requiring frequent refills, rather than supplying them with large amounts, to reduce the opportunity for a suicide attempt.

> **Special note:** Patients with depression should be prescribed a sedating tricyclic antidepressant such as Elavil® (amitriptyline), Tofranil® (imipramine), or Anafranil® (clomipramine), to be taken about one hour before bedtime. In general, these drugs are prescribed at the lowest dose and for the shortest duration needed to relieve the symptoms of insomnia. Some drugs should be tapered off gradually as the medicine is discontinued, because, if they are stopped abruptly, the insomnia may recur.

MECHANISM OF ACTION FOR THE NON-BENZODIAZEPINES

The non-benzodiazepines, a miscellaneous group, vary in characteristics depending upon the specific agent. Conventional benzodiazepines such as triazolam and fluazepam, the treatment of choice for short-term insomnia for many years, are associated with adverse effects such as rebound insomnia, withdrawal, and dependency. The newer "hypnosedatives," sometimes call the "Z" drugs, include zolpidem, zaleplon, and zopiclone. These agents are starting to be preferred over conventional BZs to treat short-term insomnia because they are considered less likely to cause significant rebound insomnia, or tolerance, and are as efficacious as the conventional benzodiazepines. They are still Class IV drugs. Since they are newer to the market, there are not as many post-market studies. More about these drugs may be known in the near future.

Ambien® (zolpidem), an imidazopyridine, acts by increasing GABA potential, but is not useful for anticonvulsant therapy or skeletal muscle relaxation. It is used mainly as a hypnotic for short-term therapy for seven to ten days, but may be used up to 28 days. A comparative study of Ambien (zolopidem, or ZLP, which selectively binds to omega-1 BZ receptor) versus Imovane® (zopiclone, or ZPC, a cyclopyrrolone, which only marginally binds to the same receptor) showed that ZLP acts more rapidly than ZPC, yet ZLP has less residual effect on sleepiness and psychomotor function the next morning.

Sonata® (zaleplon) belongs to the pyrazolopyrimidine class of hypnotics and has the same selective binding as zolopidem. Zopiclone is the racemate of eszopiclone, currently under study for transient and chronic insomnia. While triazolam and midazolam are biotransformed almost entirely via CYP3A4, the newer "Z" drugs are metabolized by several CYP isozymes, incuding CYP3A4. Therefore, the resulting hepatic enzyme inhibitors and inducers have less effect on the patient metabolism.

Noctec, or chloral hydrate, depresses the CNS and is associated with liver toxicity if combined with ulcer drugs, birth control pills, propranolol, or disulfiram because its metabolism pathway is similar to that of alcohol. Both of these drugs are Class IV substances.

TABLE 19-9   Sedatives—Hypnotics

Classification Type	Site and Mechanism of Action	Side and Toxic Effects/Special Notes	Drug Interactions
Barbiturates Controlled CII, CIII, and CIV	**SOA: Reticular formation and cerebral cortex** **MOA #1**—Low doses increase GABA, causing relaxation. **MOA #2**—High doses cause sleep and depression of CNS.	Dry mouth, **lethargy, drowsiness** OD—CV and CNS depression, kidney failure, low blood pressure, death **Note:** No known antidote	Increased effect with other CNS depressants and alcohol.
Non-Barbiturates (miscellaneous group)	**SOA and MOA vary** **Zolpidem** and **zaleplon** selectively bind to omega-1 BZ receptor, potentiating GABA, while **zopiclone** mildly binds to omega-1.	Produces less tolerance and addiction. Exception: "Z" drugs produce more dependence in patients with pre-existing substance-related addictions. (1) Zolpidem—GI and CNS disturbances, rare—delirium, nightmares, and hallucinations; may reduce memory or psychomotor function within the first 2 hours after administration of single oral dose. (2) Zaleplon does not impair memory or psychomotor function. Most common SE–H/A.	Rifampicin induces metabolism of newer hypnosedatives and decreases sedative effects. Induces metabolism: Ketoconazole, erythromycin, and cimetidine
Benzodiazepines	**SOA: Reticular formation** **MOA #1**—Low doses increase GABA, causing relaxation. **MOA #2**—High doses cause sleep and depression of CNS.	Do not cause REM rebound when discontinued. Less addictive than barbiturates, may be used a few weeks longer before tolerance builds up. Halcion® may cause rebound insomnia, nightmares, and daytime anxiety.	Decreased effect with cimetidine. Increased effect with other CNS depressants and alcohol.

TABLE 19-10	Hypnotic/Sedative Dosing		
Classification and/or Type	Trade/Generic Name	Controlled Substance Schedule	Onset and Dosing
Barbiturates		Scheduled Non-Narcotic Agents	
	Luminol® (phenobarbital) Used as a sedative and for epilepsy	CIV	
	Brevital® (methohexital)	CIV Duration 4–7 minutes	
	Pentothal® (thiopental)	CIII	**Induction:** 25–75 mg (2.5%) **Maintenance anesthesia:** 25–50 mg when **patient moves**
	Nembutal® (pentobarbital)	Intermediate acting Duration of 4–6 hrs CII	**Sedation:** 20 mg TID or QID **Hypnosis:** 100 mg HS
	Amytal® (amobarbital)	CII Intermediate acting Duration of 4–6 hrs	**Sedation:** 50–300 mg **Hypnosis:** 100–200 mg
	Seconal® (secobarbital)	CII Short acting duration 2–4 hrs	**Hypnotic:** 100 mg HS **Pre-Op:** 200–300 mg 1 hour **before surgery**
Non-Barbiturates		Scheduled Non-Narcotic Agents	
	Ambien® (zolpidem)	C IV	
	Imovane® (zopiclone)	C IV	
	Noctec® (chloral hydrate)	C IV	
	Placidyl® (ethchlorvynol)	C IV	
	Sonata® (zaleplon)	C IV	
Benzodiazepines (Used as hypnotics)		Non-Narcotic	
	Dalmane® (flurazepam)	C IV	
	Doral® (quazepam)	C IV	
	Halcion® (triazolam)	C IV	
	ProSom® (estazolam)	C IV	

Stimulants

Stimulants are drugs that increase mental alertness or the activity of the nervous system. They speed up the physiological and metabolic activity of the body and other system functions. Stimulants are a class of drugs that enhance brain activity and increase alertness, attention, and energy. In addition, they elevate blood pressure and increase respiration and heart rate. Therefore, they are used to keep people awake, for narcolepsy, attention-deficit hyperactivity disorder (ADHD), attention deficit disorder (ADD), and depression that have not responded to other treatments. They may also be used as appetite suppressants for short-term treatment of obesity, and for patients with asthma to increase breathing rate. Because of the potential for abuse and addiction, prescription stimulants are usually classified as Control Substance Schedule II drugs and reserved for treatment of only a few diseases or conditions (listed previously).

Stimulants have chemical structures similar to the neurotransmitters found in the brain called monoamines, which include norepinephrine and dopamine. Stimulants act like these compounds, increase the amount of them, or promote the synthesis or production of these chemicals in the brain. The results of the stimulation of the sympathetic nervous system are as follows:

- increase in blood pressure, heart rate
- constriction of the blood vessels (narrowing)
- increase in blood glucose
- opening up of the pathways of the respiratory system for easier breathing

In addition, the increase in dopamine is associated with a sense of euphoria that can accompany the use of these drugs. Cocaine is a stimulant that can produce this euphoric effect. Other CII stimulants are amphetamines such as Ritalin® (methylphenidate), used for ADD/ADHD, and Dexedrine® (dextroamphetamine), a synthetically altered amphetamine used for weight loss, narcolepsy, and ADD/ADHD.

Over-the-counter pharmacological stimulants include pseudoephedrine, used in cough and cold remedies, caffeine used in analgesics, and weight loss products. An example of an herbal stimulant is guarana, used in weight loss products and Brazilian soda drinks.

The many manufactures in the diet industry boast that their guarana containing diet pills have no caffeine. However the constituents of the crystalline principle, guaranine, is "identical with caffeine, which exists in the seeds, united with tannic acid, catechutannic acid starch, and a greenish fixed oil." German botanist Theodore Von Martius named the crystalline substance guaranine and later renamed it caffeine. It has been reported that "guarana seeds contain up to 4–8% caffeine, as well as trace amounts of xanthines: theophylline and theobromine." Compare this with Black tea (*Camellia sinensis*), which has 2.5–4.5 percent caffeine, coffee beans, which have 1–2.5 percent caffeine, and cocoa seed having 0.25 percent. They also contain large "quantities of alkaloids, terpenes, tannins, flavonoids, starch, saponins, and resinous substances."

ADVERSE ACTIONS OF STIMULANTS

High doses of some stimulants taken repeatedly over a short period of time may lead to feelings of paranoia, anger, or hostility. Other detrimental outcomes are fatally high body temperatures, seizures, irregular heartbeat (arrhythmias), or CV failure. Less serious side effects include headache, dizziness, diarrhea or constipation, restlessness, tremor, nervousness, anxiety, insomnia, dry mouth, unpleasant taste in the mouth, erectile dysfunction, changes in libido (sex drive), GI disturbances, and weight loss.

CONTRAINDICATIONS: DRUG–CONDITION INTERACTIONS OF STIMULANTS

Since stimulation of the sympathetic nervous system can exacerbate high intra-optic pressure (glaucoma), hypertension, coronary artery disease (CAD), or an overactive thyroid gland, patients with these conditions should not take stimulant prescriptions or over-the-counter stimulant products. Stimulants cause a fatally acute rise in BP when taken within two weeks of taking an MAO inhibitor antidepressant (such as Nardil® or Parnate®). Therefore, patients must be warned and counseled of this drug interaction. Stimulants should not be given to those with agitation or anxiety.

WITHDRAWAL TREATMENT

Addiction to prescription stimulants may first be treated with a tapering off of the drug. Withdrawal symptoms may be treated with antidepressants to help manage the symptoms of depression that occur during the early phase of abstinence from stimulants. Detoxification involves psychotherapy, which includes behavioral—learning skills for coping with daily life—and cognitive—changing the way the patient thinks about things, his future outlook, and therefore his reactions. Recovery support or 12-step groups may also be employed effectively in conjunction with psychotherapy.

ADD and ADHD

ADHD is a condition (note: NOT a disease) in which a person, child, or adult has a very short attention span and is easily distracted, excessively active, and possibly overly emotional or highly impulsive. ADD does not present the excessive movement or activity (hyperkinetic) associated with ADHD. Treatment should include psychological, educational approaches and pharmacological approaches.

STIMULANTS USED IN THE TREATMENT OF ADHD AND ADD

- Ritalin® (methylphenidate) is a *mild* central nervous system stimulant.
- Concerta® (methylphenidae) is the first once-daily treatment for ADD/ADHD with a 12-hour time-release formula of

methylphenidate. Medical studies have demonstrated that Concerta® can help children with ADHD improve focus in the classroom and even perform better on math tests. It has lower incidence of side effects than the immediate release form of methylphenidate. Taking immediate release methylphenidate, dextroamphetamine alone, or dextroamphetamine plus an amphetamine usually produces weight loss in patients. Only four percent of patients taking Concerta® reported any loss of appetite or sleep. Sustained release methylphenidate can be taken without regard to food.

- Dexedrine is all dextroamphetamine, a strong CNS stimulant, more potent than methyphenidate.

- Adderall® contains Dextroamphetamine Sulfate + Dextroamphetamine Saccharate + Amphetamine Asparate + Amphetamine Sulphate. Amphetamine is more potent than dextroamphetamine, and amphetamine sulfate is a widely abused street drug. Adderall® is used to treat ADHD, ADD, and narcolepsy. Adderall XR® is an extended-release form of Adderall®. Adderall XR® is for once-daily dosing.It has been shown to have many benefits over immediate release multiple daily dosing of methylphenidate, and a single significant benefit over the once-daily, 12-hour time-release formula of Concerta®. Adderall® and Adderall XR® may be better choices, as they last longer and are more powerful than methlyphenidate or dexedrine. Because the "speed rush" is brought about more gradually, the patient "comes down" more easily and gradually. Most people on dexedrine have a "crash" (sleep for many hours) after it wears off.

- Once a day dosing is preferable not only for convenience and patient compliance. It also allows the parent to do the medication administration from home, and eliminating the worry about a school nurse or official administering the medication and the stigma to the child associated with being medicated at school.

With the two bead system inside the capsule, the medication can be placed in applesauce or other soft food and swallowed whole, which helps when a person does not like to, or cannot swallow capsules. Above all, this long-acting formula works to control ADHD symptoms throughout the whole day—morning and afternoon—and many claim that the patient has less groggy feeling in the mornings.

In comparison, Concerta® capsule has a quick dissolving outer coat of medication and two small compartments of medication inside that release gradually. Concerta®, unlike Adderal XR®, cannot be crushed, opened, or sprinkled onto food. Concerta® provides up to 12-hour coverage and relieves more symptoms of ADHD than Ritalin. It has been reported to significantly disrupt normal sleep patterns if not taken early enough in the morning. Therefore, if the dosing time is missed, the patient is advised to *skip* that day's dose, which means the child may have focus or hyperactivity problems throughout the day.

NONSTIMULANTS USED IN THE TREATMENT OF ADHD AND ADD

Strattera® (atomoxetine), a serotonin norepinephrine reuptake inhibitor, or SNRI, is used to treat ADHD. It is the first nonstimulant drug that has been FDA-approved for attention deficit disorder. It is not a controlled substance, but rather a "regular" prescription drug (legend drug). In addition to being nonaddictive, Strattera® prescription refills can be phoned in. Strattera® is an oral capsule for once or twice a day dosing. Strattera® is not a stimulant like Concerta® or Adderal XR®, but all three drugs have once/twice a day dosing, which eliminates the need for school children to medicate during the school day. Strattera® is the only ADHD medication FDA-approved for adults.

ADVERSE REACTIONS OF STRATTERA® (ATOMOXETINE)

In addition to those mentioned for stimulants, Strattera® (atomoxetine) has the following side effects:

- mood swings
- ear infection
- influenza

Because this drug has been tested and is also used on adults with ADD and ADHD, sexual side effects in adults have been reported, as follows:

- decreased libido
- difficulty in ejaculation
- erectile dysfunction
- urination problems
- painful menstrual cycles

CONTRAINDICATIONS OF STRATTERA® (ATOMOXETINE)

Although rare, potentially serious allergic reactions (anaphylaxis) may occur with usage of Strattera® (atomoxetine). In addition to having the *same* contraindications as stimulants, Strattera® should not be given to patients with the following conditions:

- epilepsy or seizure disorders
- liver disease or kidney disease

Convulsions, Seizures, and Epilepsy

Epilepsy is a disorder of the central nervous system in which the patient may have convulsions or seizures. Convulsions are more physical and seizures are irregular electrical activity in the brain. A sudden onset of violent, uncontrollable (involuntary) contractions of the muscles, with possible uncontrollable shaking, twitching of arms or legs, characterizes convulsions and seizures. The patient may fall on the ground and lose control of bladder or bowel.

The seizures occur due to an abnormal electrical discharge of neurons, in which they fire uncontrollably. The nerves cells are said to be hyperexcitable. The seizure causes a sudden break in the stream of thought and activity and may include loss of consciousness. Brain seizures may cause a temporary lack of memory, or fainting spells. The presence of the two together is more severe than the seizure alone. Causes may be some injury to the brain, high fever possibly due to infection, head trauma, cephalic tumor, stroke, alcohol dependence, or over-intoxication. In these cases, the injury is to the neurons. Epilepsy can be diagnosed by the specific waves patterns depicted by the recording of an EEG (electroencephalogram). Many types of seizures exist.

DIFFERENT TYPES AND CLASSIFICATIONS OF SEIZURES

There are two types of seizures: partial and generalized, depending upon where it begins and ends within the nervous system and the body. Partial seizures travel short distances on one side of the brain. Generalized seizures can travel anywhere throughout the brain on both sides. These types are classified further into two more groups: simple and complex.

Simple partial seizures affect only one side, or portion of the brain, usually occuring without loss of consciousness. The patient may experience an intense emotional feeling such as elation, sorrow, or sadness. The following characteristics are associated with simple partial seizures:

- muscle contractions of a specific body part
- abnormal sensations such as numbness and tingling, especially in the hands, feet, arms, or legs
- nausea, skin flushing, sweating, or dilated pupils
- may hear noises, see things, or have other symptoms
- loss of awareness of where they are for a brief time.

A patient having a *partial complex seizure* may or may not lose consciousness. All or any of the symptoms of partial simple seizures may present, in addition to any of the following:

- being on "automatic pilot"—performance of complex behaviors (such as driving) without conscious awareness
- abnormal sensations
- changes in personality or alertness
- may or may not lose consciousness
- olfactory (smell) or gustatory (taste) hallucinations or impairments, if the epilepsy is focused in the temporal lobe of the brain
- usually a specific body movement such as smacking the lips or foot tapping, often referred to as psychomotor
- recalled or inappropriate emotions

Generalized seizures involve two sides of the brain and are further sub-classified as tonic-clonic, myoclonic, and absence seizures.

- *Tonic-clonic,* also known as Grand Mal, these affect the whole brain and are considered the most severe, causing the whole body to convulse with rhythmic, alternating, sustained contractions with relaxed muscles. Infection causing high fever may induce these seizures, called febrile seizures in small children and infants. Brought on with a light or sound, the experience will last up to several minutes, with possible difficulty breathing and/or loss of bladder/bowel.
- *Myoclonic seizures* are characterized by specific body parts or muscle groups exhibiting convulsive twitching for a brief period of time. Children with infantile spasms may present quick, "jack-knifing" muscular spasms of the head, trunk, and extremities. These seizures may become severe.
- *Absence seizures*, also known as Petite Mal, affect the whole brain. When a person is having an absence seizure, an onlooker may think that he is merely daydreaming or "zoning out." He looks like most people do when bored or distracted, with a blank stare into space. This type of seizure does not typically last longer than a few seconds to two minutes. For this reason, absence seizures are difficult to diagnose. They are rare in adults and most common in girls beginning between the ages of six and twelve. Medication usually helps, and some outgrow this type of seizure.

STATUS EPILEPTICUS

Any and all seizures that are generalized, sustained longer than five minutes, or repeated present a medical emergency called *status epilepticus*. Irregular heartbeat, lack of oxygen due to difficulty breathing, and hyper/hypotension occur because the muscle of the heart or the diaphragm may also be convulsing. Hyper/hypoglycemia, lacticacidosis, and rise in body temperature are all due to movement. Immediate administration of IV anticonvulsant/anti-epileptic medication is warranted before cerebral cortex damage or death occurs as a result of the catecholamine surge.

Treatment of status epilepticus is usually with a benzodiazepine, administered as follows:

Step 1: Uncontrolled in 2 minutes
Ativan® (lorazepam) IV—0.1 mg/kg, give 1 mg/min to a maximum of 10 mg over 10 minutes

Versed® (midazolam)—10 mg IM (0.15–0.3 mg/kg IM)

Valim® (diazepam)—0.5–1.0 mg/kg rectally, using the IV solution per rectal tube or the diazepam gel preparation

Step 2: Uncontrolled in 10 minutes
Cerebryx® (fosphenytoin)—IV–20 mg/kg, at a maximum IV rate of 150 mg/min in the average-sized adult (~3 mg/kg/min)

TABLE 19-11	Comparison of Neuronal State to Ionic Concentration	
Resting State	Hyperexcited Neuronal State	Suppressed Neuronal Activity
Outside of nerve cell: high amounts of Na$^+$, Ca^{++}, and Cl$^-$ ions Inside nerve cell: High K$^+$	Outside nerve cell: Less Na$^+$, and Ca^{++} – ions, high or normal Cl Inside nerve cell: High K$^+$ and Na$^+$, and Ca^{++} ions	Outside: Less Cl$^-$, normal to high Na$^+$, and Ca^{++} ions Inside nerve cell: High K$^+$ and Cl$^-$

Step 3: an additional dose of

1. fosphenytoin IV—10 mg/kg of over 5 minutes to a maximum total dose of 30 mg/kg (recommended treatment) or

2. phenobarbital IV—20 mg/kg, at a maximum rate of 50–100 mg/min in the average-sized adult (~1 mg/kg/min)

Step 4: an additional dose of 10 mg/kg of phenobarbital IV to a maximum total dose of 30 mg/kg, or give a 4th drug loading dose IV until the seizure ceases. Pentobarbital is the "traditional" choice when using a 4th drug—15 mg/kg (max rate of 25–50 mg/min).

TREATMENT OF SEIZURES AND CONVULSIONS

Most major drugs used to prevent or treat epilepsy or convulsions characteristically treat alternating relaxing muscles and motor contractions. Antiepileptic drugs treat the CNS neuronal hyperstate of activity. As stated before in the discussion on neurons, ionic concentration affects discharge or firing. Increasing neuronal activity is caused by an increase of specific ions traveling into the neuron or nerve cell (influx) (see Table 19-11).

Following are three specific MOAs to prevent and treat epilepsy and hyperexcitability of the neuron (see Table 19-12):

- drugs that slow down an influx of sodium ions (Na$^+$, go outside neuron)
- drugs that slow down an influx of calcium ion (Ca^{++}, stay outside neuron)
- drugs that speed up the influx of chloride ions (Cl$^-$, go inside the neuron)

Parkinson's Disease

Parkinson's disease occurs as nerve cells (neurons) in the brain that produce the chemical neurotransmitter dopamine begin to malfunction and progressively die. These neurotransmitters enable the central nervous system (cerebrum) to communicate with the body's muscles (somatic nervous system) in

TABLE 19-12 Three Major Drug Classes Used to Control Seizures

Drugs that Stimulate an Influx of Chloride Ion

Benzodiazepines	Barbiturates	Miscellaneous
clonazepam (Klonopin®)	amobarbital (Amytal®)	gabapentin (Neurontin®)
clorazepate (Tranxene®)	pentobarbital (Nembutal®)	primidone (Mysoline®)
diazepam (Valium®)	phenobarbital (Luminal®)	tiagabine (Gabitril®)
lorazepam (Ativan®)	secobarbital (Seconal®)	topiramate (Topamax®)

Drugs that Delay an Influx of Sodium

	Hydantoins	Miscellaneous
	phenytoin (Dilantin®)	carbamazepine (Tegretol®)
	fosphenytoin (Cerebyx®)	divalporex (Depakote®)
		felbamate (Felbatol®)
		lamotrigine (Lamictal®)
		valproic acid (Depakene®)
		zonisamide (Zonegran®)

Drugs that Delay an Influx of Calcium

	Succinimides	Miscellaneous
	ethosuximide (Zarontin®)	divalproex (Depakote®)
	methsuximide (Celontin®)	valproic acid (Depakene®)
	phensuximide (Milontin®)	zonisamide (Zonegran®)

order to translate thought into motion. Since the neurotransmitter dopamine acts as a chemical messenger to send signals to other parts of the brain that control movement and coordination (the cerebral medulla and cerebellum, respectively), a change in body movement would be an expected symptom of Parkinson's disease. Tremor, stiff or rigid muscles and joints, and/or difficulty in moving present. Too much or too little dopamine can disrupt the normal balance between the dopamine system and another neurotransmitter system (peripheral nervous system) that uses acetylcholine, and interfere with smooth, continuous movement. Excess dopamine that does not get bound to, or is not accepted by, the receptor of the postsynaptic neuron is broken down by a chemical in the synapse called MAO-B . This constant transmission and disintegration of dopamine to and from one neuron to another creates a homeostasis. The balance of the dopamine activity is essential to body coordination and movement. However, as more of these cells die, less and less dopamine is produced, which causes Parkinson's disease. In addition, MAO–B continues to destroy the little remaining dopamine in the synapse. The balance of dopamine to acetylcholine (Ach) is thrown off balance.

Contributing factors to the malfunction of the cells, which causes the death of the neurons that produce dopamine, are as follows:

1. high fevers at a young age, such as those that accompany viral infections

2. infections to the brain

3. injury to the brain, specifically the basal ganglia

4. Antipsychotic drugs increase dopamine activity or production or mimic dopamine.

Currently there is no way to stop the death of the cells that make dopamine. However certain drugs can help the patient to "manage" the decline in motor function and activity as the disease progresses.

NONPHARMACEUTICAL TREATMENTS OF PARKINSON'S DISEASE, OR PD

Since rigidity is a main concern and symptom of PD, regular exercise is essential for keeping the muscles strong and flexible. As the disease progresses, a physical trainer or therapist may be necessary to help move the muscles. A diet that allows the patient to keep a normal weight and avoid weight gain is necessary because excess weight can mean more work and more trouble for the muscles. In addition, some drugs require a low amount of protein, which may interfere with the absorption of the medication. Emotional and mental support can be gained by active participation in a support group. Continued medical evaluations by a doctor to assess the progression of the disease and to monitor drug therapy are necessary.

FUTURE TREATMENTS

Recent experimental procedures have had encouraging results, but limited success. One such procedure involves transplanting dopamine-producing tissue into the brains of people with Parkinson's disease. Another procedure that has been attempted is to transplant growth-factor-producing cells into the brain in hopes of regrowing damaged dopamine-producing nerve cells.

PHARMACEUTICAL TREATMENTS OF PD

Levodopa is a fat soluble substance that can cross the blood–brain barrier and then, with the help of an enzyme, be converted to dopamine in the brain. However, dopamine is a water soluble substance and cannot cross the blood–brain barrier. One of the problems with this Parkinson's disease treatment is that the enzyme is converting Levodopa before it gets a chance to cross the blood–brain barrier. Therefore, the conversion to water soluble dopamine is quick and keeps the dopamine away from the brain, where it is needed.

Sinemet® is the most commonly used agent to combat PD. Sinemet® is made from a combination of levodopa and an enzyme, carbidopa, that slows down the conversion of levodopa to dopamine. As PD progresses, more Sinemet® is required, which means more side effects occur. One way to prevent a requirement of high doses of Sinemet® is by the addition of adjunctive therapy. Two examples are (1) Parlodel®, which mimics the action of dopamine upon attaching to the post-synaptic dopamine receptor and (2) Eldepryl®, which blocks the MAO Type B that destroys dopamine (see Table 19-13).

TABLE 19-13 Drugs that Treat Parkinson's Disease

Drug Trade/Generic Name	Availability	Dosage and Administration	MOA	Side Effects and Special Notes
Sinemet® and Sinemet CR® (carbidopa and levodopa)	10/100, 25/100, and 25/250 mg tablets and CR 25–100 50–200 sustained release tablets. (carbidopa and levodopa, respectively)	Sinemet®: Start with one tablet QD, Increase to 2 tablets q.i.d. Sinemet CR®: UAD = 200–300 mg levodopa BID or TID, max: 1000 mg levodopa per day in 3–4 divided doses.	Levodopa is converted to dopamine, and carbidopa slows down the conversion so that levodopa can cross the BBB	Can be used to control symptoms for several years. As dopamine-producing cells decrease, symptoms continue to worsen, and the dose of Sinemet will often have to be increased. Ultimately, the SE at high doses of Sinemet are unacceptable, and it may need to be discontinued. Dyskinesias, involuntary muscular movements, result from an overload of Sinemet, or dopamine, in the brain.
Parlodel® (bromocriptine mesylate) and Permax® (pergolide mesylate)	Parlodel® (bromocriptine) = 2.5 mg and 5 mg tablets. Permax® (pergolide mesylate) = 0.05 mg, 0.25 mg, and 1 mg tablets	Parlodel® (bromocriptine) Start $\frac{1}{2}$ of 2.5 mg tablet QD, increase to safe amount NTE 100 mg/day. Permax® (pergolide mesylate) Start: 0.05 mg QD and increase to a max NTE 5 mg/day. UAD 3 mg/day in three divided doses.	Dopaminergics: These drugs mimic the action of dopamine by attaching to the dopamine receptor sites on the surface of the receiving neuron or postsynaptic neuron, acting like dopamine. This is a substitution-like action. Parlodel® (bromocriptine) is an ergot with dopamine receptor agonist activity. Permax® is an ergot derivative dopamine receptor agonist at both D_1 and D_2 receptor sites.	Dyskinesias are less common because dopamine itself is not being increased, only the dopamine-like action. **Side Effects of Parlodel® (bromocriptine):** N/V, abnormal involuntary movements, hallucinations, confusion, dizziness, drowsiness, fainting, asthenia, abdominal discomfort, visual disturbance, ataxia, insomnia, depression,

TABLE 19-13   Drugs that Treat Parkinson's Disease (*continued*)

Drug Trade/Generic Name	Availability	Dosage and Administration	MOA	Side Effects and Special Notes
				hypotension, shortness of breath, constipation, and vertigo. **Contraindications:** Decreased efficacy of bromocriptine mesylate with dopamine antagonists butyrophenones, phenothiazines, haloperidol, metoclopramide, pimozide. **Side effects of Permax® (pergolide):** dyskinesia, hallucinations, somnolence, and insomnia.
Symmetrel® (amantadine hydrochloride)	100 mg gel capsules	Start: 100 mg QD, UAD: 100 mg BID, NTE 400 mg QD	Allows the dopamine-producing nerve cell storage sites to open up easier and wider to release dopamine from the pre-synaptic neuron into the synapse.	Used in milder cases of Parkinson's disease. **Contraindications:** Decrease the dose in patients with CHF, peripheral edema, orthostatic hypotension, or impaired renal function.
Artane® (trihexyphenidyl HCl) and Cogentin® (benztropine mesylate)	Artane®: 2 and 5 mg tablets and 2 mg/5 ml Elixir	Artane: Start low at 1 mg with 2 mg/day increments. UAD = 6–10 mg Max = 12–15 mg QD. Daily dose is given in three divided doses, usually with a meal.	Artane®, an antispasmodic drug, inhibits the PSNS. Cogentin® is both anticholinergic and antihistaminic. Both drugs restore the dopamine/ACH balance by reducing the activity of acetylcholine in the brain.	Used in early stages of Parkinson's, to be taken in combination with Sinemet® (adjunct therapy). They successfully reduce the tremor and muscle stiffness that result from having much more ACH than D. These agents do not

TABLE 19-13   Drugs that Treat Parkinson's Disease (*continued*)

Drug Trade/Generic Name	Availability	Dosage and Administration	MOA	Side Effects and Special Notes
	Cogentin®: 0.5 mg, 1 mg, and 2 mg tablets	Cogentin®: 0.5 mg–6 mg QD. May be given at bedtime in one dose or in divided doses.		correct the problem of too little dopamine. Usually, these agents will be used in the early stages of Parkinson's disease. **Side effects of Artane®**: dryness of the mouth, blurred vision, dizziness, mild nausea, or nervousness. **Toxic effects**: delusions, hallucinations, and paranoia. **Side effects of Cogentin®**: tachycardia, constipation, dry mouth. Toxic psychosis. **Contraindications**: antipsychotic drugs and antidepressants.
Eldepryl® (selegiline hydrochloride)	5 mg tablets	Two 5 mg tabs; one at breakfast and one at lunch	Selective MAO Type B Inhibitor—Actually blocks MAO-B, the chemical in the synapse that breaks down dopamine, thus conserving the dopamine already in the brain, keeping it in the synapse, so that D can bind to the post-synaptic dopamine receptors.	**Side effects**: N/V, dizziness, abdominal pain, H/A **Contraindications**: nonselective MAOIs, TCAs, SSRIs, and meperidine. Toxic effects of these drug interactions are severe agitation, hallucinations, and death.

Dementia and Alzheimer's Disease

Dementia is a progressive brain dysfunction with a loss of cognition that leads to a gradually increasing restriction of daily activities. Patients with irreversible dementia, such as Alzheimer's disease, eventually become unable to care for themselves and may require around-the-clock care. According to the American Psychiatric Association (APA), Alzheimer's disease is the fourth leading cause of death in America.[25] The changes in the brain, which may be caused by disease or trauma, may occur gradually or quickly. How they occur may predict if the dementia is permanent or temporary. The cognitive function is the process of thinking, perceiving, and learning. Dementia may interfere with decision making, judgment, memory, thinking, reasoning, verbal communication, and spatial orientation. Behavioral and personality changes may also result, depending on the areas of the brain affected. It is believed that the changes in the brain cause a lack of ACH or acetylcholine, which is thought to be the root of Alzheimer's disease. Treating dementia quickly may result in partial or total reversal of the disease.

SIGNS AND SYMPTOMS OF DEMENTIA

Early stages are characterized by loss of recent, or short-term, memory, for example, not being able to recall shutting off the stove. As Alzheimer's progresses, the patient has trouble with abstract thinking, which shows up as having problems counting or handling money, paying bills, understanding what was just read, or organizing daily activities. In late stages of Alzheimer's, the patient becomes disoriented about times and dates, confused, and unable to describe his residence or a recently visited place.

Behavioral and personality changes may include the following:

- unable to dress without help
- unable to eat or loss of desire to eat
- toileting problems leading to incontinence
- unable to care for himself or groom himself
- abandons interests and hobbies
- unable to perform routine activities, household tasks
- personality changes, with inappropriate responses, lack of emotional control, apathy, or social withdrawal.

As the disease progresses, patients with Alzheimer's may become more irritable, agitated and quarrelsome and less neat in appearance, with diminished attention to grooming habits. In late stages of Alzheimer's, the patient stops talking, has erratic mood swings, and becomes uncooperative.

Age is the most commonly accepted contributing factor for dementia. However, according to the American Psychiatric Association, only 15–25 percent of the elderly suffer from significant symptoms of mental illness.[25] Untreated infections, metabolic disease, and substance abuse also can lead to dementia. The following disorders are risk factors leading to dementia: brain tumors, HTN, CAD, head injury, renal failure, hepatic disease, and thyroid disease. Dietary deficiencies in Vitamin B12 (cyanocobalamin), folic acid, and B1 (thiamine) have also been associated with dementia. Genetic disorders such as Huntington's, infections such as HIV/AIDS, amyotrophic lateral sclerosis (also known as Lou Gehrig's disease), and Parkinson's disease have also been associated with dementias.

Substances associated with drug induced dementias may include the following:

- anticholinergics
- barbiturates
- benzodiazepines
- cough suppressants
- digitalis medications
- monoamine oxidase inhibitors
- tricyclic antidepressants

It has been suggested that there is no sure way of diagnosing Alzheimer's and that the only absolute determination that a patient *had* Alzheimer's is via an autopsy. However, new research has shown, in the analysis of DNA in a blood sample of patients with suspected Alzheimer's, a high correlation of the ApoE4 gene, which is found in about one-third of Alzheimer's disease patients. *Electroencephalography* (EEG), which traces brain wave activity, reveals "slow" waves in Alzheimer's disease. *Imaging tests* (MRI scan or CT scan) can detect physical changes in the brain caused by stroke, blood clots, tumors, head injury, or hydrocephalus. A CT scan shows characteristic structural changes that occur with Huntington's disease. Patient history of familial dementia or Alzheimer's, stroke, and alcohol or illegal or prescription drug use are all risk factors.

The most commonly used criteria for diagnoses of dementia is the DSM-IV (Diagnostic and Statistical Manual for Mental Disorders, American Psychiatric Association).[25] The criteria consist of two parts:

1. a deterioration of recent and remote memory
2. an impairment of one or more of the following functions: aphasia, apraxia, agnosia, or executive function (see Table 19-14).

TREATMENT OF DEMENTIA

First of all, the underlying cause of the dementia must be treated. Infections such as HIV/AIDS are treated with antiretroviral agents; antibiotics and antifungals are applied for neurosyphilis dementia and other infections, antihypertensives and anithyperlipidemics are used for cardiovascular disease.

TABLE 19-14   Secondary Criteria for Diagnosing Dementia

Language impairment: aphasia	Misuse words, or unable to remember and/or use words appropriately
Motor activity impairment: apraxia	Unable to perform motor activities, even though physical ability remains intact (can walk, grasp)
Recognition impairment: agnosia	Unable to recognize objects, even though sensory (sight, touch, smell) function is intact
Executive function impairment	Unable to plan, organize, and think abstractly

The goals in treating the dementia directly are to improve the quality of life and maximize physical function. Some objectives include improvement of cognitive skills, mood, and behavior. Realistically, the goal of pharmacotherapy for irreversible conditions is plainly to control symptoms.

Tranquilizers and sedatives can modify personality changes manifested by agitation, anxiety, and aggression. Medications may be used to help manage insomnia, restlessness, and incontinence. Caretakers and family must employ safety precautions to protect the confused and disoriented patient from wandering away from home.

In 1993, the FDA approved tacrine, the first agent specifically designed for the treatment of cognitive symptoms in Alzheimer's disease. Cognex® (tacrine) is a reversible cholinesterase inhibitor and is believed to work by increasing the availability of acetylcholine in the synapses between the neurons in the brains of Alzheimer's disease patients (see Table 19-15).

TABLE 19-15 Drugs that Treat Alzheimer's Disease

Drug Trade/Generic Name	Availability	Dosage and Administration	MOA	Side Effects and Special Notes
Cognex® (tacrine)	10, 20, 30, and 40 mg capsules	Start: 10 mg Q.I.D. UAD 20 mg Q.I.D. NTE 120 and 160 mg/day Must monitor transaminase levels. Serum ALT/SGPT should be monitored QOW from at least week 4 to week 16, then decrease monitoring to every 3 months.	Parasympathomimetic Reversible Cholinesterase Inhibitor—Blocks the enzyme that destroys ACH.	N/V/D, myalgia, ataxia, and anorexia. High serum ALT/SGPT or liver damage.
Aricept® (donepezil) Use: mild to moderate Alzheimer's disease	5 and 10 mg tablets	i tablet qhs, NTE 10 mg/day	Reversible Acetylcholinesterase Inhibitor blocks the enzyme that destroys ACH.	N/V/D, insomnia, muscle cramps, fatigue, and anorexia.
Reminyl® (galantamine) Use: mild to moderate Alzheimer's disease	4, 8 and 12 g tablets and 4 mg/mL oral solution	4 mg BID, with morning and evening meals, NTE 24 mg BID	Reversible, competitive Acetylcholinesterase Inhibitor	If therapy has been interrupted, pt should restart at lowest dose. Lower dose for hepatic impairment.
Exelon® (rivastigmine)	1.5 mg, 3 mg, 4.5 mg, or 6 mg capsules	Start: 1.5 mg BID NTE 6 mg BID (12 mg/day). Take with morning and evening meals.	Reversible Acetylcholinesterase Inhibitor blocks the enzyme that destroys ACH.	Common: N/V/D, insomnia, UTI, and fatigue. Rarely—abnormal hepatic function.

Transaminase levels are the same as aspartate aminotransferase (also known as serum glutamic oxaloacetic transaminase) (AST or SGOT) and alanine aminotransferase (serum glutamic pyruvic transaminase) (ALT or SGPT). AST or SGOT enzymes are found in various tissues, including liver, heart, muscle, kidney, and brain. The ALT or SGPT enzymes are normally contained within liver cells. However, if the liver, heart, muscle, kidney, and brain are injured, the organ cells spill the enzymes into the blood, raising the serum enzyme levels and signaling the liver damage. AST or SGOT serum rises with myocardial infarctions (MIs).

Other approaches to treatment of dementias include the following:

Vitamin E, due to its antioxidant properties, "has been shown to slow nerve cell damage and death in animal models and cell culture (including damage associated with amyloid deposition), and thus possibly relevant to the development and progression of Alzheimer's disease."[25]

Eldepryl® *(selegiline)*, a selective MAO Type B inhibitor, is used in the United States for Parkinson's disease. However, it is used off label in some European countries and in this country by some doctors. According to the American Psychiatric Association, it may act as an "antioxidant or neuroprotective agent and slow the progression of Alzheimer's disease."[25]

Ergoloid mesylates, Hydergine, derived from rye, is used for dementias other than Alzheimer's disease and as an alternative when cholinesterase inhibitors, vitamin E, or selegiline prove ineffective in the Alzheimer's patient. UAD is 3 mg/day, NTE 9 mg/day. It is thought to enhance mental abilities and lengthen the period of intense mental workload by improving oxygen supply to the brain because of its ability to act as a mild vasodilator. In addition, it is believed to possess antioxidant properties that protect the brain and the heart from free radical damage, improving the number of brain dendrites and their ability to make connections.

Current research using aspirin and other NSAIDs to reduce inflammation has shown less decline over a six-month period (see Table 19-16). The outcomes of more trials and research are pending. Another supplement therapy being researched for Alzheimer's disease in postmenopausal women is estrogen replacement. Another hormone in research is melatonin, from the pineal gland, because it is a potent free radical scavenger and antioxidant. Lack of melatonin may be responsible for "Sundowners Syndrome." The herbal agent ginkgo biloba has been touted for stimulating memory improvement through its positive effect on the vascular system, especially in the cerebellum, where it relaxes constricted blood vessels so that they can deliver more oxygen to the brain. This herb also has antioxidant properties that contribute to the oxidation of free radicals and the antiplatelet effect (anticlotting effect).

Migraine Headaches

A migraine is a very painful headache that tends to recur. The patient may feel nauseated, with the urge to vomit. The pain is usually on one side of the head, and the patient may be very sensitive to any light and noise. Body movement can make the headache feel worse. There are many types of migraine headaches. The two major types are the Classic and the Common migraine headaches.

CLASSIC MIGRAINE

The major distinction is the experience of an aura preceding 10–30 minutes before the classic migraine attack. The aura may occur as flashing lights, zigzag lines, or a temporary vision loss, and may or may not be accompanied by speech difficulty, confusion, weakness of an arm or leg, and tingling of the face or hands.

The pain of a classic migraine headache is characterized by an intense throbbing or pounding forehead, temple, ear, jaw, or the entire area around the eyes. Beginning on one side of the head, it may spread to the other side. It may last one to two days.

COMMON MIGRAINE

The common migraine is the one most frequently observed in the general population. It is not preceded by an aura. A variety of vague symptoms may be experienced before onset of the headaches, such as a mental fog, mood swings, fatigue, and unusual retention of fluid. During the migraine headache phase, the patient may experience abdominal pain, polyuria, and N/V/D.

The frequency of either classic or common migraine can occur as often as several times a week or as rarely as once every few years.

The cause of the migraine may be a chemical or electrical problem in certain parts of the brain where blood flow is changed. Responding to a trigger such as stress or something eaten, heard, or smelled, the brain creates spasms in the arteries at the base of the brain, which constricts some of the arteries that supply blood, and therefore oxygen, to the brain. Flow of blood to the brain is restricted. Platelets clump together, releasing the chemical serotonin, a powerful constrictor of arteries, and this process further reduces the blood and oxygen supply to the brain. In response to the reduced blood flow and oxygen supply, certain arteries within the brain dilate to meet the brain's energy needs. Scientists believe this vasodilation causes the pain of the migraine headache.

Some known migraine triggers are the following:

- **Medicines:**
  - cimetidine
  - fenfluramine
  - nifedipine
  - indomethacin
  - NTG
  - theophylline
  - estrogens/BCPs/HRT
- **Foods:**
  - Aged food, including cheese, beer, wine, and hard liquor
  - Yeast-containing food, such as donuts and fresh breads
  - Caffeine in coffee, tea, cola, and medicines

- Citrus fruits, bananas, figs, and raisins
- Dairy products
- MSG and other seasonings
- Legumes—peas, peanuts, lima beans, and nuts
- Sulfites, aspartame, and saccharin
- Fermented foods like pickled herring

Some migraines are influenced by hormonal changes, especially in women.

Nonpharmaceutical treatments of migraine headaches include the following:

- stress reduction
- biofeedback training
- removal of certain foods from the diet
- regular exercise, such as swimming or vigorous walking, that increases endorphins and reduces stress
- reducing the inflammation of the arteries with cold packs

PHARMACEUTICAL TREATMENT OF MIGRAINE HEADACHE

Analgesics, Antipyretic, and Anti-inflammatory Agents   Analgesics relieve pain and soothe body aches that are not due to inflammation, such as headache. Analgesics work in the brain to produce a mild degree of analgesia, much less than the analgesia produced by opioid analgesics such as morphine. OTC analgesics reduce the pain threshold without disturbing consciousness. Antipyretics lower elevated body temperature to reduce fever by their action on the hypothalamus, which responds to the sensing of the thalamus in the brain (see Table 19-17). (However, these drugs will not reduce normal body temperature.)

Anti-inflammatory drugs are used to treat simple headaches, minor migraines, rheumatoid disorders and other inflammatory diseases, injuries, and body aches caused by inflammation.

This is a hypersensitivity to the ingredient, which causes a person to experience difficulty in breathing, such as shortness of breath (SOB), congestion, and narrowing of the airway passages (bronchoconstriction). The patient must get emergency help within 5 to 15 minutes or death will most likely ensue. The DOC (drug of choice) is epinephrine injectable and possibly diphenhydramine injectable. Asthmatics may or may not be allergic to these substances; in any case, they should not use Aspirin or other NSAIDs.

REYE'S SYNDROME

Reye's Syndrome is a fatal disease that results after children and teenagers ingest salicylates, found in ASA and NSAIDs, before or during influenza, other viral infections, and small pox. The disease is named after the Australian pathologist Dr. R. Douglas Reye who discovered the connection in 1963. It affects all body parts, but lethally the brain (where there is severe increase of pressure) and the

TABLE 19-16 Comparison of the Properties of Aspirin, NSAID, and Acetaminophen

Property	Aspirin	NSAIDs	Acetaminophen
Analgesic	✓	✓	✓
Antipyretic	✓	✓	✓
Anti-inflammatory	✓	✓	—
Anti-platelet	✓	✓	—
Cause GI upset	✓	✓	—
Cause liver damage	—	—	✓
Cause kidney damage	✓	✓	—
Example of generics names	Willow bark, ASA, acetylsalicylic acid or equivalent	ibuprophen, naproxen	N-acetyl P-aminophenol, acetaminophen; APAP, or paracetamol
Example of trade names	St. Joseph's®, Bayer®	Motrin®, Advil®, Aleve®, Naprosyn®, Anaprox®	Tylenol®
MOA	The MOA of salicylates is the inhibition of cyclooxygenase, COX I and II, as well as prostaglandins. The MOA of the analgesic effect of APAP is unclear, however the MOA of the antipyretic effect is that is acts directly on the hypothalamic heat-regulating center to cause vasodilation and sweating, reducing body temperature by dissipating heat through the skin. **Note:** See Chapter 9, the Musculoskeletal System.	The MOA of NSAIDs, which are in the salicylate family, is the inhibition of cyclooxygenase, COX I and II, as well as prostaglandins. The MOA of the analgesic effect of APAP is unclear, however the MOA of the antipyretic effect is that is acts directly on the hypothalamic heat-regulating center to cause vasodilation and sweating, reducing body temperature by dissipating heat through the skin. **Note:** See Chapter 9, the Musculoskeletal System.	The MOA of the analgesic effect of APAP is unclear; however, the MOA of the antipyretic effect is that it acts directly on the hypothalamic heat-regulating center to cause vasodilation and sweating, reducing body temperature by dissipating heat through the skin.
Side Effects:	(1) GI upset or ulcers, blood thinning. (2) Tinnitis (ringing in the ear). **Note:** GI upset and ulcers result from COX I inhibition, that thins out the gastrointestinal mucous protective lining, which is not necessary to inhibit for an anti-inflammatory effect.	(1) GI upset or ulcers, blood thinning. (2) Tinnitis (ringing in the ear). **Note:** GI upset and ulcers result from COX I inhibition, that thins out the gastrointestinal mucous protective lining, which is not necessary to inhibit for an anti-inflammatory effect.	(1) Rash (2) Fever (3) H/A (4) Jaundice

Property	Aspirin	NSAIDs	Acetaminophen
Toxic Effects:	(1) Salicylates may cause prophylaxis or prophylactic shock, which leads to (a) SOB, shortness of breath, with congestion and (b) Broncho-constriction. (2) Most asthmatics should not use aspirin or other NSAIDs, as it may cause anaphylaxis.	(1) Salicylates may cause prophylaxis or prophylactic shock, which leads to (a) SOB, shortness of breath, with congestion and (b) Bronchoconstriction. (2) Most asthmatics should not use aspirin or other NSAIDs, as it may cause anaphylaxis.	(1) anuria (2) neutropenia (3) leukopenia (4) pancytopenia (5) thrombocytopenia (6) hypoglycemia (7) hepatic toxicity and failure leading to the following conditions: (a) brain damage (b) acute kidney failure (c) renal tubular necrosis (d) myocardial damage
Special Information:	may cause Reye's Syndrome	may cause Reye's Syndrome	It has been determined that acetaminophen has very little anti-inflammatory effect, but does have analgesic and antipyretic properties. (Read more about acetaminophen in Chapter 9, The Musculoskeletal System.)

liver (where abnormal accumulations of fat collect). The number of deaths related to the use of ASA has declined since 1980. Vomiting is often the first sign of Reye's syndrome. Children or infants under two usually have diarrhea or hyperventilate as a first sign. Stage I is characterized by severe tiredness, belligerence due to illness (moodiness), nausea, and loss of energy. Stage II manifests personality changes, bizarre mental and physical behavior (confusion, restlessness, and irrational behavior), and lethargy or inactivity of the senses, sometimes to the point of convulsions and coma. Since health care workers in emergency rooms do not see too many cases of Reye's syndrome, it is sometimes misdiagnosed as encephalitis, meningitis, diabetes, poisoning, mental illness, or drug abuse. Pharmaceutical treatment of early diagnosed Reye's Syndrome includes barbiturates to reduce the pressure in the brain and to cool body temperature. Insulin is often given to increase glucose metabolism, and corticosteroids are administered to reduce brain swelling. Diuretics are used to increase fluid loss. Patients are NPO and fed intravenously. A breathing machine or respirator may be employed if the child has difficulty in breathing.

OTHER DRUGS

Preventative drugs used for headaches that occur several times a month include the following: methysergide, which counteracts blood vessels; propranolol, which stops blood vessel dilation; and amitriptyline, an antidepressant.

Drugs for severe migraine pain relief include ergotemine, imimtrex, Zoming, Maxalt, and Amerg.

TABLE 19-17 Antimigraine Headache Agents

Drug Trade/Generic Name	Availability	Dosage and Administration	MOA	Side Effects and Special Notes
Sansert® (methysergide)	2 mg tablet	UAD 4–8 mg QD with meals.	Ergot derivative that blocks effects of serotonin, a substance that causes vasoconstriction and also lowers pain threshold. Thus, vasodilation results, along with the ability to perceive pain differently.	**Rare:** May cause retroperitoneal fibrosis, pleuropulmonary fibrosis, and fibrotic thickening of cardiac valves in patients receiving long-term therapy.
Inderal LA® (propranolol) Used for the Prophylaxis of common migraine headache	60, 80, 120, and 160 mg LA	Dosage varies. Start 80 mg Inderal LA, UAD 160–240 mg Inderal LA QD.	Synthetic non-selective beta-adrenergic receptor-blocking agent causing vasodilation.	**Common Side Effects:** CHF, bradycardia, light-headedness, insomnia, N/V/D, agranulocytosis, **Contraindications:** Avoid reserpine containing drugs, may lead to bradycardia and hypotension.
Elavil® (amitriptyline) Unlabeled use—pain associated with migraine headaches and to reduce pain perception	10, 25, 50, 75, 100, and 150 mg tablets 10 mg/ml injection	75–300 mg/day	TCA Antidepressant that blocks neuronal reuptake of NE and serotonin. Lowering serotonin lowers pain perception and causes vasodilation.	**Common Side Effects:** Skin rash, GI upset, edema, MI, hepatic failure, coma, seizures, and hallucinations. **Drug Interactions:** Avoid cimetidine and MAOIs.
Ergotemine + caffeine	1 mg/100 mg tablets	Start: 2 tablets. May take 1 additional tablet every 1/2 hour, if needed for full relief NTE 6 tablets/attack, or 10 tablets/wk	Partial alpha adrenergic agonist and antagonist—with direct stimulating effect on smooth muscle of cranial and peripheral blood vessels, causing vasoconstriction. Added caffeine is also vasoconstrictive.	Numbness and tingling of the fingers and toes, weakness in the legs, tachycardia.

TABLE 19-17 Antimigraine Headache Agents (*continued*)

Drug Trade/Generic Name	Availability	Dosage and Administration	MOA	Side Effects and Special Notes
Imitrex® (sumatriptan) For acute onset of classic or common migraine	**PO:** 25, 50, and 100 mg tablets **Nasal Spray:** 20 mg/spray and 5 mg/spray.	**PO:** 25 to 50 mg at onset. May be repeated in 2 hrs, NTE 200 mg per day **Nasal:** 1 spray, may repeat once in 2 hr (Max 40 mg/day)	A selective 5-hydroxytryptamine$_1$ receptor subtype agonist, binds with high affinity to 5-HT$_{1D}$ and 5-HT$_{1B}$ receptors, resulting in cranial blood vessel constriction and a decrease in prostaglandin pro-inflammatory neuropeptide release.	**Common Side Effects:** Diarrhea, numbness, sinusitis, tinnitus. **Rare:** Fatal cardiac events and HTN crisis.
Zoming® (zolmitriptan) For acute onset of classic or common migraine	2.5 and 5 mg tablets **Nasal Spray:** 5 mg/spray	1, 2.5, and 5 mg in a single dose, may be repeated in 2 hrs. NTE 10 mg/24hr	A selective 5-hydroxytryptamine$_{1B/1D}$ (5-HT$_{1B/1D}$) receptor agonist, resulting in cranial blood vessel constriction and a decrease in prostaglandin pro-inflammatory neuropeptide release.	Monitor hepatic impaired pts.
Maxalt® (rizatriptan) For acute onset of classic or common migraine	5 and 10 mg tablets and 5 and 10 Oral Disintegrating	5 or 10 mg in a single dose, may be repeated in 2 hrs, NTE 30 mg/24hr	A selective 5-hydroxytryptamine$_{1B/1D}$ (5-HT$_{1B/1D}$) receptor agonist, resulting in cranial blood vessel constriction and a decrease in prostaglandin pro-inflammatory neuropeptide release.	**Common:** Chest pain, dry mouth, GI upset, N/V, paresthesia **Rare:** Fatal cardiac events and HTN crisis
Amerge® (naratriptan) For acute onset of classic or common migraine	1 and 2.5 mg tablets	1, 2.5 mg single dose, may repeat in 4 hours, NTE 5 mg/24 hr or NTE 2.5 mg/24 hr in hepatic impaired pts	A selective 5-hydroxytryptamine$_1$ receptor subtype agonist that binds with high affinity to 5-HT$_{1D}$ and 5-HT$_{1B}$ receptors, resulting in cranial blood vessel constriction and a decrease in prostaglandin pro-inflammatory neuropeptide release.	**Common:** paresthesias, dizziness, drowsiness, malaise/fatigue **Rare:** Fatal cardiac events and HTN crisis

Drug Trade/Generic Name	Availability	Dosage and Administration	MOA	Side Effects and Special Notes
Frova® (frovatriptan)	2.5 mg tablets	2.5 mg tab, may take a second dose in 2 hours, NTE 3 tab/24 hr	A selective 5-hydroxytryptamine$_1$ (5-HT$_{1B/1D}$) receptor subtype agonist, resulting in cranial blood vessel constriction and a decrease in prostaglandin pro-inflammatory neuropeptide release	**Common:** paresthesias, dizziness, drowsiness, malaise/fatigue **Rare:** Fatal cardiac events and HTN crisis
Relpax® (eletriptan)	20, 40 mg tablets	UAD 20–40 mg per 24 hr.	A selective 5-hydroxytryptamine$_1$ (5-HT$_{1B/1D}$) receptor subtype agonist, resulting in cranial blood vessel constriction and a decrease in prostaglandin pro-inflammatory neuropeptide release	**Common:** paresthesias, dizziness, drowsiness, malaise/fatigue **Rare:** Fatal cardiac events and HTN crisis
Axert® (almotriptan)	6.25 mg, 12.5 tablets	NTE 12.5– 25 mg/24 hr	A selective 5-hydroxytryptamine$_1$ (5-HT$_{1B/1D}$) receptor subtype agonist, resulting in cranial blood vessel constriction and a decrease in prostaglandin pro-inflammatory neuropeptide release	**Common:** paresthesias, dizziness, drowsiness, malaise/fatigue **Rare:** Fatal cardiac events and HTN crisis

Cancer Pain

The International Association for the Study of Pain states that pain is "an unpleasant sensory and emotional experience in association with actual or potential tissue damage, or described in terms of such damage." Approximately 30 to 50 percent of patients with cancer experience pain while undergoing treatment, and 70 to 90 percent of patients with advanced cancer experience pain.

Pain can be acute or chronic. Acute pain starts suddenly; it may be sharp and is often a signal of a quick onset of injury to the body. Sometimes other body reactions, such as sweating or an elevated blood pressure, can occur with pain.

Chronic pain is persistent pain that lasts beyond the time expected for an injury to heal or an illness to be resolved. Cancer pain can be chronic, sometimes with acute flares of pain not completely controlled by the medication or therapy. This is called breakthrough pain. Cancer pain most often can be controlled with morphine and other opioid-like compounds.

Cancer causes pain by the mere pressure of a tumor on one of the body's organs, on bone, or on nerves. When blood vessels become obstructed by the tumor, cancer can result. Chemotherapy may cause the following sources of pain:

- mouth sores (mucositis)
- peripheral neuropathy (numb and sometimes painful sensations in the feet, legs, fingers, hands, and arms)
- GI upset—constipation, diarrhea, nausea, vomiting, and abdominal cramps
- bone and joint pain from chemotherapy

Surgical treatments and other procedures (biopsies, blood draws, lumbar punctures, and laser treatments) can cause pain.

Managing cancer pain can become problematic because some physicians may not always prescribe the right medications or sufficient doses of the medication. This is mainly due to the under-estimation of the degree of pain the cancer patient is experiencing and the doctor's concerns about the potential for addiction. The use of various pain assessment scales, where "0" means "no pain at all," and "10" means "the worst pain one has ever felt before," can help the physician ascertain what drug to prescribe and in what dosage.

Pain itself is electrical and chemical in nature. When pain receptors are triggered by mechanical, chemical, or thermal stimuli, the pain signal is transmitted through the nerves to the spinal cord and then to the brain. Substance P can get into mu or opioid receptors in the brain. The most common cancer pain is from tumors that metastasize to the bone. Tumors erode the bone, forming large holes that make the bone thin and weak. Nerve endings in and around the bone send pain signals to the brain.

TREATMENT OF CANCER PAIN

Analgesics do not cure the cause of the pain and provide only temporary relief. But they make short-term pain tolerable.

Mild pain may be managed with non-opioid analgesics such as APAP and NSAIDs. About 30 percent of cancer pain can be treated with this type of OTC medication. *Severe pain* is treated with opioid analgesics such as Duragesic® (fentanyl transdermal system), which provides continuous pain relief for 72 hours. Respiratory failure, hypotension, and hypoventilation may result from an overdose. The Duragesic® patches are available as 25, 50, 75, and 100 mg doses. Duragesic® is a Class II drug and must be ordered on a DEA 222 form. Repeated administration may result in tolerance and physical and psychological dependence. Other side effects include the following:

- constipation, nausea, and vomiting
- dry mouth, excessive sweating
- excessive sleepiness (somnolence)

- high blood pressure (hypertension) or low blood pressure (hypotension)
- confusion

Oral opioids, the most convenient and the least expensive form, have a slower onset of action. Thus they may remain in the bloodstream longer than necessary, often causing intolerable side effects such as dizziness, sedation, and vomiting.

Sublingual administration (under the tongue) delays the body's absorption of the drug. This method generally is considered to be no more effective than oral administration. Cancer patients are usually opioid-tolerant and can handle much more narcotic that the average person in pain.

Oral transmucosal fentanyl citrate (Actiq®) is a lozenge attached to a plastic handle, which can take 15 minutes to dissolve. There are six lozenge strengths that range from 200 to 1600 mcg. However, the patient should not exceed four doses in a 24-hour period.

Rectal suppositories can provide rapid onset of pain relief, but the quantity or strength delivered is unpredictable, and the method may be inconvenient.

Adjuvant drugs enhance the pain relieving actions of opioid analgesics. Antidepressants used in smaller amounts than those prescribed for depression are usual choices for adjuvant drugs. Elavil is an example.

Bone pain associated with bone fracture due to metastasis can be allieviated by bisphosphonates. These bind to the areas of the destroyed bone and slow down the damage caused by cancer cells.

NONPHARMACEUTICAL PAIN RELIEF

A transcutaneous electric nerve stimulation (TENS unit) gives mild electric currents to stimulate certain nerve endings that, when activated, block pain transmissions. It is a proven safe, noninvasive, and effective method for relief of many different types of pain, including neuropathic pain.

Scheduled Narcotic Analgesics

The Controlled Substance Act categorizes addictive drugs into schedules according to addiction and abuse potential (see Table 19-18). Class or Schedule I is the most addictive and has no medicinal value in the United States. Drugs such as LSD, marijuana, heroin, peyote, and mescaline are in this class.

Class II, or Schedule II, drugs are less addictive than Class I, Class III is less addictive than Class II, Class IV is less addictive than Class III, and Class V is less addictive than Class IV.

Overdose of Narcotics   The signs of overdose are as follows:

1. pinpoint constriction of the pupils

2. shallow respirations or breathing

3. deep sleep

4. coma

5. death

TABLE 19-18   Selected Scheduled Narcotics

Drug Trade/Generic Name	Availability	Dosage and Administration	MOA	Side Effects and Special Notes
Oramorph®, MS Contin (morphine sulfate) May be used for prn pain and breakthrough pain.	15, 30, 60, 100, and 200 mg immediate or SR tablets	Immediate Release: 5–30 mg q 4 hr prn SR: Swallow whole 15–200 mg q12 hrs NTE 400 mg/day	An opioid agonist binds to the opioid mu receptor sites in the brain, producing analgesia and sedation and increasing tolerance to pain.	**Common side effects:** Constipation, dysphoria, drowsiness, N/V, respiratory depression, coma, death
Sublimaze® (fentanyl)	0.05 mg/ml	0.05–1 mg IM 30–60 minutes pre-op	An opioid agonist binds to the opioid mu receptor sites in the brain, producing analgesia and sedation and increasing tolerance to pain.	**Common side effects:** Constipation, dysphoria, drowsiness, N/V, respiratory depression, coma, death
DURAGESIC® (fentanyl transdermal system)	25, 50, 75, and 100 mcg patches	i patch Q 72 hrs	An opioid agonist binds to the opioid mu receptor sites in the brain, producing analgesia and sedation and increasing tolerance to pain.	**Common side effects:** Constipation, dysphoria, drowsiness, N/V, respiratory depression, coma, death
Dilaudid® (hydromorphone) May be used for prn pain and breakthrough pain	1, 2, 3 and 4 mg tablets 3 mg Rectal Supp Single Dose Ampules for Injection 1 mg/1 ml 2 mg/1 ml 4 mg/1 ml Multiple Dose Vials for injection: 2 mg/mL–20 ml	PO: 2 mg every 4 to 6 hours prn	An opioid agonist binds to the opioid mu receptor sites in the brain, producing analgesia and sedation and increasing tolerance to pain.	**Common side effects:** Constipation, dysphoria, drowsiness, N/V, respiratory depression, coma, death
Oxycontin® (oxycodone) for continuous ATC pain,	10, 20, 40, 80, and 160 mg CR tablets	10 mg CR to 160 mg CR q12h Must be swallowed	An opioid agonist binds to the opioid mu receptor sites in	**Common side Effects:** Constipation, dysphoria,

TABLE 19-18   Selected Scheduled Narcotics (*continued*)

Drug Trade/Generic Name	Availability	Dosage and Administration	MOA	Side Effects and Special Notes
chronic/cancer pain		whole	the brain, producing analgesia and sedation and increasing tolerance to pain.	drowsiness, N/V, respiratory depression, coma, death
Numorphan® (oxymorphone) Use for prn pain	1 mg/1 ml × 1 ml SD ampule and 1.5 mg/1 ml × 5 ml injectable MVD vials Rectal Supp: 5 mg	1–1.5 mg q4–6 hr prn	A semi-synthetic opioid agonist	**Common side Effects:** Constipation, dysphoria, drowsiness, N/V, respiratory depression, coma, death
Demerol® (meperidine) Post-operative and pre-op pain Obstetrical Analgesia, *not* for long-term pain management	**PO:** 50 and 100 mg tablets **Injections** 25 mg/1 ml, 50 mg/1 ml, 75 mg/1 ml and 100 mg/1 ml **PO:** 50 mg/5 ml syrup	50 mg–150 mg IM, SC or PO Q 3–4 hrs prn	An opioid agonist binds to the opioid mu receptor sites in the brain, producing analgesia and sedation and increasing tolerance to pain.	**Common side Effects:** Constipation, dysphoria, drowsiness, N/V, respiratory depression, coma, death **Drug Interactions:** phenothiazines and many other tranquilizers increase the action of meperidine.
Codeine Use as antitussive, mild to severe prn pain	15, 30, and 60 mg tablets 30 and 60 ml injection 15 mh/5 ml PO solution	**PO, SC, IV or IM:** 15–60 mg Q4–6 hrs NTE 360 mg/day	Centrally active analgesic	**Common side Effects:** Constipation, dysphoria, drowsiness, N/V, respiratory, depression, coma, death

Narcotic overdose can be reversed with the injection of Narcan® (naloxone), which "knocks out" or displaces the narcotic opioid in the mu receptors. Narcan® (naloxone) will not work on overdoses of barbiturates or stimulants (cocaine) because those drugs do not bind to the mu receptors.

The Peripheral Nervous System

The nervous system is divided into two parts, the central nervous system and the peripheral nervous system. The peripheral nervous system, or PNS, consists of all nerves that are not located in the brain and spinal cord. The PNS is further divided into two parts, the somatic and the autonomic nervous systems. The somatic nervous system controls the nerves that connect to the skeletal muscles and voluntary movement of the whole body. The autonomic nervous system, or ANS, controls the nerves that connect to smooth and cardiac muscles and involuntary movement of intricate functions that a person does not have to consciously think about. The cerebrum has made a decision to allow the PNS to "maintain" certain musculoskeletal (somatic) and visceral (organ/trunk, ANS) duties. The visceral duties are those that an individual does not consciously decide to do, such as digest food, breath-, or dilate and constrict arteries and veins. The ANS is subdivided into two nervous systems called the sympathetic and the parasympathetic.

The sympathetic nervous system, or SNS, is governed by the neurotransmitter, norepinephrine, or NE; while the parasympathetic nervous system, or PSNS, is governed by acetylcholine, or ACH. The opposite of what occurs in the SNS occurs in the PSNS. Motor neurons carry nerve impulses and signals from the axon part of the neuron in the CNS to the body, glands, organs, and skeletal muscles (the PNS). Sensory neurons carry nerve impulses and signals from the dendrite part of the neuron in the sensory organs of the body (PNS) to various areas of the brain (CNS). The motor neurons are considered efferent in response, while the sensory neurons are considered afferent in sensing environmental change.

The SNS prepares the body for energetic tasks, stressful situations, and the "fight or flight" response. The adrenergic receptors are the ones controlled and regulated by the brain stem—Beta-1 in the heart, Beta-2 in the lungs, and Alpha-1 and 2 in the blood vessels, PNS, and the cranium, respectively. When NE is inside the receptors of these organs, it stimulates the organs to "rev them up." The heart rate, breathing rate, blood pressure, and vasoconstriction go up; while the bronchoconstriction, vasodilation, gastrointestinal (GI), and genitourinary (GU) go down.

The PSNS activates the body for sleep under nonstressful periods and effects the "rest and relaxation" (R and R) response. When NE is not present inside the receptors of the heart, lungs, or blood vessels—or if ACH is high—then the organs are depressed, or slowed down. ACH is released from the finger-like ends, called the ganglia, of presynaptic neurons in many different locations within the body, and it also activates the sweat glands. The unusual association of ACH with the sweat glands "crosses over" the responsibility of the SNS in the "fight or flight" response. The R and R response decreases heart rate, breathing rate, blood pressure, and vasoconstriction; while bronchoconstriction; vasodilation, GI, and GU go up.

Note: Understanding what each neurotransmitter does to each of the branches of the ANS is essential to understanding disease states and how they are treated.

SUMMARY

The nervous system is a very complex system that interacts with every other system in the body to ensure homeostasis, and to regulate the body's responses to internal and external stimuli. The nervous system communicates to all cells in the body through nerve impulses that are conducted from one part of the body to another through the transmission of chemicals called neurotransmitters.

The nervous system is divided into two parts, the central nervous system and the peripheral nervous system. The central nervous system includes the brain, the spinal column, and their nerves. The peripheral nervous system is divided into two parts: the somatic nervous system which controls voluntary movement of the body through muscles, and the autonomic nervous system which controls involuntary motor functions, and affects such things as heart rate and digestion.

Neuropharmacology, or pharmacology related to the nervous system is one of the most diverse and complicated areas of pharmacology. By completing this chapter, you will gain an understanding of the common diseases affecting the nervous system, and the pharmaceutical treatments associated with these diseases.

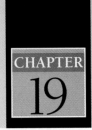

CHAPTER REVIEW QUESTIONS

1. What is the name of the condition affecting the immune system that was caused by the original atypical antipsychotic, Clozaril? (This condition resulted in a reluctance on the part of psychiatrists to prescribe Clorazil as often as they once did.)
   a. agranulomunity
   b. granulocytosis
   c. grancytology
   d. agranulocytosis

2. What are the two main reasons a psychiatrist would prescribe a conventional antipsychotic drug?
   a. Convenience in taking the drug enhances compliance.
   b. The patient does not want to take an atypical antipsychotic drug.
   c. The patient is doing well on the older treatment.
   d. The doctor has had great success with other patients using conventional antipsychotics.
   e. a and c
   f. a and d
   g. none of the above

3. Neurons have dendrites and axons. Explain the function of each.

4. List the three main parts of the nervous system.

5. The brain sends electrical signals through what channel?
   a. spinal cord
   b. neurons
   c. left half of the brain to the right half
   d. heart

6. The neurons produce electrochemical hormones known as:

   a. sympathetic nerves
   b. ions
   c. neurotransmitters
   d. receptors

7. An excess of neurotransmitters reabsorbed into the proximal nerve, which may lead to a shortage of neurotransmitters such as serotonin, norepinephrin, and dopamine, can result in what condition?
   a. depression
   b. anxiety
   c. compulsive–obsessive disorder
   d. hyperactivity

8. Carrying proteins transport the neurotransmitters back to the axon from which they originally came, by a process called:
   a. reuptake
   b. thinking
   c. psychosis
   d. osmosis

9. List the four symptoms of alcohol dependency.

10. Which of the following are more likely to be used to treat depression?
    a. psychotherapy
    b. medication
    c. hypnosis
    d. both a and b
    e. both a and c

11. The disorder that is characterized by peaks and valleys of severe highs (mania) and lows (depression) is known as:
    a. manic–depressive disorder
    b. obsessive–compulsive disorder

c. bipolar disorder (BD)

d. both a and c

12. Explain why an alcohol-dependent patient needs vitamins, such as folate, while undergoing treatment. (Note: you may need to do a bit of research.)

13. What happens when an antipsychotic drug attaches to the dopamine D2 receptor site?

    a. Serotonin levels decrease.

    b. Neurotransmitters increase in activity.

    c. Dopamine activity decreases.

    d. Both a and b.

14. ADHD is a disease in which a person, child or adult, has a very short attention span and is easily distracted, excessively active, and possibly overly emotional or highly impulsive.

    a. true

    b. false

15. Any and all seizures that are generalized and sustained longer than five minutes, or repeated, present a medical emergency called:

    a. Grand Mal

    b. Status Epilepticus

    c. Tonic Clonic

    d. Myoclonic

16. What is the main neurotransmitter that is lacking in the patient with Parkinson's disease?

    a. serotonin

    b. norepinephrine

    c. phenytoin

    d. dopamine

17. What is the mechanism of action of Sinemet for Parkinson's disease?

    a. Blocks dopamine at presynaptic neuron

    b. Blocks dopamine at post-synaptic neuron

c. Blocks serotonin at synapse

d. Facilitates delay of conversion of levodopa to dopamine in the brain until after it crosses the blood brain barrier

18. Which of the following drugs used for migraine headaches may cause agranulocytosis?

    a. beta-blocker, propranolol

    b. naratriptan, selective 5-hydroxytryptamine$_1$ receptor subtype agonist that binds with high affinity to 5-HT$_{1D}$ and 5-HT$_{1B}$

    c. methysergide, which blocks serotonin effects

    d. none of the above

19. The contolled substances most commonly used for pain are:

    a. stimulants

    b. dopaminergics

    c. parasympathetics

    d. narcotics

20. Narcotics used most often for cancer pain are:

    a. opioids and stimulants

    b. dopaminergics that release serotonin

    c. opioid transdermal fentanyl systems that bind to the mu receptors

    d. IM injectable opioids that bind to mu receptors

21. If a patient has glaucoma, would you give him an anticholinergic drug?

    a. No, because it would cause more mitosis.

    b. No, because it would cause more parasympathomimetic response.

    c. No, because it would cause more ACH.

    d. No, because it would cause more NE, mydriasis, and sympathomimetic response.

22. If a patient has HTN, would you give him a parasympatholytic agent?

    a. Yes, because it will increase NE.

b. Yes, because it will increase ACH.

c. No, because it will relatively increase NE.

d. No, because it will lower ACH.

23. A patient comes into the retail pharmacy to get a script for Corgard. The patient:

    a. needs a sympatholytic drug to lower BP.

    b. needs an adrenergic non selective beta blocker to lower BP.

    c. needs an Alpha-1 selective adrenergic blocker to lower BP.

    d. needs a parasympatholytic drug to keep BP at homeostasis.

24. The same patient comes into the retail pharmacy with the same prescription, and the profile shows that he is also taking Cogentin® for Parkinson's disease. What do you do?

    a. Inform the pharmacist to check out the possibility of a drug interaction, on the basis of the fact that Cogentin® may speed up movement and the heart rate, while Corgard may slow it down.

    b. Inform the pharmacist to check out the possibility of a duplicate drug therapy, on the basis of the fact that both Cogentin® and Corgard® may speed up the heart rate.

    c. Inform the pharmacist to check out the possibility of a drug interaction, on the basis of the fact that Cogentin® may slow down the movement and the heart rate, while Corgard® may speed it up.

    d. Do and say nothing to the pharmacist because you are a technician, and it is not your responsibility to catch potential errors.

25. A patient is on Elavil® for depression. She walks into the retail pharmacy with a prescription for Cogentin®.

    a. This is an example of a contraindication.

    b. This is an example of duplicate therapeutics.

    c. This is an example of a side effect.

    d. This is an example of a drug interaction.

Resources and References

1. Schizophrenia Information
   http://www.schizophrenia.com/newsletter/buckets/hypo.html

2. Mechanism of Action of Atypical Antipsychotic Drugs: Critical Analysis
   http://www.ncbi.nlm.nih.gov/entrez/query.fcgi?cmd=Retrieve&db=PubMed&list_uids=8935797&dopt=Abstract

3. Anxiety Disorders Association of America (ADA)
   http://www.adaa.org/

4. Doctor's Guide. Effexor XR Approved in the U.S. for anxiety, March 12, 1999
   http://www.pslgroup.com/dg/ebe9a.htm
   http://www.docguide.com/dgc.nsf/ge/Unregistered.User.545434?OpenDocument

5. Research to practice: adoption of naltrexone in alcoholism treatment. Thomas CP, Wallack SS, Lee S, McCarty D, Swift R
   http://www.ncbi.nlm.nih.gov/entrez/query.fcgi?cmd=Retrieve&db=PubMed&list_uids=12646325&dopt=Abstract

6. Alcohol Related Emergencies
   http://www.vh.org/adult/provider/emergencymedicine/Psychiatry/AlcoholWithdrawal.html

7. National Institute on Drug Abuse
   http://www.drugabuse.gov/ResearchReports/Prescription/prescription4.html

8. National Institute of Mental Health
   http://www.nimh.nih.gov/publicat/medicate.cfm

9. Twenty-Nine Medical Causes of "Schizophrenia," by Carl C. Pfeiffer, Ph.D., M.D.
   http://www.alternativementalhealth.com/articles/causesofschizophrenia.html

10. Atypical antipsychotics: mechanism of action
    http://www.ncbi.nlm.nih.gov/entrez/query.fcgi?cmd=Retrieve&db=PubMed&list_uids=11873706&dopt=Abstract

11. The Merck Manual of Diagnosis and Therapy, Section 15. Psychiatric Disorders, Chapter 189. Mood Disorders—Treatment
    http://www.merck.com/mrkshared/mmanual/section15/chapter189/189d.jsp

12. Common Pharmacological Treatments of Bipolar Disorder and Subtypes: A Review, by David Cox
    http://itech.fgcu.edu/&issues/vol2/issue1/bipolar.htm

13. Internet Mental Health—Monograph for Lamotrigine
    http://www.mentalhealth.com/drug/p30-l06.html#Head_1

14. Bipolar Disorder Sanctuary, by Paul J. Markovitz, M.D., Ph.D
    http://www.mhsanctuary.com/bipolar/bipolardr/208.HTM

15. Neuroland, by Charles Tuen M.D., Neurologist at Methodist Medical Center in Dallas, Texas
    http://neuroland.com/psy/anxiety.htm

16. Doctor's Guide Citalopram Therapy Effective in Treating Social Anxiety Disorder and Comorbid Major Depressive Disorder, 07/04/2003, by Jill Taylor
    http://www.docguide.com/dgc.nsf/ge/Unregistered.User.545434

17. The Crime Prevention Group: Tobacco Addiction Data, 1527 to 1998
    http://medicolegal.tripod.com/tobaccoaddiction.htm

18. American Family Physician: Smoking Cessation: Integration of Behavioral and Drug Therapies, by Robert Mallin, M.D.
    http://www.aafp.org/afp/20020315/1107.html

19. Family Practice Notebook, Smoking Cessation—Tobacco Cessation
    http://www.fpnotebook.com/PSY52.htm

20. The effects of zolpidem and zopiclone on daytime sleepiness and psychomotor performance, Abstract by Uchiumi M, Isawa S, Suzuki M, Murasaki M
http://www.biopsychiatry.com/zolpidemvzopiclone.htm

21. Tropical Plant Database Guaraná (*Paullinia cupana*)
http://www.rain-tree.com/guarana.htm

22. Botanical.com a Modern Herbal, by Mrs. M. Grieve, 1931
http://www.botanical.com/botanical/mgmh/g/guaran43.html

23. Mental Health—Matters Concerta, by Jeannine Virtue
http://www.mental-health-matters.com/articles/article.php?artID=436

24. Adoption Library: Strattera, the Newest ADHD Medication, by Jeannine Virtue
http://library.adoption.com/Attention-Deficit-Hyperactive-Disorder-ADHD/Strattera-The-Newest-ADHD-Medication/article/2250/1.html

25. American Psychiatric Association
http://penta.ufrgs.br/edu/telelab/3/dementia.htm
http://www.psych.org/public_info/elderly.cfm

26. Holland, Norman and Michael Patrick Adams. *Core Concepts in Pharmacology*. Upper Saddle River, NJ: Pearson Education, 2003.

27. Adams, Michael Patrick, Dianne L. Josephson, and Leland Norman Holland, Jr. *Pharmacology for Nurses—A Pathophysiologic Approach*. Upper Saddle River, NJ: Pearson Education, 2005.

Things to do

28. Watch video on neurotransmission.
http://www.utexas.edu/research/asrec/neurotr_copy01a.movr_0.mov

29. Hear the way "hypothalamus" and "corpus callosum" are pronounced.
http://faculty.washington.edu/chudler/wav/hypot.wav

30. Find out about many more brain disorders.
http://faculty.washington.edu/chudler/disorders.html

31. The Merck Manual of Diagnosis and Therapy.
http://www.merck.com/mrkshared/mmanual/section15/chapter189/189d.jsp

32. Watch video on depression.
http://www.depression.com/understanding_depression.html

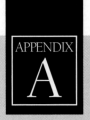

Terminology

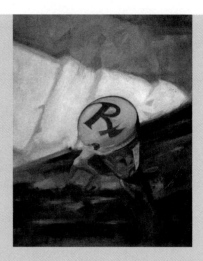

abstinence The act of refraining from

acetylcholine A white crystalline derivative of choline, $C_7H_{17}NO_3$, that is released at the ends of nerve fibers in the somatic and parasympathetic nervous systems and is involved in the transmission of nerve impulses in the body

ACTH Adenocorticotropic Hormone, Prolactin (which is related to pregnancy as the delivery of breast milk), TSH, or the thyroid stimulating hormone

actin A filamentous protein involved in muscle contraction

acute Severe state of being, begins all of a sudden, sharp onset or attack

addiction Pattern of compulsive drug use characterized by a continued craving for an opioid and the need to use the opioid for effects other than pain relief, such as psychological or physical

adipose Fat

adverse effect A general term that applies to an instance of an undesirable and potentially hazardous experience after the ingestion of a drug; this occurs when a person takes a drug for a specific reason, but other unexpected effects occur within the body

affinity The ability of the agonist to actually bind to the cell receptor structure

agonist A drug or other chemical that can combine with a receptor on a cell to produce a physiologic reaction typical of a naturally occurring substance

alveoli A small cell containing air in the lungs

amylase An enzyme that breaks down carbohydrates into monosaccharides, the building blocks of sugars and starches

anaesthetic A drug that decreases all sensation causing unarousable sleep for surgery

analgesic   A drug that selectively suppresses pain, but is non-sedating

anaphylactic   Damaging effect

anhydrase   An enzyme that catalyses the removal of water from a compound

antagonist   A chemical substance that interferes with the physiological action of another, especially by combining with and blocking its nerve receptor

antibacterial   A substance that destroys bacteria or suppresses their growth or reproduction

antibiotic   Drug used to treat infection by killing or inhibiting the growth of disease causing bacteria

antibodies   Any of numerous protein molecules produced by the B-cells as a primary immune defense

antidepressant   Decreases depression

antigen   A substance that induces the production of antibodies

antihistamines   A drug used to counteract the physiological effects of histamine

antipsychotic   A drug which decreases psychoses or psychotic episodes, such as schizophrenia. Production in allergic reactions and colds

anxiolytic   A drug which decreases anxiety, aka anti-anxiety

arrhythmia   Any variation from the normal rhythm of the heart

arteries   Vessels in the body that supply oxygenated blood to the tissues

asthma   A disease process characterized by narrowing of the bronchi

asymptomatic   Without obvious signs or symptoms of disease

atrophy   Waste away

autoimmune   A condition in which an individual's immune system starts reacting against his or her own tissues

B Cell   A type of white blood cell, B lymphocyte, that develops in the bone marrow, matures into plasma cells and produces antibodies, known as immunoglobulins

bactericidal   Bacteria killing

bacteriostatic   An adjective used to describe a drug that inhibits the growth of bacteria, but does not kill them

bioavailability   The degree to which a drug becomes available to tissue after administration

bioequivalence   The condition of two different drugs having the same potency

bronchodilators   A medicine given to open up the airways to ease breathing

buffers   Substances that prevent change of other substances

bronchitis   Inflammation of one or more bronchi

cadence   Rhythm

calculi   Microscopic hard crystals that remain in the kidney

Canal of Schlemm   The passageway for the aqueous fluid to exit the eye

catalyst   A substance that accelerates a chemical reaction, but is not consumed or changed in the process

capillaries   The smallest vessels that carry oxygentated blood

carbon dioxide   A colorless, odorless, incombustible gas

cataracts   An ocular opacity or obscurity in the lens of the eye

catecholamines Include adrenaline, noradrenaline, and dopamine, with roles as hormones and neurotransmitters

cellulitis Painful, red (erythemia) infection of deep skin tissue with poor marked perimeter or borders

cervix The neck or opening of the uterus (the womb)

chamber An area in the heart where blood pumping takes place

chelator An organic chemical that removes free metal ions from solutions

chemical name The chemical composition that defines a specific drug. In contrast to, for example, the word Zantac, the chemical name is quite foreign to most people and would have no use to people other than chemists

chloride A binary compound of chlorine

chronic Recurring condition or disease that must be treated with maintenance therapy

cilia Small, hair-like organelles

coagulation The process of clot formation

complement A large group of proteins that activate in sequence when cells are exposed to an antigen (foreign substance). After activation, they form the membrane attack complex (MAC), resulting in the death of cells. In general, they complement, amplify, or enhance the effects of antibodies and inflammation

corticosteroids A group of synthetic hormones such as prednisone

contraindications This term is used when a specific drug or combination of drugs should not be used in a person or a certain class of people, for any number of reasons. Typically, the use of the drug will or might have a dangerous and possibly fatal effect

controlled substance A scheduled drug that is classified according to potential for abuse

controlled Substance Act of 1970 Designed to regulate how pharmaceuticals are handled, how they are dispensed, and how they are directed by physicians

COPD Chronic Obstructive Pulmonary Disease–A progressive disease process that most commonly results from smoking. COPD is characterized by difficulty breathing, wheezing, and a chronic cough

cornea The outermost layer of the eye. Light passes through the cornea

corpus luteum or yellow body In effect, a tiny and "temporary" endocrine gland that continues to secrete reduced amounts of estrogen, which return the cervix and mucus to their naturally infertile state. The cervix closes and hardens, while the mucus dries up

cystic fibrosis A chronic pulmonary disease of the exocrine glands

cytokines Nonantibody proteins secreted by inflammatory leukocytes, and some nonleukocytic cells, that act as intercellular mediators

dendrites The threadlike extensions of the cytoplasm of a neuron

dependency State of being dependent

depressed Lowering of spirits

dextrose A syrupy form of sugar

diasystole The time when the heart is at rest

disease   An abnormal state in which part or all of the body is not properly adjusted or is incapable of performing normal functions

diuretic   An agent that promotes the excretion of urine

dopamine   A catecholamine neurotransmitter and hormone

dose   The exact amount of a drug to be administered to a specific person to produce a desirable effect. Typically, giving a person less than the dose will have no effect, or the drug will not work as well as expected. An overdose has the potential for causing many problems

drug   Any chemical substance that, when ingested, injected, applied to the skin, or used in any other fashion that will admit it into the bloodstream, will cause a specific change in the body

drug indication   The exact reason for the use of a drug; in other words, each drug or compound has a specific reason, and this describes the indication for the drug

ED50   A name that is applied to exactly one-half of the maximum dose of a drug, so that, when the maximum is used, the exact effects will be known. This term is more of a scientific one that has no real clinical applications; however, knowing the term is essential to understanding other aspects of pharmacology

edema   Swelling of the peripheral areas of the body and of the skin with an excess of water or other fluid

efferent nerves   Conductors of motor impulses from the CNS to effector organs and tissues

efficacious   Producing or capable of producing a desired effect

ejaculation   The ejection of semen through the penis, usually during sexual activity

electrolytes   Substances that dissociate into two ions to some extent in water

emesis   The act of vomiting

endocytosis   The process in which cells take up fluids, particles, and other substances by pinching off the plasma to form an intracellular vesicle

endometrium   The mucous membrane lining of the uterus

enteric   Relating to the intestine

epididymis   A set of coiled tubes that lie alongside of and connect the testes with the vas deferens

epiglottis   Small, leaf-shaped cartilage attached to thyroid cartilage, lying behind the tongue and in front of the entrance to the larynx

erythema   Redness of the skin

erythrocytes   Red blood cells

ester   Drug salt

estrogen   The female sex hormone responsible for the development and maintenance of female reproductive organs, especially the breasts and uterus, and the secondary sex characteristics such as distribution of fat and hair patterns

eukaryotes   Cells that have a complex nucleus of several chromosomes separated from the compartmentalized cytoplasm by a double membrane. The organelles each play a role in support, metabolism, or genetics. Protozoa are eukaryotes

exogenous   Made outside the body and used by the body. For example, calcium is found outside of the body and utilized by the body to make bones and teeth

extrinsically   Originating from the outside

Federal Drug Administration (FDA)   The U.S. Agency responsible for regulation of biotechnology food products. The FDA has been responsible for the creation of such major laws as the Food, Drug, and Cosmetic Act and the Public Health Service Act

follicle   A small secretory sac that surrounds the ovum in the ovary

folliculitis   A papular or pustular inflammation of hair follicles

FSH or Follicle Stimulating Hormone   A hormone released from the pituitary gland that stimulates cells in the ovaries to secrete estrogens; also assists the mature ovum to be released from ovary, a process known as ovulation

formularies   Lists of drugs

GABA   Also known as Gamma-aminobutyric acid, the major inhibitory neurotransmitter of the nervous system

gene expression   The majority of genes are expressed as the proteins that they encode. The process occurs in two steps called transcription and translation. Transcription is the process of changing DNA to RNA, while translation is the process of changing RNA to protein. Working together, they compose the central theme of biology, in which DNA $\rightarrow$ RNA $\rightarrow$ protein

generic name   Drugs are released into market with two names, the generic name and the nongeneric name. The generic name is more appropriately used for the exact name of the drug, as it defines the class and something about its use

genitals   Organs of the reproductive system

genome   The complete hereditary material or code of an organism; genome of HIV contains nine genes

glaucoma   A group of eye diseases characterized by an increase in intraocular pressure

glossitis   Inflammation of the tongue

gonads   The male and female sex organs: testes and ovaries

gradient   A rate of inclination

H2 blocker   A class of anti-ulcer medication that works through the inhibition of basal and nocturnal gastric acid secretion by competitive inhibition of the action of histamine at histamine H2 receptor sites on the parietal cells

health maintenance organizations   Organized systems for providing comprehensive, prepaid health care

hematopoiesis   The formation and development of blood cells

hemoglobin   Protein chemical that carries iron

Hippocrates   Greek physician who laid the foundation of scientific medicine by freeing medical study from the constraints of philosophical speculation and superstition

hives   Raised, whitish patches, often called "welts," that may look like large mosquito bites and may be pink in color, accompanied by pruritus

homeostasis   A tendency for stability in the normal body states

hordeolum   A swelling of the eyelid that results from the plugging of an eye gland

hormone A chemical substance produced by an organ, gland, or special cells that is carried through the bloodstream to regulate the activity of certain organs

humidify To make high amounts of water present

hyperlipidemia A general term for elevated concentrations of any or all of the lipids in the plasma

hypertension High arterial blood pressure

hyperuricemia Excess uric acid in the blood

hypnotic Induces sleep

hypotension Abnormally low blood pressure

hypothalamus A portion of the brain that lies beneath the thalamus and secretes substances which control metabolism by exerting an influence on pituitary gland function

infection The invasion or colonization of pathogens in the body. An infection occurs when a pathogenic microbe is able to multiply in the tissues where it lodges

intoxicated To excite by the action of a chemical substance such as alcohol

intra-arterial Injected directly into the bloodstream

intramuscular Within the substance of a muscle

intraocular Within the eye

intravenous Within a vein or veins

intrinsically Situated within or belonging solely to the organ or body part on which it acts

ionized To convert or be converted totally or partially into ions

ischemia The condition that results when blood stops moving toward tissue or source

isotonicity The quality of processing and maintaining a uniform tone

ketones A byproduct of fat metabolism

lesions Sores

leukocytes White blood cells

lipase Enzyme that breaks down fats into the nutrients of fatty acids and glycerol, the building blocks of lipids or fats

lipid Fat, helps in lubrication, warmth, and padding of the body, along with stored energy

lipid soluble Able to dissolve in fat

lipophilic Having an affinity for fat; pertaining to or characterized by lipophilia

loading dose A dose normally given once to bring a certain level up

lymphocytes The cells that attack bacteria in the blood

macrophage A large and versatile immune cell that acts as a microbe-eating phagocyte, due to its lysosomes, as it polices for invaders and foreign matter. It is an antigen-presenting cell and an important source of immune secretions. It alerts the entire immune system by producing neopterin. It produces Interleukin 1, involved in inflammation. Macrophages are also responsible for the breakdown of worn-out red blood cells

manubrium A handle-like process or part; especially, the anterior segment of the sternum or presternum

marrow　The tissue that fills the cavities of the bones

mechanism of action　A term that explains essentially how a drug works and produces its desirable (and sometimes undesirable) effects

melanocyte　A releasing hormone

menopause　The termination of the menstrual cycle in women usually in midlife between the ages of 40 and 55 years. It also refers to one year after the last period

menstruation　Is the term given to the periodic discharge of blood, tissue fluid, and mucus from the endometrium that lasts from 3-7 days. It is caused by a sudden reduction in estrogens and progesterone. Can also be referred to as the menstrual phase or menstrual cycle, or menses

metabolism　The process of the transforming of energy

metabolites　Any substance produced by the metabolic process

mitigation　Steps taken to minimize negative impact

molecular　A very small mass or matter of molecule size

monosaccharides　Simple sugars such as glucose or lactose, the building blocks of carbohydrates

motility　The contractions of the colon which are unsynchronized (non-peristaltic) and constitute the movement of waste through the GI tract

mucopurulent　Containing both mucous and pus

myocardial infarction　Term used to describe irreversible injury to heart muscle, heart attack

myocardium　Heart muscle

myosin　The most common protein in muscle cells, responsible for the elastic and contractile properties of muscle

myringotomy　a surgical insertion of ventilation tubes into the middle ear

mucosa　The lubricated inner lining of the mouth, nasal passages, vagina and urethra, any membrane or lining which contains mucous secreting glands

mucous membranes　The lubricated inner lining of the mouth, nasal passages, vagina and urethra, any membrane or lining which contains mucous secreting glands

narcotic　Produces deep sleep, relieves pain, may also be used colloquially for illegal drugs, however narcotics are related to opium and bind to the opioid receptors (mu) in the brain

nephrons　Microscopic kidney cells

neurological　Of or pertaining to neurology

neurotransmitters　In its most general sense, the term includes not only messengers that act directly to regulate ion channels, but also those that act through second messenger systems

nomenclature　Description or group of definitions relating to a specific subject

opiate　A remedy derived from or containing opium, a sedative

osmotic　Pertaining to the nature of osmosis

ossicle　A small bone, particularly in the ear

oxygenated　Containing oxygen

ovary   A female gland that produces hormones and the female reproductive, or germ, cell (ova)

ovulation   The release of a fertile ovum, or egg, from the ovary into the fallopian tube

ovum (plural) or **Ova** (singular)   The female reproductive, egg, or germ cell

over-the-counter (OTC) drugs   Drugs available to the public without a prescription. These drugs will change from time to time, as the FDA will commonly permit drugs to be released to the public after the potential dangers have been eliminated

palliative treatment   Use of drugs and procedures to offer symptomatic relief and comfort care, but without a cure

parenteral   An injection through a particular route such as SQ, IM, IV, and so on

pathogenic   Term used to describe a disease-causing agent such as bacteria or virus

penis   Male reproductive organ that transfers sperm to the female

phagocyte   A type of white blood cell that is able to engulf, break down, and digest protozoa, foreign particles, cell debris, and disease-producing microorganisms in the body. These cells play a very important part in the immune system

pharmacodynamics   The processes by which drugs produce their effects

pharmacokinetics   Mathematical descriptions of drug response based on time

pharmacology   This is the study of drugs, how they work, how they are metabolized and secreted from the body

pharmacotherapeutics   This is a major study in the realm of pharmacology; it is concerned with how drugs are used in the treatment of disease within the human body, and, as medicine progresses, there is no doubt that the amount of medications will only increase

pharmacy   This is an actual science, and not merely a place where people go to retrieve their medications. This is the study of preparing the dispensing medications. One might think that the only issues involved in getting a prescription ready is to count pills or fill a bottle, but there are many instances when medications are *compounded* into different chemicals, creating a new formula, which is then used by physicians to treat any array of ailments

pituitary gland   A small, oval shaped gland sitting at the base of the brain with the production of bone

platelets   Small cells in the bloodstream

posoly   Although you will probably not be exposed to this facet of pharmacy to the degree that others might, it is the study of the exact amount of a drug that is needed in order to produce a therapeutic effect. You will see this science throughout this text, but in other ways, as a pharmacist and a pharmacy technician should always be prepared to calculate the exact amount of drug that is needed to take care of a problem. Most times, physicians don't do the calculations for the pharmacist—who is left to do the math so that the patient is given the amount that is needed, no less and no more

potassium   An alkali element necessary for the human body

prokaryotes   A microorganism with a simple nucleus and one chromosome attached to it. Bacteria are prokaryotes

prophylactically   Preventive measure

prostate gland   A structure surrounding the ejaculatory ducts that produces some of the components of sperm

protease   Enzyme that breaks down proteins into the building blocks of amino acids

potency   The power of a medicinal agent to produce the desired effects

precursor   A biochemical substance, such as an intermediate compound in a chain of enzymatic reactions, from which a more stable or definitive product is formed

protein binding   A process in which some drugs are either transported by a means of attraction to these proteins, or freely floating through the blood

pruritus   A skin inflammation that causes itching

PTT or Partial Thromboplastin Time   Used to detect the primary means by which the body conducts homestasis. PT or Prothrobin Time is used to detect the secondary means of homeostasis

pupil   A "hole" or aperture of the colored iris that allows light to enter the eye

osteoblasts   Cells that arise from fibroblasts and which, as they mature, are associated

osteoporosis   A condition that results from the reduction in the amount of bone mass

oxytocin   A peptide hormone from the hypothalamus

reabsorption   Regarding kidneys, the act of transporting ions back into the blood

receptor   A specialized cell or group of nerve endings that responds to sensory stimuli

rosacea   A facial skin disorder accompanied by chronic inflammation and/or acne

sarcomere   One of the segments into which a fibril of striated muscle is divided

scaling   An excess amount of keratin or protein in the dermal layer

Schedule I Drug   The class of drugs that have the highest potential for abuse and, because of their actions, have no acceptable medical applications; in other words, they are illegal, even in the laboratory

Schedule II Drug   The class of drugs that do have acceptable medical use, but they are also extremely addictive. Because of the laws of individual states as well as federal laws, as a pharmacy technician, you will probably not be exposed to these drugs, except under the direct supervision of the pharmacist. Federal laws demand that pharmacies be highly accountable for these drugs and, if even one is missing, the federal or state government can actually close the doors of the pharmacy

Schedule III Drugs   The class of drugs that are addictive, but the potential for abuse is considerably less than other schedules. There is a moderate potential for abuse, and, therefore, you will probably not be exposed to these drugs unless for exceptional purposes

Schedule IV Drugs   The class of drugs with a very limited degree of potential for abuse. You will probably have some contact with them and thus be able to become a good adjunct to your pharmacist

Schedule V Drugs   The class of drugs that have the most limited degree of abuse, they are typically handled by both pharmacists and pharmacy technicians

sclera   The white of the eye. The conjunctiva is a clear membrane that covers the white of the eye (sclera)

scrotum   Pouch-like structure that contains the testes

sedative   A tranquilizer that promotes a calming effect and causes a decrease in all reactions and emotions

seminal fluid   A whitish fluid that mixes with sperm to form semen

seminal vesicles   Sac-like structures attached to the vas deferens that provide fluids to lubricate the duct system and nourish the sperm

seminiferous tubules   The tiny coiled tubes in the testes that produce sperm

semi-permeable   Partly able to penetrate

serotonin   An organic compound, $C_{10}H_{12}N_2O$, formed from tryptophan and found in animal and human tissue, especially the brain, blood serum, and gastric mucous membranes, and active as a neurotransmitter and in vasoconstriction, stimulation of the smooth muscles, and regulation of cyclic body processes

side effect   An effect that a drug has on the body that is unexpected and undesirable, but not specifically deemed harmful. An example would be an upset stomach after taking a prescription medication for a headache

sinoatrial (SA) node   Provides energy in the form of electricity to the heart

site of action   The location (at the cellular level) where a drug will typically be expected to exert its effect, that is, at the cellular level

sperm   The male sex cells, the male reproductive or germ cell

solubility   The ability to dissolve into

sphincter   A muscle that acts to close or contract an opening or orifice of the body

spina bifida   Spina bifida means cleft spine, which is an incomplete closure in the spinal column

staphylococcus   A spherical gram-positive parasitic bacterium causing infection

stenosis   Narrowing of a duct or canal

stimulant   Increase alertness, or stimulates reticular formation

stomatitis   Inflammation of the mouth

subcutaneous   Under the skin

sympathetic   One of the two divisions of the vertebrate autonomic nervous system

synapses   The side-by-side association of homologous paternal and maternal chromosomes during the first prophase of meiosis

systole　The time at which ventricular contraction occurs

T Cell　White blood cells, which include helper, killer, suppressor, and memory cells, critical to the immune response

target cell　Referring to a large number of cells, all of which are probably quite similar such as the nerve cells

teratogenic　Tending to produce anomalies of formation or teratism

testicle　A structure in males in which sperm are produced (plural: testes). There are two testes

testosterone　Major male sex hormone

thrombocytopenia　A decrease in the number of platelets in the blood

tinnitus　Ringing in the ears

tolerance　The ability to endure large amounts of drug

toxicology　This is the study of drugs that is concerned with whatever harmful effects any specific or any number of drugs have on living human tissue. The study is toxicology, although sometimes behind the scenes, is an important and sometimes overlooked aspect of pharmacology. For the pharmacy technician, it is important to understand that all drugs, to one extent or another, can have a toxic effect, just as water, as vital as it is to life, can cause one to drown

trachea　Wind pipe

trade name　Brand or proprietary name of a developed drug

ulcers　An open sore

urethra　Organ that carries both sperm through the penis and urine from the bladder and ureters

uterus　A hollow, muscular organ in females that is the site of menstruation, implantation, development of the fetus, and labor. Also called the womb

uvula　The fleshy piece of muscle, tissue, and mucous membrane that hangs down from the palate that flips up and helps close off the nasal passages when we swallow

vas deferens　A muscular tube that passes upward alongside the testes and transports the sperm

vasoconstrictor　Something which causes narrowing of the blood vessels

vasomotor　Effecting the calibre of a vessel

vein　Blood vessel that returns blood from the microvasculature to the heart

venules　The smallest of veins

vessels　A duct, canal, or other tube that contains or conveys a body fluid: *a blood vessel*

vestibular nuclei　This section introduces the location and appearance of the four vestibular nuclei and the fiber tracts that originate with them and that send signals to motoneurons in the brainstem and spinal cord that mediate reflexive eye, head, and neck movement

virus　Obligate intracellular parasites of living but noncellular nature, consisting of DNA or RNA and a protein coat

zygote　The fertilized ovum; a combination of egg and sperm

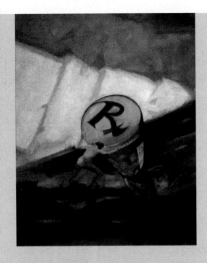

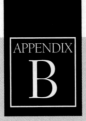

Answers

CHAPTER 1
Introduction to Pharmacology

ANSWERS TO CHAPTER REVIEW QUESTIONS

1. d. pharmacodynamics
2. b. false
3. Answer will vary.
4. a. true
5. drug indication

CHAPTER 2
The Realm of Pharmacology

ANSWERS TO CHAPTER REVIEW QUESTIONS

1. a. according to the way they affect the body
2. **Class I**—highly addictive, no medical reasons and are not used in medicine for any reason
   Class II—highly addictive. In most states, they cannot be released other than through a specific route (must be a prescription with no refills)
   Class III—These are prescriptions that have less addictive value

Class IV—These are prescriptions that have less addictive value
Class V—because of specific qualities, are addictive, but the potential is very rare.
3. Highest—Class I, Lowest—Class V
4. c. FDA
5. c. the Controlled Substance Act of 1970
6. b. H_2 blocker
7. a. an organ
8. Topical; Rectal and Vaginal; Parenteral Administration
9. Answers will vary.
10. Answers will vary.

CHAPTER 3
The Body and Drugs

ANSWERS TO CHAPTER REVIEW QUESTIONS

1. c. 4
2. b. heart attack
3. a. capillaries
4. d. sodium-potassium pump
5. d. oxygen and carbon dioxide
6. a. mid 20s

7. c. COPD
8. b. kidneys
9. c. renal dysfunction
10. d. the mouth
11. Answers will vary.

CHAPTER 4
Pharmacodynamics

ANSWERS TO CHAPTER REVIEW QUESTIONS

1. b. receptors
2. Mechanism of action essentially explains how a drug works and how it produces its desirable (and sometimes undesirable) effects.
3. a. red eyes, runny nose
4. c. hormone
5. An opiod helps interrupt the pathway between the central nervous system and the peripheral nervous system. (Answers will vary.)
6. An agonist is a specific type of drug that, when it binds to the correct receptor to which it was designed, produces a certain, predicted action. An antagonist is a drug that, when it binds to a specific receptor on cell, does not produce any noticeable or desirable effect; however, it may or may not have any predictable side effects.
7. a. affinity and efficacy
8. Answers will vary.
9. d. dose–response curve
10. c. rat poison

CHAPTER 5
Pharmacokinetics

ANSWERS TO CHAPTER REVIEW QUESTIONS

1. a. for the medication to become absorbed into the body
2. b. specialized transport mechanisms
3. b. affinity
4. Answers will vary.

5. Answers will vary.
6. b. *Physician's Desk Reference*
7. d. ionized
8. Answers will vary.
9. d. both a and b
10. b. false

CHAPTER 6
Drug Distribution and Metabolism

ANSWERS TO CHAPTER REVIEW QUESTIONS

1. a. protein binding
2. c. diabetes
3. b. affinity and number of available sites on cells
4. d. 80%
5. Ingredients such as fillers may interfere with their body metabolism. (Answers will vary.)
6. c. a loading dose
7. b. false

CHAPTER 7
Addiction

ANSWERS TO CHAPTER REVIEW QUESTIONS

1. a. disease
2. b. dependency
3. a. dopamine
4. Answers will vary.
5. b. synapses

CHAPTER 8
Drug Dependency

ANSWERS TO CHAPTER REVIEW QUESTIONS

1. Answers will vary.
2. Answers will vary.

CHAPTER 9
The Skin

ANSWERS TO CHAPTER REVIEW QUESTIONS

1. 1. c   2. a   3. b
2. a. protection   b. maintenance of body temperature   c. excretion   d. perception of stimuli
3.

Skin Disease	Symptoms	Drug Used to Treat
Chronic plaque psoriasis	d	b
Eczema	a	e
Cellulitis	f	a
Athlete's foot	c	c
Acne	g	d
Lice	e	g
Rosacea	b	f

4. a. 1   b. 2   c. 3   d. 4.
5. Answers will vary.

CHAPTER 10
Eyes and Ears

ANSWERS TO CHAPTER REVIEW QUESTIONS

1. b.   glaucoma
2. c.   both a and b
3. c.   use OTC drugs without consulting their doctor
4. a.   otitis media
5. b.   an inflammation and infection of the middle ear
6. c.   retina
7. When blood vessels constrict over a long period of time, they become tired and after the drug wears off, the body tries to make up for the earlier long term constriction as it overcorrects, making the same blood vessels dilate even more.
8. a.   the Organ of Corti within the scala media of the cochlea
9. d.   ototoxicity
10. Answers will vary.

CHAPTER 11
The Gastrointestinal System

ANSWERS TO CHAPTER REVIEW QUESTIONS

1. Teeth   Tongue
   Salivary Glands   Liver
   Gall Bladder   Pancreas
2. Liver - bile   Pancreas - enzymes
3. b. emulsification
4. c. 55%
5. a. true
6. When a pt refuses to eat (anorexia or depression)
   A pt is unable to eat
   A pt should not eat
   A pt requires more nutrition than what the average person can eat
   A pt is unable to absorb or digest nutrients properly
   *** Also—A pt has a disease state causing bowel obstruction A pt has severe weight loss or GI fistula
7. a. 50 cc/hr for 4–6 hours
8. Calcium
   Phosphorus
9. 1. carbohydrates   2. proteins   3. fats
   4. vitamins   5. minerals   6. water
10. a. jejunum, duodenum, ileum
11. 1. Cecum   2. Ascending colon   3. Transverse colon   4. Descending colon   5. Sigmoid colon   6. Rectum   7. Anus
12. b. high amplitude propagating contraction
13. a. 24 hours

CHAPTER 12
The Musculoskeletal System

ANSWERS TO CHAPTER REVIEW QUESTIONS

1.

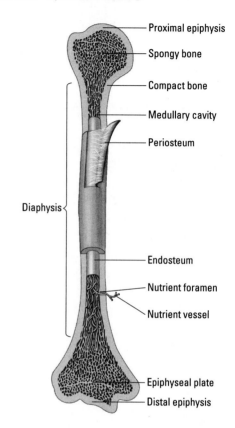

- Proximal epiphysis
- Spongy bone
- Compact bone
- Medullary cavity
- Periosteum
- Diaphysis
- Endosteum
- Nutrient foramen
- Nutrient vessel
- Epiphyseal plate
- Distal epiphysis

2. b. produce red blood cells, some white blood cells, and platelets, as well as acting as storage area for fat
3. a. true
4. b. false
5. d. all of the above
6. d. a and b only
7. b. false
8. e. all of the above
9. e. all of the above
10. d. a and b only
11. e. a and d only
12. f. a, b, c, and d only
13. b. block Cycoloxygenase II, the enzyme that produces the prostaglandins that contribute to inflammation

14. b. bisphosphonates, which inhibit bone resorption and osteoclast activity
15. a. true
16. a. true
17. d. all of the above
18. c. Lioresal®
19. f. a and c

CHAPTER 13
The Respiratory System

ANSWERS TO CHAPTER REVIEW QUESTIONS

1. nasal cavity, paranasal sinuses, pharynx, larynx, trachea, lungs, main and secondary bronchi, bronchioles, alveolar ducts, alveoli
2. Answers will vary. Respiratory disease states include the common cold, allergies, anaplylactic shock, and chronic obstructive diseases such as emphysema and asthma.
3. Answers will vary and include chronic and acute bronchopulmonary disease and acetaminophen overdose.
4. a. 2   b. 5   c. 6   d. 8   e. 7   f. 3   g. 4   h. 1
5. a. 3   b. 8   c. 5   d. 2   e. 7   f. 4   g. 6   h. 1
6. a. 4   b. 3   c. 5   d. 6   e. 2   f. 1
7. histamine
8. H-1 receptors
9. a. Cystic fibrosis
10. a. mantain fluids   b. provide respiratory immune defense   c. remove inhaled solid material/microorganisms
11. d. nitrogen 78%, oxygen 21%, carbon dioxide .03%
12. c. aveoli
13. To push carbon dioxide out of the lungs
14. b. false
15. a. leukotrienese   b. histamines

CHAPTER 14
The Cardio, Circulatory, and Lymph Systems

ANSWERS TO CHAPTER REVIEW QUESTIONS

1. a. 4,300
2. To deliver oxygen rich blood to every cell in the body
3. d. 5.6 liters
4. electrocardiogram
5. b. atrial fib
6. Right
7. The actual stiffening of the arteries themselves
8. Low potassium levels in the serum
9. No
10. Break down blood clots by reversing the clotting order and interfering with the synthesis of various clotting factors
11. a. one to two quarts

CHAPTER 15
The Immune System

ANSWERS TO CHAPTER REVIEW QUESTIONS

1. a. antibodies and complement
2. c. 1844
3. b. methylene blue
4. b. to kill invading cells
5. 1. airborne   2. digestive tract   3. blood or other bodily fluids
6. b. diplococcus
7. a. parasites   b. bacteria   c. rickettsia (or viruses)
8. c. stage 3
9. a. toxoid
10. Bladder, breast, colon, rectal, prostate, skin, or others listed on p. 311

CHAPTER 16
The Renal System

ANSWERS TO CHAPTER REVIEW QUESTIONS

1.

a. Kidney

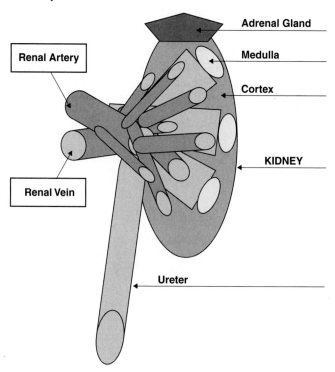

b. Renal system

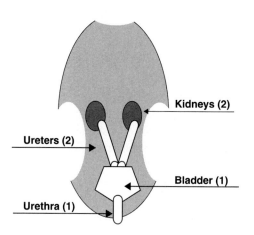

c. Nephron

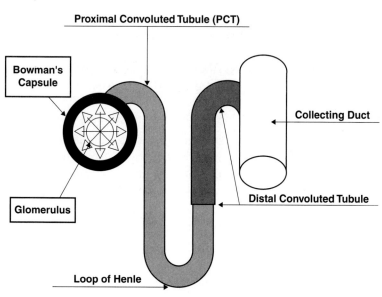

2.
1. Filtering the "waste" known as urine from the blood.
2. Removal of urine from the body.
3. Maintains water balance
4. Maintains electrolyte balance
5. Maintains acid-base balance

3. About 25% of the blood from the heart enters the Kidney where it is filtered by glomerulus of the small kidney cells called nephrons. Toxins are flushed out of the tubules of the nephrons into the collecting ducts, then along with some water, sodium and chloride the waste known as urine enters the ureters. The ureters bring the urine to the bladder. When the bladder reaches a 'fullness' there is a spasm that signals the person that it is time to release the urine. Some sodium and chlorine, and therefore water, will stay on the outer side of the ureter or cross the tubule membrane. This is called reabsorption. The person will retain water. At other times, the sodium and chlorine, attracting water will stay inside the tubule and flow to the collecting ducts as urine. This balance of retention of water or elimination of water is called homeostasis. If the kidneys loose their ability to filter toxins the person will die. In the process of removal of water potassium can also be eliminated. This important electrolyte is needed for nerve and muscular function, in particular the heart. In addition the loss of H^+ Na^+ and K^+ can lead to a change in pH making it more acidic. Homeostasis allows for a balance in changes in water retention water elimination, ph changes and ionic changes. (Answers will vary.)

4.

Disease State	Causative Factor (s)	Rx Treatment
Urinary Tract Infection	Pseudomonas	Quinolones: ciprofloxacin
Acute prostatitis	P. mirabilis	Cephalosporins: cefazolin
Urinary Tract Infection	group D streptococcus	Augmentin®
Complicated and recurrent upper UTI's	P. aeruginosa,	Aminoglycosides: tobramicin, gentamycin
Urinary Tract Infection	Klebsiella, Staphylococcus	Tetracyclines
Urinary Tract Infection	Staphylococcus, Klebsiella	Sulfonamides: sulfamethoxazole/ trimethoprim
Urinary Tract Infection	E. faecalis, P. mirabilis	Amoxicillin- a specific penicillin

5. f. all of the above
6. b. false
7. e. a and c only
8. a. true
9. f. all of the above
10. a. true
11. g. all of the above, except f
12. a. true
13. f. only a–d

CHAPTER 17
The Endocrine System

ANSWERS TO CHAPTER REVIEW QUESTIONS

1. hypothalamus and pituitary gland
2. A systematic process that the body uses to maintain the body's physical and chemical processes with pre-set limits. An example is the calcium being taken up by the blood and deposited into the bone, by the homeostasis of calcitonin and parathyroid hormone.
3. c. growth
4. Somatropin
5. b. mineralcorticoids and glucocorticoids

6. So that the patient will not dehydrate

To maintain pH balance in the body

To assist in the electrical function of the nerves and muscles

7. less

8. a. increases HDL and lowers LDL

9. a. true

10. to stimulate the development of male sex organs

to maintain the secondary sex characteristics.

11. d. adrenal

12. d. acromegaly

CHAPTER 18
The Reproductive System

ANSWERS TO CHAPTER REVIEW QUESTIONS

1. c. mid-cycle, usually day 12–14

2. d. a and b only

3. d. a and c only

4. a. FSH

5. a. Major pre-fertilization mechanisms such as ovulation and thickening of the cervical mucus to provide a barrier to sperm, reducing likelihood of implantation

6. a. true

7. c. epididymis

8. a. Gonadotropin-releasing hormone (GnRH) in the hypothalamus

9. b. age

10. d. all of the above

11. c. Alpha blockers

12. b. H/A, dizziness, hypotension

13. b. prevent the conversion of testosterone to the hormone dihydrotestosterone (DHT)

14. a. finasteride (Proscar®) and dutasteride (Avodart™)

15.

Male Reproductive System	Female Reproductive System
Anatomy • Penis • Testes • Scrotum • seminiferous tubules • Prostate gland • Cowper's glands • Epididymis • Vas Deferens • seminal vesicles • Urethra	**Anatomy** • Two ovaries • Two fallopian tubes • Uterus • Vagina • Cervix
Description of the System 1. Adult male produces several million sperm cells every day in the testicles within a system of tubes called seminiferous tubules. 2. During sexual stimulation, a whitish fluid called seminal fluid is produced by the prostate and the seminal vesicles to mix with sperm to form semen. 3. The tissues in the penis fill with blood and it becomes erect and rigid. 4. During the stimulation of the erect penis, the muscles around the reproductive organs contract and force the semen epididymis)through the duct system (vas deferens and the urethra.	**Description of the System** 1. Cycle is about 28 days 2. Day on is the period or mensus begins. After the period ends one egg from one ovary will mature. 3. At approximately Day 14 ovulation in which the matured egg is released from the ovary. 4. If the egg is penetrated inside the later section of the fallopian tube a single sperm may penetrate it causing conception. 5. If the lining of the uterus is intact and nourished the fertilized egg will attach to the wall or implant.

Male Reproductive System	Female Reproductive System
Description of the System	Description of the System
5. Semen is expelled or ejaculated from the body through the urethra inside the penis. The ejaculate, of about 1/5 of a teaspoon, will contain about 100 million sperm. 6. The movement of the tails or flagella of the sperm along with the uterine contractions aid the sperm in 'swimming' to the cervix and fallopian tubes to find the egg and penetrate it to deposit the DNA contained in the head of the sperm.	6. Gestation period is about 9 months. 7. If penetration of the sperm to the egg does not occur the egg and sperm will disintegrate/die. And the lining will be shed, once again known as the period or mensus. 5. Semen is expelled or ejaculated from the body through

CHAPTER 19
The Nervous System

ANSWERS TO CHAPTER REVIEW QUESTIONS

1. d. agranulocytosis
2. e. a and c
3. Dendrites bring information to the cell body from the CNS
   Axons take information away from the cell body to the CNS.
4. brain, spinal cord, and nerves
5. b. neurons
6. c. neurotransmitters
7. a. depression
8. a. reuptake
9. Craving for alcohol
   Loss of control
   Physical dependence
   Tolerance
10. d. both a and b
11. d. both a and c
12. Excessive alcohol use depletes the body of nutrients. Also, the alcoholic patient normally does not eat well and does not receive the RDA of vitamins

while abusing alcohol. A deficiency of Folate can lead to anemia. Inadequate dietary intake, intestinal malabsorption, and impaired folate storage in the liver all contribute to folate deficiency.

13. c. dopamine activity decreases.
14. b. false
15. b. Status Epilepticus
16. d. dopamine
17. d. Facilitates delay of conversion of levodopa to dopamine in the brain until after it crosses the blood brain barrier
18. a. beta-blocker, propranolol
19. d. narcotics
20. c. opioid transdermal fentanyl systems that bind to the mu receptors
21. d. No, because it would cause more NE, mydriasis, and sympathomimetic response.
22. c. No, because it will relatively increase NE.
23. b. needs an adrenergic nonselective Beta blocker to lower BP.
24. a. Inform the pharmacist to check out the possibility of a drug interaction, on the basis of the fact that Cogentin® may speed up movement and the heart rate, while Corgard may slow it down.
25. d. This is an example of a drug interaction.

Index

A

Aancobon® (flucytosine), 284, 285, 286
AAT, 210
Abacavir (Ziagen®), 278, 289
Abbokinase®, 249
Abciximab, 246
Abdominal aorta, 319
Abdominal pain, 28
Abilify® (aripiprazole), 426
Abitrate®, 255
Abortion, spontaneous, 385
Abraham, E.P., 326
Abreva® (docosanol), 87
Absence seizures (Petite Mal), 436
Absorption, 30, 49–50, 57, 60, 61
    buccal and sublingual, 15–16
Abstinence syndrome, 76
Acarbose (Precose©), 361, 370
Accessory organs, 124, 125
Accolate® (zafirlukast), 86, 219, 220
Accupril®, 242
Accutane® (isotretinoin), 86, 142
Acebutolol, 244
ACE inhibitors, 241–242
Acellular vaccines, 305
Aceon®, 242
Acetaminophen (Tylenol®), 70, 176,
        449–450, 454
    with codeine, 328
    overdose of, 211, 212
Acetate, 151
Acetazolamide (Diamox®), 109, 33
N-Acetyl P-aminophenol, 449
Acetylcholine (ACH), 38, 135, 177, 216,
        233, 443, 458
Acetylcysteine, 211, 212
Acetylsalicylic acid, 246, 449
Achromycin V®, 179
Aciphex®, 136, 137
Acne, 81, 83, 86
Acoustic meatus, 117
Acquired immune deficiency syndrome.
        See HIV/AIDS
Acromegaly, 343, 358, 359, 369

ACTH, 31, 338, 344, 346–347, 365, 366,
        368, 370
Actifed®, 203
Actin, 159, 160
Acting®, 205
Actinic keratosis (AK), 84
Actinomycin, 238
Action
    mechanism of, 4, 39
    site of, 5
Action potential, 400, 401
Actiq® (fentanyl citrate), 455
Activase®, 249
Activated partial thromboplastin time
        (aPTT), 251
Activella®, 354
Active transport, 50, 51
Actonel® (risedronate), 182
Actos© (pioglitazone), 361
Acular®, 102
Acute angina, 240
Acute myeloid leukemia (AML), 314
Acyclovir, 9, 99, 289
Acyclovir triphosphate, 304
Adalat®, 257, 258
Adalimumab (Humirara®), 82, 87, 92
Adderall®, 433
Adderall XR®, 433
Addiction, 64–73
    to alcohol, 68–71
        brain and, 69–71
        treatment for, 71
    brain and, 67, 68, 69–71
    causes of, 66–67
    characteristics of, 66
    criteria for, 67
    defined, 66, 75
    dependency vs., 66, 71, 77
    as disease, 65–66
    to other drugs, 69–71
    roots of drug abuse, 68
    to street drugs, 66
    symptoms of, 65
    websites on, 77
Addictive drugs, classification of, 11

Addison's disease (hypocortisolism), 349,
        365–366, 371
Adenohypophysis, 338, 343
Adenoma, pituitary, 359, 365
Adenosine triphosphate (ATP), 158
ADHD and ADD, 432–434
    nonstimulants for, 434
    stimulants for, 432–433
Adipose (fat) tissue, 80, 253, 339
Adjunctive therapy, 439
Adjuvant drugs, 455
Administration, rate of, 60
Adrenal cortex, 339, 345
Adrenal gland, 31, 337, 339, 340,
        345–347
    abnormalities of, 364–371
Adrenaline (epinephrine), 216, 243, 339,
        345
Adrenal medulla, 339, 345
Adrenal tumors, 365
Adrenergic agonists, 107
Adrenergic neuronal blocker, 244
Adrenergic receptors, 458
Adrenocorticosteroids, 252
Adrenocorticotropic hormone (ACTH),
        31, 338, 344, 346–347, 365, 366,
        368, 370
Adriamycin PFS™, 313
Adriamycin RDF®, 313
Adrucil®, 314
Advair Diskus®, 216, 218
Adverse effect, defined, 3
Advil®, 70, 449
Aerobid®, 218
Aerosols, 16
Afferent (sensory) function, 396
Affinity, 40, 49
African Americans, 329
Afrin Children's®, 205
Afrin Topical Decongestant®, 205
Age
    dementia and, 443
    infertility and, 385
Agenerase® (amprenavir), 278, 289, 355
Aggrastat®, 246, 258

Agnosia, 444
Agonists, 3, 40–41
Agranulocytosis, 425
Air, oxygen vs., 194
Airbron, 211
Air sacs (alveoli), 50, 192, 194–195, 209–210
Alamast®, 102
Alanine, 141
Alanine aminotransferase (ALT), 446
Alavert®, 202
Albumin, 59
Albuterol, 208, 215, 217
Alcohol
    metronidazole and, 286–287
    muscle relaxants and, 179
    ulcers and, 135
    use with medications, 68–69, 70
Alcoholics Anonymous (AA), 71
Alcoholism, 68–71
    brain and, 69–71
    treatment for, 71
    withdrawal, 420–422
Alcohol (solution), 88
Aldactazide, 240
Aldactone® (spironolactone), 240, 331, 389
Aldara® (imiquimod), 82, 87, 88, 93
Aldomet®, 244
Aldosterone, 320, 339, 341, 348, 365, 371
Alefacept (Amevive®), 81–82, 86, 92, 281
Alendronate (Fosamax®), 182
Alertness, degree of, 404
Alesse®, 378
Aleve®, 449
Alfuzosin (UroXatral™), 390
Alkaloids, 135, 313
Alkylamines, 203
Alkylating antineoplastic agents, 311–312
Allegra® (fexofenadine), 202, 389
Allerest®, 103
Allergen, 208
Allergic asthma, 208, 219
Allergic conjunctivitis, 98
Allergic rhinitis, 199, 208, 213
Allergies, 38, 212–214
    antihistamines for, 201, 202, 212–213
    food, 147
    mast cell stabilizers for, 213–214
Allergy shots, 208
Allermed®, 203
Allopurinol, 185, 328
All-or-nothing principle, 43
Almotriptan (Axert®), 453
Alomide®, 102
Alora® estradiol, 352
Alpha 1-antitrypsin (AAT), 210
Alpha-adrenergic agonists, 203, 323
Alpha blockers, 390

Alphagan®, 107
Alpha-glucosidase inhibitors, 361, 370
Alpha Keri Lotion®, 88
5-Alpha reductase inhibitors, 390
Alprazolam (Xanax®), 70, 179, 409, 423
Altace®, 242
Alteplase, 249
Altretamine (Hexalen®), 313
Alupent®, 216
Alveolar ducts, 192
Alveoli (air sacs), 50, 192, 194–195, 209–210
Alzheimer's disease, 442–446
    drugs for, 445
Amantadine, 289, 304
Amantadine hydrochloride (Symmetrel®), 441
Amaryl© (glimeprimide), 361
Ambien® (zolpidem), 407, 409, 428, 430
Amebicides, 284–287, 289
Amebic infections, 289
Ameboids, 272
Amerge® (naratriptan), 450, 452
American Cancer Society (ACS), 310
American Psychiatric Association (APA), 422, 443
American Society of Addiction Medicine, 69
Amevive® (alefacept), 81–82, 86, 92, 281
Amickin®, 119
Amidate®, 179
Amikacin IV, 119
Amikacin sulfate (Amikin®), 300
Amines, 340
Amino acids, 127, 128, 140–141
Aminocaproic acid, 251
Aminoglutethimide, 365, 370
Aminoglycosides, 8, 100, 118, 166, 238, 289, 300
    for urinary tract infections, 325
Aminopenicillins, 295, 296
Aminophylline, 60, 217
Amiodarone (Cordarone), 257, 258
Amitriptyline (Elavil®), 322, 415, 428, 451, 455
Amlodipine, 242, 257
Amobarbital (Amytal®), 430, 438
Amoxicillin, 15, 87, 97, 120, 136, 137, 296, 297, 325, 326
Amoxicillin sulfisoxazole, 120
Amoxil®, 120, 296, 325
Amphetamine asparate, 433
Amphetamines, 70
Amphotec®, 285
Amphotericin B (Fungizone®), 88, 285, 286
Ampicillin, 296, 297
Amprenavir (Agenerase®), 278, 289, 355
Amygdala, 80

Amyloid-beta, 174
Amylopsin, 127
Amytal® (amobarbital), 430, 438
Anabolic drugs, 9
Anabolic steroids, 354, 389
Anafranil® (clomipramine), 409, 415–416, 428
Analgesics, 8, 15, 201, 448, 454
    anti-inflammatory, 184
    narcotic, 455–457
Anal warts, 87
Anaphylactic reaction, 18
Anaprox®, 175, 449
Anastrozole (Arimidex®), 313
Ancef® (cefazolin), 87, 298
Androderm®, 355
AndroGel®, 355
Androgens, 9, 312, 339, 350, 355, 357–358
Androstenedione, 376
Anectine®, 178
Anemia, 33, 144, 168, 355
    pernicious, 145, 282
Anesthesia, 39
    muscle relaxants and, 179
Angina pectoris, 234, 240, 243
Angioedema, 355
Angiotensin, 341
Angiotensin converting enzyme inhibitors (ACEIs), 241–242
Angiotensin II receptor blockers, 242
Angiotensin receptor blockers (ARBs), 244–245
Anistreplase, 249
Anitvert®, 131
Ankle (tarsals), 165
Ansaid®, 175
Antabuse® (disulfiram), 71, 287, 355, 421, 422
Antagonists, 3, 40–41, 76
Anterior chamber, 95, 104
Anthra-Derm® (anthralin), 281
Anthrax, 307
Antianxiety drugs, 9, 423
Antiarrhythmics, 118, 179
Antiasthmatics, 10
Antibacterials, 100, 293, 295–304
    aminoglycosides, 8, 100, 118, 166, 238, 289, 300, 325
    cephalosporins, 9, 289, 293, 295–298
    MOA of,298
    fluoroquinolones, 99, 294, 300–301
    macrolides, 9, 289, 294, 299
    penicillins (PCNs), 171, 289, 293, 295, 378
    allergy to, 120
    groups of, 295, 296–297
    MOA of, 295

other antibacterials related to, 297–298
    penicillinase resistant, 292
    for urinary tract infections, 325
  for renal system, 318
  sulfonomides (sulfa drugs), 301, 325
  tetracyclines (TCNs), 9, 179, 289, 292, 293–294, 295, 299, 326
  for tuberculosis, 302–304
Antibiotic resistance, 290–291
Antibiotics, 282, 378
  antitumor, 313
  colds and, 201
  in eye treatments, 100
  hearing loss from, 119
  male infertility and, 389
  muscle relaxants and, 179
  oral contraceptives and, 292
  for otitis media in children, 120
  pregnancy classification of, 10–11
  sulfur-containing, 294
  in treatment of eye, 97, 98, 99
  for yeast infections, 283
Antibodies (immunoglobulins), 140, 266–267, 271, 311, 386
Antibody-mediated response, 270, 271
Anti-cancer drugs, 118, 119
Anti-cholinergic effects, 201
Anticholinergics, 135–136, 215, 216, 217
Anticoagulants, 9, 258
  antidotes for overdose of, 250–251
  for CAD, 245–248, 250–251, 258
Anticonvulsants, 10, 378, 418
  for bipolar disorder, 418, 419, 420
Antidepressants, 9, 409, 410, 411–412
  for cancer pain, 455
  in smoking cessation, 423
Antidiarrheals, 9, 135
Antidiuretic hormone (ADH), 321, 338, 340, 341, 342, 362, 369
Antiemetics, 130, 131–132
Antiestrogenic non-steroidal antiestrogen, 386
Antifungals, 8, 284, 285–286, 289, 378
Antigens, 82, 270
Antihelix, 117
Antihistamines, 10, 38, 98, 101
  for allergies, 201, 202, 212–213
  as antiemetics, 131–132
  for common cold, 201–203
  degree of sedation of, 203
  male infertility and, 389
Antihyperlipidemics, 9, 251, 255
Antihypertensives, 9
Anti-infectives (antimicrobials), 8–9, 288, 289
  comparison overview of, 293–294
  mechanisms of action of, 292
  side effects of, 292, 293–294

Anti-inflammatories, 102, 201, 215, 216–217, 281, 448
Anti-leukotrienes, 215, 219–221
Antimetabolites, 312
Antimetics, 9
Antimicrobial resistance, 290
Antinauseants, 130, 131
Antineoplastics, 9, 118, 119
Antioxidants, 145
Antiplatelets, 258
  antidotes for overdose of, 250–251
  for CAD, 245, 246, 250–251, 258
Antiprotozoals, 284–287, 289
Antipsychotics, 9, 421, 425–426
  atypical, 424–425, 426
  mechanism of action of, 424
Antipyretics, 201, 448
Antirheumatics, 8
Antiseptics, 9
Antispasmodics, 135
Antitussives, 206
Antivert®, 202
Antivirals, 9, 101, 304
Antrum, 126
Anturane®, 185
Anuria, 323
Anus, 124, 128, 129, 375
Anvil (incus), 116, 117
Anxiety, 405–408
  risk factors for, 405
  treatments for, 407–408, 409–410, 412
    benzodiazepines, 407–408, 409
    buspirone, 408, 409
  types of, 405, 406
Anzemet®, 132
Aorta, 24, 227, 228
Aortic arch, 196, 228
Aortic disease, 25
Aortic valve, 23, 228
APAP. See Acetaminophen (Tylenol®)
Aphasia, 444
ApoE 4 gene, 444
Appendix, 29, 124, 129
Appetite, 80
Apraclonidine, 107
Apraxia, 444
Apresoline®, 241
Aquatag®, 330
Aquatensin®, 330
Aqueous chamber, 96
Aqueous humor, 96, 104
Arachnoid, 402
Aralen®, 119, 309
Arava® (leflunomide), 170, 171–172
Arcuate vein, 348
Aredia® (pamidronate), 182
Argatroban, 251
Arginine, 141
Aricept® (donepezil), 445

Arimidex® (anastrozole), 313
Aripiprazole (Abilify®), 426
Aristocort® (triamcinonide), 88, 218, 349
Arivan® (lorazepam), 421
Arrhythmias, 25, 234–237
  cardiac, 243
  characteristics of, 235
  lethal, 329
  treatments for, 255–256, 258
  types of, 234–237
Artane® (trihexyphenidyl HCL), 441–442
Arterial blood, 230, 231
Arteries, 24, 192, 228
  hardening of, 237
  pulmonary, 230
Arterioles, 228, 348
Arteriosclerosis, 237
Arthritic psoriasis, 87
Arthritis, 168–172, 314
  gouty, 169–170
  leeches in treating, 176
  osteoarthritis, 169
  psoriatic, 81
  rheumatoid, 81, 82, 169, 170, 171, 279–280, 282
  treatment of, 170–172
Articular capsule, 164
Articular cartilage, 161, 164
Articular cavity, 164
Articulating bone, 163
ASA, 449
Asacol®, 281
Ascending colon, 29, 124, 127, 128, 129
Ascorbic acid (vitamin C), 145–146, 152, 207
Aseptic technique, 288
Asparagine, 141
Aspartate aminotransferase (AST), 446
Aspartic acid, 141
Aspart (Novolog), 361
Aspergillus fungi, 283
Aspermia, 388
Aspirin, 39, 70, 118, 133, 173, 184, 246, 258, 446
  properties of, 449–450
Astelin NS®, 202
Asthma, 26, 27, 40, 207–209
  allergic, 208, 219
  bronchoconstriction, 208, 212
  coughing and, 199
  symptoms of attack, 208
  treatment of, 208–209, 215, 217
Asthmatics, 448
Atacand®, 242
Atarax®, 202

Atazanavir (Zrivada®), 278
Atenolol (Tenormin®), 22, 244, 410
Atherosclerosis, 112, 237, 245
Athlete's foot (*Tinea pedis*), 83, 88, 283, 307
Ativan® (lorazepam), 409, 418, 421, 438
Atomoxetine (Strattera®), 434
Atorvastatin, 252
Atovaquone, 289, 309
ATP, 158
ATPase, 160
Atracurium, 178
Atria, 23, 24, 196, 227, 229
Atrial fibrillation (AFib), 234
Atrial flutter, 235
Atrial-natriuretic peptide (ANP), 338
Atrioventricular (AV) node, 227, 232
Atrioventricular bundle (Bundle of His), 227, 232
Atromid-S®, 255
Atropine, 219
Atrovent®, 217
Attenuated vaccines, 305
Atypical antipsychotics, 424–425, 426
Auditory nerve, 117
Augmentin®, 120, 297, 326
Auracle, 115
Autoantibodies, 388
Autoimmune diseases, 169, 186, 279–282
    list of common, 280–282
Autonomic nervous system (ANS), 209, 233, 396, 458
Autorhythmicity, 232
Avalide®, 242
Avandia© (rosiglitazone), 361
Avapro®, 242
Aventyl® (nortriptyline), 416
Aversion therapy, 422
AV node, 227, 232
Avodart™ (dutasteride), 390
Axert® (almotriptan), 453
Axillary nerve, 398
Axons, 399, 400, 401
Aygestin® (norethindrone acetate), 353, 354
Azactam®, 298
Azathioprine (Imuran®), 279, 281, 313
Azelastine, 202
Azithromycin (Zithromax®), 87, 99, 120, 299
Azmacort®, 218
Azoles, 286
Azoospermia, 388
Azopt®, 109
Aztreonam, 298
AZT (zidovudine), 277, 278, 289
Azulfidine® (sulfasalazine), 86, 171, 281, 282, 389

B

Bacampicillin, 296
Bacillus, 273
Bacillus Calmette-Guerin (BCG), 312–313
Bacitracin, 87
Bacitracin/polymyxin B, 98
Bacitracin zinc ointment, 100
Baclofen, 187
Bacteria, 272–273
    antibiotic-resistant, 291
    gram staining for, 287–288
    nosocomal, 290
Bacterial conjunctivitis, 98–99
Bacterial diseases, treatments for, 289
Bacterial gastroenteritis, 131
Bacterial skin infections, 82–83, 93
Bacterial vaginosis, 382
Bactrim®, 120, 325
Bactrim DS®, 301
Balsalazide (Colazal®), 281
Banophen®, 202
Barbiturates, 407, 427–428, 429, 430, 438
Barrel chest, 210
Bartholin's gland, 375
Basal cell carcinoma, 84
Basal ganglia, 403
Basophils, 209
Bayer®, 449
B-cells, 267, 270, 271
BCG vaccine, 305
Beclomethasone, 218
Beclovent®, 218
Belladonna alkaloids, 135
Benadryl® (diphenhydramine), 2, 70, 88, 202, 203, 427
Benazepril, 242
Bendroflumethiazide (Naturetin®), 330
Benemid®, 185
Benicar®, 242
Benign prostatic hypertrophy (BPH), 314, 323, 389–391
    non-pharmaceutical treatment of, 37, 391
    pharmaceutical treatment of, 390–391
Benign tumors, 83–84
Benzalkonium chloride (Zephiran®), 88
Benzedrex Inhaler®, 205
Benzimidazoles, 289
Benzocaine (Solarcaine®), 88
Benzodiazepines, 407–408, 409, 418, 421, 428
    for insomnia, 428, 429, 430
    muscle relaxants and, 179
    for seizures, 436–437, 438
    in smoking cessation, 423
Benzoyl peroxide, 86, 88
Benzthiazide, 330
Bepridil (Vascor®), 257

Beriberi, 143
Beta-2 receptors, 203, 209
Beta-adrenergic blockers, 243–244, 256, 407, 410
Beta adrenergic inhalers, 215, 216
Beta blockers, 9, 107, 240, 257, 258
Betacarotene, 142
Betagan®, 107
Beta hydroxy acids, 88
Beta-lactamase, 295
Beta-lactamase inhibitors, 292, 295, 297
Betamethasone (Celestone®), 86, 88, 349
Betapace® (sotalol), 257, 258
Betaxolol HCl solution, 107
Betimol®, 107
Betoptic®, 107
Betoptic-S®, 107
Biaxin®, 120, 299
Bicalutamide (Casodex®), 313
Bicarbonate, 127, 129
Bicarbonate ion, 320–321
Bicillin®, 296
Bicuspid (mitral) valve, 23, 228, 231
Biguanides, 361, 370
Bile, 124, 127
Bile ducts, 124
Bilirubin, 322
Bimatoprost ophthalmic solution, 111
Binary fission, 272
Binding, 401
Binding sites on receptors, 40
Bioavailability, 53, 60
Biochemical mediators, 209
Bioequivalence, 247
Biological response modifiers (BRMs), 311, 312
Biotin, 152
Biphosphonates, 180
Bipolar disorder (BD), 412–420
    anticonvulsant drugs for, 418, 419, 420
    causes of, 417–418
    lithium carbonate for, 418, 420
    rapid-cycling, 418
Birth control pills (oral contraceptives), 292, 378–379
Bismuth subsalicylate (Pepto Bismol®), 136, 137
Bisoprolol, 244
Bisphosphonates, 180, 182–183
Bitolterol, 216
Bladder, 28, 319, 320, 321–322, 375, 387
Bladder infections, 28
Bleeding, excessive, 250
Blepharitis, 98
Bleth—10®, 100
Blocadren®, 244
Block K⁺ efflux, 257
Blood, 32–33, 229. *See also* Clots and clotting; Heart

arterial, 230, 231
  flow of, 229–231
  fungal infections of, 283
  pumping of, 228–229
  venous, 229, 231
Blood brain barrier (BBB), 404–405
Blood cells, formation of, 164
Blood-forming (hemopoietic) stem cells, 267
Blood glucose, 150
Blood pressure, 22–23, 27, 28, 40
  high (hypertension), 22, 27, 67, 105, 239, 243, 328, 404
    CAD and, 237, 244–245
Bloodstream, 49
Blood vessels, 192–193
Body, structure of, 21–36
  cardiovascular system, 22–25. *See also* Heart; Lymphatic system
  endocrine system. *See* Endocrine system
  gastrointestinal (GI) system. *See* Gastrointestinal (GI) system
  hematologic system, 32–34
  renal system. *See* Renal system
  respiratory system. *See* Respiratory system
Body lice, 83
Body movement, 159
Body of stomach, 126
Bolus, 125
Bonding, coreceptor, 275, 276
Bone(s), 160–161
  cancellous, 161
  compact, 161
  defined, 163
  functions of, 163–164
  long, 160–161
  spongy, 161, 163
  tumors of, 454
Bone density, 167
Bone fractures, 167
Bone marrow, 33, 161–163, 166
  disorders of, 168–170, 313
  hematopoiesis in, 164
  nutrient storage in, 164
Bone pain, 455
Bone resorption, 180, 181
Bone resorption inhibitors, 182
Boniva® (ibandronate), 182
Bony orbit, 95
Booker, Steven L., 77
Bovine spongiform encephalopathy ("mad cow disease"), 287
Bowman's (glomerular) capsule, 320, 348
Brachial plexus, 398

Brachiocephalic artery, 228, 231
Brachiocephalic vein, 196
Bradycardia, 235
Brain, 396, 402–405
  addiction and, 67, 68, 69–71
  blood brain barrier (BBB), 404–405
  cancers of, 313
  cerebellum, 402, 403
  cerebrum, 402–403
  degenerative disorders of, 287
  glucose and, 396
  limbic system, 404
  neurons in, 399
  reticular formation, 404
Brain stem, 403–404
Brand names, 12
Breakthrough drugs, 81
Breast bone (sternum), 165
Breast cancer, 183, 312, 313, 314
  endocrine therapy for, 357–358
  estrogen and, 351
Breathing (respiration), 191, 193, 194–196
  definition of, 25
Brethine®, 216
Bretyllium (Bretylol), 257
Brevibloc® (esmolol), 244, 257
Brevital® (methohexital), 179, 430
Bricanyl®, 216
Brimonidine, 107
Brinzolamide solution, 109
Brittle diabetic, 151
Bromocriptine mesylate (Parlodel®), 358, 385, 389, 439, 440
Brompheniramine, 202, 203
Bronchi, 25, 192, 193, 195–196
Bronchial congestion, 207
Bronchiectasis, 27
Bronchiole congestion, 207
Bronchioles, 192, 195–196
Bronchitis, 27
Bronchoconstriction, 208, 212
Bronchodilation, 209
Bronchodilators, 208, 215
Bronkodyl®, 217
Bronkosol®, 216
Broviac®, 154
"Bubble gum" medicine, 15
Buccal absorption, 15–16
Budesonide (Entocort EC®), 218, 280
Buffers, 52, 60
Bulbourethral gland, 387
Bumetanide (Bumex®), 119, 239, 330
Bundle branches, 227
Bundle of His (atrioventricular bundle), 227, 232
Bupropion, 414, 415, 423

Burns, 85, 88
Bursa-equivalent structure, 267
Bursitis, 168
Buspirone (Buspar®), 407, 408, 409
Busulfan (Myleran®), 313
Busulfex®, 313
Butoconazole nitrate (Femstat 3®), 284

C

Cabergoline, 358
Cadence, 159
Caffeine, 404, 431, 451
Calan® (verapamil), 242, 257, 258
Calcifediol, 180
Calciferol (vitamin D 3), 339
Calcipotriene (Dovonex®), 281
Calcitonin, 181, 338, 344
Calcitonin-polypeptide hormone, 182
Calcitriol, 180
Calcium, 146, 151, 153, 160, 166, 180
  cardiac influx/efflux of, 228–229
  delaying influx of, 438
  scleroderma and, 282
Calcium channel blockers, 9, 240, 256, 257, 258, 389
Calcium ions, 238
Calcium pyrophosphate, 169
Calculi, 327, 328
Calvulanic acid, 297
Canal of Schlemm, 105, 106
Cancellous bone, 161
Cancer(s), 183, 310–314
  brain, 313
  breast, 183, 312, 313, 314, 351, 357–358
  colon, 183
  DNA and, 168
  drugs for, 311–314
  endocrine therapy for, 357–358
  endometrial, 314, 351, 358
  estrogen and, 351
  lung, 27
  metastatic, 311
  ovarian, 313
  pain from, 453–455
    nonpharmaceutical relief of, 455
    treatment for, 454–455
  prostate, 312, 313, 314, 358
  skin, 84, 88, 93
  testicular, 313
  thyroid, 343
  treatment methods, 118, 119, 311
  uterine, 183
Cancerous growths, 83–84
Candesartan, 242
Candida albicans, 217
Candida fungi, 283
Candida glabrata, 283

Canker sores, 283
Capecitabine (Xeloda®), 313
Capillaries, 22–23, 24, 192, 228
Capoten®, 241, 242
Capozide®, 242
Capsules, 15
Captopril, 241, 242
Carac™, 314
Carbachol solution, 108
Carbamazepine (Tegretol®), 187, 378, 419, 438
Carbamide peroxide (Murine Ear Drops®), 117
Carbapenums, 295, 297
Carbastat®, 108
Carbenicillin, 296
Carbidopa, 440
Carbohydrates, 138–139, 347
    complex, 128
    in TPN, 149
    types of, 138
Carbon dioxide, 22, 25, 194–195, 231
Carbonic anhydrase inhibitors, 109, 331
Carbonic anhydrase system, 320
Carboplatin, 119
Cardene® (nicardipine), 257
Cardiac cycle, 232
Cardiac depression, 193
Cardiac glycosides, 238
Cardiac muscle, 159
Cardiac sphincter, 124, 125, 126
Cardiac tumors, 25
Cardiovascular drugs, 9
Cardiovascular events, Cox inhibitors and, 134
Cardiovascular system, 22–25. See also Heart; Lymphatic system
    diseases of, 24–25
    nervous system and, 397
Cardizem® (diltiazem), 242, 257, 258
Cardura® (doxazosin), 390
Carisoprodol, 177
Carotenosis, 142
Carotid artery, 196, 228, 231
Carpals (wrist), 165
Carrier protein, 51
Carteolol HCl solution, 107
Cart fill procedures, 2
Cartilage, 160, 163, 195
    articular, 161
    smooth, 163
Cartilage (chondrocyte) function, 174, 176
Cascading effect of blood coagulation, 32
Casodex® (bicalutamide), 313
Catabolic patient, 152–153
Catapress, 44
Cataract, 105, 106
Catecholamines, 40, 67, 345

Catheter
    Foley, 323
    TPN, 154
Cauda equina, 398
CCR5, 275, 276
CD4, 275, 276
Ceclor®, 298
Cecum, 29, 124, 127, 128, 129
Cedax®, 120
Cedilanid-D®, 238
Cefaclor, 298
Cefadroxil, 298
Cefamanadole nafate, 298
Cefazolin (Ancef®), 87, 298
Cefdinir, 298
Cefepime, 298
Cefixime, 298
Cefonicid sodium, 298
Cefotaxime sodium, 298
Cefpodoxime proxetil, 120
Cefprozil, 120, 298
Ceftibuten, 120
Ceftin®, 120, 298
Ceftriaxone sodium, 120, 298
Cefuroxime axetil, 120
Cefuroxime sodium, 298
Cefzil®, 120, 298
Ceiling, 42
Celebrex©, 133, 134
Celecoxib, 176
Celestone® (betamethasone), 86, 88, 349
Celexa® (citalopram), 410, 413
Cell body, 399
Cell-mediated response, 270
Cell membrane, 49–50, 52, 271
    transport mechanisms through, 50–52
Cells, target, 41
Cellulitis, 83, 87
Cell wall, 49–50, 53, 292
    protein synthesis, 83
Celontin® (methsuximide), 438
Cenestin®, 353
Centocor®, 246
Central nervous system (CNS), 396, 401–430, 458
    brain, 396, 402–405
        addiction and, 67, 68, 69–71
        blood brain barrier (BBB), 404–405
        brain stem, 403–404
        cancers of, 313
        cerebellum, 402, 403
        cerebrum, 402–403
        degenerative disorders of, 287
        glucose and, 396
        limbic system, 404
        neurons in, 399
        reticular formation, 404
    cancer pain, 453–455
        nonpharmaceutical relief of, 455

        treatment of, 454–455
    convulsions, seizures, and epilepsy, 434–437
    diseases affecting
        alcohol withdrawal, 420–422
        anxiety, 405–408, 409–410, 412
        bipolar disorder (manic-depressive disorder), 412–420
        dementia and Alzheimer's disease, 70–71, 442–446
        depression, 408–412, 413–417, 428
        insomnia, 425–430
        Parkinson's disease, 403, 437–442
        psychosis, 423–425, 426
        smoking withdrawal and cessation, 422–423
    drugs affecting, 9
    migraine headaches, 446–448
        classic, 447
        common, 447–448
        pharmaceutical treatment of, 448, 449–450, 451–453
    Reye's Syndrome, 174, 448–450
    scheduled narcotic analgesics, 455–457
Central nervous system (CNS) depressants, 71
Central vein occlusion, 112
Cephalexin (Keflex®), 87, 298, 326
Cephalosporins, 9, 289, 293, 295–298
    MOA of, 298
Cerebellum, 402, 403
Cerebral cortex, 402
Cerebral hemispheres, 398, 402
Cerebral medulla, 403
Cerebral palsy, 186
Cerebrospinal fluid (CSF), 116, 402
Cerebrum, 402–403
Cerebyx® (fosphenytoin), 438
Cervical caps, 381
Cervical nerve, 398
Cervical roots, 403
Cervical spine, 162
Cervical vertebrae (neck), 165, 401
Cervicitis, 383
Cervix, 375, 385
Cetaphil®, 88
Cetirizine (Zyrtec®), 202, 389
Chain, Ernst, 325
Chambers, cardiac, 227
Channel blockers, 282
Chelator, 171
Chemical dependency, 65, 69
Chemical names, 3, 12, 13
Chemistry, 39
Chemoreceptors, 80
Chemoreceptor trigger zone (CTZ), 130, 173
Chemotactic factor, 267
Chemotherapy, 311, 454

nausea/vomiting due to, 132–133
Chewable forms of medications, 14
Chibroxin, 99, 100
Childbirth, 383–384
Children
    asthmatic, 26
    otitis media in, 120
Chlamydia, 99, 308, 323, 383, 385
Chlamydia trachomatis, 382
Chlonazepam, 70
Chloral hydrate (Noctec®), 428, 430
Chlordiazepoxide (Librium®), 177, 409, 421
Chloride, 23, 53, 151, 329
Chloride ions, 320, 321
Chlorinated fluorocarbons (CFCs), 221
Chloroquine, 119, 287, 289, 309
Chlorothiazide (Diuril®), 239, 330
Chlorpheniramine, 202
Chlorpromazine (Thorazine®), 405, 425
Chlorpropamide, 370
Chlor-Trimeton®, 202
Chlorzoxazone, 177
Chlropheniramine, 203
Chocolate, 217
Choecalciferol, 180
Cholecystokinin (CCK), 338
Choledyl®, 217
Cholera, 307
Cholesterol, 139, 180, 251
    estrogens and, 351
    heart disease and, 252–255
    synthesis of, 252
Cholestyramine, 255
Cholinergic agents, 108
Chondrocyte (cartilage) function, 174, 176
Chordae tendineae, 23
Choroid, 96
Chromium, 152
Chronic adrenal insufficiency, 366
Chronic angina, 240
Chronic myeloid leukemia (CML), 314
Chronic obstructive pulmonary disease (COPD), 26, 27, 197, 209, 210, 215–221
    anticholinergics for, 216, 217
    anti-inflammatories for, 215, 216–217
    anti-leukotrienes for, 215, 219–221
    bronchodilators for, 215
    mast cell stabilizers for, 215, 217–219, 220
    xanthines for, 215–216, 217
Chylomicrons, 253
Chyme, 126, 127
Cialis® (tadalafil), 367, 371, 389
Cilia, 115, 194
Ciliates, 272
Ciloxan, 99, 100

Cimetidine (Tagamet®), 70, 136, 389
Ciprofloxacin (Cipro®), 301, 327
Circulatory system, 227, 258. See also Heart
    autoimmune diseases and, 282
    lymphatic system and, 269
Circumcision, 324
Circumflex (Cx) artery, 228
Cirrhosis, 71, 152, 253
Cisplatin (Platinol®), 119, 313
Citalopram (Celexa®), 410, 413
Citrus fruit, 328
Claforan®, 298
Clarithromycin, 120, 136, 137, 299
Claritin-D®, 202
Claritin® (loratidine), 86, 202, 389
Class I drugs, 11
Class II drugs, 11
Class III drugs, 11
Class IV drugs, 11
Class V drugs, 11
Classic migraine, 447
Clavicle (collarbone), 165
Clavulanate, 326
Clavulanate potassium, 120
Clavulanic acid, 297, 326
Clearance, 61
Clear Eyes®, 103
Clemastine, 202, 203
Cleocin®, 120, 179
Climara®, 182
Climara TDP, 353
Clindamycin, 120, 166, 179
Clinical depression, 408, 411
Clinoril®, 175
Clitoris, 375
Clofazimine (Lamprene®), 289
Clofibrate, 255
CLOMID®, 386
Clomiphene, 386
Clomipramine (Anafranil®), 409, 415–416, 428
Clonazepam, 418, 438
Clonazepine, 419
Clonidine, 44
Clopidogrel, 246
Clorazepate (Tranxene®), 438
Closed angle glaucoma, 104
Clostridia, 292
Clostridium difficile, 292
Clostridium tetani, 273
Clotrimazole, 87, 88, 284, 286, 289
Clots and clotting, 32, 351
    snowballing, 245
    stages of formation of, 249–250
    in veins, 234
    vitamin K and, 142–143
Clotting factors, 266
    anabolic steroids and, 357

Cloxacillin, 296
Clozapine (Clozaril®), 425, 426
Clubbing of fingernails, 26
CNS. See Central nervous system (CNS)
Coagulation, 32, 33–34
Coal tars, 281
Cocaine, 68, 70, 431
Coccobacillus, 273
Coccus, 272–273
Coccygeal spine, 162
Coccyx (tail bone), 165, 375
Cochlea, 115, 116, 117, 118
Cocoa plant, 68
Coconut oil, 140
Codeine, 206, 457
Cognex® (tacrine), 445
Colazal® (balsalazide), 281
Colbenemid®, 184, 185
Colchicine, 184, 185, 389
Cold remedies, 105
Colds, 197–207, 273
    cold virus and, 198
    cough as symptom and complication of, 198–200
    cough medications for, 201, 205, 206–207
    decongestants for, 201, 203–205
    drug treatments of, 200–205
        antihistamines, 201–203
        cough medications, 201, 205, 206–207
        decongestants, 10, 103, 113, 201, 203–205
    flu vs., 198
    nondrug treatment of, 205–207
Colesevelam, 255
Colestid®, 255
Colestipol, 255
Colic flexure, 29
Colitis
    pseudomembranous, 292
    ulcerative, 281
Collagen, 80, 85
Collarbone (clavicle), 165
Collecting tubule, 348
Colon, 29, 124, 125, 127, 128–129, 375
Colon cancer, 183
Combivent®, 216, 217
Combivir®, 278, 289
Common carotid artery, 196
Common cold. See Colds
Common migraine, 447–448
Common peroneal nerve, 398
Compact bone, 161
Compazine®, 132
Competitive inhibition, 213, 244–245
Complement, 266, 267
Complex carbohydrates, 138
Conception, 377

Concerta® (methylphenidae), 432
Concha (bowl), 117
Condoms, 379, 380–381
Conducting airways, 195–196
Conductive hearing loss, 118, 119
Cones, 95
Congestive heart failure (CHF), 24, 233–234, 237–244
  ACE inhibitors for, 241–242
  arrhythmias, 234–237, 255–256
  beta-adrenergic blockers for, 243–244, 256, 257, 258
  cardiac glycosides for, 238
  complications of, 234
  diuretics for, 238–240
  phosphodiesterase inhibitors for, 237, 244
  right-sided vs. left-sided, 236
  vasodilators for, 240–241
Conjunctiva, 95
Conjunctivitis, 97, 98–99
Contact dermatitis, 81
Contraceptives, 377–382
  contraindications, 379
  devices, 380–381
  diaphragms and cervical caps, 381
  dosage forms, 377–378
  intrauterine devices (IUDs), 382
  oral (birth control pills), 292
    drug-drug and drug-herb interactions with, 378–379
  topical, 380
Contractility, 228
Contraction
  labor, 383
  lack of force of, 233
  myocardial, 238
  premature ventricular, 235
Contraindications, 4
Controlled Substances Act of 1970, 11–12, 75, 455
Controlled substances (scheduled medications), 10, 11
  dependency and, 75–77
Convulsions, 434–437
COPD. See Chronic obstructive pulmonary disease (COPD)
Copper, 152
Cordan® (flurandrenolide), 88
Cordarone® (amiodarone), 257, 258
Coreceptor bonding, 275, 276
Corgard®, 244
Coricidin®, 206
Cornea, 95
Coronary arteries, 228
Coronary artery disease (CAD), 24, 237, 245–249
  adrenocorticosteroids for, 252

anticoagulants for, 245–248, 250–251, 258
antihyperlipidemics for, 251
antiplatelet agents for, 245, 246, 250–251, 258
arteriosclerosis, 237
atherosclerosis, 112, 237, 245
hypertension and, 237, 244–245
hypolipidemics for, 251
new direct thrombin inhibitors (DTIs) for, 251
tissue plasminogen activators (t-PA), 248–249
triglycerides and, 253–255
Corona viruses, 197
Corpus luteum, 339, 376, 383, 384, 386
Cortef®, 349
Corticaine® (hydrocortisone), 86, 88, 218, 349
Corticosteroids, 9, 98, 105, 209, 215, 216, 218, 279, 281, 341, 389
Corticotrophs, 368
Corticotropin, 341
Corticotropin-releasing hormone (CRH), 338, 365
Cortisol, 344, 346, 347, 364–366, 370
Cortisone, 144
Cortisporin®, 87
Cosopt®, 109
Cough
  chronic, 200
  medications for, 201, 205, 206–207
  nonproductive, 200, 205, 206–207
  productive, 200, 206–207
  psychogenic, 199
  smokers', 200
  as symptom and complication of colds, 198–200
Coumadin®, 142, 151, 247, 248, 258
Cox (cyclooxygenase), 133
Cox-2, 173
Cox-2 inhibitors, 174–176
Cozaar®, 242
Crabs, 382
Cranberry juice, 325
Cranial cavity, 192
Cranial nerve, 95
Cranium (skull), 165, 401, 402
Craving, 67
Creams, 16
Cretenism (hypothyroidism), 253, 366, 369
Creutzfeldt-Jakob disease, 287
Crixivan® (indinavir), 277, 278, 289
Crohn's disease, 280
Crolom®, 102, 213
Cromolyn sodium. See Sodium cromolyn
Cryptococcal meningitis, 307
Cryptococcus neoformans, 307

Cryptorchidism, 389
Crystodigin®, 238
Curare, 178
Cushing's disease, 365, 370
Cushing's syndrome (hypercortisolism, hyperadrenocortism), 364–365, 370
Cuticle layer (scarfskin), 80
Cuts, 87
CXCR4, 275, 276
Cyanocobalamin, 145
Cyclobenzaprine, 177
Cyclooxygenase (Cox), 133
Cyclophosphamide, 279, 282, 313
Cycloplegic drugs, 113
Cyclosporin, 86, 279, 281
Cyclosporine, 170, 282
Cycoloxygenase I, 174–176
Cycoloxygenase II, 174
Cycrin®, 353
Cyproheptadine, 202
Cysteine, 141
Cystic fibrosis (CF), 26, 27, 199, 211–212
Cystitis, 324
Cytarabine (Cytosar-U®), 313
Cytochrome P–450, 284
Cytokines, 81, 209, 282, 312
Cytomegalovirus, 304
Cytoplasm, 271
Cytotec®, 135
Cytoxan®, 313

D

D4T, 289
Dalmane® (flurazepam), 179, 430
Dalteparin, 248
Dantrium®, 177, 187
Dantrolene, 177, 351
Dapsone, 289
Daypro®, 175
DDAVP (desmopressin), 363, 364
Debrox®, 117
Decadron®, 219, 349
Declomycin®, 299
Decongestants, 10, 103, 113, 201, 203–205
Deep peroneal nerve, 398
DEET insect repellent, 309
"Definition of Addiction, The" (Booker), 77
Delatestryl®, 355
Delavirdine (Rescriptor®), 278, 289
Delsym®, 206
Deltasone®, 218
Demadex® (torsemide), 119, 239, 330
Demeclocycline hydrochloride, 299
Dementia, 70–71, 442–446
  signs and symptoms of, 443–444

treatment of, 444–446
Demerol® (meperidine), 457
Dendrites, 79, 399, 400
Denial of addiction, 66
Depakene® (valproic acid), 418, 419, 438
Depakote® (divalproex), 418, 419, 438
Department of Health and Human
    Services (DHHS), 137, 147
Dependency, 74–78
    addiction vs., 66, 71, 77
    chemical, 65, 69
    controlled medications and, 75–77
    defined, 66
    problem of, 75
Depolarization of axon, 401
Depo-Provera®, 353, 377
Depressants, 68
    central nervous system (CNS), 71
Depression, 408–412, 413–417
    addiction and, 67
    causes of, 408, 411
    clinical, 408, 411
    hypnotics and sedatives and, 428
    risk factors for, 411
    treatments for, 411–412, 413–417
    types of, 410
Dermis, 80
Descending colon, 29, 124, 127, 128, 129
Desipramine (Norpramin®), 416
Deslanoside, 238
Desmopressin (DDAVP), 363, 364
Desoxycholate (Fungizone®), 285
Destasone®, 349
Desyrel® (trazedone), 414
Dexamethasone, 101, 218, 349
Dexamethasone sodium phosphate, 219
Dexone®, 218
Dextroamphetamine (Dexedrine®), 431,
    433
Dextroamphetamine saccharate, 433
Dextroamphetamine sulfate, 433
Dextromethorphan, 206
Dextrose, 18, 149, 154
DHODHase, 172
DHT (dihydrotestosterone), 390
Diabeta©, 361
Diabetes, 324, 359–364, 369, 370
    brittle diabetic, 151
    diabetes insipidus, 362–364, 369
    diabetes mellitus, 362, 363–364, 370
      kidneys and,328–329
    insulin for, 361–362
    oral hypoglycemics for, 360–361
    types of, 360, 361, 363–364
    uncontrolled, 253
    yeast infections and, 283
Diabetic nephropathy, 329
Diabetic retinopathies, 112
Diabinese®, 370

Diagnostic and Statistical Manual of Mental
    Disorders, 4th rev. ed. (DSM-IV-
    TR), 422, 444
Diamox® (acetazolamide), 109, 331
Diaphragmatic spasm, 194
Diaphragm (contraceptive), 381
Diaphragm (muscle), 129, 195, 196
Diaphysis, 160–161
Diapid® (lypressin), 364
Diarrhea, 30, 135
    Shigella, 291
Diastole, 232
Diasystole, 22
Diazepam (Valium®), 70, 177, 179, 187,
    421, 438
Diclofenac, 175, 328
Diclofenac sodium (Solaraze®), 88
Dicloxacillin (Dynapen®), 87, 97, 296
Didanosine (Videx®), 278, 289
Didronel® (etidronate), 182
Diet, urolithiasis and, 327
Dietary Reference Intake (DRI), 138
Dietitian, TPN and, 149
Diffusion
    facilitated, 51
    passive (passive transport), 50, 51
Diflucan® (fluconazole), 245, 284, 285,
    286, 378
Diflunisal, 175
Difumarate, 101
Digestive aids, 9
Digestive enzymes, 337
Digestive function, 125
Digestive juices, 124
Digestive process, 28–29
Digestive system. See also Gastrointestinal
    (GI)
    system
    lymphatic system and, 268
    nervous system and, 397
Digitalization, 238
Digital nerve, 398
Digitoxin, 238
Digoxin, 238
Dihydrotestosterone (DHT), 390
Dilantin® (phenytoin), 70, 187, 378, 389,
    438
Dilaudid® (hydromorphone), 456
Diltiazem (Cardizem®), 242, 257, 258
Dimenhydrinate, 131
Dimetapp®, 202, 206
Diovan®, 242
Diphedryl®, 202
Diphenhydramine (Benadryl®), 2, 70, 88,
    202, 203, 427
Diphenhydramine class, 38
Diphtheria, 305, 306
Diphtheria/Tetanus/Pertussis (DTaP), 200
Diploccocus, 273

Diprivan®, 179
Diptheria, 307
Dipyridamole, 246
Direct thrombin inhibitors (DTIs), 251
Dirithromycin, 299
Disease(s). See also Infectious disease(s);
    specific diseases
    addiction as, 65–66
    autoimmune, 169, 186
    of cardiovascular system, 24–25
    of eyes, 97
    gastrointestinal, 29–30
    of lungs, 26
    of respiratory system, 27, 197
    sexually transmitted, 288,
      382–383
    of skin, 81–85
      pharmaceutical treatment for,85–88
    spastic, 186–187
    of spleen, 260–261
Disease modifying anti-rheumatic drugs
    (DMARDs), 170, 282
Disopryamide (Norpace®), 257, 258
Distal convoluted tubule (DCT), 320, 348
Distribution, drug, 50
    volume of, 57, 60–61
Disulfiram (Antabuse®), 71, 287, 355,
    421, 422
Diucardin®, 330
Diurese®, 330
Diuretics, 8, 9, 238–240, 318, 328, 329–330
    osmodic, 110, 329–330
Diuril® (chlorothiazide), 239, 330
Divalproex (Depakote®), 418, 419, 438
DNA, 271, 284
    cancer and, 168
    spontaneous mutation, 291
Docosanol (Abreva®), 87
Docusate sodium, 15
Dolasetron mesylate, 132
Dolobid®, 175
Dolophine® (methadone), 389
Domagk, Gerhard, 325
Dominique®, 381
Donepezil (Aricept®), 445
Donnatal®, 135
Dopamine, 66–67, 69–70, 338, 349–350,
    424, 431,
    437–438
    disintegration of, 437–439
Dopamine receptor antagonists, 130
Doral® (quazepam), 430
Dornase alpha (rhDNase), 212
Doryx®, 299
Dorzolamide hydrochloride, 109
Dose
    defined, 4, 42
    loading, 61
    maintenance, 61

Dose–response curve, 41–43
    ED 50, 4, 42–43
    potency, 42
Douching, 380
Dovonex® (calcipotriene), 281
Doxazosin (Cardura®), 390
Doxorubicin (Rubex®), 313
Doxy®, 299
Doxycycline, 87, 99, 309
Doxycycline hyclate (Periostat®), 87, 299
Doxylamine, 203, 427
Dramamine®, 131
Dristan 12-Hr, 205
Drixoral®, 203, 206
Drug(s)
    classification of, 8–12
        controlled substances (scheduled
            medications), 10, 11
        methods of, 8
        pregnancy categories, 10–11
        universally accepted, 8–10
    defined, 4
    names of, 12–13
    routes of administration, 13–18
        buccal and sublingual absorption,
            15–16
        inhalation, 17–18
        nasogastral, 18
        oral, 13–15
        parenteral, 18
        rectal and vaginal, 17, 50
        topical, 16–17
Drug abuse, 64
Drug dependency. See Dependency
Drug distribution and metabolism, 50,
        56–63. See also
        Pharmacokinetics
    absorption, 30, 49–50, 57, 60,
        61
    clearance, 61
    equilibrium, 59
    half life, 42, 61–62
    information resources on, 62
    path of, 57–58
    plasma binding protein and,
        58–59
    rate of administration, 60
    two-compartment model, 61
    volume of distribution, 57,
        60–61
Drug-drug interactions, 2, 43–45
Drug indication, 4
Drug-receptor complex, 38–39
Drug resistance, 290
DSM-IV-TR, 422, 444
Ductus deferens, 387
Duggar, Benjamin, 326
Duodenal ulcer, 29, 127, 133, 136, 155
Duodenum, 124, 126, 129

Duragesic® (fentanyl transdermal system),
        454, 456
Dura matter, 402
Durex®, 381
Duricef®, 298
Dutasteride (Avodart™), 390
Dwarfism, pituitary, 343, 358–359, 369
Dyazide®, 240
Dynabac®, 299
Dynacin®, 299
DynaCirc® (isradipine), 257
Dynapen® (dicloxacillin), 87, 97,
        296
Dyrenium®, 240
Dyscrasias, 174
Dysentery, 307
Dyslipidemia, 254
Dysspermia, 388
Dysthymia, 411
Dysuria, 324

E

E. coli, 324
E2 glycoprotein, 197
Ear, 115–120
    anatomy and physiology of, 115–117
        cochlea, 115, 116, 117, 118
        Eustachian tube, 116, 117
        vestibular labyrinth, 116
    complications of earwax buildup, 117
    hearing loss, 118–119
    otitis media, 119–120, 208
    websites on, 122
Eardrum (tympanic membrane), 115–116,
        117
Ear lobes, 115
Ebastine, 389
Eby, George, 205
Echothiophate iodide ophthalmic
        solution, 108
Ectopic ACTH Syndrome, 365
Ectopic (tubal) pregnancy, 376
Eczema, 81, 87
ED50, 4, 42–43
Edecrin® (ethacrynic acid), 119, 330
Edema, 239, 328
    peripheral, 369
    pulmonary, 234
Efalizumab (Raptiva®), 82, 86, 92
Efavirenz (Sustiva®), 278, 289
Efferent arteriole, 348
Efferent (motor) function, 396
Effexor® (venlafaxine), 410, 414
Effexor XR, 407
Efficacy
    of agonists, 40
    liver function and, 57–58
Eflone®, 102

Eflornithine, 289, 371
Efudex®, 314
Ejaculation, 387
    retrograde, 388–389
Ejaculatory duct, 387
Elastin, 80, 85
Elavil® (amitriptyline), 322, 415, 428,
        451, 455
Eldepryl® (selegiline), 417, 439, 442, 446
Elderly patients, 44
Electrical bridge, 232
Electrical systems, cardiovascular, 22,
        232–233
Electrocardiogram, 232
Electroencephalogram (EEG), 402, 444
Electrolyte balance, 348
Electrolytes, 10, 23, 30, 53, 146, 150, 151,
        153
Elements, trace, 146, 152
Eletriptan (Relpax®), 453
Elidel® (pimecrolimus), 81, 82, 86, 87, 92
Elimination, rate of, 61
Elixirs, 15
Ellence® (epirubicin), 314
Emadine®, 101, 202
Emedastine, 101, 202
Emergency drugs, 18
Emesis, 8
Eminase®, 249
Emphysema, 27, 209–210
Emptying time, 130
Emtricitabine (Emtriva®), 278
Emulsification, 127
Emulsifier, 16
Enalapril, 242
ENBREL® (etanercept), 81, 86, 92
End buttons, 399
Endocardium, 226
Endocrine drugs, 9
Endocrine system, 30–31, 336–373, 395
    adrenal gland, 31, 337, 339, 340,
        345–347
        abnormalities of, 364–371
    anatomy of, 337
    autoimmune diseases and, 281
    disorders of, 358–371
        acromegaly, 343, 358, 359, 369
        Addison's disease
            (hypocortisolism), 349,
            365–366, 371
        cretenism (hypothyroidism), 366,
            369
        Cushing's syndrome
            (hypercortisolism,
            hyperadrenocortism), 364–365,
            370
        diabetes. See Diabetes
        erectile dysfunction, 367, 371
        goiter, 371

Grave's disease (thyroid eye disease, thyroid orbitopathy), 281, 366–367, 370
hirsutism, 371
myxedema (secondary hypothyroidism), 366, 369
peripheral edema, 369
pituitary dwarfism, 343, 358–359, 369
pituitary gigantism, 343, 358, 369
estrogen replacement therapy and menopause, 323, 351–354
contraindications, 354
drug choices, 352–354
indications for, 351
glands, organs, and secretions, 336, 338–340
glandular disease states, 357–358
gonads, 337, 340, 349
hormones, 336, 337, 338, 340–341
female sex, 349–350
glucocorticoids, 216, 339, 345, 346, 347, 366
male sex (androgens), 9, 312, 339, 350, 355, 357–358
mineralcorticoids, 339, 345, 348–349
thyroxine (T4), 146, 253, 338, 344, 345
triiodothyronine (T3), 253, 338, 344, 345
hypothalamus, 31, 337, 338, 340, 342, 343, 368, 403
lymphatic system and, 269
nervous system and, 397
pancreas, 29, 31, 124, 125, 127, 129, 253, 337, 340
parathyroid, 31, 180, 337, 338, 340, 343–345
pineal body, 340
pituitary gland (hypophysis), 31, 337, 338, 340, 342, 343, 368, 403
testosterone hormonal replacement, 354–357
contraindications, 355
precautions, 357
side effects of anabolic steroids, 356–357
thalamus, 39, 343, 403
thymus, 31, 260, 267, 337, 340
thyroid, 31, 180, 253, 337, 338, 340, 343–345, 366
websites on, 372–373
Endocrinology, 336
Endocytosis, 275, 276
Endometrial cancer, 314, 351, 358
Endometrial hyperplasia, 351
Endometriosis, 385
End stage renal disease (ESRD), 329

Enduron®, 330
Enflurane, 179
Enfuvirtide (Fuzeon®), 275, 277
Enoxaparin, 248
Enteric coated medications, 14
Enterobacter, 324
Enterococcus faecium, 291
Entocort EC® (budesonide), 218, 280
Enzymes, 124, 140, 400
digestive, 337
Eosinophilic chemotactic factor of anaphylaxis (ECF-A), 209
Eosinophils, 209
Ephedra, 203
Ephedrine, 215
Epidermis, 80
Epididymis, 387
Epilepsy, 434–437
Epinephrine (adrenaline), 216, 243, 339, 345
Epiphysis, 160–161
Epirubicin (Ellence®), 314
Epivir® (lamivudine), 9, 277, 278, 289
Eprosartan, 242
Epstein-Barr virus, 260
Eptifibatide, 246
Epzicom®, 278
Equilibrium, 59
Erectile dysfunction, 367, 371
Ergocalciferol (vitamin D), 152
Ergoloid mesylates, 446
Ergosterol, 284
Ergotemine, 450, 451
Ertapenem, 297
Eryhromycin®, 45
Erythema, 85
Erythrocytes (red blood cells), 28, 33, 229
Erythromycin (E-mycin®, Erythrocin®), 97, 99, 100, 295, 299
Erythropoietin (EPO), 339, 341
Eskalith®, 418
Esmolol (Brevibloc®), 244, 257
Esophagus, 29, 124, 126, 129, 196
Essential fatty acids, 140
Essential proteins, 140
Estazolam (ProSom®), 430
Ester, 60
Estrace®, 352
Estradiol cypionate, 377
Estradiol, 352, 354, 375–376
Estratab®, 353
Estriol, 376
Estrogel®, 352
Estrogen, 166, 312, 341, 349, 376
overload of, 385
during pregnancy, 384
Estrogen replacement therapy (ERT), 180, 323, 351–354, 446

contraindications, 354
drug choices, 352–354
indications for, 351
Estrogens, 339, 375
Estrogensprogestins, 9
Estrone, 351, 375–376
Etanercept (ENBREL®), 81, 86, 92
Ethacrynic acid (Edecrin®), 119, 330
Ethambutol, 289, 303
Ethanolamines, 203
Ethchlorvynol (Placidyl®), 430
Ethinyl estradiol, 378
Ethosuximide (Zarontin®), 378, 438
Ethrane®, 179
Etidronate (Didronel®), 182
Etomidate, 179
Etonogestrel, 378
Etoposide, 314
Eustachian tube, 116, 117
Evista®, 182
Excitation coupling contraction, 160
Excitatory fibers, 404
Excretion, 57
Executive function impairment, 444
Exelon® (rivastigmine), 445
Exna®, 330
Expectorants, 205, 206
Expiration, 196
Extended-spectrum penicillins, 295, 296
External exchange, 193, 194–195
External gas exchange, 234
External hordeolum, 97
External ocular nerve, 403
Extraocular muscles, 95
Eyes, 95–115
anatomy and physiology of, 95–96
cycloplegic drugs for, 113
diseases of, 97
disorders affecting vision, 104–113
cataract, 105, 106
drugs for, 107–111
glaucoma, 104–106
vascular retinopathies retinopathy, 106–113
infections of, 97–103
blepharitis, 98
conjunctivitis, 97, 98–99
ophthalmics used for, 100–103, 113–115
stye, 97
lubricants for, 113
mydriatic drugs for, 113
websites on, 122
workings of, 96–97
Eye socket (orbit), 165
Ezetimibe, 254, 255

F

Facial nerve, 403
Facilitated diffusion, 51
Factor VIII, 250–251
Factor IXa, 251
Fagerstrom test score, 422–423
Fallopian (tubal, ectopic) pregnancy, 376
Fallopian tubes, 375, 385
False gout (pseudoarthritis), 169
Famciclovir, 289, 304
Famvir, 9
Fat(s)
   dietary, 138, 139–140, 141
   lipids, 128, 140, 151, 251
   orbital, 95
Fat (adipose) tissue, 80, 253, 339
Fat-soluble vitamins, 142
Fatty acids, 127, 128, 139
FDA, 39, 85, 290
Federal Drug Administration, 8
Feedback, 340
   negative, 342, 347
Felbamate (Felbatol®), 438
Feldene®, 175
Felodipine (Plendil®), 242, 257
Female condom®, 381
Female reproductive system, 375–386
   anatomy and physiology of, 375–376
   contraceptives, 377–382
      contraindications, 379
      devices, 380–381
      diaphragms and cervical caps, 381
      dosage forms, 377–378
      drug-drug and drug-herb
         interactions with birth control
         pills, 378–379
      intrauterine devices (IUDs), 382
      oral, 292
      topical, 380
   fertility, 383–384
   infertility, 384–386
   causes of, 385–386
   pharmaceutical treatment of, 386
mammary glands and childbirth, 375,
   383–384
menstrual cycle, 375, 383–384, 386
sexually transmitted diseases (STDs), 288,
   382–383
      treatment and prevention of, 383
   websites on, 393–394
Femara® (letrozole), 314
Femcap®, 382
Femidom®, 381
Femoral nerve, 398
Femstat 3® (butoconazole nitrate), 284
Femur (thigh bone), 164
Femy®, 381
Fenesin®, 206

Fenofibrate, 255
Fenoprofen, 175
Fentanyl citrate (Actiq®), 455
Fentanyl (Sublimaze®), 456
Fentanyl transdermal system
      (Duragesic®), 454, 456
Fertility, female, 383–384
Fetal risk, 11
Fexofenadine (Allegra®), 202, 389
Fibrates, 253
Fibrillation
   atrial (AFib), 234
   ventricular, 234–235, 256
Fibrin, 250
Fibrinogen, 250
Fibrinolysin, 248
Fibroblasts, 80
Fibrolysin, 250
Fibula, 165
Filaments of muscles, 159–160
Filtration, 50
Fimbria, 375
Finasteride (Proscar®), 314, 390
Fingernails, clubbing of, 26
Firing of neurons, 400
First pass effect, 57–58
5FU (fluorouraci) cream, 88
5-HT$_3$ antagonists, 132, 133
Flagella, 387
Flagyl® (metronidazole), 70, 87, 136, 137,
   284–287, 289
Flaps, 115
Flat bones, 160
Flaxedil®, 178
Flecainide (Tambocor®), 257
Fleming, Alexander, 325
Flexeril®, 177
Flora, natural, 266
Florey, Howard, 325
Florinef® (fludrocortisone acetate), 348,
   349, 366, 371
Flovent®, 218
Flowmax® (tamsulosin hydrochloride),
   390
Floxin®, 301
Flu, colds vs., 198
Fluazepam, 428
Fluconazole (Diflucan®), 245, 284, 285,
   286, 378
Flucytosine (Aancobon®), 284, 285, 286
Fludrocortisone, 349, 371
Fludrocortisone acetate (Florinef), 348,
   349, 366, 371
Flufoxamine (Luvox®), 410, 413
Flumazenil (Romazicon®), 408
Flunisolide, 218
Fluocinolone (Synalar®), 88
Fluocinonide (Lidex®), 88
Fluorometholone, 98, 102

Fluoroquinolones (quinolones), 9, 99,
   100, 289, 294, 300–301, 327
Fluorouracil (Fluoroplex®), 314
Fluothane®, 179
Fluoxetine (Prozac®), 409, 413
Fluoxymesterone, 355
Fluphenazine (Permitil®), 425
Flurandrenolide (Cordan®), 88
Flurazepam (Dalmane®), 179, 430
Flurbiprophen, 175
Flushers, 153
Fluticasone, 86, 216, 218
Flutter, atrial, 235
Fluvastatin, 252
FML Liquifilm®, 102
FML S.O.P 0.1% ointment®, 102
Foam cells, 252
Foams, 15, 16
   spermicidal, 380
Folex® (methotrexate), 279, 282, 314,
   389
Foley catheter, 323
Folic acid, 145, 152, 282
Follicle-stimulating hormone (FSH), 338,
   341, 342, 344, 349, 368, 375,
   376, 384, 387
Follicular cells, 344
Food, Drug, and Cosmetic Act of 1938,
   327
Food allergies, 147
Food and Nutrition Board of National
   Academy of Sciences, 138
Food guide pyramid, 147, 148
Food intolerance, 147
Food pipe, 196
Foradil®, 216
Forane®, 179
Forearm, 165
Formoterol, 216
Formularies, 13
Forrestier, Jacques, 171
Forte Liquifilm®, 102
Forteo®, 182
Fortovase®, 278
Fosamax® (alendronate), 182
Fos amprenivir (Lexiva®), 278
Foscarnet, 289
Fosinopril, 242
Fosphenytoin (Cerebyx®), 438
4-Way Fast, 205
Fovea, 95
Fractures, bone, 167
Fragmin®, 248
Freon inhalation, 68
Frontal bone, 165
Frontal lobe, 402
Frontal sinus, 192
Frovatriptan (Frova®), 453
5-FU (5-flourouracil), 284

Fulvicin® (griseofulvin), 87, 285
Fumarate, 87
Fundus, 126
    of stomach, 29
    of uterus, 375
Fungal diseases, treatments for, 289
Fungal skin infections, 83
Fungizone®, 88, 285, 286
Fungus, 283–287
    antifungals, 9, 284, 285–286, 289, 378
    yeast, 83, 283–284
Furosemide (Lasix®), 119, 239, 330
Fusion, 275, 276
Fuzeon® (enfuvirtide), 275, 277

G

G6PD deficiency, 308
Gabapentin (Neurontin®), 419, 438
Gabitril® (tiagabine), 438
Galactorrhea, 350
Galantamine (Reminyl®), 445
Gallamine, 178
Gallbladder, 29, 124, 125, 129
Gamma-aminobutyric acid (GABA), 407,
        408, 420, 423
Gancicovir, 289, 304
Gantanol®, 301
Gantrisin®, 301
Garamycin®, 119, 300, 325
Garamycin Ophtalmic®, 100
Gases, exchange of, 193, 194–195
Gastric emptying difficulties, 13
Gastric esophageal reflux disease (GERD),
        129–130, 183, 199
Gastric mucosa, 134
Gastric ulcers, 133, 134, 136
Gastrin, 338
Gastrocrom®, 213
Gastroenteritis, 131
Gastrointestinal (GI) system, 28–30,
        123–157
    anatomy and physiology of, 124–125
    autoimmune diseases and, 281
    drug absorption via, 52
    drugs for, 9
    food allergies, 147
    food guide pyramid, 147, 148
    function of digestion, 125
    GERD (gastric esophageal reflux
        disease), 129–130, 183, 199
    large intestine (colon), 29, 124, 125,
        127, 128–129, 183, 375
    mouth, 28–29, 124, 125–126
    nausea and/or vomiting, 130–133
        chemotherapy and, 132–133
        post-operative, 131, 132
    nutrition, 137–147

carbohydrates, 128, 138–139, 149,
        347
    fats, 138, 139–140, 141
    macronutrients, 138
    micronutrients, 138, 141–147
    minerals, 138, 146
    protein, 138, 140–141
    vitamins, 138, 141–146
    water, 138, 147
small intestine, 125, 127–128
stomach, 28–30, 124, 125, 126–127,
        129, 338
total parenteral nutrition (TPN),
        147–155
    compatibility of, 153
    contraindications of, 154–155
    indications, 148–149
    solutions for special disease state
        dietary needs, 152–153
    stability of, 153–155
    types of lines, 150–152
ulcers, 124, 133–137
    causes and treatments of, 135–137
    duodenal (peptic), 29, 127, 133,
        136, 155
    gastric, 133, 134, 136
    nonsteroidal antiinflammatory
        drugs (NSAIDs) and, 10,
        133–134, 135–136, 172
Gels, 16, 17
Gemfibrozil, 255
Gemtuzumab ozogamicin (Mylotarg™),
        314
Genaphed®, 203
Generalized anxiety disorder (GAD), 405,
        406
Generalized seizures, 435, 436
Generic drugs, 60
Generic names, 4, 12, 13
Genital herpes, 383
Genital warts, 87, 308, 382
Genoptic®, 100
Gentamicin (gentamycin), 98, 99, 100,
        300
Gentamicin IV, 119
Gentamicin sulfate, 300
Geocillin®, 296
Geodon®, 426
Germinal centers, 268
Gestational diabetes, 360
Gigantism, pituitary, 343, 358, 369
Ginger root, 133
Ginkgo biloba, 446
Glans, 387
Glargine (Lantus), 361
Glaucoma, 104–106
    closed angle, 104
    open angle, 105
    secondary, 105

Gleevec™ (Imatinib), 314
Glimepride (Amaryl©), 361
Glipizide (Glucotrol©), 361
Global Fund, 275
Globulins, 59
Glomerular (Bowman's) capsule, 320, 348
Glomerulus, 320, 348
Glossopharyngeal nerve, 403
Glucagon, 339, 341
Glucocorticoids, 216, 339, 345, 346, 347,
        366
Glucocorticosteroids, 346
Glucophage© (metformin), 70, 361, 370
Glucose, 138–139, 329, 347
    blood, 150
    brain and, 396
    metabolism of, 153
Glucotrol© (glipizide), 361
Glutamic acid, 141
Glutamine, 141
Glyburide (Micronase©), 70, 361
Glycerin anhydrous, 110
Glycerol, 128
Glycine, 141
Glycogen, 139, 147
Glycoprotein II/IIIa, 246
Glycoproteins, 368
Glycosides, cardiac, 238
Glyset© (miglitol), 361, 370
G-mycin®, 300
Goiter, 371
Gold (Ridaura®), 171
Gold therapy, 282
Gonadotrophs, 368
Gonadotropin, 356, 376
Gonadotropin-releasing hormone
        (GnRH), 338, 387, 388, 389
Gonads, 337, 340, 349
Gonorrhea, 308, 382, 383, 385
    penicillin-resistant, 291
Gout, 169–170, 184–185
gp, 120, 275, 276
Gradients, 51
Gram, Hans Christian, 287
Gram staining, 287–288
Grand Mal (tonic-clonic) seizures, 436
Granisetron HCI, 132
Grave's disease (thyroid eye disease,
        thyroid orbitopathy), 281,
        366–367, 370
Griseofulvin, 70, 87, 285, 289
Griseofulvin ultramicrosize, 285
Gris-Peg, 285
Groshongs®, 154
Ground substance, 80
Growth hormone (GH), 338, 341, 343,
        344, 358–359, 368, 369
Growth hormone-releasing hormone
        (GHRH), 338

Growth hormone replacement therapy, 359
Guaifenesin, 206
Guanadrel, 244
Guanethidine, 244
Guarana, 431
Guaranine, 431
Guarded filtration procedure, 105
Gustatory sense organs, 80
Gynecomastia, 350
Gyne-Lotrimin® (clotrimazole), 284
Gyrase, 301

H

H⁺-ATPase Enzyme System, 136
H-1 antagonists, 202
H1 receptor sites, 132
H2 blocker, 12
H2 receptor antagonist therapy, 136, 137
Habitrol, 422
Haemophilus influenzae B (HIB) vaccine, 305, 306
Hair, 80
Hair cell depolarization, 116
Hair follicle, 80
Hair root, 80
Halcion® (triazolam), 179, 428, 430
Half life, 42, 61–62
Halofantrine (Halfan), 309
Haloperidol (Haldol®), 421, 425
Halotestin®, 355
Halothane, 179
Hammer (malleus), 116, 117
Hard palate, 192
HCL acid, 127
Headaches, migraine, 446–448
    classic, 47
    common, 447–448
    pharmaceutical treatment of, 448, 449–450, 451–453
Head lice, 83
Health maintenance organizations (HMOs), 13
Hearing. See Ear
Heart, 22–23, 159, 192, 226, 227–233, 338
    anatomy of, 227–228
    blood flow through, 229–231
    conduction (electrical) system of, 22, 232–233
    function of, 228–231
    nerve supply to, 233
    nervous system and, 397
    thyroid and, 345
Heart attack (myocardial infarction), 22, 134, 234, 248, 252
    massive, 237
Heartbeat rate, 40

Heart block, 236
Heartburn. See Gastric esophageal reflux disease (GERD)
Heart disease(s), 24, 183, 233–252
    cholesterol and, 252–255
    congestive heart failure (CHF), 24, 233–234, 237–244
        ACE inhibitors for, 241–242
        arrhythmias, 234–237, 255–256
        beta-adrenergic blockers for, 243–244, 256, 257, 258
        cardiac glycosides for, 238
        complications of, 234
        diuretics for, 238–240
        phosphodiesterase inhibitors for, 237, 244
        right-sided vs. left-sided, 236
        vasodilators for, 240–241
    coronary artery disease (CAD), 24, 237, 245–249
        adrenocorticosteroids for, 252
        anticoagulants for, 245–248, 250–251, 258
        antihyperlipidemics for, 251
        antiplatelet agents for, 245, 246, 250–251, 258
        arteriosclerosis, 237
        atherosclerosis, 112, 237, 245
        hypertension and, 237, 244–245
        hypolipidemics for, 251
        new direct thrombin inhibitors (DTIs) for, 251
        tissue plasminogen activators (t-PA), 248–249
        triglycerides and, 253–255
    coughing and, 199
    diabetes and, 360
    polyunsaturated fatty acids and, 139
    symptoms of, 237
    websites on, 262–263
Heart failure, 234, 329
Heart rate, 232, 233
Heart valve transplant, 32
Helicobacter pylori, 133, 134, 135, 136–137
Helix, 117
Helper T-cells, 270
Hematological drugs, 9
Hematologic system, 32–34
Hematopoiesis, 164
Hematuria, 324
Hemoglobin, 146
Hemophilia, 250–251
Hemopoietic (blood-forming) stem cells, 267
Hemorrhage, 251
Hemorrhagic disease, vitamin K-related, 143
Hemorrhagic effect, 173

Hemostatics, 9
Henry VIII, King, 170
Heparin, 247, 251
Heparin flush, 153
Heparin sodium, 248
Hepatamine, 152
Hepatic cirrhosis, 152
Hepatic flexure, 124
Hepatitis, 303, 306, 382
Hepatitis B vaccine, 305
Herbal preparations, 70
Herbs, contraceptives and, 378–379
Herpes, 323, 382, 383
    treatments for, 289
Herpes cold sore, 87
Herpes simplex virus, 99
Herpes viruses, 304
Herplex®, 101
Hexadrol®, 349
Hexalen® (altretamine), 313
Hiccups, 194
Hickman® catheters, 154
High amplitude propagating contraction (HAPC), 128–129
Highly active anti-retroviral therapy (HAART), 277
Hip (ilium), 165
Hippocampus, 80
Hirsutism, 371
Histamine, 424
Histamine-1 (H-1), 201, 212–213
Histamine-2 (H-2), 136
Histidine, 141
Histone deacetylases (HDACs), 216
Histoplasmosis, 307
HIV/AIDS, 273, 274–278, 382, 383
    contraceptives and, 379
    drug treatments for, 276–279, 289, 304
    progression of, 275
    retroviral replication, 275–276
    transmission of, 275
    types of, 274
    vaccine for, 275
Hives (urticaria), 81, 86
Hivid® (zalcitabine), 278, 289
Hlatky, Mark A., 379
HMG-CoA reductase, 255
Homeostasis, 28, 320, 342, 365
    nervous system and, 397
Hordeolum, 97
Hormonal therapy, 180, 311
Hormone replacement therapy, 182–183.
        See also Estrogen replacement
        therapy (ERT); Testosterone
        hormonal replacement
Hormones, 30–31, 40, 140, 395
    cancer and, 312
    endocrine, 336, 337, 338, 340–341
        female sex, 349–350

glucocorticoids, 216, 339, 345, 346, 347, 366
male sex (androgens), 9, 312, 339, 350, 355, 357–358
mineralcorticoids, 339, 345, 348–349
thyroxine (T4), 146, 253, 338, 344, 345
triiodothyronine (T3), 253, 338, 344, 345
infertility and, 385
pituitary, 368
tropic, 342, 344
Hot flashes, 181, 351
Humalog (Lispro), 361
Human chorionic gonadotrophin (HCG), 339
Human immunodeficiency virus. *See* HIV/AIDS
Human intestinal parasitic worms, 271–272
Human papilloma virus (HPV), 82, 84, 93
Human placental lactogen (HPL), 384
Humatin®, 300
Humatrope®, 359
Humerus, 165
Humibid®, 206
Humibid LA®, 206
Humirara® (adalimumab), 82, 87, 92
Humoral immunity, 267
Humulin, 361
Hycodan®, 206
Hydantoins, 438
Hydergine, 446
Hydralazine, 241
Hydrex®, 330
Hydrochlorothiazide (HCTZ®), 170, 239, 240, 242, 330
Hydrocodone, 70, 206
Hydrocortisone (Corticaine®), 86, 88, 218, 349
Hydrocortisone cream, 50
Hydrocortone®, 349
Hydrodiuril®, 239, 330
Hydroflumethiazide, 330
Hydrogenated fats, 139, 140
Hydrogen ions, 320, 321
Hydromorphone (Dilaudid®), 456
Hydromox® (quinethazone), 330
Hydroxychloroquine (Plaquenil®), 171, 282, 309
Hydroxychloroquine sulfate, 309
Hydroxyzine, 202
Hylorel®, 244
Hyperbaric oxygen therapy (HBO), 166
Hypercalcemia, 179, 180, 238, 327
Hypercholesterolemia, 254

Hypercortisolism (hyperadrenocortism, Cushing's syndrome), 364–365, 370
Hyperglycemia, 154
Hyperkalemia, 238
Hyperkeratosis, 84, 88
Hyperlipidemia, 252, 253
Hypernatremia, 327
Hyperosmolity, 405
Hyperparathyroidism, 328
Hyperplasia, 85
Hyperprolactinaemia, 350
Hypertension (high blood pressure), 22, 27, 67, 105, 239, 243, 404
CAD and, 237, 244–245
edema and, 328
Hypertensive retinopathy, 113
Hyperthyroidism, 328
Hyperuricemia, 169, 170
Hypnosedatives (Z drugs), 428
Hypnotics, 9, 427–428, 429–430
Hypoalbunemia, 253
Hypocortisolism (Addison's disease), 349, 365–366, 371
Hypodermis, 80
Hypoglossal nerve, 403
Hypoglycemia, 154
Hypoglycemics, oral, 360–361
Hypogonadism, 388
Hypokalemia, 238
Hypolipidemics, 251
Hypophysis (pituitary gland), 31, 337, 338, 340, 342, 343, 368, 403
Hypopigmentation, 84
Hypoproteinemia, 253
Hypotension, postural, 44
Hypothalamic-pituitary axis, 31
Hypothalamus, 31, 39, 337, 338, 340, 342, 343, 368, 403
Hypothyroidism (cretenism, myxedema), 253, 366, 369
Hypouricemic agents, 184
Hytrin® (terazosin), 390
Hyzaar®, 242

I

Ibandronate (Boniva®), 182
Ibuprofen, 10, 133, 174, 175, 184
Idoxuridine, 99, 101
IIb/IIIa inhibitors, 245, 246
Ileocecal valve, 124, 128, 129
Ileum, 29, 124, 127
Ilium (hip), 165
Ilotycin®, 100
Imaging tests, 444
Imatinib (Gleevec™), 314
Imidazoles, 284, 287, 289
Imimtrex, 450

Imipenemcilastatin, 297
Imipramine (Tofranil®), 323, 409, 416, 428
Imiquimod (Aldara®), 82, 87, 88, 93
Imitrex® (sumatriptan), 452
Immune cells, 80
Immune modulators, 281
Immune system, 264–317
anatomy and physiology of, 265–267
autoimmune diseases, 169, 186, 279–282
list of common, 280–282
cell structure and function and, 271
HIV/AIDS, 273, 274–278, 382, 383
contraceptives and, 379
drugs against, 276–279, 289, 304
progression of, 275
retroviral replication, 275–276
transmission of, 275
types of, 274
vaccine for, 275
infectious organisms, 271–278. *See also* Pathogens
amebicides/antiprotozoals, 284–287, 289
animal microorganisms, 271–273
Gram staining for, 287–288
methods of transmission of, 288
lymphocytes, 259, 267–270
nervous system and, 397
nonspecific defense mechanism vs., 265–266
plant microorganisms and, 283–287
antifungals, 9, 284, 285–286, 289, 378
fungus, 283–287
yeast, 83, 283–284
prions and, 287
as specific defense mechanisms 266–267, 270–271
tuberculosis and, 302–304
websites on, 316–317
Immune thrombocytopenic purpura (ITP), 245
Immunity, mucosal, 275
Immunoglobulins (antibodies), 140, 266–267, 271, 311, 386
Immunosuppressants, 279, 281, 282
Immunosuppressed patient, 266
Immunosuppression, 170
Imovane® (zopiclone), 428, 430
Impetigo, 87
Implanted ports, 154
Impotence, 367
Imuran® (azathioprine), 279, 281, 313
Inactivated (killed) vaccines, 305
Inamrinone, 244
Incomplete proteins, 140
Incontinence, 322–323

Incus (anvil), 116, 117
Indapamide (Lozol®), 330
Inderal® (propranolol), 40, 243, 244, 257, 258, 407, 410, 451
Indinavir (Crixivan®), 277, 278, 289
Indocin®, 175
Indomethacin, 175, 185
Infants, projectile vomiting in, 131
Infection(s)
  amebic, 289
  bacterial, 82–83, 93
  bladder, 28
  of eyes, 97–103
    blepharitis, 98
    conjunctivitis, 97, 98–99
    ophthalmics used for, 100–103
    stye, 97
  fungal, 83, 283
  kidney, 324
  parasitic, 83, 88
  in pelvic area, 323
  pneumococcal, 261
  preventive medications, 88
  protozoal, 272
  sexually transmitted (STDs), 288, 382–383
  urinary tract, 324–327
  vaginal yeast, 283–284, 307, 382, 383
  viral, 82, 198
  yeast, 217
Infectious disease(s), 306–310
  malaria, 289, 306–310
    diagnosis of, 306
    treatment of, 118, 308–310
    types of, 306
    origin of, 307–308
Inferior concha, 192
Inferior lobe, 193
Inferior maxillary nerve, 403
Inferior vena cava, 23
Infertility, 384–386
  causes of, 385–386
  in males, 387–389
    causes of, 387–388
    medications contributing to, 389
    treatment of, 389
  pharmaceutical treatment of, 386
Inflammation, 266, 279, 347
  of musculoskeletal system, 172–176
    Cox-2 inhibitors, 174–176
    nonsteroidal anti-inflammatory drugs (NSAIDs), 174, 175
    salicylates for, 173–174
Infliximab (Remicade®), 81, 87, 92, 280, 281
Influenza, 131
Infusaport®, 154
Inhalation, highs from, 68
Inhalation administration, 17–18

Inhaled medications, 50
Inhibition, competitive, 213, 244–245
Inhibitors, cancer, 311
Inhibitory fibers, 404
INH (isonizaid), 289, 302–303
Injections, 50
Innohep®, 248
INR, 247
Insomnia, 425–430
  characteristics of, 425–426
  chronic, 427
  non-benzodiazepines for, 428
  rebound, 428
  risk factors for, 426–427
  treatments for, 427–428, 429–430
Inspiration, 196
Insulin, 151, 339, 340, 341, 360–362, 370. See also Diabetes
Insulin-like growth factor, 339
Intal®, 213, 214, 217, 220
Integrase, 275
Integrase inhibitors, 275, 276, 278
Integratative (CNS) function, 396
Integrilin®, 246
Integumentary system. See also Skin
  autoimmune diseases and, 281, 282
  lymphatic system and, 268
  nervous system and, 397
Intercostal nerve, 398
Interferon, 312
Interleukins, 209
Intermediary nerve, 403
Intermediate-density lipoprotein (IDL), 255
Internal exchange, 193, 231
Internal hordeolum, 97
Internal nares, 192
Internal thoracic vein, 196
International Association for Study of Pain, 453
International Union of Pure and Applied Chemistry (IUPAC), 13
Internet sites, 62. See also Websites
Interstitial fluid, 259
Interstitial space, 259
Interventricular septum, 227
Intestinal cholesterol, 251
Intestinal parasitic worms, human, 271–272
Intestinal transit time, decreased, 13
Intestines, 29, 30, 338
  large, 29, 124, 125, 127, 128–129, 183, 375
  small, 29, 30, 125, 127–128
Intoxication, 67
Intoxification, verminous, 272
Intramuscular injection, 18
Intraocular pressure, 104, 105
Intrapulmonary pressure, 194

Intrarectal steroids, 10
Intrauterine devices (IUDs), 382
Intravenous (IV) administration, 18
Intrinsic factor (IF), 145
Invanz®, 297
Invirase®, 278
Iodine, 146, 344, 345
  radioactive, 281
Iodoquinol, 289
Ionic concentration to neuronal state, comparison of, 437
Ionization, 53
Ionocor®, 244
Iopidine®, 107
Ipratropium bromide, 217
Irbesartan, 242
Iris, 95
Iron, 146
Iron compounds, 322
Iron level in blood, 33
Irregular bones, 160
Ischemia, 112, 153, 193, 234
Ischemic stroke, 248
Ischium, 165
Islets of Langerhans, 339
Ismelin®, 244
Isocarboxazid (Marplan®), 417
Isoetharine, 216
Isoflurane, 179
Isoleucine, 141
Isonizaid (INH), 289, 302–303
Isoproterenol, 40, 216
Isoptin®, 257, 258
Isoptocarpine®, 108
Isordil®, 241
Isorsorbide dinitrate, 241
Isosorbide, 70
Isotonicity, 348
Isotretinoin (Accutane®), 86, 142
Isradipine (DynaCirc®), 257
Isthmus, 343
Isuprel®, 216
Itch medications, 88
Itraconazole (Sporanox), 284, 286
IV (intravenous) administration, 18

J

Jejunum, 29, 127
Jenamicin®, 300
Jenner, Edward, 305
Jock itch (Tinea cruris), 307
Joint capsule, 163
Joints, 163, 164
Jugular vein, 196

K

Kaletra® (lopinavir/ritonavir), 278
Kanamycin, 300
Kantrex®, 300
Kasbikinase®, 249
Keflex® (cephalexin), 87, 298, 326
Kefurox®, 298
Kefzol®, 298
Kegel exercises, 322
Kenalog®, 88, 349
Keratin, 84
Keratinized layer, 80
Keratinocytes, 281
Ketalar®, 179
Ketamine, 179
Ketoconazole (Nizoral), 283, 284, 285, 365, 370
Ketones, 322
Ketoprofen, 175
Ketorolac, 102
Ketotifen fumarate, 103, 202
Kidneys, 27–28, 42, 319, 339
    diabetes mellitus and, 328–329
    infection of, 324
Kidney stones (urolithiasis), 170, 327–328
Killed (inactivated) vaccines, 305
Killer T-cells, 270, 271
Kilocalories (kcal), 138
Kinetics, 159
Kinins, 198
Klebsiella, 324
Klonopin®, 418, 419, 438
Knee cap (patella), 165
Knee joint, 164, 169
Korsakoff's syndrome, 80
Krebs cycle, 25
Kwell® (lindane), 83, 88
Kytril®, 132

L

Labetolol, 244
Labia majora, 375
Labia minora, 375
Labor contractions, 383
Lactation, 384
Lacteals, 128
Lactobacilli, 283
Lactose intolerance, 147
Lamivudine (Epivir®), 9, 277, 278, 289
Lamotrigine (Lamictal®), 419, 438
Lamprene® (clofazimine), 289
Lamsil (terbinafine), 286
Lanoxin®, 238
Lanreotide, 358
Lansoprazole, 10, 137
Lantus (glargine), 361

Large intestine (colon), 29, 124, 125, 127, 128–129, 375
    cancer of, 183
Lariam™, 310
Laryngopharynx, 192
Larynx (voice box), 25, 124, 192, 193, 194
Lasix® (furosemide), 119, 239, 330
Latanaprost solution, 111
Lateral femoral cutaneous nerve, 398
Laxatives, 9
Leeches, 176
Leflunomide (Arava®), 170, 171–172
Leflunomide D-penicillamine, 282
Left anterior descending (LAD) artery, 228
Lens, 95
Leprosy, treatments for, 289
Leptin, 339
Letrozole (Femara®), 314
Leucine, 141
Leukemia, 168, 313
Leukocytes (white blood cells), 170, 229
Leukotriene inhibitors, 215, 219–221
Leukotrienes, 209, 219
Levaquin®, 301
Levitra® (vardenafil), 367, 371, 389
Levlen®, 378
Levobunolol HCl solution, 107
Levocabastine suspension, 102
Levodopa, 322, 439, 440
Levofloxacin, 301
Levonorgestrel, 377, 382
Lexiva® (fos amprenivir), 278
Lexxel®, 242
Leydig cells, 387
Librium® (chlordiazepoxide), 177, 409, 421
Lice, 83, 382
Lidex® (fluocinonide), 88
Lidocaine (Xylocaine®), 88, 179, 257, 258
Lifestyles®, 381
Ligaments, 163
Limbic system, 404
Lincosamides, 289
Lindane (Kwell®), 83, 88
Lingual frenulum, 126
Lioresal®, 187
Lipids, 128, 140. *See also* Fat(s)
    plasma levels of, 251
    in TPNs, 151
Lipid-soluble drug, 52
Lipophillic barrier, 17
Lipoproteins, 141
Lips, 126
Lisinopril, 242
Lispro (Humalog), 361
Lithium carbonate, 418, 420
Lithobid®, 418
Lithotabs®, 418

Liver, 29, 42, 124, 125, 127, 143, 339
    cholesterol in, 251
    cirrhosis of, 71, 152, 253
    drug efficacy and, 57–58
Liver disease
    chronic, 152
    estrogens and, 351
Livostin™, 102
Loading dose, 61
Lbes of lung, 196
Lock and key theory, 136
Lodoxamide solution, 102
Lomotil®, 105
Long-acting lanreotide LAR®, 359
Long bones, 160–161
Loop diuretics, 118, 119, 239, 330
Loop of Henle (LOH), 239, 320, 330, 348
Lo/Ovral®, 378
Lopid®, 255
Lopressor®, 244
Lorabid®, 120
Loracarbef, 120
Loratidine (Claritin®), 86, 202, 389
Lorazepam (Ativan®), 409, 418, 421, 438
Losartan, 242, 245
Lotensin®, 242
Lotions, 16, 17
Lotrel®, 242, 257
Lotrimin® (clotrimazole), 87
Lovastatin, 252
Lovenox®, 248
Low density lipoproteins (LDLs), 252, 253, 254
Lower esophageal sphincter (LES), 125, 126, 129–130
Low molecular weight heparins (LMWH), 247
Lozenges, 15
Lozol® (indapamide), 330
Lubricants for eyes, 113
Ludiomil® (maprotiline), 416
Lumbar spine, 162
Lumbar vertebrae, 165, 401
Lumbosacral plexus, 398
Lumen, 195
Lumigan®, 111, 122
Luminal® (phenobarbital), 187, 378, 430, 438
Lunelle®, 377
Lung cancer, 27
Lungs, 24, 25–26, 192, 193, 195–196
    lymphatic system of, 193
Lung tumors, 365
Lupus, 279, 282
Luteal phase, 386
Luteinizing hormone (LH), 338, 341, 344, 349, 368, 376, 384, 387
Luvox® (flufoxamine), 410, 413

Lyme disease, 87
Lymph, 259
Lymphatic duct, 259
Lymphatic system, 256–260
    of lungs, 193
    lymphatic route, 259–260
    nervous system and, 397
    relationships between body systems
        and, 268–270
    spleen, 29, 124, 259–261
    structural components, 256–259
Lymph node, 268
Lymphocytes, 259, 267–270
Lymphokines, 270–271
Lymphoma, Non-Hodgkin's, 314
Lymphotoxin, 267
Lypressin (Diapid®), 364
Lysine, 141
Lysozyme, 265

M

Macrodantin® (nitrofuantoin), 378
Macrolides, 9, 289, 294, 299
Macronutrients, 138
Macrophage activating factor, 267
Macrophages, 252, 259, 260, 265–266,
    270
Macula, 95, 96
"Mad cow disease" (bovine spongiform
        encephalopathy), 287
Mafenide acetate (Sulfamylon®), 88
Magnesium, 146, 151
Magnum®, 381
Ma huang, 203
Maintenance dose, 61
Major minerals, 146
Malabsorption, 142
Malaria, 289, 306–310
    diagnosis of, 306
    treatment of, 118, 308–310
    types of, 306
Malarone™, 309
Male reproductive system, 386–391
    anatomy of, 386–387
    benign prostatic hypertrophy, 314, 323,
        389–391
        non-pharmaceutical treatment of,
            37, 391
        pharmaceutical treatment of,
            390–391
    infertility, 387–389
        causes of, 387–388
        medications contributing to, 389
        treatment of, 389
    websites on, 393–394
Malignant melanoma, 84
Malleus (hammer), 116, 117
Mamillary body, 403

Mammary glands, 375, 383–384
Mammotrophs, 368
Mandible, 165
Manganese, 152
Manic-depressive disorder. See Bipolar
        disorder (BD)
Mannitol, 110
Manubrium, 33
MAO-B, 438
Maprotiline (Ludiomil®), 416
Marplan® (isocarboxazid), 417
Marrow, 161
Martius, Theodore Von, 431
Masculinizing hormones, 350
Mast cells, 207, 209, 389
Mast cell stabilizers, 102
    for allergies, 213–214
    for COPD, 215, 217–219, 220
Mastication, 125
Mastoid process, 117
Mavik®, 242
Maxair®, 216
Maxalt® (rizatriptan), 450, 452
Maxilla, 165
Maximpime®, 298
Maxitrol®, 100
Measles, 305, 306
Mechanism of action, 4, 39
Meclizine, 131, 202
Meclofenamate, 175
Meclomen®, 175
Median nerve, 398
Mediator-release inhibitors. See Mast cell
        stabilizers
Medrol®, 218, 349
Medrol Dosepak®, 218
Medroxyprogesterone, 377
Medroxyprogesterone acetate (MPA), 353,
    377
Medulla, lymphatic, 268
Medulla oblongata, 398, 403, 404
Medullary cavity, 161
Mefloquine, 310
Megestrol acetate (Megace®), 314, 357,
    358
Meglitinides, 361
Meglitinides Prandin®, 370
Meibomianitis, 97
Meibomitis (meibomian gland
        dysfunction), 98
Melanin, 84
Melanocytes, 80, 84
Melanoma, malignant, 84
Melatonin, 338, 446
Mellaril® (thioridazine), 389, 425
Meloxicam (Mobicox®), 176
Membrane transport mechanisms, 50–52
Membranous urethra, 387
Memory, 80

Memory B-cells, 271
Memory cells, 267
Menaquinones, 143
Menest®, 353
Meninges, 265, 402
Meningitis, 307
    cryptococcal, 307
Meniscus, 164
Menopause, 166, 384
    estrogen replacement therapy and,
        351–354
        contraindications, 354
        drug choices, 352–354
        indications for, 351
    osteoporosis in, 182
Menstrual cycle, 375, 383–384, 386
Menstruation, 375, 383–384
Meperidine (Demerol®), 457
Mepron®, 309
Merck Sharpe Dome, 275
Meropenem, 297
Merrem®, 297
Merthiolate, 88
Mesalamine, 281
Metabolic drugs, 9
Metabolism
    of glucose, 153
    hormone regulation of, 347
Metabolites, 44
Metacarpals, 165
Metahydrin®, 330
Metalyse®, 249
Metamucil©, 50
Metaprel®, 216
Metaproterenol, 216
Metatarsals, 165
Metformin (Glucophage©), 70, 361, 370
Methadone (Dolophine®), 389
Methamphetamine, 70, 204
Methionine, 141
Methocarbamol, 177
Methohexital (Brevital®), 179, 430
Methotrexate (Folex®), 279, 282, 314,
    389
Methoxyflurane, 179
Methsuximide (Celontin®), 438
Methylclothiazide, 330
Methyldopa, 244
Methylphenidate, 404, 431, 432–433
Methylprednisolone, 86, 218, 219, 349
Methyltestosterone, 355
Methyl xanthines, 217
Methysergide (Sansert®), 450, 451
Meticorten®, 218
Metipranololet axolol HCl solution, 107
Metoclopramide, 130
Metolazone, 330
Metoprolol, 244

Metronidazole (Flagyl®), 70, 87, 136, 137, 284–287, 289
Metyrapone, 365, 370
Mevolonate pathway, 180
Mexiletine (Mexitil®), 257
Mezlin®, 297
Mezlocillin, 297
Miacalcin Nasal Spray®, 181, 182
Micardis®, 242
Miconazole, 88, 284, 286, 289
Microaneurysms, 112
Microbicides, 379
Micronase© (glyburide), 70, 361
Micronutrients, 138, 141–147
    minerals, 10, 138, 146
    vitamins, 10, 138, 141–146
        fat-soluble, 139, 142
        in TPNs,152
        water-soluble,143
    water, 138, 147
Microorganisms
    infectious. See also Pathogens
        animal®, 271–273
        plant, 283–287, 289
    natural, 266
Micturition reflex, 321
Midazolam, 428
Middle concha, 192
Middle ear, 116
Middle lobe, 193
Mifeprex®, 136
Miglitol (Glyset©), 361, 370
Migraine headaches, 446–448
    classic, 447
    common, 447–448
    pharmaceutical treatment of, 448, 449–450, 451–453
Mildews, 283
Milk production in humans, 383
Milontin® (phensuximide), 438
Milrinone, 244
Mineralcorticoids, 339, 345, 348–349
Minerals, 10, 138, 146
Minipills, 377
Minipress® (prazosin), 241, 390
Minocin®, 299
Minocycline azathioprine, 282
Minocycline hydrochloride, 299
Minor minerals, 146
Miostat®, 108
Miotics, 108
Mirtazapine (Remeron®), 416
Miscarriage, 384
Misoprostol, 135
Mitomycin-C, 313
Mitotane, 365, 370
Mitral (bicuspid) valve, 23, 228, 231
Mivacron®, 178
Mivacurium, 178

Mobicox® (meloxicam), 176
Moexipri, 242
Molds, 283
Molecular structure, 30
Molluscum, 382
Monistat 7® (miconazole), 284
Monoamine oxidase inhibitors (MAOIs), 417, 423
Monoamine oxidases, 408
Monoamines, 431
Monobactams, 298
Monocid®, 298
Monoclonal antibodies, 312
Monodox®, 299
Mononucleosis, 260–261
Monopril®, 242
Monosaccharides, 125, 128
Monounsaturated fats, 139
Montagu, Lady Mary Wortley, 305
Montelukast (Singulair®), 86, 219, 220
Mood, alcohol and, 69–70
Mood disorders, 408–420
    bipolar disorder (BD), 412–420
        anticonvulsant drugs for, 418, 419, 420
        causes of, 417–418
        lithium carbonate for, 418, 420
        rapid-cycling, 418
    depression, 408–412, 413–417
        addiction and, 67
        causes of, 408, 411
        clinical, 408, 411
        hypnotics and sedatives and, 428
        risk factors for, 411
        treatments for, 411–412, 413–417
        types of, 410
Mood swings, 412
Morphine, 328, 454
Morphine sulfate (MS Contin), 456
Mother-child bonding, 383
Motility, 128, 135
Motion sickness, 131
Motor (efferent) function, 396
Motor neurons, 458
Motrin®, 175, 449
Motrin IB®, 175
Mouth, 28–29, 124, 125–126
MS Contin (morphine sulfate), 456
Mucociliary elevator (MCE), 212
Mucolytics, 211
Mucomyst, 211
Mucoprotein, 211
Mucopurulent discharge, 98–99
Mucosa, 124
    gastric, 134
    respiratory, 195
Mucosal immunity, 275
Mucous membranes, 16
Mucus, 198, 200, 211, 265

Multifocal atrial tachycardia, 236
Multiple sclerosis (MS), 186, 280
Mumps, 305, 306
Murine Ear Drops® (carbamide peroxide), 117
Murine Plus®, 103
Muscarinic receptor antagonists, 135
Muscle(s), 158
    action of, 159–160
    anatomy of, 159
    cardiac, 159
    extraocular, 95
    filaments of, 159
    nervous system and, 397
    skeletal, 159
    smooth, 124, 159
    visceral, 159
Musculoskeletal system, 158–190
    anatomical vocabulary, 163
    anatomy of muscles, 159
    autoimmune diseases and, 282
    bone marrow, 32–33, 161–163, 166
        disorders of, 168–170, 313
        hematopoiesis in, 164
        nutrient storage in, 164
    bones, 160–161
        cancellous, 161
        compact, 161
        defined, 163
        functions of, 163–164
        long, 160–161
        tumors of, 454
    disorders of, 164–168
        anemia, 33, 144, 145, 168, 282, 355
        arthritis, 81, 82, 168–172, 176, 279, 282, 314
        bursitis, 168
        gout, 169–170, 184–185
        leukemia, 168, 313
        myalgia, 168
        osteomyelitis, 165–166
        osteoporosis, 166, 178–184, 351
        Paget's disease, 168, 180
        tendonitis, 168
    inflammation of, 172–176
        Cox-2 inhibitors, 174–176
        nonsteroidal anti-inflammatory drugs (NSAIDs), 174, 175
        salicylates for, 173–174
    lymphatic system and, 269
    muscle action, 159–160
    skeletal muscle relaxants (SMRs), 176–178
        adverse actions of, 178
        drugs interacting with,179
    spastic diseases, 186–187
    websites on, 190
Myalgia, 168

Myasthenia gravis, 280
Mycifradin®, 300
Mycobacterium tuberculosis, 302, 305
Mycodone®, 206
Mycoplasma, 324
Mycoses, 83
Mydriatic drugs, 113
Myelin, 186
Myelin sheath, 280
Myfemy®, 381
Mykrox®, 330
Myleran® (busulfan), 313
Mylotarg™ (gemtuzumab ozogamicin), 314
Myocardial disease, 25
Myocardial infarction (heart attack), 22, 134, 234, 248, 252
   massive, 237
Myocardium, 159, 228, 233, 329
Myoclonic seizures, 436
Myofibrils, 160
Myosin, 159, 160
Mysoline® (primidone), 378, 438
Myxedema (hypothyroidism), 253, 366, 369

N

N-9 spermicides, 379
Nabumetone, 175
Nadolol, 244
Nafcil®, 296
Nafcillin, 87, 166, 296
Naftifine 1%, 88
Nalfon®, 175
Nalidixic, 327
Naloxone (Narcan®), 41, 457
Naltrexone (Revia®), 421–422
Naphazoline HCl, 103
Naphazoline HCl/pheniramine maleate, 98, 103
Naphcon®, 103
Naphcon-A®, 103
Naprelan® Controlled Release, 175
Naprosyn®, 175, 449
Naproxen, 175, 449
Naproxen sodium, 133, 175
Naqua®, 330
Naratriptan (Amerge®), 450, 452
Narcan® (naloxone), 41, 457
Narcotics (opioids), 8, 40, 67, 76, 455
   overdose of, 455–457
   scheduled, 455–457
Nardil® (phenelzine), 417, 432
Nasahist B®, 202
Nasal cavity (nose), 192
Nasal Crom®, 213, 214, 220
Nasal Spray®, 205
Nasogastral administration, 18

Nasopharynx, 116, 192
Nateglinide (Starlix©), 361
National Institute of Mental Health, 405
Native Americans, 329
Natural pacemaker, 232
Natural PCNs, 295, 296
Nature's Way®, 203
Naturetin® (bendroflumethiazide), 330
Nausea, 130–133, 173
   chemotherapy and, 132–133
   post-emetogenic, 132–133
   post-operative, 131, 132
Navane® (thiothixene), 425
Navelbine® (vinorelbine), 314
Nebcin®, 119, 300, 325
Neck (cervical vertebrae), 165, 401
Nedocromil, 213, 214, 217, 220
Nefazodone (Serzone®), 410, 414
Negative feedback, 342, 347
Nelfinavir (Viracept®), 278, 289
Nembutal® (pentobarbital), 430, 438
Neomycin, 87, 100, 179
Neomycin sulfate, 300
Neonatal inclusion conjunctivitis, 99
Neosar®, 313
Neosporin®, 87
Neo-Synephrine 4-Hr®, 205
Neovascularization, 112
Nephritis, 324
Nephrons, 319–320, 348
Nephropathy, 253, 329
Nerve(s). *See also specific nerves*
   auditory, 117
   cardiac, 233
   cranial, 95
   hyperexcitable, 435
   olfactory, 80
   optic, 95, 96
   touch, 80
   vestibular, 117
Nerve cells. *See* Neurons
Nervous system, 395–464
   ADD and ADHD, 432–434
   anatomy of, 396
   autoimmune diseases and, 280
   central. *See* Central nervous system (CNS) depressants
   functions of, 396–398
   homeostatic effects of, 397
   lymphatic system and, 270
   neurotransmission and receptors, 395, 400–401
   peripheral, 396, 458
   stimulants for, 431–432
   thyroid and, 345
   websites on, 462–464
Netilmicin sulfate, 300
Netromycin®, 300
Neural hearing loss, 118

Neuroadaptation, 70
Neurohypophysis, 338, 342, 343
Neurological system, 22
Neuromuscular drugs, 10
Neuromuscular junction (NMJ), 177
Neuronal state to ionic concentration, comparison of, 437
Neurons, 79, 396, 399–400, 402
   firing of, 400
   motor, 458
   replacement of, 174
   sensory, 458
Neurontin® (gabapentin), 419, 438
Neuropeptide Y, 339
Neurotoxic effects, 70–71
Neurotransmission, 395, 400–401
Neurotransmitters, 40, 66–67, 69–70, 144, 395, 400, 401, 408
Neutrophils, 212
Nevirapine (Viramune®), 278, 289, 304
New England Journal of Medicine, 291
Nexium, 137
Niacin, 143, 144, 253
Niacinamide, 152
Niazide®, 330
Nicardipine (Cardene®), 257
Nicoderm CQ, 422
Nicorette (nicotine polacrilex), 422
Nicotine gum, 422
Nicotine inhaler, 422
Nicotine nasal spray, 422
Nicotine patch, 422–423
Nicotinic-II receptors, 177
Nicotrol Inhaler®, 422
Nicotrol NS®, 422
Nifedipine (Procardia®), 257, 258, 282
Nimodipine (Nimotop®), 257
Nipride®, 241
Nitrates, 240
Nitrobid®, 240, 241
Nitro-Dur®, 241
Nitrofuantoin (Macrodantin®), 378
Nitrogenous waste, 324
Nitroglycerin SL, 241
Nitrol®, 241
Nitroprusside, 241
Nitrostat®, 241
Nizatidine, 70
Nizoral (ketoconazole), 283, 284, 285, 365, 370
"N" (nodal point), 96
Noctec® (chloral hydrate), 428, 430
Nolvadex® (tamoxifen), 183, 314, 357
Nomenclature guidelines, 13
Non-Hodgkin's lymphoma, 314
Nonnucleoside reverse transcriptase inhibitors (NNRTIs), 277, 278, 289
Nonoxynol– 9, 380

Nonphenothiazines, 132
Nonproliferative (simple) retinopathies, 112
Nonspecific defense mechanism, 265–266
Nonsteroidal antiinflammatory drugs (NSAIDs), 10, 133–134, 135–136, 172, 174, 175, 446
   properties of, 449–450
Non-tunneled catheters, 154
Noradrenaline, 233, 243, 244, 339, 431, 458
Norcuron®, 178
Nordette®, 378
Norelgestromin, 378
Norepinephrine (NE), 233, 243, 244, 339, 431, 458
Norethindrone, 377
Norethindrone acetate (Aygestin®), 353, 354
Norflex®, 177
Norfloxacin, 100
Norgestrel, 377
Normal saline, 18
Normodyne®, 244
Norpace® (disopryamide), 257, 258
Norplant®, 377
Norpramin® (desipramine), 416
Nortriptyline (Aventyl®), 416
Norvasc®, 257
Norvir®, 278
Nose (nasal cavity), 192
Novamine, 152
Novolin, 361
Novolog (Aspart), 361
NSAIDs. See Nonsteroidal antiinflammatory drugs (NSAIDs)
NTG, 70
Nucleoside analogs, 277
Nucleoside reverse transcriptase, 278
Nucleoside reverse transcriptase inhibitors, 289
Nucleotide analog reverse transcriptase inhibitors, 289
Nucleus, 399
Numorphan® (oxymorphone), 457
Nupercainal, 88
Nurse, TPN and, 149
Nutrients, 128, 158
   storage in bone marrow, 164
Nutrition, 137–147
   carbohydrates, 128, 138–139, 149, 347
   fats, 138, 139–140, 141
   macronutrients, 138
   micronutrients, 10, 138, 141–147
   minerals, 138, 146
   protein, 138, 140–141
   vitamins, 138, 141–146
   water, 138, 147

Nutritional drugs, 10
Nutrition and Your Health: Dietary Guidelines for Americans, 137
NuvaRing®, 378
Nytol®, 427

O

Oblique muscles, 95
Obsessive-compulsive disorder (OCD), 405, 406
Obturator nerve, 398
Occipital bone, 165
Occipital lobe, 402, 403
Octreotide, 358, 359
OcuClear®, 103
OcuDose®, 107
Ocuflox, 99, 100
Oculomotor nerve, 403
Ocupress®, 107
Odors, 80
Ofloxacin, 100
Ofoxacin, 301
Ogen®, 353
Ointments, 16, 17, 114
Olanzapine (Zyprexa®), 426
Olfactory bulb, 403
Olfactory nerve, 80, 403
Olfactory tract, 403
Oligospermia, 388
Oliguria, 323, 324
Olmesartan, 242
Olopatadine, 102
Omega 3 and Omega 6 fatty acids, 140
Omeprazole, 10, 137
Omnicef®, 298
Omnipen®, 296, 325
Oncovin®, 314
Onxol™, 314
Oophoritis, autoimmune, 281
Open angle glaucoma, 105
Ophthalagen, 110
Ophthalmics, 10, 100–103
   applying ointments, 114
   basics of using, 113–114
   instilling solutions, 114–115
Opiates, 76
Opioids (narcotics), 8, 40, 67, 76, 455
   overdose of, 455–457
   scheduled, 455–457
Opthalmic groove, 403
Opthalmic nerve, 403
Optic nerve, 95, 96, 403
Opticrom®, 213
OptiPranolol®, 107
Oral administration, 13–15
Oral cavity, 192
Oral contraceptives, 292, 378–379

Oral Fluid Based Rapid HIV Test Kit (OraQuick®), 274
Oral thrush (thrush mouth), 217
Oraminic II®, 202
Oramorph®, 456
OraQuick® (Oral Fluid Based Rapid HIV Test Kit), 274
Orasone®, 349
Orbit, 95, 165
Orbital fat, 95
Orchitis, autoimmune, 281
Oreton®, 355
Organic Acid Diuretics, 239
Organic loop diuretics, 330
Organidin NR®, 206
Organ of Corti, 116, 300
Orgasm, 387
Orinase, 370
Ormeloxifene, 181
Oropharynx, 192
Orphenadrine, 177
OrthoCyclen®, 378
Ortho-est®, 353
Ortho Evra Patch®, 378
Ortho-Micronor®, 377
Ortho-Novum 7/7/7®, 378
OrthoTriCyclen Lo®, 378
Orudis®, 175
Oruvail® capsules, 175
Osmitrol, 110
Osmodic diuretics, 110, 329–330
Osmotic gradient, 320
Ossicles, 115, 116
Osteoarthritis, 169
Osteoblasts, 161, 349
Osteoclasts, 180, 181
Osteomalacia, 142
Osteomyelitis, 165–166
Osteoporosis, 166, 178–184, 351
   bisphosphonates for, 180
   calcitonin for, 181
   selective estrogen receptor modulators (SERMs) for, 181
   treatments for, 178–184
      in menopause, 182
      nonpharmacologic, 181–184
Otic drugs, 10
Otitis media, 119–120, 208
   in children, 120
Ototoxicity, 118
Outer ear, 115
Ova, 337
Ovarian cancer, 313
Ovarian follicle, 339
Ovaries, 31, 337, 340, 375, 383–384, 385
Over-the-counter (OTC) drugs, 4
Ovrette®, 377
Ovulation, 375, 376
Oxacillin, 87, 166, 296

Oxalodinones, 289
Oxandrin, 355
Oxandrolone, 355
Oxaprozin, 175
Oxazepam (Serax®), 409, 421
Oxidants (Oxygen-Free Radicals), 388
Oxtriphylline, 217
Oxycodone (Oxycontin®), 64, 70, 456
Oxygen, 22, 25, 158
    air vs., 194
Oxygen deprivation, 234
Oxygen-Free Radicals (Oxidants), 388
Oxymetazoline, 103, 205
Oxymetholone, 355
Oxymorphone (Numorphan®), 457
Oxytetracycline, 299
Oxytocin, 338, 341, 342, 349, 383, 384

P

Pacemaker, natural, 232
Paclitaxel (Taxol®), 314
Paget's disease, 168, 180
Pain
    acute, 453
    cancer, 453–455
        nonpharmaceutical relief of,
            455
        treatment of, 454–455
    chronic, 453–454
    mild, 454
    severe, 454
Pain medication, 75–76, 88
Palatine tonsil, 126
Palatoglossal arch, 126
Palm oil, 140
Pamelor®, 416
Pamidronate (Aredia®), 182
Pancreas, 29, 31, 124, 125, 127, 129, 253,
    337, 340
Pancreatitis, 253
Pancuronium, 178
Panic disorder, 405, 406
Pantothenic acid, 144, 152
Paracetamol, 449
Paracetamol, N-Acetyl
        P-Aminophenol, 176
Parafollicular cells, 344
Parafon Forte DSC®, 177
Paranasal sinuses, 25, 192
Paraplatin®, 119
Parasites, 271–272
Parasitic infections, 83, 88
Parasympathetic nervous system (PNS),
        233, 396, 458
Parathyroid gland, 31, 180, 337, 338, 340,
        343–345
Parathyroid hormone (PTH), 180,
        182–183, 338, 341

Parenteral administration, 18
Parenteral glycoprotein, 246
Parietal bone, 165
Parietal cells, 127, 133
Parietal lobe, 402
Parietal pleura, 196
Parkinson's disease, 403, 437–442
    dopamine disintegration and, 437–439
    future treatments for, 439
    nonpharmaceutical treatments of, 439
    pharmaceutical treatments of, 439–442
    symptoms of, 438
Parlodel® (bromocriptine mesylate), 358,
        385, 389, 439, 440
Parnate® (trancypomine), 417, 432
Paromomycin sulfate, 300
Parotid duct, 29
Parotid gland, 29
Paroxetine (Paxil®), 410, 414
Partial complex seizure, 435
Partial seizures, 435
Partial thromboplastin time (PTT), 33–34
Passive transport (passive diffusion), 50,
        51
Patanol®, 102
Patches, 16, 17, 50
Patella (knee cap), 164, 165
Path, metabolic, 57–58
Pathogens, 271
    animal, 271–274
        bacteria, 272–273, 287–288, 290,
            291
        parasites, 271–272
        rickettsia, 273, 307
        viruses, 198, 273
    anti-infectives, 8–9, 288, 289
        comparison overview of, 293–294
        mechanisms of action of, 292
        side effects of, 292, 293–294
    methods of transmission of, 288
    plant, 283–287
        antifungals, 284, 285–286, 289
        fungus, 283–287
        yeast, 283–284
    resistance in, 288–292
Patient(s)
    catabolic, 152–153
    elderly, 44
    GI medication for, 30
    immunosuppressed, 266
Patient profile, 44
Pavalon®, 178
Paxil® (paroxetine), 410, 414
Pediculosis, 307
Pellagra, 144
Pelvic area, infections in, 323
Pelvic Inflammatory Disease (PID), 323,
        382, 383, 385
Pemirolast potassium, 102

Pen G benzathine, 296
Pen G potassium, 296
Pen G sodium, 296
Penicillamine, 171
Penicillinase-resistant penicillins, 166,
        292, 295, 296
Penicillinases, 295
Penicillins (PCNs), 9, 289, 290, 293, 295
    groups of, 166, 292, 295, 296–297
    MOA of, 295
    other antibacterials related to, 297–298
    for urinary tract infections, 325
Penicillin V, 325
Penile urethra, 387
Penis, 350
Pentamidine, 287, 289
Pentasa®, 281
Penthrane®, 179
Pentobarbital (Nembutal®), 430, 438
Pentothal® (thiopental), 179, 430
Pen Vee K®, 296, 325
Pepcid®, 136
Pepsin, 127
Peptic ulcers, 29, 127, 133, 136, 155
Peptides, 340
Pepto Bismol® (bismuth subsalicylate),
        136, 137
Pergolide mesylate (Permax®), 440–441
Periactin, 202
Pericardial cavity, 226
Pericardial disease, 25
Pericardium, 196, 226
Perilymph, 116
Perimeter effect, 266
Perindopril, 242
Periostat (R)® (doxycycline hyclate), 87,
        299
Periosteum, 161
Peripheral edema, 369
Peripheral nervous system (PNS), 396,
        458
Peripheral vascular disease, 25
Peripheral venous nutrition (PVN), 150
Peristalsis, 124, 126, 127, 130
    excessive, 135
Peritubular capillaries, 348
Permax® (pergolide mesylate), 440–441
Permitil® (fluphenazine), 425
Pernicious anemia, 145, 282
Perphenazine (Trilafon®), 425
Persantine®, 246
Pertussin®, 206
Pertussis (whooping cough), 200, 305,
        306, 308
Peruvian Indians, 68
Petite Mal (absence seizures), 436
Pfeiffer, Carl C., 424
PGE, 136

Phagocytes, 170, 252, 265–266. *See also* Macrophages
Phalanges, 165
Pharmaceuticals, kinds of, 2–3
Pharmacist, TPN and, 149
Pharmacodynamics, 5, 37–47
  agonists and antagonists, 3, 40–41, 76
  dose-response curve, 41–43
    ED50, 4, 42–43
    potency, 42
  mechanism of action, 39
  mechanisms in, 43–45
  receptor complex, 38–39
  receptor site, 39–40
  site of action, 39
  time-response curve, 43
Pharmacokinetics, 5, 48–55
  absorption, 15–16, 30, 49–50, 57, 60, 61
  clearance, 61
  definition of, 48
  drug distribution, 50
    volume of, 57, 60–61
  equilibrium, 59
  half life, 42, 61–62
  ionization, 53
  membrane transport mechanisms, 50–52
  plasma concentration (Cp), 49
  rate of administration, 60
  solubility, 52
Pharmacological classification, 8
Pharmacology, 1–6
  basic terminology of, 3–5, 465–475
  defined, 1, 4
  major areas of, 5
  studying, 2–3
Pharmacotherapeutics, 5, 34
Pharmacy (science), 5
Pharyngotympanic tube, 192
Pharynx (throat), 25, 29, 124, 192
Phenazopyridine (Pyridium), 322, 325
Phenelzine (Nardil®), 417, 432
Phenergan®, 132, 202
Pheniramine, 203
Phenobarbital (Luminal®), 187, 378, 430, 438
Phenothiazines, 132
Phensuximide (Milontin®), 438
Phenylalanine, 141
Phenylephrine, 205
Phenylpropanolamine (PPA), 205
Phenytoin (Dilantin®), 70, 187, 378, 389, 438
Phlebitis, 234
Phobias, 405, 406
Phosphate, 151, 153
Phosphodiesterase inhibitors, 237, 244
Phosphodiesterase (PDE), 216, 367

Phospholine Iodide®, 108
Phosphorus, 146
Photophobia, 99
Photoreceptors, 95
Physical dependence. *See* Dependency
Physician, TPN and, 149
Physician's Desk Reference, 52
Pia matter, 402
Pigmention disorders, 84
Pilocar®, 108
Pilocarpine ophthalmic gel, 108
Pimecrolimus (Elidel®), 81, 82, 86, 87, 92
Pineal body, 340
Pineal gland, 31, 337, 338
Pinkeye, 98, 99
Pinna, 115
Pinocytosis, 51–52
Pinolol, 244
Pinworms, 271–272
Pioglitazone (Actos©), 361
Piperacillin, 179, 297
Pipracil®, 179, 297
Pirbuterol, 216
Piroxicam, 175
Pitocin, 383
Pitressin® (vasopressin), 321, 338, 340, 341, 342, 362, 364, 369
Pituitary abnormalities, 358–359
  acromegaly, 343, 358, 359, 369
  dwarfism, 343, 358–359, 369
  gigantism, 343, 358, 369
Pituitary adenoma, 359, 365
Pituitary gland (hypophysis), 31, 337, 338, 340, 342, 343, 368, 403
  hormones of, 368
Placenta, 337, 339, 384
Placidyl® (ethchlorvynol), 430
Plan B®, 377
Plant microorganisms, 283–287
  antifungals, 284, 285–286, 289
  fungus, 283–287
  yeast, 283–284
Plant (vinca) alkaloids, 313
Plaque, 237, 252
Plaquenil® (hydroxychloroquine), 171, 282, 309
Plaque psoriasis, chronic, 81, 82
Plaques, 281
Plasma binding protein, 58–59
Plasma cells, 267
Plasma concentration (Cp), 49
Plasmapheresis, 280
Plasma proteins, 50
Plasmid, 291
Plasmodium, 306, 308
Plasters, 16
Platelet aggregating substance thromboxane A 2, 173

Platelet aggregation inhibitors. *See* Antiplatelets
Platelets, 32, 173
Platinol® (cisplatin), 119, 313
Plavix®, 246, 258
Plendil® (felodipine), 242, 257
Pleura, 25
PMS, 376
Pneumococcal infections, 261
Pneumococcal vaccine, 306
Pneumococci, resistant, 120
Pneumococcus (streptococcus pneumoniae), 291
Pneumonia, 307
Pneumonitis, 27
Poliomyelitis vaccine, 306
Polycystic ovarian syndrome (PCO), 358, 385
Polydipsia, 362
Polymixin B sulfate, 87, 98, 99, 100
Polyphagia, 362
Polythiazide (Renese®), 330
Polytrim®, 87, 98, 99, 100
Polyunsaturated fats, 139
Polyuria, 362
POMC, 368
Pons, 403, 404
Port-A-Cath®, 154
Portal vein, 128, 259
Posology, 5
Posterior chamber, 95, 96
Postmenopausal women, 181
Postnasal drip (PND), 199
Post-traumatic stress disorder (PTSD), 405, 406
Postural hypotension, 44
Potassium, 23, 146, 151, 325
Potassium citrate, 328
Potassium (K+) ions, 256, 320, 321
Potassium sparing diuretics, 239, 240, 330–331
Potency, 42
Powders, 16
Prandin© (repaglinide), 361, 370
Pravastatin, 252
Praziquantel, 289
Prazosin (Minipress®), 241, 390
Prealbumin (transthyretin), 142
Precose© (acarbose), 361, 370
Pred forte®, 103
Pre-diabetes, 360
Prednisolone, 98
Prednisolone acetate, 103
Prednisone, 86, 218, 279, 349, 364
Pregnancy, 131, 376, 384
Pregnancy categories for drugs, 10–11
Premarin®, 182, 352
Premature ventricular contraction, 235

Premenstrual syndrome (PMS), 376–377
Presbycusis, 118–119
Pressure, intrapulmonary, 194
Prevacid, 137
Prilosec, 137
Primacor®, 244
Primaquine, 308, 310
Primaxin®, 297
Primidone (Mysoline®), 378, 438
Prinatene Mist®, 216
Prinivil®, 242
Prinizide®, 242
Prions, 287
Proanthocyanidins, 325
Probenecid, 184, 185
Procainamide (Procanbid®), 257, 258
Procan®, 258
Procardia® (nifedipine), 257, 258, 282
Prochlorperazine, 132
Professional relationships, 15
Progesterone, 339, 340, 341, 349, 350,
       376
   in contraceptives, 382
   infertility and, 386
   during pregnancy, 384
Progesterone deficiency, 385
Progestin, 378
Progestins or progestin-only (POPs)
       contraceptives, 377–378
Projectile vomiting in infants, 131
Prolactin (PRL), 31, 338, 341, 344,
       349–350, 368, 383, 384
   elevated, 385
Proliferative retinopathies, 112
Proline, 141
Prolixin®, 425
Promethazine, 132
Prometrium®, 353
Propacil®, 367, 370
Propafenone (Rhythmol®), 257, 258
Propanolol, 244
Propecia®, 314
Prophylactic drugs. See Mast cell
       stabilizers
Prophylactic therapy for gout, 184
Propioni bacterium, 83
Propofol, 179
Propoxyphene HCL, 328
Propranolol (Inderal®), 40, 243, 244, 257,
       258, 407, 410, 451
Proprietary names, 12
Propylhexedrine, 205
Propylthiouracil (PTU), 180, 281, 367,
       370
Proscar® (finasteride), 314, 390
ProSom® (estazolam), 430
Prostaglandins, 110, 133–134, 135, 173,
       174–176, 209
Prostamides, 110

Prostaphlin®, 296
Prostate cancer, 312, 313, 314, 358
Prostate gland, 319, 386, 387
   enlargement of, 323, 324
   progesterone and, 350
Prostatic stents, 391
Prostatic urethra, 387
Prostatismurinary problems, 390
Prostatitis, 383
Protamine sulfate, 251
Protease boosting, 277
Protease inhibitors, 276, 277, 278, 289
Protein(s), 128, 138, 140–141, 266
   in blood, 32
   carrier, 51
   essential, 140
   incomplete, 140
   plasma, 50
   plasma binding, 58–59
Protein synthesis, 83
Proteinuria, 253
Proteus, 324
Prothrombin, 249
Prothrombin time (PT), 33–34, 247
Protonix, 137
Proton pump inhibitors, 10, 136
Protopic® (tacrolimus), 81, 86, 87, 92,
       170
Protopin®, 359
Protozoa, 272
Protozoal diseases, treatments for, 289
Provera®, 353
Proximal convoluted tubule (PCT), 320,
       348
Prozac® (fluoxetine), 409, 413
Pseudoarthritis (false gout), 169
Pseudoephedrine, 203–204, 323, 431
Pseudomembranous colitis, 292
Pseudomonas, 99, 324
Psoriasis, 81, 82, 86, 93, 281, 314
   arthritic, 87
Psoriatic arthritis, 81
Psuedoephedrine, 202
Psychogenic cough, 199
Psychogenic vomiting, 131
Psychological dependence. See Addiction
Psychosis, 423–425, 426
Ptyalin, 125
Pubic lice, 83
Pubis, 165
Pulmicort®, 218
Pulmonary arteries, 23, 24, 230
Pulmonary circuit, 24
Pulmonary edema, 234
Pulmonary hypertension, 27
Pulmonary rehabilitation, 210
Pulmonary semilunar valve, 23
Pulmonary valve, 228
Pulmonary veins, 23, 24, 230

Pulmozyme®, 212
Pulse dosing, 300
Pumps, electrolytic, 30
Pupils, 95
   dilated, 105–106, 113
Purine, 284
Purkinje fibers, 227, 232
Purodigin®, 238
P-wave, 232
Pyazinamide, 303
Pyelonephritis, 324
Pyloric sphincter, 124, 126, 130
Pyloric stenosis, 131
Pylorus, 29, 126
Pyrantel, 289
Pyrazinamide, 289, 303
Pyrethrins (RID®), 83, 88
Pyridium (phenazopyridine), 322, 325
Pyridoxine, 143, 144
Pyridozine HCl (vitamin B 6), 143,
       144–145, 152, 328
Pyrilamine, 203
Pyrimadine, 284
Pyrimethamine, 287
Pyuria, 324

Q

QRS wave, 232
Quantal dose-response curve (ED 50), 43
Quazepam (Doral®), 430
Quelicin®, 178
Questran®, 255
Questran Light®, 255
Quetiapine (Seroquel®), 426
Quinaglute®, 257
Quinaglute Dura-tabs®, 119
Quinalones, 295
Quinapril, 242
Quinethazone (Hydromox®), 330
Quinidex Extentab®, 119
Quinidine (Quinadex®), 119, 257
Quinine, 119, 287
Quinolones (fluoroquinolones), 9, 99, 100,
       289, 294, 300–301,
       327

R

Rabies, 308
Radial nerve, 398
Radiation therapy, 311, 367
Radius, 165
Raloxifene, 181, 182, 183
Ramilpril, 242
Ranitidine, 12
Ranitidine bismuth citrate, 136
Raptiva® (efalizumab), 82, 86, 92

Rash, 81
Rate of administration, 60
Reality®, 381
Rebound effect, 204
Receptor(s), 4, 37, 38, 76, 80, 337, 395, 400–401
    adrenergic, 458
    binding sites on, 40
Receptor antagonists, 246
Receptor complex, 38–39
Receptor site, 39–40
Recombinant Human Deoxyribonuclease I (rhDNase, Dornase alpha), 212
Recommended Dietary Allowances (RDA), 138
    vitamin recommendations, 141–146
Rectal administration, 17, 50
Rectal lining, 379
Rectal suppositories, 455
Rectum, 29, 124, 128, 129, 319, 375, 387
Rectus muscles, 95
Red blood cells (erythrocytes), 28, 33, 229
Red bone marrow, 161
Redeye, 98
Reglan®, 130
Relafen®, 175
Relationships, professional, 15
Relaxants. See Skeletal muscle relaxants (SMRs)
Relaxation, 427
Releasing factors, 342, 343
Relpax® (eletriptan), 453
Remeron® (mirtazapine), 416
Remicade® (infliximab), 81, 87, 92, 280, 281
Reminyl® (galantamine), 445
Renal artery and vein, 319
Renal failure, 152
Renal system, 27–28, 318–335
    anatomy and physiology of, 319–321
    bladder and urine, 28, 319, 320, 321–322, 375, 387
    diseases and treatment of, 322–329
        antibacterials, 318
        diabetes mellitus and the kidneys, 328–329
        diuretics, 318, 328, 329–330
        edema and hypertension, 328
        kidney stones (urolithiasis), 170, 327–328
        urinary incontinence, 199, 322–323
        urinary retention, 323–324
        urinary tract infections, 324–327
    lymphatic system and, 269
    nervous system and, 397
    websites on, 335
Renamine®, 152
Renese® (polythiazide), 330
Renin, 339, 341

ReoPro®, 246
Repaglinide (Prandin©), 361, 370
Replacement therapy
    estrogen, 180, 323, 351–354, 446
        contraindications, 354
        drug choices, 352–354
        indications for, 351
    growth hormone, 359
    testosterone, 354–357
        contraindications, 355
        precautions, 357
        side effects of anabolic steroids, 356–357
Replication, retroviral, 275–276
Reproductive cycle, 375–376, 383
Reproductive system, lymphatic system and, 269–270. See also Female reproductive system; Male reproductive system
Rescriptor® (delavirdine), 278, 289
Rescula®, 111
Reserpine, 244
Resistance
    pathogenic, 288–292
    solutions to, 291–292
Respiration (breathing), 191, 193, 194–196
    definition of, 25
Respiratory drugs, 10
Respiratory mucosa, 195
Respiratory smooth muscle relaxants, 215
Respiratory system, 25–27, 191–225
    allergies, 38, 212–214
        antihistamines for, 201, 202, 212–213
        mast cell stabilizers to prevent, 213–214
    anatomy of, 192
    asthma, 26, 27, 40, 207–209
        allergic, 208, 219
        bronchoconstriction, 208, 212
        treatment of, 208–209, 215, 217
    breathing (respiration), 191, 193, 194–196
        definition of, 25
    colds, 197–207, 273
        antihistamines for, 201–203
        cold virus and, 198
        cough as symptom and complication of, 198–200
        cough medications for, 201, 205, 206–207
        decongestants for, 201, 203–205
        flu vs., 198
        nondrug treatment of, 205–207
        treatment with drugs, 200–205
    COPD treatment, 215–221
        anticholinergics, 216, 217

    anti-inflammatory agents, 215, 216–217
    anti-leukotriene drugs, 215, 219–221
    bronchodilators, 215
    mast cell stabilizers, 215, 217–219, 220
    xanthines, 215–216, 217
    cystic fibrosis (CF), 26, 27, 199, 211–212
    diaphragm, 129, 195
    diseases of, 27
    disease states of respiratory tract, 197
    emphysema, 27, 209–210
    function of, 192–195
    lung and conducting airways, 24, 25–26, 192, 193, 195–196
    lymphatic system and, 269
    nervous system and, 397
    websites on, 223–225
Resting tone, 130
Restoril (terbutaline sulfate), 12
Retention, urinary, 323–324
Reticular formation, 404
Retina, 94, 95, 96
Retinal artery occlusion, 112
Retin-A® (retinoic acid, tretinoin) cream, 86
13-cis-Retinoic acid (isotretinoin), 142
Retinoic acid (Retin-A®) cream, 86
Retinoid, 281
Retinol binding protein, 142
Retinol (vitamin A), 142, 152
Retinopathy(ies), 106–113
    diabetic, 112
    hypertensive, 113
    sequence of events for, 112
    solar, 112
    syphilitic, 113
    types of, 112
Retinyl palmitate, 142
Retiplase, 249
Retivase®, 249
Retrovir® (zidovudine), 278, 289
Retroviral replication, 275–276
Reuptake, 401
    excessive, 408–409
Reverse transcriptase, 277
Reverse transcriptase inhibitors, 275, 276, 278
Revia® (naltrexone), 421–422
Reye, R. Douglas, 448
Reye's Syndrome, 174, 448–450
Rheumatoid arthritis, 81, 82, 169, 170, 171, 279–280, 282
Rheumatoid Factor, 342
Rheumatrex®, 314
Rhinitis, 197
    allergic, 199, 208, 213

Rhinoviruses, 197
RHO-ROCK interaction, 174
RhuMAb-E 25, 219
Rhythmol® (propafenone), 257, 258
Ribavirin, 289, 304
Riboflavin (vitamin B 2), 143–144, 152
Ribs, 165
Rickets, 142
Rickettsia, 273, 307
Ridaura® (gold), 171
RID® (pyrethrins), 83, 88
Rifabutin, 289
Rifampin, 245, 289, 303, 378
Rifapentine, 289
Right coronary artery (RCA), 228
Rimantadine, 289, 304
Ringworm, 87, 283, 307
Risedronate (Actonel®), 182
Risperdal® (risperidone), 426
Risperidone (Risperdal®), 426
Ritalin® (methylphenidate), 404, 431, 432
Ritonavir, 278, 289
Rituximab (Rituxan®), 314
Rivastigmine (Exelon®), 445
Rizatriptan (Maxalt®), 450, 452
RNA, 271, 284
Robaxin®, 177
Robitussin®, 206
Robitussin-DM®, 206
Rocephin®, 120, 298
Rocky Mountain Spotted Fever, 307
Rocuronium, 178
Rods, 95
Romazicon® (flumazenil), 408
Rosacea, 85, 87, 93
Rosea, 81
Rosiglitazone (Avandia©), 361
Round ligament, 375
Roundworms, 271–272
Rowasa®, 281
RU486, 136
Rubella, 305, 306
Rubex® (doxorubicin), 313
Rugae, 126
Rythmol®, 258

S

Sacral spine, 162
Sacral vertebrae (sacrum), 165, 375, 401
St. John's Wort, 378
St. Joseph's®, 449
Salicylamide, 173
Salicylates, 173–174
Salicylic acids, 88
Saline, normal, 18
Saliva, 265
Salivary glands, 29, 125
Salk poliomyelitis vaccine, 305

Salmeterol, 215, 218
Salmonella typhi (typhoid fever), 308
Salt forms, 60
Saluron®, 330
Sandostatin®, 359
Sansert® (methysergide), 450, 451
Saphenous nerve, 398
Saquinavir, 278, 289
Sarcina arrangement, 273
Sarcoidosis, 27
Sarcomere, 160
Sarcoplasmic reticulum (SR), 228–229
Saturated fat, 139, 140
Scabbing, 266
Scabies, 83, 307
Scala tympani, 116
Scapula (shoulder blade), 165
Scarfskin (cuticle layer), 80
Scarlet fever, 307
Schedule I drugs, 4
Schedule II drugs, 4
Schedule III drugs, 4
Schedule IV drugs, 4
Schedule V drugs, 4
Scheduled medications (controlled
        substances), 10, 11
Schizomycetes bacteria, 273
Schizophrenia, 423–424
Sciatic nerve, 398
Sclera, 58, 95
Scleroderma (systemic sclerosis), 279, 282
Scoplamine, 131
Scrotum, 350, 387
Scurvy, 146
Seasonale®, 378
Sebaceous gland, 80, 97
Seborrheic blepharitis, 98
Secobarbital (Seconal®), 430, 438
Secondary glaucoma, 105
Secondary hypothyroidism (myxedema),
        366, 369
Secondary sex characteristics, 349
Secretin, 338
Sectral®, 244
Sedatives, 427–428, 429–430
    muscle relaxants and, 179
Seizures, 434–437
    Status epilepticus, 436–437
    treatment of, 437, 438
    types and classifications of, 435–436
Selective estrogen receptor modulators
        (SERMs), 181, 182–183
Selective serotonin reuptake inhibitors
        (SSRIs), 70, 413
Selegiline (Eldepryl®), 417, 439, 442, 446
Selenium, 146, 151
Semen, 387
Semicircular canals, 117
Seminal vesicles, 350, 387

Seminiferous tubules, 387
Semi-permeable barrier, 50
Sensory (afferent) function, 396
Sensory hearing loss, 118
Sensory neurons, 79, 458
Septra®, 120, 325
Septra Bactrim®, 301
Septum, 227
Serax® (oxazepam), 409, 421
Serevent®, 216
Serine, 141
Serophene®, 386
Seroquel® (quetiapine), 426
Serotonin, 70, 425
Serotonin receptors, 132–133, 407
Serotonin secretion re-uptake inhibitors
        (SSRIs), 70
Serous bags, 164
Serous otitis media (SOM), 116
Serpasil®, 244
Sertraline (Zoloft®), 410, 414
Serum glutamic oxaloacetic transaminase
        (SGOT), 446
Serum glutamic pyruvic transaminase
        (SGPT), 446
Serzone® (nefazodone), 410, 414
Sesamoid bones, 160
Set-point, 342
Sexually transmitted diseases (STDs), 288,
        382–383
    treatment and prevention of, 383
Shigella diarrhea, 291
Shingles, 308
Short bones, 160
Shortness of breath (SOB), 234
Shoulder blade (scapula), 165
Side effect(s), 40
    defined, 4
    websites on, 62
Sight. See Eyes
Sigmoid colon, 124, 127, 128, 129
Sildenafil (Viagra®), 367, 371, 389
Silver sulfadiazine (Silvadene®), 85, 88
Simple carbohydrates, 138
Simple (nonproliferative) retinopathies,
        112
Simple partial seizures, 435
Simvastatin, 252
Sinemet®, 439, 440
Sinemet CR®, 440
Singulair® (montelukast), 86, 219, 220
Singultus, 194
Sinoatrial (SA) node, 227, 232
Sinuses, lymphatic, 268
Sinusitis, 199, 208
    coughing and, 199
Site of action, 5, 39
6-MP, 281

Skeletal muscle relaxants (SMRs), 10,
  176–178
  adverse actions of, 178
  drugs interacting with, 179
Skeletal muscles, 159
Skeletal system, nervous system and, 397
Skelid® (tiludronate), 182
Skin, 17, 79–93, 265, 339
  anatomy of, 80
  diseases and conditions of, 81–85
  drugs versus cosmetics for, 85
  pharmaceutical treatment for, 85–88
  websites on, 92, 93
Skin cancer, 88, 93
Skin test, 302
Skull (cranium), 165, 401, 402
Sleep wake cycle, 346
Slo-Bid®, 217
Small intestines, 29, 30, 125, 127–128
Small pox, 308
Smell, 80
Smokers' cough, 200
Smoking
  COPD and, 210
  erectile dysfunction and, 367
  ulcers and, 135
  withdrawal and cessation, 422–423
Smooth cartilage, 163
Smooth muscle, 124, 159
Social anxiety disorder (SAD), 405, 406
Social worker, TPN and, 149
Sodium, 23, 53, 146, 151, 329, 348
  delaying influx of, 438
Sodium cromolyn, 102, 213, 214, 217,
  220
Sodium flush, 153
Sodium ions, 320, 321
Sodium-potassium pump, 23
Sodium salicylates, 173
Sodium sulfacetamide, 87
Soft palate, 192
Solaraze® (diclofenac sodium), 88
Solarcaine® (benzocaine), 88
Solar keratosis, 84
Solar retinopathy, 112
Solubility, 52
SoluCortef®, 218
SoluMedrol®, 219, 349
Solutions, 15
Soma®, 177
Somatic nervous system, 396, 458
Somatomammotrophs, 368
Somatostatin, 338, 339, 359
Somatotropin, 343, 359
Somatrem, 359
Somatropin, 359
Somatuline LA®, 359
Sominex®, 427
Sonata® (zaleplon), 407, 409, 428, 430

Sotalol (Betapace®), 257, 258
Sparfloxacin, 301
Spasm, diaphragmatic, 194
Spastic diseases, 186–187
Spectrobid®, 296
Sperm, 337, 386–387
  antibodies to, 386
Spermicides, 380
Sphenoid sinus, 192
Spider veins, 85
Spinal cord, 401–402, 403
  degenerative disorders of, 287
Spinal cord fluid, 265
Spinal nerve, 403
Spine, 162
Spiral bacteria, 273
Spirillium arrangement, 273
Spirochete arrangement, 273
Spirometry breathing test, 208
Spironolactone (Aldactone®), 240, 331,
  389
Spleen, 29, 124, 259–261
Splenectomy, 261
Splenic artery, 259
Splenic flexure, 124
Spongy bone, 161, 163
Spontaneous abortion, 385
Sporanox (Itraconazole), 284, 286
Sporotrichosis, 307
Sporozoans, 272
Sprays, 16
Squamous cell cancer, 84
SRS-A, 209
Stanozolol, 355
Stapes (stirrup), 116, 117
Staphcillin®, 296
Staphylococcus, 97, 324
Staphylococcus arrangement, 273
Staphylococcus aureus, 166, 273, 290, 291
Starches, 138
Starlix© (nateglinide), 361
Statins, 252, 255
Status epilepticus, 436–437
Stavudine (Zerit®), 278, 289
Steapsin, 127–128
Stelazine® (trifluoperazine), 425
Stem cells, hemopoietic (blood-forming),
  267
Stenosis, 237, 248
Stents, prostatic, 391
Sterling-Winthrop, 327
Sternum (breast bone), 165
Steroids, 340
  anabolic, 354, 389
  intrarectal, 10
  therapeutic, 349
  topical, 347
Stevens-Johnson Syndrome, 286

Stimulants, 9
Stimuli, 400
Stirrup (stapes), 116, 117
Stomach, 28–30, 124, 125, 126–127, 129,
  338
Strattera® (atomoxetine), 434
Street drugs, 11, 64, 65, 66
Strepase®, 249
Streptobacillus, 273
Streptococcus, 273
Streptococcus pneumoniae
  (pneumococcus), 291
Streptokinase, 248, 249
Streptomyces griseus, 325
Streptomycin, 289, 303
Streptomycin sulfate, 300
Stress, hormone release and, 346
Stress incontinence, 323
Stroke, 32, 134, 234
  ischemic, 248
Strychnos Castelnaei, 178
Strychnos toxifera, 178
Stye, 97
Subactam, 297
Subclavian arteries and veins, 196, 228,
  231
Subcutaneous injection, 18
Subcutaneous layers, 80
Sublimaze® (fentanyl), 456
Sublingual absorption, 15–16
Sublingual administration, 455
Submandibular, 126
Substance abuse, 66
Subunit vaccines, 305
Succinimides, 438
Succinylcholine, 178
Sucostrin®, 178
Sudafed®, 203
Sugars, 138
Sulbactam, 297
Sulfacetamide, 100
Sulfacetamide sodium 10%, 99
Sulfadiazine, 301
Sulfa drugs (sulfonomides), 28, 301, 325,
  378
Sulfamethoxazole, 301, 325
Sulfamylon® (mafenide Acetate),
  88
Sulfanilamide, 327
Sulfasalazine (Azulfidine®), 86, 171, 281,
  282, 389
Sulfinpyrazone, 185
Sulfisoxazole, 301
Sulfmethoxazole, 289

Sulfonomides (sulfa drugs), 28, 301, 325, 378
Sulfonylureas, 361, 370
Sulindac, 175
Sumatriptan (Imitrex®), 452
Sumycin®, 326
Sundowners Syndrome, 446
Super-aspirins, 245
Superficial peroneal nerve, 398
Superior concha, 192
Superior lobe, 193
Superior maxillary nerve, 403
Superior vena cava, 23, 196, 227
Suppositories, 16, 17
Suprarenal gland, 319
Supraventricular tachycardia (SVT), 236, 256
Suprax®, 298
Sustiva® (efavirenz), 278, 289
Swallowing, 196
Sweat gland, 80
Symmetrel® (amantadine hydrochloride), 441
Sympathetic nervous system (SNS), 233, 345, 396, 458
Symphysis pubis, 375
Synalar® (fluocinolone), 88
Synapse, 70, 400
Synovial fluid, 163, 169
Synovial membrane, 163
Syphilis, 69, 308, 382
Syphilitic retinopathy, 113
Syrups, 15
Systemic circuit, 24, 228
Systemic lupus erythematosus, 282
Systemic sclerosis (scleroderma), 279, 282
Systole, 22, 232–233

T

Tablets, 13–14
Tachycardia, 235, 236, 256
Tacrine (Cognex®), 445
Tacrolimus (Protopic®), 81, 86, 87, 92, 170
Tadalafil (Cialis®), 367, 371, 389
Tagamet® (cimetidine), 70, 136, 389
Tail bone (coccyx), 165, 375
Tambocor® (flecainide), 257
Tamonade, 154
Tamoxifen (Nolvadex®), 183, 314, 357
Tamsulosin hydrochloride (Flowmax®), 390
Tannins, condensed, 325
Tape worms, 271–272
Tardive dyskinesia (TD), 424
Target cells, 41
Tarka®, 242
Tarsals (ankle), 165

Taste buds, 80
Tavist–1, 202
Taxol® (paclitaxel), 314
Tazarotene, 281
Tazobactam, 297
TCAs, 415
T-cells, 267, 270, 271, 281
Tea, 217
Tears, 265
Teczem®, 242
Teeth, 124, 125
Tegopen®, 296
Tegretol® (carbamazepine), 187, 378, 419, 438
Telangiectasia, 85
Telmisartan, 242
Temazepam, 70
Temporal bone, 117, 165
Temporal lobe, 402
Tendonitis, 168
Tendons, 163
Tenecteplase, 249
Tenofovir (Viread®), 278, 289
Tenormin® (atenolol), 22, 244, 410
TENS unit, 455
Teratogenic drugs, 11
Terazosin (Hytrin®), 390
Terbinafine (Lamsil), 286
Terbutaline, 215, 216
Terbutaline sulfate (Restoril), 12
Teriparatide, 182
Terminology, 3–5, 465–475
Terramycin®, 299
Testes (testicles), 337, 339, 340, 350, 386–387
Testicular cancer, 313
Testim®, 355
Testis, 31, 387
Testoderm®, 355
Testoderm TTS®, 355
Testosterone, 312, 339, 340, 350, 356, 358
  production of, 387
Testosterone hormonal replacement, 354–357
  contraindications, 355
  precautions, 357
  side effects of anabolic steroids, 356–357
Tetanus, 305, 306, 308
Tetany, 180
Tetracyclic agents, 416
Tetracycline(s) (TCNs), 9, 87, 97, 136, 137, 179, 289, 292, 293–294, 295, 299, 378
  for urinary tract infections, 326
Tetracycline hydrochloride, 299
Tetrad arrangement, 273
Tetrahydrozoline, 103
Tevetan®, 242

Thalamus, 39, 343, 403
Theodur®, 217
Theophylline, 60, 216, 217
Therapeutic classification, 8
Therapeutic window, 418
Thermogenesis, 345
Thiamin, 143
Thiamine (vitamin B 1), 143, 152
Thiazide and thiazide-like diuretics, 330
Thiazide diuretics, 239
Thiazolidinediones, 370
Thick filaments, 159–160
Thienopyrindines, 245, 246
Thigh bone (femur), 165
Thin filaments, 159–160
Thiopental (Pentothal®), 179, 430
Thiopental sodium, 179
Thioridazine (Mellaril®), 389, 425
Thiothixene (Navane®), 425
Thonzylamine, 203
Thoracic duct, 259
Thoracic spine, 162
Thoracic vertebrae, 165, 401
Thoracic vein, 196
Thorazine® (chlorpromazine), 405, 425
3TC, 289
Threonine, 141
Throat (pharynx), 25, 29, 124, 192
Thrombin, 249–250
  direct inhibitors, 251
Thrombin IIa, 251
Thrombocytopenia, 82
Thrombolytic enzyme, 251
Thrombolytics, 248–249
Thrombophlebitis, 234
Thromboplastin, 249
Thrombopoietin, 339
Thrombosis, 154
Thrombotic thrombocytopenic purpura (TTP), 245
Thrush, 307
Thrush mouth (oral thrush), 217
Thymectomy, 280
Thymidine kinase, 101
Thymus gland, 31, 260, 267, 337, 340
Thyroid cancer, 343
Thyroid drugs, 9
Thyroid eye disease (thyroid orbitopathy, Grave's disease), 281, 366–367, 370
Thyroid gland, 31, 180, 253, 337, 338, 340, 343–345, 366
Thyroid hormone (TH), 341, 366, 369, 370
Thyroid-stimulating hormone (TSH), 31, 338, 341, 342, 344, 366, 368
Thyrotrophs, 368
Thyrotropin-releasing hormone (TRH), 338

Thyroxine (T 4), 146, 253, 338, 344, 345
Tiagabine (Gabitril®), 438
Tiamate®, 257
Tiazem®, 257
Tibia, 164
Tibial nerve, 398
Ticar®, 296
Ticarcillin, 296, 297
Ticlid®, 245, 246, 258
Ticlopidine, 246
Tigan®, 132
Tilade®, 213, 214, 217, 220
Tiludronate (Skelid®), 182
Timentin®, 297
Time-response curve, 43
Timolol®, 107, 122, 244
Timolol maleate, 109
Timoptic-XE®, 107
Tinctures, 15
Tinea cruris (jock itch), 307
Tinea pedis (Athlete's Foot), 83, 88, 283, 307
Tinidazole, 287
Tinnitus, 118, 173
Tinzaparin, 248
Tioconazole (Vagistat®), 284
Tirofiban, 246
Tissue plasminogen activators (t-PA), 248–249
Tissues, 5
Tobradex®, 101
Tobramycin, 99, 100, 101, 325, 326
Tobramycin IV, 119
Tobramycin sulfate, 300
Tobrex®, 100
Tocainide (Tonocard®), 257
Tofranil® (imipramine), 323, 409, 416, 428
Tolbutamide, 370
Tolectin®, 175
Tolerance to drugs, 66, 67
Tolmetin, 175
Tolnaftate 1%, 88
Tongue, 29, 124, 125, 126
Tonic-clonic (Grand Mal) seizures, 436
Tonic water, 119
Tophi, 170, 184
Topical administration, 16–17
Topical drugs, 10
Topical medications, 50
Topical steroids, 347
Topiramate (Topamax®), 419, 438
Toposar®, 314
Tornalate®, 216
Torsade De Pointes, 421
Torsemide (Demadex®), 119, 239, 330
Total Nutrient Admixture (TNA), 149
Total parenteral nutrition (TPN), 147–155
    compatibility of, 153

contraindications of, 154–155
    indications, 148–149
    solutions for special disease state
        dietary needs, 152–153
    stability of, 153–155
    types of lines, 150–152
Touch nerve, 80
Toxicology, 5
Toxic Shock Syndrome, 308
Toxoid vaccines, 305
Toxoplasmosis, 307
TPN. *See* Total parenteral nutrition (TPN)
Trabecular meshwork, 106
Trace elements, 146, 152
Trachea (wind pipe), 25, 124, 192, 193, 194, 196
Tracrium®, 178
Trade names, 12–13
Trancypomine (Parnate®), 417, 432
Trandolapril, 242
Tranexamic acid, 251
Tranilast, 389
Tranquilizers, muscle relaxants and, 179
Transcutaneous electric nerve stimulation (TENS unit), 455
Trans Dermal Patch, 241
Transdermal patch, 355, 378
Transderm Scop®, 131
Transduction, 401
Trans-fatty acids, 139–140
Transformation, 291
Transthyretin (prealbumin), 142
Transverse colon, 29, 128, 129
Tranxene® (clorazepate), 438
Travatan®, 111
Trazedone (Desyrel®), 414
Trelstar™ Depot (triptorelin), 314
Tretinoin cream, 86
Trexall™, 314
Triamcinonide (Aristocort®), 88, 218, 349
Triaminic®, 206
Triamterene, 240
Triazolam (Halcion®), 179, 428, 430
Triazole antifungals, 284
Trichlormethiazide, 330
Trichomonas, 382
Trichomonas vaginalis, 272
Trichomoniasis, 383
Tricor®, 255
Tricuspid valve, 23, 227
Tricyclic antidepressant, 44, 428
Trifluoperazine (Stelazine®), 425
Trifluridine solution, 99, 101
Trigeminal nerve, 403
Triglycerides, 253–255
Trihexyphenidyl HCL (Artane®), 441–442
Triiodothyronine (T 3), 253, 338, 344, 345

Trilafon® (perphenazine), 425
Trilostane, 365, 370
Trimethobenzamide, 132
Trimethoprim, 301, 325
Trimethoprim/polymyxin B, 99
Trimethoprim-sulfamethoxazole (SMX TMP), 120
Trimethoprim sulfate, 99, 100
Trimox®, 120
Triphasil- 28®, 378
Triple Antibiotic® ointment, 87
Triprolidine, 203
Triptorelin (Trelstar™ Depot), 314
Trivora®, 378
Trizivir®, 278, 289
Troches, 15
Trochlear nerve, 403
Trojan®, 381
Tropic hormones, 342, 344
Tropomyosin, 160
Troponin, 160
Trovoprost solution, 111
Truspot®, 109
Truvada®, 278
Trypsin, 127
Tryptophan, 141, 144
Tubal (ectopic) pregnancy, 376
Tuberculosis, 302–304, 308
    treatments for, 289
Tubular reabsorption, 320
Tubules, renal, 28
Tumor Necrosis Factor (TNF), 81
Tumors, 83–84
    adrenal, 365
    bone, 454
    cardiac, 25
    lung, 365
Tumor vaccines, 312
Tunica albuginea, 387
Tunneled catheters, 154
Tussigon®, 206
T-wave, 232
12-Step group support program, 421
Tylenol # 3, 130
Tylenol® (acetaminophen), 70, 176, 211, 449–450
Tympanic membrane (eardrum), 115–116, 117
Type1 diabetes, 360, 361
Type2 diabetes, 360
Typhoid fever (*Salmonella typhi*), 308
Typhoid vaccine, 305
Tyrosine, 141

U

Ulcer(s), 124, 133–137
    causes and treatments of, 135–137

Ulcer(s) (*cont.*)
Cox-2 inhibitors and, 176
duodenal (peptic), 127, 133, 136, 155
gastric, 133, 134, 136
nonsteroidal antiinflammatory drugs
(NSAIDs) and, 133–134,
135–136
Ulcerative blepharitis, 98
Ulcerative colitis, 281
Ulna, 165
Ulnar nerve, 398
Ultracef®, 298
Unasyn®, 297
Understanding Asthma, 209
Unfractionated heparin (UFH), 247
Unipen®, 296
Uniretic®, 242
Unisom®, 427
U.S. Department of Agriculture (USDA),
137, 147
Univasc®, 242
Unoprostone isopropyl solution, 111
Unsaturated fat, 139
Uptake, 401
Uremia, 324
Ureters, 319
Urethra, 319, 323, 375, 387,
389–390
Urethral orifice, 387
Urethritis, 383
Uric acid, 169–170, 184
Uricosuric agents, 184
Urinary incontinence, 199, 322–323
Urinary retention, 323–324
Urinary system. *See* Renal system
Urinary tract infections, 324–327
antiinfectives for, 325–327
Urination
difficulties in, 390
excessive, 362
Urine, 320, 321–322
pH of, 322
specific gravity of, 322
Urobilinogen, 322
Urokinase, 249
Urolithiasis (kidney stones), 170,
327–328
UroXatral™ (alfuzosin), 390
Urticaria (hives), 81, 86
Uterine cancer, 183
Uterine lining, 375, 376
Uterine tube, 375
Uterus, 375, 385
Uvula, 126

V

Vaccination, 271
Vaccines, 306–307

cancer, 311
tumor, 312
Vagina, 265, 375
infection of, 272
spermicides and, 379
Vaginal administration, 17, 50
Vaginal dryness, 351
Vaginal rings, 378
Vaginal yeast infections, 283–284, 307,
382, 383
Vaginosis, bacterial, 382
Vagistat® (tioconazole), 284
Vagus nerve, 403
Valacyclovir, 289, 304
Valine, 141
Valisone®, 88
Valium® (diazepam), 70, 177, 179, 187,
421, 438
Valproic acid (Depakene®), 418, 419, 438
Valsartan, 242
Valves, cardiac, 227–228
Vanceril®, 218, 349
Vancomycin, 289, 291
Vaniqatm®, 371
Vantin®, 120
Vardenafil (Levitra®), 367, 371, 389
Varicella, 306
Variolation, 305
Vascor® (bepridil), 257
Vascular retinopathies retinopathy,
106–113
Vas deferens, 387
Vaseretic®, 242
Vasoconstriction, 203
Vasoconstrictors, 98, 103, 113, 204
Vasodilators, 240–241
Vasopressin (antidiuretic hormone), 321,
338, 340, 341, 342, 362, 364,
369
Vasotec®, 242
V-Cillin K®, 296
Vectrin®, 299
Vecuronium, 178
Veetids®, 325
Veins, 24, 192, 228
clots in, 234
portal, 128
pulmonary, 230
spider, 85
Velosulin, 361
Venae cavae, 24
Venlafaxine (Effexor®), 410, 414
Venogram, 154
Venous blood, 229, 231
Ventricles, 22, 23, 24, 196, 227, 402
Ventricular fibrillation, 234–235, 256
VePesid®, 314
Verapamil (Calan®), 242, 257, 258
Verelan®, 258

Verminous intoxification, 272
Vertebrae, 401
Vertebral column, 265
Vertigo, 131
Very low density lipoprotein (VLDL), 253,
255
Vessels, 22
Vestibular labyrinth, 116
Vestibular nerve, ganglia of, 117
Vestibule, 117, 192
Vestibulocochlear nerve, 403
V-fend® (voriconazole), 284, 286
Viagra® (sildenafil), 367, 371, 389
Vibramycin®, 299
Vibrio arrangements, 273
Vicks Formula 44®, 206
Vicodin, 130
Vidarabine ointment, 99, 101
Videx® (didanosine), 278, 289
Villi, 128
Vinblastine, 313
Vinca alkaloids, 313
Vincasar PFS® (vincristine), 313, 314
Vinorelbine (Navelbine®), 314
Vioxx®, 134
Vira-A®, 101
Viracept® (nelfinavir), 278, 289
Viral conjunctivitis, 99
Viral diseases, treatments for, 289
Viral gastroenteritis, 131
Viral infections, 82
Viramune® (nevirapine), 278, 289, 304
Viread® (tenofovir), 278, 289
Viroptic®, 101
Virus(es), 273. *See also* HIV/AIDS
cold, 198
Visceral muscle, 159
Visine®, 103
Visine LR®, 103
Vision, 94, 96. *See also* Eyes
disorders affecting, 104–113
cataract, 105, 106
drugs for, 107–111
glaucoma, 104–106
vascular retinopathies retinopathy,
106–113
Visken®, 244
Vistaril®, 202
Vistazine®, 202
Vistraril®, 202
Vitamin A, 142, 152
Vitamin B, 322
Vitamin B1, 143, 152
Vitamin B2, 143–144, 152
Vitamin B3, 144
Vitamin B5, 144
Vitamin B6, 143, 144–145, 152, 328
Vitamin B9, 145
Vitamin B12, 145, 152, 153, 282

Vitamin C (ascorbic acid), 145–146, 152, 207
Vitamin D, 142, 166, 180
Vitamin D3 (calciferol), 339
Vitamin D (ergocalciferol), 152
Vitamin E, 142, 152, 446
Vitamin K, 34, 142–143, 150–151, 250
Vitamins, 10, 138, 141–146
    fat-soluble, 139, 142
    in TPNs, 152
    water-soluble, 143
Vitiligo, 84, 282
Vitreous humor, 95, 96
Voice box (larynx), 25, 124, 192, 193, 194
Voltaren®, 175
Voltaren-XR®, 175
Volume of distribution, 57, 60–61
Vomiting, 130–133, 173
    chemotherapy and, 132–133
    post-operative, 131, 132
Voriconazole (V-fend®), 284, 286
VZV eye disease, 99

W

Waksman, Selman, 325
Warfarin®, 32, 34, 45, 70, 151, 247, 248, 258, 351
    overdose of, 250–251
Warts, 84, 87, 308
    genital, 382
Waste, 320, 402
    digestive, 128–129
    elimination of, 28
    nitrogenous, 324
Water, 30, 138, 147
Water-soluble medications, 52
Water-soluble vitamins, 143
Websites, 62
    on addiction, 77
    on circulatory system, 262–263
    on ears, 122
    on endocrine system, 372–373
    on eyes, 122
    on immune system and immune diseases, 316–317
    on musculoskeletal system, 190

    on nervous system, 462–464
    on reproductive system, 393–394
    on respiratory system, 223–225
    on skin and skin treatments, 92, 93
    on urinary system, 335
Weicke-Korsakoff's syndrome, 70–71
Weight, infertility and, 385
Welchol®, 255
Wellbutrin® (bupropion), 414, 415, 423
White blood cells (leukocytes), 170, 229
Whooping cough (pertussis), 200, 305, 306, 308
Willow bark, 449
Wind pipe (trachea), 25, 124, 192, 193, 194
Winstrol®, 355
Withdrawal, 71, 75
    alcohol, 420–422
    from stimulants, 432
    symptoms of, 66, 67
    tapered, 76, 77
World Health Organization, 275
Worm infestations, 289
Worms, human intestinal parasitic, 271–272
Wound healing, 347
Wrinkles, 85
Wrist (carpals), 165
Wymox®, 120

X

Xalatan®, 111
Xanax® (alprazolam), 70, 179, 409, 423
Xanthine oxidase, 184
Xanthines, 215–216, 217
Xeloda® (capecitabine), 313
Xylocaine®, 88, 179, 257, 258

Y

Yasmin®, 378
Yawns, 195
Yeast infection, 217
Yeasts, 83, 283–284
Yellow fever, 308
Yellow marrow, 161, 162

Z

Zaditen®, 202
Zaditor®, 103
Zafirlukast (Accolate®), 86, 219, 220
Zagam®, 301
Zalcitabine (Hivid®), 278, 289
Zaleplon (Sonata®), 407, 409, 428, 430
Zanamivir, 289
Zantac®, 12, 136
Zarontin® (ethosuximide), 378, 438
Zaroxolyn®, 330
Z drugs (hypnosedatives), 428
Zebeta®, 244
Zeldox® (ziprasidone), 426
Zemuron®, 178
Zephiran® (benzalkonium chloride), 88
Zerit® (stavudine), 278, 289
Zestoretic®, 242
Zestril®, 242
Zetia®, 254
Ziagen® (abacavir), 278, 289
Zidovudine (AZT, Retrovir®), 278, 289
Zileuton, 220
Zinacef®, 298
Zinc, 146, 151, 152
Zinc lozenge, 205–207
Ziprasidone (Zeldox®), 426
Zithromax® (azithromycin), 87, 99, 120, 299
Zofran®, 132
Zoledronic acid, 182
Zolendronate (Zomig®), 182
Zolmitriptan (Zoming®), 450, 452
Zoloft® (sertraline), 410, 414
Zolpidem (Ambien®), 407, 409, 428, 430
Zometa®, 182
Zonegran® (Zonisamide), 438
Zooflagelates, 272
Zopiclone (Imovane®), 428, 430
Zosyn®, 297
Zrivada® (atazanavir), 278
Zyban® (bupropion), 415, 423
Zyflo®, 219, 220
Zyloprim®, 185
Zyprexa® (olanzapine), 426
Zyrtec® (cetirizine), 202, 389